The Century Biological Series
Robert Hegner, Editor

PARASITOLOGY

WITH SPECIAL REFERENCE TO MAN
AND DOMESTICATED ANIMALS

BY

ROBERT HEGNER, Ph.D.

PROFESSOR OF PROTOZOÖLOGY
THE JOHNS HOPKINS UNIVERSITY

FRANCIS M. ROOT, Ph.D.

LATE ASSOCIATE PROFESSOR OF MEDICAL ENTOMOLOGY
THE JOHNS HOPKINS UNIVERSITY

DONALD L. AUGUSTINE, Sc.D.

ASSISTANT PROFESSOR OF HELMINTHOLOGY
HARVARD UNIVERSITY

AND

CLAY G. HUFF, Sc.D.

ASSOCIATE PROFESSOR OF PARASITOLOGY
UNIVERSITY OF CHICAGO

D. APPLETON–CENTURY COMPANY
INCORPORATED
NEW YORK   LONDON

This book is a general revision of
Animal Parasitology, copyright 1929, by
THE CENTURY CO.

PREFACE

Since 1929, when *Animal Parasitology* was published, rapid progress has been made in the field of parasitology. Both the authors and the teachers who use the book have for some time felt that a revised edition would be desirable. Owing to the death of Dr. Francis M. Root it was necessary to obtain the help of someone else to revise the section on Medical Entomology. One of his former students, Dr. Clay G. Huff, consented to do this. The title of this section has been changed to "Arthropods of Parasitological Importance," since this more clearly describes the material contained in it.

The title of the first edition, namely, *Animal Parasitology,* appears to be misleading, giving the impression that the parasites of man are not considered. For this reason we have changed the title to *Parasitology.*

No radical departures have been made. Every chapter has been carefully revised so as to include the results of additions to our knowledge that have been made during the past nine years. Changes have been made wherever possible as the result of the criticisms of teachers, students and colleagues. Many new figures have been used to replace old ones and others have been improved. The bibliography has been brought up-to-date. We hope this edition will meet with the approval of teachers and students of parasitology, and veterinarians and practicing physicians, for whom it was originally written.

THE AUTHORS.

PREFACE TO "ANIMAL PARASITOLOGY"

This textbook has been prepared for the use of students in colleges, universities, medical schools, schools of hygiene and public health, schools of tropical medicine, and similar institutions. It is hoped that it will also be of use to veterinarians and practising physicians.

There is, at the present time, no textbook of parasitology in the English language that includes the many recent additions to our knowledge of this subject. Since the war, parasitology, especially those phases of the subject that concern the parasites of man, has practically been revolutionized. Many new species of parasites have been described and established and many others have been found to be of doubtful validity or identical with previously described species and hence have been dropped from the list. Much new information regarding the life-cycles of common parasites has been published within the past few years, and a more definite attack on the subject of host-parasite relations has been organized than ever before.

Because of space limitations it has been necessary to practise rigid selection with respect to the material included in this book. The parasites of man are emphasized throughout; those of domesticated animals are described wherever possible, since they are relatively easy to obtain for study and are of practical importance; and parasites of other lower animals are included because of their availability or their value for teaching purposes.

The book is divided into an Introduction and three Sections. The Introduction was prepared by the senior author, and the three Sections are the exclusive work of the author to whom they are credited, although each author has benefited by the advice of the others. The writers are indebted to their several colleagues for advice and criticism, especially to Dr. Justin Andrews, who read the Section on Protozoa, and Dr. W. W. Cort, who read the Introduction and the Section on Helminthology.

CONTENTS

PAGE

Preface v
Preface to "Animal Parasitology" vii

INTRODUCTION

By Robert Hegner

PARASITISM 1

I. *Animal Habitats* 1
II. *Types of Association* 2
III. *Types of Parasitism* 2
IV. *Effects of a Parasitic Existence on the Parasite* . . . 4
V. *Parasitism in the Animal Kingdom* 5
VI. *Host-Parasite Specificity* 6
VII. *Host-Parasite Relations* 10
VIII. *Origin and Evolution of Parasitism* 17
IX. *Parasitism and the Geographical Distribution and Evolution of Hosts* 18
X. *The Protozoa of Man and Monkeys* 20
XI. *Rules of Nomenclature* 22

SECTION I

PROTOZOÖLOGY

By Robert Hegner

CHAPTER I

THE BIOLOGY OF THE PROTOZOA 27

I. *Morphology* 27
II. *Classification* 30
III. *Maintenance of the Individual* 31
IV. *Maintenance of the Race* 33
V. *Protozoa of Man* 36
VI. *Protozoa of Lower Animals Easily Obtained for Study* 38

ix

CHAPTER II

PAGE

INTRODUCTION TO THE SARCODINA 42

I. *Classification* 42
II. *Amœba proteus* 44
III. *Parasitic Sarcodina in General* 45

CHAPTER III

AMŒBÆ LIVING IN MAN 46

I. *Generic and Specific Characteristics* 46
II. *Incidence of Infection* 47
III. *Endamœba histolytica* 48
    1. HISTORICAL 48
    2. LIFE-CYCLE 48
    3. MORPHOLOGY 49
    4. HOST-PARASITE RELATIONS 50
    5. PREVENTION AND CONTROL 58
    6. HOST-PARASITE SPECIFICITY 58
IV. *Endamœba coli* 59
V. *Endamœba gingivalis* 61
VI. *Endolimax nana* 63
VII. *Iodamœba williamsi* 65
VIII. *Dientamœba fragilis* 67
IX. *Doubtful Species of Amœbæ Reported from Man* . . 68
X. *Coprozoic Amœbæ* 69
XI. *Methods of Obtaining and Preparing Amœbæ for Study* 70
XII. *Methods of Cultivating Amœbæ* 74
XIII. *Pseudoparasites in Human Feces* 77
XIV. *Differential Diagnosis of Human Amœbæ* 79

CHAPTER IV

AMŒBÆ OF LOWER ANIMALS 80

I. *Amœbæ of Monkeys* 80
II. *Amœbæ of Domesticated Mammals and Birds* . . . 81
III. *Amœbæ of Other Animals* 84

CHAPTER V

PAGE

INTRODUCTION TO THE MASTIGOPHORA . . . 87

I. Classification 87
II. Euglena 88
III. Parasitic Mastigophora in General 90
   1. PARASITIC PLANT-LIKE FLAGELLATES 90
   2. TRYPANOSOMIDÆ, EXCLUSIVE OF THE GENERA TRY-
      PANOSOMA AND LEISHMANIA 92
   3. PARASITIC ANIMAL-LIKE FLAGELLATES 94
   4. INTESTINAL FLAGELLATES OF TERMITES . . . 96

CHAPTER VI

HÆMOFLAGELLATES OF MAN AND LOWER ANIMALS . . 98

I. The Genus Trypanosoma 98
II. The Genus Leishmania 110

CHAPTER VII

INTESTINAL FLAGELLATES OF MAN AND LOWER ANIMALS . 116

I. Classification and Diagnosis 116
II. Chilomastix in Man 117
III. Chilomastix in Lower Animals 119
IV. Trichomonas hominis 119
V. Trichomonas (buccalis) elongata 122
VI. Trichomonas vaginalis 123
VII. Trichomonas in Lower Animals 124
VIII. Retortamonas (Embadomonas) intestinalis 126
IX. Retortamonas in Lower Animals 126
X. Enteromonas hominis 127
XI. Giardia lamblia 127
XII. Giardia in Lower Animals 130

CHAPTER VIII

SPOROZOA IN GENERAL AND GREGARINES IN PARTICULAR . 133

I. Classification 133
II. Life-Cycles 134
III. Gregarines 136

CHAPTER IX

PAGE

COCCIDIA 140

I. *General Characteristics* 140
II. *Coccidia in Man* 140
III. *Coccidia in Lower Animals* 144
IV. *Hæmogregarines* 145

CHAPTER X

HÆMOSPORIDIA EXCLUSIVE OF MALARIAL PARASITES . 149

I. *The Genus Hæmoproteus* 149
II. *The Genus Leucocytozoön* 150
III. *Babesidæ (Piroplasmidæ)* 151
IV. *Doubtful Species of Hæmosporidia* 155

CHAPTER XI

MALARIAL PARASITES OF MAN 157

I. *Introduction* 157
II. *The Discovery of the Malarial Parasites in Man and
    Mosquito* 157
III. *The Asexual Cycle of the Malarial Parasites in Man* . 158
        1. PLASMODIUM VIVAX 158
        2. PLASMODIUM MALARIÆ 162
        3. PLASMODIUM FALCIPARUM 162
IV. *The Sexual Cycle of the Malarial Parasites in the Mos-
    quito* 164
V. *Host-Parasite Relations* 166
VI. *Treatment, Prevention and Control* 170
VII. *Therapeutic Malaria* 171
VIII. *Methods of Obtaining and Preparing Malarial Parasites
    for Study* 172

CHAPTER XII

MALARIAL PARASITES OF LOWER ANIMALS . . . 174

I. *Malarial Parasites of Monkeys* 174
II. *Malarial Parasites of Birds* 175
III. *Malarial Parasites of Other Animals* 177

CHAPTER XIII

PAGE

CNIDOSPORIDIA 178

I. *Myxosporidia* 178
II. *Microsporidia* 180
III. *Sarcosporidia and Haplosporidia* 182

CHAPTER XIV

PARASITIC INFUSORIA OF LOWER ANIMALS . . . 185

I. *General Characteristics and Classification* 185
II. *Nyctotherus cordiformis* 186
III. *Ectoparasitic Ciliates* 188
IV. *The Family Opalinidæ* 190
V. *Ciliates of Mosquito Larvæ* 192
VI. *Entozoic Ciliates of Cattle* 193
VII. *Ciliates of Monkeys* 195
VIII. *The Genus Balantidium* 196
IX. *Other Ciliates of Lower Animals* 199
X. *Parasitic Suctoria* 199

CHAPTER XV

PARASITIC CILIATES OF MAN 201

I. *Balantidium coli* 201
II. *Doubtful Ciliates of Man* 206

SECTION II

HELMINTHOLOGY

By Donald L. Augustine

CHAPTER XVI

INTRODUCTION TO THE HELMINTHS 211

I. *General Classification* 211
II. *Distribution and Incidence* 212
III. *Effects Produced by Helminths on the Host* . . . 214

CHAPTER XVII

PAGE

CLASS TREMATODA 219

I. *General Characteristics of the Class* 219
II. *Collection and Preservation of Trematodoes* . . . 234
III. *Classification* 235

CHAPTER XVIII

THE DIGENETIC TREMATODES 238

I. *The Order Prosostomata, Monostomata* 238

CHAPTER XIX

THE DIGENETIC TREMATODES (continued) . . . 240

I. *The Order Prosostomata* (continued), *Distomata* . . 240
   I. THE FAMILY FASCIOLIDÆ 240
   2. THE FAMILY OPISTHORCHIIDÆ 250
   3. THE FAMILY DICROCOELIIDÆ 260
   4. THE FAMILY PLAGIORCHIIDÆ 265
   5. THE FAMILY ECHINOSTOMATIDÆ 268
   6. THE FAMILY HETEROPHYIDÆ 270
   7. THE FAMILY TROGLOTREMATIDÆ 276

CHAPTER XX

THE DIGENETIC TREMATODES (continued) . . . 286

I. *The Order Prosostomata* (concluded), *Amphistomata* 286
   I. THE FAMILY GASTRODISCIDÆ 286
   2. THE FAMILY PARAMPHISTOMIDÆ 288
   3. AMPHISTOME LIFE CYCLES 289

CHAPTER XXI

THE DIGENETIC TREMATODES (concluded) . . . 292

I. *The Order Strigeatoidea* 292
   I. THE SUBORDER STRIGEATA 292
   2. THE SUBORDER BUCEPHALATA 292
   3. THE SUBORDER SCHISTOSOMATA 294

CHAPTER XXII

CLASS CESTOIDEA 311

I. *General Characteristics of the Class* 311
II. *Collection and Preservation of Tapeworms* 322
III. *Classification* 323

CHAPTER XXIII

THE PSEUDOPHYLLIDEAN TAPEWORMS . . . 325

I. *The Order Pseudophyllidea* 325
   1. DIPHYLLOBOTHRIUM LATUM 325
   2. DIPHYLLOBOTHRIUM ERINACEI 332
   3. OTHER SPECIES OF THE GENUS DIPHYLLOBOTHRIUM 333
   4. SPARGANUM PROLIFERUM 334
   5. THE GENUS DIPLOGONOPORUS 335

CHAPTER XXIV

THE CYCLOPHYLLIDEAN TAPEWORMS . . . 336

I. *The Order Cyclophyllidea* 336
   1. THE FAMILY TÆNIIDÆ 336
   2. THE FAMILY DAVAINEIDÆ 363
   3. THE FAMILY ANOPLOCEPHALIDÆ 365
   4. THE FAMILY HYMENOLEPIDIDÆ 366
   5. THE FAMILY DILEPIDIDÆ 371

CHAPTER XXV

CLASS NEMATODA 374

I. *General Characteristics of the Class* 374
II. *Collection and Preservation of Nematodes* 384
III. *Classification* 385

CHAPTER XXVI

NEMATODE PARASITES 386

I. *The Order Ascaroidæ* 386
   1. THE FAMILY ASCARIDÆ 386
   2. THE FAMILY HETERAKIDÆ 394
   3. THE FAMILY OXYURIDÆ 398
   4. THE FAMILY RHABDITIDÆ 402

CHAPTER XXVII

PAGE

NEMATODE PARASITES (continued) 411

I. *The Order Strongyloidea* 411
   1. THE FAMILY STRONGYLIDÆ 411
   2. THE FAMILY ANCYLOSTOMIDÆ 418
   3. THE FAMILY METASTRONGYLIDÆ 438

CHAPTER XXVIII

NEMATODE PARASITES (continued) 443

I. *The Order Filarioidea* 443
   1. THE FAMILY FILARIIDÆ 443
   2. THE FAMILY PHILOMETRIDÆ 457
   3. THE FAMILY SPIRURIDÆ 461
   4. THE FAMILY CAMALLANIDÆ 467
   5. THE FAMILY CUCULLANIDÆ 468
   6. THE FAMILY GNATHOSTOMIDÆ 468

CHAPTER XXIX

NEMATODE PARASITES (continued) 470

I. *The Order Dioctophymoidea* 470
   1. THE FAMILY DIOCTOPHYMIDÆ 470

CHAPTER XXX

NEMATODE PARASITES (continued) 473

I. *The Order Trichinelloidea* 473
   1. THE SUBFAMILY TRICHINELLIDÆ 473
   2. THE SUBFAMILY TRICHURINÆ 483
   3. THE SUBFAMILY TRICHOSOMOIDINÆ 486

CHAPTER XXXI

NEMATODE PARASITES (concluded) 487

I. *Appendix to Nemathelminthes* 487
   1. THE GORDIACEA 487
   2. THE ACANTHOCEPHALA 489

SECTION III

ARTHROPODS OF PARASITOLOGICAL IMPORTANCE

By Francis M. Root. Revised by Clay G. Huff

CHAPTER XXXII

INTRODUCTION . . . . . . 493 PAGE

   I. *Arthropods of Parasitological Importance* 493
  II. *External Structure of Insects* 495
 III. *Internal Structure of Insects* 496
 IV. *Life Histories of Insects* 498
  V. *Relationship to Disease* 499

CHAPTER XXXIII

THE DIPTERA (FLIES, MOSQUITOES, ETC.) . . . 502

   I. *Importance* 502
  II. *Characteristics* 502
 III. *Classification* 503

CHAPTER XXXIV

FAMILY CULICIDÆ—SUBFAMILY CULICINÆ—TRUE MOSQUITOES . 508

   I. *Characteristics* 508
  II. *Structure of Adult* 508
 III. *Life History* 511
 IV. *Structure of Larvæ* 512
  V. *Structure of Pupæ* 513
 VI. *Classification of Mosquitoes* 513

CHAPTER XXXV

TRIBE ANOPHELINI—THE MALARIAL MOSQUITOES . . 515

    I. *Characteristics* 515
   II. *Classification of Anophelini* 521
  III. *Geographical Distribution of Anopheles* 521
  IV. *Identification of American Species of Anopheles* . . 522
   V. *Identification of Anopheles Larvæ* 526
  VI. *Notes on Groups and Species of American Anopheles* . 531
 VII. *Malaria Carriers in Other Parts of the World* . . . 534
VIII. *Vectors of Simian Malaria* 537

CHAPTER XXXVI

PAGE

MALARIA AND MOSQUITO SURVEYS 538

I. The Prevalence of Malaria 538
II. Anopheline Surveys 540
III. Anopheline Breeding-Places 542
IV. Determination of the Dangerous Vectors of the Locality 542
V. Dissection of Anopheline Mosquitoes 544

CHAPTER XXXVII

EPIDEMIOLOGY AND CONTROL OF MALARIA . . . 546

A. EPIDEMIOLOGY 546
B. CONTROL 548

I. Measures of Defense 548
II. Measures of Attack 549

CHAPTER XXXVIII

CULICINE MOSQUITOES 556

I. Tribe Megarhinini 556
II. Tribe Culicini 556
III. Comments on Some of the Genera of the Tribe Culicini 561

CHAPTER XXXIX

CULICINE MOSQUITOES IN RELATION TO DISEASE . . 565

I. Yellow Fever 565
II. Dengue Fever 567
III. Relation of Mosquitoes to Other Filterable Virus Diseases 567
IV. Avian Malaria 568
V. Filarial Diseases 568
VI. Nuisance Mosquitoes 570
VII. Biology and Control of Important Culicine Mosquitoes 571

CHAPTER XL

OTHER BLOOD-SUCKING NEMATOCERA (FAMILIES CERATOPOGONIDÆ, PSYCHODIDÆ, SIMULIIDÆ). . . 577

I. Ceratopogonidæ 577

PAGE

II. *Psychodidæ* 582
III. *Simuliidæ* 587

CHAPTER XLI

SUBORDER ORTHORRHAPHA, SECTION BRACHYCERA,
FAMILY TABANIDÆ 590

I. *Characteristics* 590
II. *Life History* 592
III. *Classification* 592
IV. *Notes on Some Genera of Tabanidæ* 593
V. *Tabanids as Disease Carriers* 594

CHAPTER XLII

THE HIGHER DIPTERA—STRUCTURE, LIFE HISTORY
AND CLASSIFICATION 597

I. *Tribe Acalyptratæ* 597
II. *Tribe Calyptratæ* 598

CHAPTER XLIII

BLOOD-SUCKING MUSCIDÆ AND HIPPOBOSCIDÆ . . 609

I. Stomoxys calcitrans. *The Biting Stable-Fly* . . . 609
II. Hæmatobia irritans. *The Horn-Fly* 610
III. *Genus* Glossina, *the Tsetse Flies* 611
IV. *Pupiparous Flies—Especially the Family Hippoboscidæ* 613

CHAPTER XLIV

NON-BLOODSUCKING FLIES CONCERNED IN THE
TRANSMISSION OF DISEASE 615

I. *"Eye-Flies" or Frit Flies* 615
II. *Domestic Flies* 615
III. *Control of Domestic Flies* 617

CHAPTER XLV

MYIASIS AND THE IDENTIFICATION OF FLY LARVÆ . 621

I. *Myiasis* 621
II. *Identification of Fly Larvæ* 626
III. *The Use of Maggots in Surgery* 629

CHAPTER XLVI

PAGE

ORDER SIPHONAPTERA—FLEAS 631

I. Characteristics 631
II. Structure of Adult Flea 631
III. Life History of Fleas 633
IV. Classification 633
V. Family Hectopsyllidæ 635
VI. Family Pulicidæ 636
VII. Family Dolichopsyllidæ 639
VIII. Family Hystrichopsyllidæ 639
IX. Fleas as Disease-Carriers 639

CHAPTER XLVII

ORDER ANOPLURA—LICE 644

I. Mallophaga 644
II. Siphunculata 645
III. Species of Lice Found on Man 648
IV. Lice as Disease-Carriers 649
V. Louse Control 650

CHAPTER XLVIII

ORDER HEMIPTERA—TRUE BUGS 652

I. Family Cimicidæ—Bedbugs 653
II. Family Reduviidæ—"Assassin-Bugs" 656

CHAPTER XLIX

THE CLASS ARACHNIDA AND THE ORDER ACARINA . . 658

CHAPTER L

THE TICKS (SUPERFAMILY IXODIDEA) . . . 666

I. Family Argasidæ—Soft Ticks 668
II. Family Ixodidæ—Hard Ticks 670

CHAPTER LI

PARASITIC MITES 682

I. Superfamily Parasitoidea 682
II. Superfamily Trombidoidea 683

PAGE

III. *Superfamily Hydrachnoidea* 685
IV. *Superfamily Tarsonemoidea* 685
V. *Superfamily Tyroglyphoidea* 686
VI. *Superfamily Sarcoptoidea* 686
VII. *Superfamily Demodecoidea* 688

CHAPTER LII

MISCELLANEOUS ARTHROPODS OF PARASITOLOGICAL INTEREST   689

I. *Arthropods which Produce Symptoms by their Direct
    Action on the Host* 689
II. *Arthropods Serving as Intermediate Hosts of Miscel-
    laneous Helminths* 693

CHAPTER LIII

NOTES ON COLLECTING, PRESERVING, AND REARING
ARTHROPODS OF PARASITOLOGICAL IMPORTANCE   . . .   696

I. *Collecting* 696
II. *Preserving* 697
III. *Rearing* 699

Bibliography 701

Index of Authors 783

Index of Subjects 793

PARASITISM

Parasitology is the science or study of parasitism. Parasitism may be defined as the relation that exists between parasites and their hosts. A parasite is an organism that lives on, or within and at the expense of some other living organism. This book is limited in subject-matter to parasitism in man and other animals. In the Introduction certain subjects are discussed that have a bearing on the phenomena of parasitism in general. In later chapters parasitism among the protozoa, worms and insects, is described and illustrated in detail.

I. *Animal Habitats*

The major habitats available on the earth for animals as usually recognized are (1) terrestrial, (2) fresh water and (3) marine. A fourth habitat should be added to these, namely, parasitic. Parasites have often been considered as living in the same habitats as their hosts but it is obvious that the environment of most of them is in reality radically different from that of the animals on or within which they live. For this reason it seems advisable to recognize a fourth major habitat with the characteristics common to those situations in which organisms live a parasitic existence. It is often assumed that parasites differ from free-living organisms in some more fundamental respect than habitat and very little attention is paid to this group of organisms in most textbooks and courses in zoölogy. As a matter of fact, as has been shown elsewhere (Hegner, 1926), the principles that govern the structure, life-cycles, habitats and activities of free-living and parasitic animals are really the same.

The activities of all animals may be separated into (1) those necessary for the maintenance of the individual and (2) those necessary for the maintenance of the race. The individual must be able to protect itself in its environment, to escape enemies, to reach a favorable situation in which to live, to find, capture, ingest, digest and assimilate food, to egest undigested material, to secrete pro-

1

tective substances, digestive juices and the like, to carry on respiration and to excrete waste products. Races are maintained by the asexual reproduction of the individuals of which they are composed, or by sexual reproduction or by both of these processes.

A comparison of any parasitic protozoön, worm or insect with nearly related free-living organisms will reveal the fact that both types of organisms are related in a similar way to their physical and biological environments. The relations between parasites and their hosts should, therefore, be studied as biological phenomena just as we are accustomed to study the relations between free-living organisms and their environment.

II. *Types of Association*

Living organisms, as just pointed out, must meet both physical and biological factors in their habitats. All living organisms are thus associated with other living organisms belonging both to the same species and to different species. Many types of association might be listed. Some of these are accidental or temporary, whereas others are invariable and permanent. Some of these types of association may be presented as follows:

(1) The two members of the association may be mutually and approximately equally benefited. For example, termites and their intestinal flagellates (p. 97).

(2) One member may secure an advantage from the association without the other undergoing any disadvantage. For example, *Trichodina pediculus* on *Hydra* (p. 190).

(3) One member may live more or less at the expense of the other without causing any injury to it. For example, bird lice.

(4) One member may injure the body of the other but not enough to produce clinical symptoms unless present in large numbers. For example, hookworms in man.

(5) One member may be distinctly pathogenic to the other, that is, may give rise to a diseased condition. The disease produced may be mild and only a contributory cause of death or may be severe and the direct cause of death. For example, *Endamœba histolytica* in man (p. 56).

III. *Types of Parasitism*

The term *parasitism* may be used in either a broad or a narrow sense. In a broad sense the word parasitism may be applied to any association in which one species lives on or within the body of another species. In a more restricted sense parasitism involves an obvious injury by the parasite to the other member of the association, the host.

Symbiosis is a term that is frequently employed to describe a certain type of association between two species of organisms. This term was proposed by deBary in 1879. Etymologically, symbiosis means simply "living together," and hence should include parasitism and other types of association. Usually, however, symbiosis is used to imply the permanent association of two specifically distinct organisms so dependent on each other that life apart is impossible.

Commensalism is another term in common use. It indicates an association in which one partner is benefited whereas the other is neither injured nor benefited; the former is the commensal and the latter the host.

Various types of parasites and hosts have been recognized by biologists. Some of these and certain terms commonly used by parasitologists are defined in the following list.

Host. An organism which harbors a parasite.

> Definitive host. The host which harbors the adult stage of the parasite.
>
> Intermediate host. The host which harbors the larval stages of the parasite.
>
> First intermediate host. The first host parasitized by the larval stages of the parasite.
>
> Second intermediate host. The host parasitized by the larval stages at a later period in the life-cycle.

Infection. The establishment of parasites within a host.

Infestation. A term used in connection with external, and in most cases, visible agents, for example, dogs infested with fleas. (See Journal of Parasitology, 23 : 325, 1937.)

Mutualism. An association of two organisms by which both are benefited.

Parasite. A plant or animal that lives upon or within another organism and feeds at its expense.

> Endoparasite. A parasite that lives within the body.
>
> Ectoparasite. A parasite that lives on the outside of the body.
>
> Erratic parasite. A parasite that wanders into an organ in which it does not usually live.
>
> Facultative parasite. An organism that is capable of living either free or as a parasite.
>
> Incidental parasite. A parasite that establishes itself in a host in which it does not usually live.

Obligatory parasite. An organism that depends for its existence on its host.

Periodic parasite. A parasite that makes short visits to its
host to obtain nourishment or other benefits.

Permanent parasite. A parasite that is parasitic throughout its
entire life-cycle.

Temporary parasite. A parasite that is free-living during a
part of its life-cycle.

Pathogenic parasite. An organism that may bring about harmful
modifications that can be demonstrated in the living or dead host, but
are not necessarily accompanied by symptoms.

Pseudoparasite. An object that is mistaken for a parasite.

IV. *Effects of a Parasitic Existence on the Parasite*

The parasitic mode of existence has brought about modifications
in structure and function and life-cycles among parasites that may
be either characteristic of parasites in general or peculiar to particular
groups, genera or species. These modifications may take the form of
both simplification and complication. Frequently the terms degeneration or degradation are applied to changes that are brought about
by a parasitic existence. Simplification and adaptation are better terms
to use to describe the phenomena observed.

Changes in the organs of locomotion, nutrition and reproduction
are rather general among parasitic organisms. For example, parasites
are ordinarily transported from place to place by the host and frequently are transmitted from one host to another without any effort
on their part. It is, therefore, not strange that the locomotor organs
of parasites should become simplified or should be in some cases
absent entirely. Organs of nutrition are also often modified or lost,
since the normal condition for parasites is life in an organic medium
from which food is absorbed through the surface of the body. The
reproductive organs of parasites, on the other hand, are frequently
larger and more complicated than those of free-living relatives, and
the number of eggs produced by parasites is in general many times
as great as that of nearly related free-living species. This must
necessarily be so, because the chances of an egg of a parasite producing an offspring which will succeed in establishing itself on or
within another host are very slender indeed.

The structural or physiological modifications of parasites may be
characteristic of groups, genera or species, as stated above. Modifi-

cations of this type will be noted in the descriptions of the various species dealt with in later chapters of this book.

V. *Parasitism in the Animal Kingdom*

Almost every large group in the animal kingdom contains parasitic species. There are very few of these, however, in certain phyla and large numbers in other phyla. A survey of the animal kingdom shows clearly that the parasites of principal importance are included in the phylum PROTOZOA, several phyla of worms and the phylum ARTHROPODA. The following list presents in abbreviated form the phyla of the animal kingdom and the groups that contain parasitic species.

Phylum I. PROTOZOA. Unicellular animals.

Class 1. SARCODINA. Free-living and parasitic. Parasitic amœbæ in man and lower animals.

Class 2. MASTIGOPHORA. Free-living and parasitic. Intestinal and blood-inhabiting parasites of man and lower animals.

Class 3. SPOROZOA. Parasitic. Coccidia and malaria parasites in man; parasites in intestine, blood and tissues of lower animals.

Class 4. INFUSORIA. Free-living and parasitic. *Balantidium coli* in man; various species in lower animals.

Phylum II. PORIFERA. Sponges. Very few parasites.

Phylum III. CŒLENTERATA. Polyps, jellyfishes, sea-anemones and corals. Very few parasites.

Phylum IV. PLATYHELMINTHES. Flatworms. Free-living and parasitic.

Class 1. TURBELLARIA. Mostly free-living; e.g., *Planaria*.

Class 2. TREMATODA. Parasitic. Flukes.

Class 3. CESTODA. Parasitic. Tapeworms.

Phylum V. NEMATHELMINTHES. Round worms. Free-living and parasitic in man and lower animals; e.g., hookworms, ascarids and trichinas.

Groups of Uncertain Systematic Position.

1. ACANTHOCEPHALA. Spineheaded worms. Parasitic in man and lower animals.

2. GORDIACEA. Hair worms. Parasitic in insects.

Phylum VI. ECHINODERMATA. Starfishes, sea-urchins. Free-living.

Phylum VII. ANNELIDA. Segmented worms. Free-living and parasitic; e.g., earthworms (free-living) and leeches (parasitic).

Phylum VIII. MOLLUSCA. Snails, clams, squids. Mostly free-living.

Phylum IX. ARTHROPODA. Crayfishes, insects, spiders, centipedes. Free-living and parasitic; many species act as intermediate hosts of parasitic PROTOZOA and worms.

Class 1. CRUSTACEA. Crayfishes, etc.; many parasites of fish.

Class 2. MYRIAPODA. Centipedes.

Class 3. INSECTA. Insects. Many parasitic and many intermediate hosts.

Class 4. ARACHNIDA. Spiders, scorpions, mites, ticks. Many parasitic.

Phylum X. VERTEBRATA. Fish, amphibians, reptiles, birds, mammals. Mostly free-living, but each group contains species that may be classed as parasites in a broad sense.

VI. *Host-Parasite Specificity*

The term *host-parasite specificity* is used here to indicate the relations between hosts and parasites regarding the degree of susceptibility of the host and the degree of infectivity or powers of infestation of the parasite. For example, man is susceptible to infection or infestation with certain species of protozoa, worms and arthropods and his degree of susceptibility differs more or less for each species; rats are susceptible to certain of the same species and to different species as well. This is host-parasite specificity viewed from the standpoint of the host.

On the other hand, host-parasite specificity when applied to the parasites refers to their degree of infectivity or powers of infestation. For example, *Endamœba histolytica* is known to be able to live in man, monkeys, dogs, cats and rats, but infects certain species of hosts more readily than others and varies with respect to its pathogenicity in the different hosts.

A committee of the American Society of Parasitologists recently criticized this term (see Jour. Parasit., 23: 326, 1937) but apparently did not understand the way in which the writer meant it to be used.

I. HOST SUSCEPTIBILITY

Parasitologists have long recognized different types of hosts with respect to their susceptibility to various parasites. Thus if a host is easily parasitized by a certain species it is said to be tolerant, whereas if it is difficult to parasitize it is classed as refractory. A host that is frequently found parasitized by a certain species in nature is known as a natural host; whereas one that does not become so parasitized may be considered a foreign host. If a species of parasite that habitually lives in or on a certain host species is found in or on a host that is very seldom infected that host is spoken of as an accidental or casual host. A host may become infected but throw off the infection after a short time, in which case it is known as a provisional or transitory host; or it may serve as a host for a short stage in the life-cycle of a parasite, thus becoming a temporary host.

Frequently it is possible to infect species of hosts in the laboratory that do not become infected, as a rule, in nature, either because their habits are such that they do not come into proper relations with the parasites or because they are refractory except when large numbers of parasites are present or when these are administered to them in certain definite ways not usually possible in nature.

Whether or not a susceptible species of animal becomes infected with a particular species of parasite in nature depends primarily on three factors: (1) animal and parasite must live in the same geographical region, (2) the habits of the animal must be such as to bring it into proper relations with the infective stage of the parasite and (3) the life-cycle of the parasite must be such that its infective stage is reached when and where the host is available to be parasitized.

The first factor mentioned is so obvious that little discussion is necessary. The absence of certain diseases from certain regions is frequently due not to the absence of susceptible hosts but to the absence of the parasites. This, for example, may account for the absence of malaria from countries where susceptible human hosts and the proper species of anopheline mosquitoes exist but where the malarial parasites have never been introduced. On the other hand, many cases might be cited of diseases that have appeared in various regions previously free from them because of the introduction of the causative parasite.

The other two factors are really the same considered from the two standpoints of host and parasite respectively. If the life-cycle of a parasite and the activities of its natural host are studied side by side it will appear as though both host and parasite were actually trying to bring about a situation favorable for infection. For example, the gametocytes of the malarial organisms live in the peripheral blood where they cannot fail to reach the stomach of the mosquito that sucks up the blood; the infective sporozoites congregate in the salivary glands of the mosquito where they seem to lie in wait to be inoculated into a new host. The mosquito feeds on the blood of man and thus enables the parasites to enter the blood stream; whereas it might feed on fruit juices as it is able to do in the laboratory. The infective mosquito bites usually at night when the host is asleep and is thus able to inoculate the sporozoites successfully during an uninterrupted meal. A change in any one of these conditions might easily bring about the annihilation of the race of parasites; for example, if the gametocytes were localized in the internal organs of man or if the sporozoites did not reach the salivary glands of the mosquito there would be no spread of malaria and the disease would soon die out.

An infection that involves injury to the host may be acute, malignant, fulminating, chronic or benign, but the evidence does not indicate that the susceptibility of the host to an infection has any bearing on the character of the infection induced. That is to say, a host may be more susceptible to infection, and probably usually is, by a species of parasite that never calls forth symptoms than by a pathogenic or lethal species.

2. PARASITE INFECTIVITY

If a host is easily parasitized by a species, the parasite is said to be highly infective. How much its infectivity is due to the host and how much to the parasite it is impossible to say. Several of the terms noted above with respect to hosts are also commonly used to designate different types of parasites. Thus, we speak of natural parasites, accidental parasites, and provisional, transitory or temporary parasites. Parasites are also classified according to the necessity of existence within a certain host, as facultative, when this is not required, and obligate, when the parasite is unable to live in any other host. The invasive powers of a parasite are indicated by such terms as virulent or aggressive, and the degree of infectivity with respect to the effects on the host as pathogenic, sublethal and lethal.

That the hosts differ in susceptibility to a given parasite has been abundantly demonstrated. The differences may be racial, familial or individual, i.e., susceptibility may be inherited. It would be interesting to study this subject with hybrids between susceptible and non-susceptible hosts. Sex and age may also have a profound effect on host-parasite specificity. In general young animals are more susceptible to infection than adults.

The physiological state of the hosts may have an important bearing on its susceptibility. Frequently a refractory host may become infected if his resistance is lowered by overwork, by previous infection with other parasites, by malnutrition, intoxication, by exposure to wet and cold, by trauma or by shock. Changes in physiological state no doubt also take place in parasites which raise or lower their powers of infectivity. Other factors that cause no inconvenience to the host may be unfavorable for the parasite.

The origin of host-parasite specificity is really synonymous with the evolution of parasitism. It is obvious that parasitism cannot exist unless the hosts and parasites involved are present in the same region and behave in such a way as to come frequently into contact. If these conditions are fulfilled, the factors that make it possible for the parasite to live and reproduce within the host present themselves for consideration. Thus it seems certain that man often takes in with his food the infective stages of many parasites of lower animals. These organisms are not able to remain in the body of man because man does not tolerate them.

But what factors are responsible for tolerance or refractoriness and how have these conditions arisen in the course of evolution? Some of the factors involved have been discussed above, and, as we have seen, are still very obscure. We must base our studies on the conditions of host and parasite as we find them to-day without much consideration of how the present status has been reached. There can be little doubt, however, but that long association has brought about changes in both host and parasite which make it possible for them to live together in harmony except under special conditions. An increase in the virulence of the parasites might disturb the equilibrium established and bring about pathological conditions in the host; a decrease in the resistance of the host might have the same effect; or a decrease in the aggressivity of the parasite might prevent infection; and an increase in the resistance of the host might also prevent infection.

3. PROBLEMS IN HOST-PARASITE SPECIFICITY

The subject of host-parasite specificity offers many problems for investigation. Material for study can be obtained easily and results promise to be of great importance to the subject of host-parasite relations. Some of these problems may be stated as follows:

(1) To what extent does the behavior of the host and that of the parasite determine host-parasite specificity?

(2) Do species of parasites that are restricted to one species of host gain access to other species of hosts?

(3) What factors within a host enable natural parasites to bring about an infection and prevent foreign parasites from doing so?

(4) How may we account for laboratory infections in foreign hosts?

(5) What conditions are responsible for differences in susceptibility between young and adult animals?

(6) What host-parasite interactions terminate an infection or bring about periods of latency and relapse?

VII. *Host-Parasite Relations*

In general, the series of events that constitute the relations of host and parasite may be considered as beginning with the transmission of the parasite from one host to another. Then follow the distribution and localization of the parasite on or within the host, the growth or multiplication of the parasite, the resistance of the host to the parasite and of the parasite to the host, the method of attack of the parasite, changes in the host brought about by the parasite and those in the parasite due to residence in the host, host-parasite adjustments during the infection, the escape of infective stages of the parasite from the host and the recovery or death of the host. These will now be considered in order for parasites in general and a similar method of presentation will be used in the case of specific parasites in later chapters with modifications necessitated by the peculiarities characteristic of each species.

I. EPIDEMIOLOGY OF TRANSMISSION

Infective stage. The stage in the life-cycle of a parasite that escapes from the body of the host is either infective to fresh hosts or develops to the infective stage outside of the body. During this period the parasites are usually subjected to external environmental factors and most of the parasites perish, but as long as a race continues it is obvious that a certain number survive and set up infections in fresh hosts. At one time it was supposed that disease-producing organisms might multiply outside of the body of the host and bring about foci of infection in soil or water, but we now know that in most cases there is no reproduction of the parasite during its life in the outer world. (See *Strongyloides stercoralis*, p. 404.)

Avenues of infection. Reaching and invading a new host is

certainly one of the most serious problems in the entire life-cycle of a parasite and only the smallest proportion of the total number of infective organisms reach a susceptible animal in or on which to live. Only the almost inconceivable fecundity of the parasites prevents the various species from dying out.

Transmission by contamination is a very effective method for a parasite to reach a new host. The organism while outside of the body may reach the food or drink of man by contamination because of unsanitary conditions due to neglect on the part of the host or through the agency of flies and other animals. Many parasites are protected by resistant walls in the cyst or egg stage which keep them viable until they are ingested by a new host.

Another method of transmission is by "contagion" or direct transference from one host to another. Thus parasites that live in the human mouth may be transferred from one person to another by kissing.

A third method of transmission is that by inoculation through the agency of an intermediate host. The mosquito, as we shall find later, is one of the most efficient vectors of parasites since mosquitoes are the transmitting agents of the organisms of malaria and filariasis and other parasites.

The so-called "hereditary" method of transmission is not known to occur in any parasites that live in man, but certain species that parasitize lower animals make their way into the eggs of these animals and hence parasitize the new generations that develop from these eggs.

Prenatal transmission occurs rather frequently, especially in the case of parasitic worms.

One interesting fact that is made clear by the study of the epidemiology of transmission is that in most cases the parasite is passive during its transfer from one host to another and transmission is almost entirely due to the activity of the host or of intermediate hosts. Simple sanitary measures, such as the prevention of soil pollution and protection against mosquitoes, are usually all that are necessary to protect human hosts from infection with such organisms as intestinal protozoa and worms and the parasites of malaria and filariasis.

2. CLINICAL AND PARASITOLOGICAL PERIODS DURING THE COURSE OF A NATURAL INFECTION

The relations of host and parasite during what may be called a natural infection, as distinguished from the invasion of a host by foreign parasites or infections complicated in various ways, may be divided into two types of periods—periods that refer to the reactions of the parasite in the host and periods descriptive of the reactions of the host to the parasite. These periods are presented in diagrammatic form in Figure 1. They may be defined briefly as follows:

PARASITOLOGICAL PERIODS. The *Prepatent Period* extends from the time the infective parasites enter the body of the host until their eggs, cysts or other stages in their life-cycle can be recovered by specified laboratory methods. The length of this period obviously depends to some extent on the character of the laboratory technique employed.

The *Patent Period* covers the interval during which the parasites can be demonstrated by the technique employed. In the PROTOZOA the parasite number usually undergoes a rise during this period, reaches a peak, and then suffers a fall. The patent period ends when the parasites can no longer be recovered. In worms the patent period lasts as long as the parasite continues to lay eggs.

In many protozoan infections the patent period is followed by a *Subpatent Period* of indefinite length. During this period parasites cannot be recovered by the usual laboratory methods but their presence can be proved in various ways depending on the species of parasite.

The subpatent period may be followed by a second patent period during which the parasite number rises, reaches a peak, and falls, but often does not rise as high as in the primary attack.

CLINICAL PERIODS. The *Incubation Period* extends from the time of entrance of the parasites until symptoms appear. This period is usually longer than the prepatent period, but may be shorter.

The *Period of Symptoms* begins when the incubation period ends and ends of course with the cessation of symptoms. In helminth diseases the symptoms induced are chronic.

The *Convalescent Period* is represented in protozoan diseases as beginning at the point of maximum symptoms and ending with the recovery of the host.

In diseases characterized by relapses one or more *Latent Periods* may be present. During these periods the causative organisms are too few in number to bring about symptoms, but, after intervals of indefinite length, some change occurs in parasite, or host or in both that results in an increase in parasite number and a reappearance of symptoms.

The reappearance of symptoms following a latent period is known as the *Period of Relapse*.

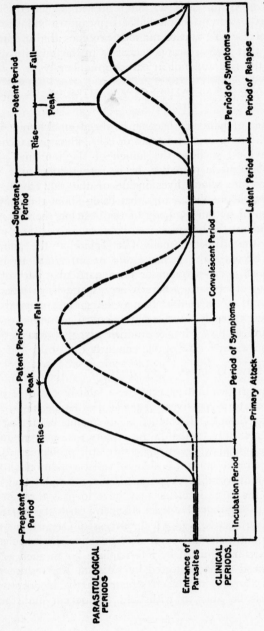

Fig. 1.—Parasitological and clinical periods, especially in protozoan infections. This illustration is intended to represent by means of curves the parasitological and clinical periods in the course of infections, especially with pathogenic protozoa. It represents in a general diagrammatic way the course of natural infections, consisting of a primary attack followed by apparent recovery of the host. This completes both the parasitological and clinical manifestations of disease in cases such as oriental sore in which one attack gives immunity. In other diseases, however, such as amoebic dysentery and malaria, the primary attack is often followed by a symptomless period when the parasites are latent. Eventually the parasite number again increases, symptoms reappear and the host is said to suffer a relapse. The terms used are fully described in the text. (From Hegner)

The curves as given probably do not represent actual conditions in any specific protozoan infection but are meant to indicate that in general the increase in parasite number precedes the appearance of symptoms and that increases and decreases in the severity of the symptoms follow the rise and fall in parasite number.

3. DISTRIBUTION AND LOCALIZATION OF PARASITES ON OR WITHIN THE HOST

Different species of parasites become localized on different parts of the body or in different organs, tissues or cells. Thus parasites may be localized in cavities, such as the lumen of the intestine, or in tissue, for example, muscle parasites, or be intracellular as is true of the malaria parasite which lives inside of the red blood cells. We know something about the factors that bring about the distribution of parasites on or within the body of the host but there is much still to be learned about this subject.

The attack of the parasite usually takes place at the point of localization. This becomes the *primary site of infection*. In many cases a parasite does not remain in or on a particular part of the body but spreads to other parts where it begins attacks at what are called *secondary sites of infection*. It may be said in general that distribution is due primarily to the physiological activities of the host and localization to host-parasite interactions, the parasites setting up an infection wherever favorable conditions exist.

4. THE PASSIVE RESISTANCE OF HOST AND PARASITE

The host characteristics that prevent the establishment of a parasite may be referred to as passive resistance. Each type of parasite encounters various obstacles that must be overcome before a host can be invaded successfully. Some of the factors that prevent infection are easily determined whereas others are still problematical.

The invading parasite must be able to resist conditions in the host that may be unfavorable. A parasite, for example, that sets up an infection in the large intestine may have to pass through the preceding sections of the digestive tract. In many cases the organism is surrounded by a protective wall which successfully resists adverse conditions in the mouth, stomach and small intestine. Blood-inhabiting parasites that are transmitted by intermediate hosts, such as the mosquito, do not need to be protected by resistant walls since they are inoculated directly into the blood stream. In the blood stream, however, they must be able to withstand the serum and escape phagocytosis.

5. THE PARASITE'S METHOD OF ATTACK

Having reached the primary site of infection the true infection of the host begins. Each parasite has its own particular method of attack and the different types of parasitism are distinguished largely on this basis. In most cases of parasitism the parasite is able to live and reproduce for many years within the host without apparent injury to it. It is obvious that the degree of injury depends on which organs or tissues are invaded and on the degree and rapidity of tissue destruction or on the production of toxic substances. Slight injuries inflicted slowly are usually repaired by the host as they occur, whereas serious injuries that are quickly produced lead to symptoms. If the host develops severe symptoms both it and the parasites are in danger and if the host dies the parasites usually die with it. This type of parasitic attack is unusual and is considered to represent a comparatively recent association since most parasites live in harmony with their hosts—a condition that is supposed to have developed during the course of evolution.

6. CHANGES IN THE HOST CAUSED BY THE PARASITE

Parasites that injure their hosts are pathogenic. If the injuries are so severe as to interfere radically with the normal functions of the organs of the host, symptoms appear. The host may build up an active resistance against such an attack, which we call immunity. The pathology of most parasitic diseases is well known, but very little is known about the genesis of the conditions observed. Likewise, the symptomatology of the parasitic diseases of man has been thoroughly described, but the way in which the functions of the organs are disturbed is still obscure. There is no doubt that the human host builds up an immunity against certain parasites. This subject, however, is one that needs further study.

7. CHANGES IN THE PARASITE DUE TO RESIDENCE IN THE HOST

Since parasites are living organisms, they also are probably capable of building up active resistance against the attacks of the host. It is obviously difficult to demonstrate such a parasite immunity, although "fastness" among the PROTOZOA may be due to such a phenomenon. Whether changes in virulence may occur in a strain of parasites while residing in a host is still an open question.

8. HOST-PARASITE ADJUSTMENTS DURING AN INFECTION

Carriers. The continued increase in numbers of parasites, due to reproduction or reinfestation without check, would obviously result in the death of the host. As stated above, parasites do not destroy their hosts in most cases. Frequently in protozoan infections, the host, by means of acquired resistance, is able to destroy most but not all of the parasites and hence to bring about what is known as the carrier condition. Such a carrier is a host in which parasites live and by which they are disseminated but which exhibits no visible symptoms of infection. Carriers may be divided into two types, contact carriers, who are parasitized but have never exhibited symptoms, and convalescent carriers, who have recovered from a parasitic disease but are still infected. Certain species of hosts are almost universally infected in nature by certain species of parasites and a parasitized condition might almost be considered the normal state of such a species. Carriers are frequently spoken of as reservoirs since they are storehouses for the parasites that are responsible for the spread of the infection to new hosts. Certain parasites are infective both to man and to lower animals and one or both kinds of hosts may serve as reservoirs.

Latency. Parasites are said to be latent when they are present in a host but do not make themselves manifest. The infected host may show no symptoms or may have recovered from symptoms and still harbor parasites. In either case, the condition is known as latency. Certain changes in host or parasite may bring on symptoms in a host that had never previously exhibited evidence of infection. Such a case might be considered only an extended incubation period.

Relapse. When a host that had previously shown symptoms but had apparently recovered again exhibits symptoms following a period of latency, the condition is known as a relapse. Relapses are of frequent occurrence in many parasitic diseases. They must be due to some change in the relation between the host and parasite but just what changes are responsible for the increase in the number of parasites and the reappearance of symptoms is known in very few cases.

9. ESCAPE OF PARASITES FROM THE HOST

Parasites obviously must escape from the host in which they are produced in order to bring about the infection of new hosts and thus prevent the race from dying out. The different types of parasites follow different routes in escaping from their hosts. Many of them attack parts of the host from which natural channels lead to the outside; for example, intestinal parasites pass out with the feces. Other species are extracted from a host by blood-sucking vectors. The method of escape of each type of parasite considered in this book will be described in an appropriate place in later chapters.

VIII. *Origin and Evolution of Parasitism*

We really know nothing definite about the origin and evolution of parasitism, since no one has ever observed a free-living species become parasitic, but there are many known facts that are of value in any attempt to work out lines of descent.

(1) In the first place, the parasitic habit must be more recently evolved than the free-living habit, since free-living forms must have existed before the parasites could obtain hosts on which to live.

(2) Ectoparasites probably evolved before endoparasites, because the change from a free-living existence to that of ectoparasitism does not appear to be so difficult as to that of endoparasitism.

(3) Inasmuch as there are free-living as well as parasitic species in many large groups of animals, it is evident that the parasitic habit has arisen independently in each of these groups and this phenomenon may therefore be considered of rather common occurrence during the course of evolution.

(4) Most parasites belong to groups that are more primitive than their hosts, i.e., are lower in the scale of life. PROTOZOA cannot be parasitized by animals more primitive than themselves, but may be parasitized by plant organisms.

(5) Certain ectoparasites are not limited to one species of host; others have been observed on only one species; and certain ectoparasites are confined to a definite part of the body of the host. These are supposed to be stages in the evolution of ectoparasitism. A species that is able to migrate from one species of host to another is probably in a more primitive stage of parasitism than one that is limited to one host, and the latter condition has probably originated from the former. The third type of ectoparasite mentioned represents a still further specialization, the parasite being limited to a single organ of the host.

(6) The relations between ectoparasitism and endoparasitism, and commensalism and symbiosis furnish much material for speculation. Do commensalism and symbiosis lead to parasitism? Many students believe that they do. For example, a species that takes its meals in a state of mutualism with another species might develop

into a food robber and from this into an actual parasite; or, symbiotic relations might become disturbed and instead of a more or less mutual association one member might develop gradually into a pathogenic parasite.

(7) Endoparasites may be limited to one species of host or may pass through part of their life-cycle in one host and part in another. How did endoparasitism arise and which of the two conditions mentioned is the more primitive? Endoparasitism may have arisen from ectoparasitism, from commensalism or from symbiosis. If an endoparasite is restricted to one species of host it probably adopted the parasitic habit within this species and is therefore no older phylogenetically than its host. Any changes that have taken place in the parasite have probably proceeded coincident with changes in its host. When an endoparasite occurs in several species of hosts, the parasite is probably older than its hosts, having adapted itself to hosts that evolved after it became a parasite.

(8) Parasites that have intermediate hosts have probably evolved from parasites with only one species of host. This condition may have arisen because of the ability of the parasite to adapt itself to changed conditions, at first simply tolerating the second host but later actually establishing itself within it. The entrance of exogenous stages of parasites into other animals is very widespread in nature, and plenty of opportunity exists for parasitism to arise.

IX. *Parasitism and the Geographical Distribution and Evolution of Hosts*

One of the most interesting phases of parasitism is that involving its bearing on the geographical distribution and genetic relationships of hosts. Von Jhering in 1902 was among the first to discuss this problem in cases of parasitic worms. He argues that two species of hosts are of common descent if they are parasitized by the same species or nearly related species of parasites. He believes that the close relationship of the parasites indicates that they come from a common ancestor and that the different species of hosts involved descended from an ancestral host that was infected by the ancestral parasite. Similar arguments were employed by Zschokke (1904) to account for the distribution of certain cestodes in marsupial mammals.

How the migration of salmon may be inferred from the character of its helminthic parasites is also pointed out by Zschokke (1903). The original home of the salmon is not necessarily indicated by the present path of its migration nor by the locality of its breeding ground, but the fact that a large proportion of its endoparasites are those of marine animals seems to prove that the ancestral home of this type of fish was the sea and not its present breeding ground, which is in fresh water. "Each parasitic fauna," says Zschokke, "comes to be to some extent a mirror image of the biology of the host, of its habits of life and especially of its relations to those creatures that share the habitat with it. Each change of nourishment and residence of an animal finds its echo in the changes in the helminthic condition."

The best work of this type on PROTOZOA is that done by Metcalf (1923). Metcalf discusses, for example, the distribution of the family LEPTODACTYLIDÆ. These are "frogs" characteristic of two widely separated geographical regions, (1) tropical and semi-tropical America and (2) Australia and Tasmania; they have been reported from no other parts of the world. There are two hypotheses that may account for this discontinuous distribution: (1) there may have been a former connection between Patagonia and Australia by way of Antarctica over which these frogs were continuously distributed, or (2) resemblances of the frogs of America and Australia may be due to convergent or parallel evolution.

Frogs of the family LEPTODACTYLIDÆ contain, in the rectum, opalinid parasites of the genus *Zelleriella*. These parasitic ciliates are present in the frogs of this family living in both America and Australia. They are so nearly alike in the frogs of the two regions that they can be separated specifically only with difficulty. It is possible that either the frogs or the opalinid ciliates may have arisen by convergent or parallel evolution. It seems very improbable, however, that both the frogs and opalinids arose in this way. The conclusion is reached that the first hypothesis is correct and that a former land connection existed between Patagonia and Australia by means of which frogs of this family, together with their opalinid parasites, migrated to Australia.

Practically all parasites lend themselves to studies of this type. Kellogg (1905) has used the method in his work on bird lice; Johnston (1914) has studied problems of evolution and zoögeography by the use of trematodes and cestodes, and Darling (1920) has studied the migrations of human races from data of hookworm distribution. In this way parasitology has proven itself a valuable aid in the study of geographical distribution and evolution.

X. *The Protozoa of Man and Monkeys*

The comparison of the protozoa that live in monkeys with those that live in man has led to results of evolutionary significance (Hegner, 1928).

For many years most of the monkey protozoa examined came from animals that had been kept in captivity, where they might have become contaminated with human protozoa. But many wild monkeys have been studied during the past few years and have yielded just as many parasites as their imprisoned relatives. Where these wild monkeys got their protozoa is an intriguing problem. Infections at the present time are no doubt transmitted from one parent to another and from parents to offspring much as human protozoa are distributed among the members of a family. This method of transmission can likewise be imagined to have occurred generation after generation for thousands of years. If we believe in organic evolution, the probability seems unquestionable that the protozoa of a living species of monkey must have been thrust upon it by the species out of which it evolved. This must also apply equally to man.

At the present time we do not know of any structural characteristics that can be used to distinguish between most of the species of human and monkey protozoa. This applies to the ameba and flagellate of the mouth, the giardia flagellate of the small intestine, the five species of amebas, three of the species of flagellates and a ciliate that live in the large intestine, the trichomonad flagellate that inhabits the genital tract, and two of the trypanosome flagellates and the three malaria parasites that live in the blood.

This means that eighteen of the twenty-five species of protozoa that are known to live in man (Fig. 2) are indistinguishable from eighteen of those that have been reported from monkeys. The other seven human species may live in monkeys somewhere but have not yet been discovered. Besides the eighteen species mentioned, monkeys are known to be parasitized by a large ciliate, *Troglodytella,* by two or three other species of ciliates and by several other species of protozoa whose specific identity is still somewhat in doubt. Thus about seven monkey species do not live in man and about the same number of human species do not live in monkeys.

Whether the protozoa of monkeys and man that cannot be distinguished from one another really belong to the same species is difficult to decide. Recent studies of the balantidial ciliates of pig, guinea-pig, and chimpanzee suggest that differences may exist that are very obscure. Balantidia from time to time conjugate two by

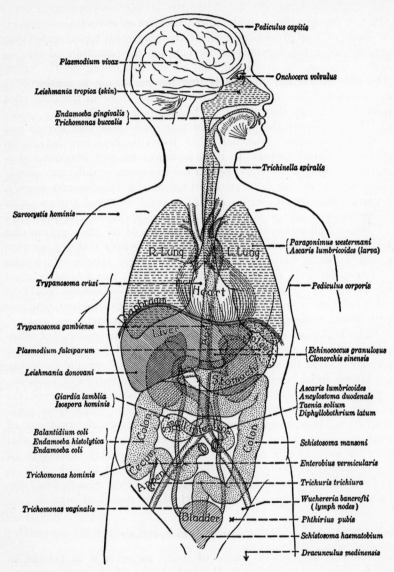

FIG. 2.—Diagram showing the localization of some of the parasites that live in the human body. On the left are protozoa and on the right are worms and insects. (From Hegner)

two much as paramecia do. After the conjugants separate a complicated reorganization of the nuclei takes place in each exconjugant.
A study of this process of nuclear reorganization has revealed differences of a fundamental nature between the balantidia of the pig
and chimp, on the one hand, and of the guinea-pig on the other.
The only conclusion possible is that the guinea-pig is inhabited by
balantidia that are specifically different from those in the other two
animals, although they appear to be alike superficially.

If we compare the protozoa of man with those that live in any
wild or domesticated animal other than monkeys, we behold an
entirely different picture. In most instances we may encounter protozoa belonging to the same genera but to obviously different species.
Thus in the rat we note an intestinal ameba (*Endamœba muris*),
a giardia flagellate (*Giardia muris*), several intestinal trichomonads
(*Trichomonas muris, T. parva* and *T. minuta*) and a trypanosome
(*T. lewisi*) all visibly different from species of the same genera that
inhabit man, as well as species belonging to genera that are not represented among human protozoa, such as three species of coccidia
(*Eimeria miyairii, E. separata,* and *E. carinii*), and a blood-inhabiting sporozoön (*Hepatozoön muris*). Similar comparisons could be
made with other species of animals, not only with mammals but also
with birds, reptiles, amphibians, fish and even invertebrates.

The biological significance of this situation seems evident when
we consider the fact that animals closely related, according to their
arrangement in the animal series on the basis of organic evolution,
are known to be inhabited by similar genera and species of parasites.
Or, stated in another way, the greater the similarity between the
parasites the more closely related are the hosts in which these parasites live. The extraordinary resemblance between the protozoa of
monkeys and man can lead to but one conclusion, and that is, that
men are more closely related to monkeys than to any other type of
lower animal. Parasitism may therefore be added to such subjects
as classification, comparative anatomy, embryology, geographical distribution and paleontology in support of the theory of organic evolution.

XI. *Rules of Nomenclature*

The correct scientific name of many parasites is at present in
doubt. This is due in part to the failure of certain investigators to
follow the rules of nomenclature in describing new species and in
part to the tendency in many cases to name new genera and species
without sufficient study of the organism or of the group to which it

belongs. In 1898 the International Congress of Zoölogy organized an International Commission on Zoölogical Nomenclature which has served since that time and has prepared a set of International Rules of Zoölogical Nomenclature. These rules apply to family, subfamily, generic, subgeneric, specific and subspecific names. They cover the formation, derivation, and orthography of zoölogical names, the author's name, the law of priority and its application and the rejection of names. According to these rules, zoölogical and botanical names are independent, hence the same genus and species name may be applied to both an animal and a plant, although this is not recommended; scientific names must be Latin or Latinized; family names are formed by adding -*idæ* to the stem of the name of the type genus; generic names should consist of a single word, written with a capital initial letter and italicized; specific names are adjectives agreeing grammatically with the generic name, substantives in the nominative in apposition with the generic name, or substantives in the genitive, and should be italicized; the author of a scientific name is the person who first publishes the name with a definition or description of the organism given. If a new genus is proposed, the type species of the genus should be designated. Type species should be deposited some place where they are accessible and a statement regarding their location included in the publication in which they are described. The list of International Rules of Zoölogical Nomenclature was published in pamphlet form in the *Proceedings of the Biological Society of Washington*, vol. xxxix, 1926, pp. 75-104, and also in Wenyon's *Protozoölogy*, vol. ii, 1926, pp. 1336-1349. These are complete except for an amendment published in *Science*, vol. lxvi, 1928, pp. 17-18.

Section I

PROTOZOÖLOGY

BY

ROBERT HEGNER

CHAPTER I

THE BIOLOGY OF THE PROTOZOA

As noted in the Introduction, a large number of parasitic animals belong to the Phylum PROTOZOA. In this section attention will be directed primarily to this type of PROTOZOA. However, much of what we know regarding the morphology, physiology and reproduction of the PROTOZOA has been learned by the study of free-living species. To understand the nature and activities of parasitic species it is, therefore, necessary to know something about the biology of the entire group. For this reason Section I on PROTOZOÖLOGY is introduced by this chapter on the Biology of the Protozoa.

The study of the biology of the PROTOZOA involves first of all a knowledge of these organisms sufficient to enable one to recognize the class, order, genus and species to which the various members of the Phylum belong. To gain this knowledge one must study the morphology and classification of PROTOZOA in general. This having been done one may then proceed to inquire in what types of habitats PROTOZOA live, how they maintain themselves in their various habitats and how races of PROTOZOA are maintained.

I. *Morphology*

PROTOZOA are usually designated unicellular animals to distinguish them from the METAZOA which are many-celled animals. Most PROTOZOA possess in fact the characteristics of a single cell (Fig. 3). The body consists of protoplasm which is of two principal types, cytoplasm and nucleoplasm, but there are almost countless variations in the shape and size of the body and in details of structure. As regards size, PROTOZOA are all small as compared with METAZOA, most of them being invisible to the naked eye. They can, therefore, be studied successfully only with the help of a microscope. Each species of protozoön has a characteristic shape, a feature which is of particular value in the identification of species. Even amœbæ, which have been defined as shapeless masses of protoplasm, can usually be separated into genera and species on the basis of body shape.

The cytoplasm of the protozoan body is usually divisible into two parts, a clear thin layer of ectoplasm at the surface and a more fluid, granular inner portion, the endoplasm. The ectoplasm at the periphery is in contact with the environment of the organism and it is, therefore, not strange that locomotor organs, skeletal and supporting structures and organs of attachment should be formed of this substance. In the endoplasm are various inclusions, the most important of which are nuclei, food vacuoles, contractile vacuoles, plastids and various other bodies concerned in reproduction and other vital activities.

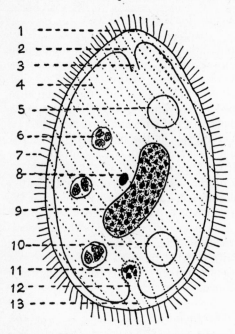

The organs of locomotion of PROTOZOA are of particular interest because of their functions both of locomotion and food capture and their use in separating the PROTOZOA into classes. It is customary to characterize the classes of PROTOZOA on the basis of the presence or absence of locomotor organs and the nature of these when present. Pseudopodia are characteristic of the Class SARCODINA, flagella of the Class MASTIGOPHORA, cilia of the Class INFUSORIA and the fourth Class, the SPOROZOA, is characterized by the absence of organs of locomotion. Different species of amœbæ differ with respect to the shape and size of their pseudopodia and the method of their formation. Flagella are fine thread-like organelles that consist, in at least some cases, of two parts, a central axial filament capable of contraction, and a surrounding elastic sheath. The diameter, length and number of flagella are constant for each species of mastigophoron and hence of considerable value in identifying species. Cilia are really small flagella, being usually shorter and thinner but structurally sim-

FIG. 3.—Diagram of a protozoon (*Balantidium coli*) designed to show the structure of a member of this phylum.

1—Peristome	8—Micronucleus
2—Cystostome	9—Macronucleus
3—Cytopharynx	10—Contractile vacuole
4—Striation	11—Excretory vacuole
5—Contractile vacuole	12—Excretory canal
6—Food vacuole	13—Cytopyge
7—Cilium	

ilar. They are ordinarily more numerous, and definitely arranged on the surface of the body according to the species. Cilia may become fused together to form membranelles or into spine-like structures known as cirri. Cirri are especially characteristic of hypotrichous ciliates, where they occur on the ventral surface and are used much like legs in walking or running.

In many PROTOZOA there is a definite region of the ectoplasm known as the peristome in which there is a funnel-shaped depression or tube, the cytopharynx, the opening of which is known as the cytostome or mouth. Such a structure is characteristic of many of the INFUSORIA and serves to transport food into the endoplasm. At

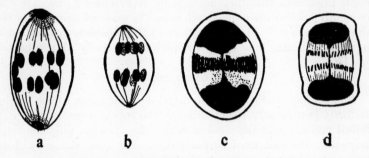

a   b   c   d

FIG. 4.—Nuclei of various species of SARCODINA in mitosis (x 4000).
(From Kofoid and Swezy)

a. *Endamœba coli.* (After Swezy)
b. *Endamœba histolytica.* (After Kofoid and Swezy)
c. *Amœba diplogena.* (After Bĕlař)
d. *Vahlkampfia diplomitotica.* (After Aragão)

the so-called posterior end of the body there may be a less complex opening in the ectoplasm, the cytopyge, through which undigested particles are cast out.

Skeletal and supporting structures are present in many species of PROTOZOA. These are formed by the protoplasm of the organism or by the acquisition of minute foreign bodies such as sand crystals or diatoms. The common fresh water genus *Arcella* possesses an external shell formed by the organism, whereas its near relative, *Difflugia,* builds its external skeleton of minute sand grains. Some of the SARCODINA, especially the HELIOZOA, RADIOLARIA and FORAMINFERA construct elaborate internal skeletons of silica or calcium carbonate. Skeletal and supporting structures other than peripheral membranes and cyst walls are not common among parasitic PROTOZOA.

Most of the PROTOZOA possess a single nucleus (Fig. 4). The INFUSORIA, however, are characterized by the presence of two nuclei of different sizes, a large macronucleus and a smaller micronucleus. Certain members of each of the four classes of PROTOZOA are provided with more than one nucleus; in some the number may reach into the hundreds. Besides the nucleus, several types of vacuoles may occur in the endoplasm: more or less permanent vacuoles filled with fluid, food vacuoles containing ingested solid particles and contractile vacuoles which periodically expel liquid to the outside through the ectoplasm. Plastids of various types may also occur in the bodies of PROTOZOA. The location, morphology and functions of these will be discussed in later chapters. Examination of the morphology of the PROTOZOA very quickly convinces one that these animals are not the simple organisms that they are usually represented to be. They are frequently said to resemble a cell, being "a mass of protoplasm containing a nucleus." The illustration of *Diplodinium ecaudatum* on page 194 indicates how really complicated the body of a protozoön may be.

II. *Classification*

In a book on Parasitology no detailed classification of the Phylum PROTOZOA is necessary since, although the species considered are described according to the class in which they belong, only the larger taxonomic divisions need be recognized. The four classes with examples of common species are as follows:

Class 1. SARCODINA. PROTOZOA with pseudopodia; usually without a cuticular cell wall; often with a shell or skeleton. Free-living examples: *Amœba proteus* (Fig. 6), *Pelomyxa palustris* (Fig. 5), *Actinophrys sol, Globigerina bulloides*. Parasitic examples: *Endamœba histolytica, Endolimax nana, Iodamœba williamsi.*

Class 2. MASTIGOPHORA. PROTOZOA with flagella; many colonial. Free-living examples: *Euglena viridis, Mastigamœba invertens, Chilomonas paramœcium* (Fig. 21), *Dinobryon sertularia*. Parasitic examples: *Trichomonas hominis, Streblomastix strix* (Fig. 25), *Trypanosoma gambiense.*

Class 3. SPOROZOA. PROTOZOA without locomotor organs; spore production a characteristic of the life-cycle. Examples: *Monocystis agilis, Isospora hominis, Hepatozoön muris, Plasmodium vivax.*

Class 4. INFUSORIA. PROTOZOA with cilia; usually with two nuclei, a macronucleus and a micronucleus. Free-living examples: *Paramœcium caudatum, Spirostomum ambiguum, Euplotes patella, Podophrya collini*. Parasitic examples: *Opalina ranarum, Balantidium coli, Nyctotherus ovalis, Trichodina pediculus.*

III. *Maintenance of the Individual*

PROTOZOA in their active stages live in a fluid medium. This may be fresh water, salt water or the body fluids of other organisms, either plants or animals. Here they are subjected to various physical and biological factors such as changes in temperature, changes in the chemical composition of the medium, movements of the medium and the like. Only a small proportion of the individuals succeed in their struggle with their environment, but a sufficient number grow to maturity and produce offspring to perpetuate the race. The principal activities necessary for the maintenance of the individual protozoön are discussed in the following paragraphs.

1. PROTECTION

PROTOZOA must protect themselves from competitors, other animals and plants and from physical agents. Many of their devices are similar to those of higher animals. Some of them resemble their surroundings in shape and color and hence escape detection. They may be protected from physical agents by a firm cuticle, resistant wall or external skeleton. With the aid of their pseudopodia, flagella or cilia they are able to move out of an unfavorable location into a satisfactory environment. Some PROTOZOA possess weapons of defense or offense such as the trichocysts of *Paramœcium*. Secretions and excretions that are repellent in nature serve as a protection for certain species, and finally, if molar agents in the medium bring about mechanical injury, the powers of regeneration of the organism frequently are such as to bring about a reformation of the complete animal.

2. RESPONSE TO STIMULI

Because of that fundamental property of protoplasm, irritability or excitability, PROTOZOA respond to various stimuli. Some of these are external and others originate within the body of the animal. Due to these responses to stimuli, which, taken together, constitute what is known as the behavior of the organism, the protozoön is able to find food, to locate an optimum habitat, and to avoid injurious environments. Many parasitic PROTOZOA exhibit a sort of affinity for definite tissues. This may be due largely to the results of responses to stimuli.

3. MOTION AND LOCOMOTION

The possession of powers of motion and of locomotion makes it possible for PROTOZOA to take advantage of the stimuli received by them. Certain species may remain attached, and, by movements of the body, create currents which bring to them a constant supply of oxygen and of food particles, and that carry away from them the products of excretion and respiration. Other species appear to go in search of food and to flee from enemies, and no doubt the dispersion of the species is due largely to the powers of locomotion of individuals.

4. NUTRITION

PROTOZOA do not use as food every type of organic material that they encounter any more than do higher animals, but practice rather definite food-selection. Thus one species may feed on bacteria and prefer certain types of bacteria, whereas others may feed on other PROTOZOA or, in the case of parasites, on red or white blood corpuscles. Free-living PROTOZOA in most cases ingest solid particles. These are usually obtained with the aid of pseudopodia, flagella or cilia. Frequently, as noted above, there is a special apparatus for the purpose of ingestion. The ingested food particles are suspended in liquid in a food vacuole into which the surrounding endoplasm secretes digestive enzymes. The products of digestion are liberated into the cytoplasm where assimilation occurs. Undigested particles are egested either through the general surface of the body or through a specialized opening, the cytopyge. Many PROTOZOA, especially among the parasitic species, do not ingest solid particles but absorb food directly through the surface of the body from the medium in which they live.

5. CIRCULATION

There is in the protozoan body no elaborate circulatory system, such as exists in certain higher animals, but movements occur in the protoplasm which serve to carry the digested food from one part of the body to another, and in some cases, for example, in *Paramœcium* and *Balantidium* a definite path is followed by the food vacuoles in their movements within the protoplasm. Protoplasmic movements no doubt also carry the injurious products of metabolism to the surface where they are expelled through the peripheral layer of ectoplasm.

6. RESPIRATION

Definite organs of respiration are also lacking in PROTOZOA, but oxygen is taken in through the surface of the body and carbon dioxide is expelled through the surface of the body, no elaborate structures being required for these purposes in such minute organisms.

7. SECRETION AND EXCRETION

Various secretion products of value are produced by PROTOZOA, such as material for the formation of skeletal and supporting structures, and enzymes for the digestion of food. As in higher animals, PROTOZOA must rid themselves of the excretory products of metabolism or they become poisoned. The excretory products are cast out either through the general body surface or in some species by the contractile vacuoles.

In the maintenance of the individual it is evident that the protozoön carries on all of the physiological processes characteristic of higher organisms. Jennings says of the simplest of all of the PROTOZOA, "If Ameba were a large animal, so as to come within the every day experience of human beings, its behavior would at once call forth the attribution to it of states of pleasure and pain, of hunger, desire, and the like, on precisely the same basis as we attribute these things to the dog."

IV. *Maintenance of the Race*

1. REPRODUCTION

The power of reproduction is a fundamental property of protoplasm and successful reproduction is, of course, necessary for the maintenance of races of PROTOZOA. Although comparatively simple in structure and minute in size, the powers of reproduction of many PROTOZOA are exceedingly great. For example, it has been estimated that the ciliate *Paramœcium,* under favorable circumstances, could produce by binary fission from a single specimen 268,000,000 offspring in one month. This, no doubt, never happens since there are checks to multiplication, just as in higher organisms, which we designate by the phrase "the struggle for existence." Lack of space and of food and injurious physical and biological factors in the environment serve to keep down the numbers of specimens so that ordinarily a sort of equilibrium exists between any particular species of protozoön and the rest of the world.

Reproduction in the PROTOZOA is brought about by cell division. This may occur without the intervention of any sexual process, in which case it is known as asexual reproduction, or may involve the more or less intimate union of gametes which is characteristic of sexual reproduction.

2. ASEXUAL REPRODUCTION

Asexual reproduction may take place by binary fission, by schizogony or by budding. During binary fission the organism usually divides into two approximately equal daughters, each of which possesses one-half of the cytoplasm and one-half of the nucleus of the parent. Other organelles that may be present may arise anew in the daughter cells or the organelles of the parent may divide, one-half of each going to each daughter, or the parent organelle may go to one daughter and a similar organelle arise anew in the other daughter.

Nuclear division during binary fission is similar in most cases to mitosis in the cells of METAZOA but often occurs in what appears to be a more simple form (Fig. 4). Thus one type of nuclear division is called promitosis. In this type the entire process takes place within the nuclear membrane; the karyosome divides into two, one passing to each end of the elongated nucleus and one-half of the chromosomes, which may or may not become arranged in an equatorial plate, likewise migrate to each end of the nucleus. Then the nuclear membrane constricts in the center and the daughter nuclei finally separate. Mesomitosis is applied to a type of nuclear division that has probably evolved from promitosis. A mitotic figure and chromosomes occur but no polar caps are formed. Division takes place entirely within the nuclear membrane. In metamitosis all or most of the nuclear membrane breaks down. Amitosis, during which the chromatin in the nucleus appears to be simply constricted into two daughter nuclei without the formation of chromosomes, may occur in certain PROTOZOA, for example, in the case of the macronuclei of ciliates, but is not as prevalent in the PROTOZOA as formerly believed.

Budding is a type of asexual reproduction that occurs in certain PROTOZOA, particularly in the Class INFUSORIA. It has even been described in amebas. The budding process involves the unequal division of a protozoön, one daughter being much smaller than the other. This difference in size is usually due to a difference in the quantity of the cytoplasm, since the nuclei of parent and bud are approximately of equal size.

The term schizogony is applied to a process which involves the repeated division of the nucleus without immediate cell division. This results in a multinucleate individual which eventually breaks up into a number of smaller uninucleate cells known as merozoites. This type of reproduction is particularly common among the SPOROZOA. The term schizogony is restricted to the formation of merozoites by a trophozoite, which is called a schizont. A type of multiple division resembling schizogony occurs also during sexual reproduction in certain SPOROZOA when sporozoites are produced by a zygote following the fertilization process.

Many PROTOZOA have a cyst stage in their life-cycle during which the single original nucleus may divide into two, four or more nuclei. Just what happens when these cysts hatch is not fully known in many species, but presumably as many daughter cells are formed as there are nuclei present. This is a type of asexual reproduction which may be called binary or multiple fission within a cyst wall.

3. SEXUAL REPRODUCTION OR SYNGAMY

Sexual processes frequently interrupt multiplication by asexual reproduction in the life-cycle. Syngamy is not really a type of multiplication but precedes certain types of reproduction. It involves either a temporary or permanent union of two cells which may be called gametes. A useful outline of the various methods by which syngamy is accomplished is given by Wenyon (1926) as follows:

1. Copulation: Complete union of two individuals

   (1) Two individuals having the characters of the ordinary reproducing forms unite.
      (a) The uniting forms are equal in size (isogamy).
      (b) The uniting forms are unequal in size (anisogamy).
   (2) Two individuals (gametocytes) give rise to a number of smaller forms (gametes) which unite in pairs.
      (a) The gametes produced by the gametocytes are equal in size and characters (isogamy).
      (b) The gametes produced by one individual are unlike those produced by the other (anisogamy).
         (i) The number of gametes produced by the gametocytes are equal, or approximately equal, in number.
         (ii) One gametocyte (macrogametocyte) gives rise to one large gamete (macrogamete), while the other

(microgametocyte) gives rise to a variable number of small motile gametes (microgametes).

2. Conjugation: Two individuals (conjugants) associate, their nuclei divide, and exchange of daughter nuclei takes place, after which the conjugants separate.
   (1) The conjugants are equal in size.
   (2) The conjugants are unequal in size, one, a small one (microconjugant), associating with a large one (macroconjugant). In some cases, after interchange of nuclei the microconjugant degenerates.

These various types of syngamy will be referred to in later chapters in descriptions of the life-cycles of various species.

It has been shown briefly in this chapter how PROTOZOA maintain themselves and the race. PROTOZOA are able to live in all the major habitats. Free-living species are exceedingly abundant. Parasitic PROTOZOA are likewise extremely rich in number of species since almost every other pecies of animal has its own species of PROTOZOA living on or within it. Both free-living and parasitic PROTOZOA are also extremely rich in numbers of individuals. If we accept numbers of species and numbers of individuals as criteria of the success of any group of organisms we must acknowledge the superiority of the PROTOZOA in the struggle for existence among animals.

V. *Protozoa of Man*

For convenience it seems desirable to present at this point a list of the PROTOZOA known to live in man. These species are recognized by most protozoölogists as valid.

A. Intestinal PROTOZOA. These appear to be world-wide in their distribution. They are located within the body as indicated.

MOUTH	Percentage of population infected
1. *Endamœba gingivalis* (ameba)	50
2. *Trichomonas (buccalis) elongata* (flagellate)	10-30

SMALL INTESTINE

3. *Giardia lamblia* (flagellate)	10
4. *Isospora hominis* (coccidium)	Rare

LARGE INTESTINE

5. *Endamœba histolytica* (ameba)   10
6. *Endamœba coli* (ameba)   50
7. *Endolimax nana* (ameba)   25
8. *Iodamœba williamsi* (ameba)   10
9. *Dientamœba fragilis* (ameba)   Rare
10. *Trichomonas hominis* (flagellate) 5-20
11. *Chilomastix mesnili* (flagellate) 10
12. *Retortamonas (Embadomonas) intestinalis* (flagellate)   Rare
13. *Enteromonas hominis* (flagellate) Rare
14. *Balantidium coli* (ciliate)   Rare

VAGINA OR URINARY TRACT

15. *Trichomonas vaginalis* (flagellate)   10-50 (women)

B. Blood-inhabiting PROTOZOA. These are restricted to certain rather definite areas as indicated.

RED BLOOD CORPUSCLES

16. *Plasmodium vivax* (tertian malaria)   Tropics and subtropics
17. *Plasmodium malariæ* (quartan malaria)   Tropics and subtropics
18. *Plasmodium falciparum* (estivo-autumnal malaria)   Tropics and subtropics

BLOOD PLASMA

19. *Trypanosoma gambiense* (Gambian sleeping sickness)   Tropical Africa
20. *Trypanosoma rhodesiense* (Rhodesian sleeping sickness)   Nyasaland, Rhodesia, etc.
21. *Trypanosoma cruzi* (Chagas' disease)   Tropical America

BLOOD AND BODY CELLS

22. *Leishmania donovani* (kala-azar)   Asia and Mediterranean
23. *Leishmania tropica* (oriental sore)   Asia and Mediterranean
24. *Leishmania braziliensis* (uta)   South and Central America

C. PROTOZOA of muscle tissue. Only one apparently aberrant species is known to occur in man.

25. *Sarcosystis* sp. (sporozoön)   Rare

VI. *Protozoa of Lower Animals Easily Obtained for Study*

One who is just beginning the study of protozoölogy must know where he may expect to find examples of the various types for examination. The following list contains some of the most easily acquired hosts and a few of the PROTOZOA that are contained in them. The PROTOZOA mentioned are those that are usually the most abundant.

1. EARTHWORM.

Intestine. *Anoplophrya marylandensis* (ciliate)
Seminal vesicles. *Monocystis* sp. (sporozoön)

2. COCKROACH

Intestine. *Endamœba blattæ* (ameba)
Balantidium blattarum (ciliate)
Nyctotherus ovalis (ciliate)
Lophomonas blattarum (flagellate)
Retortamonas blattæ (flagellate)
Gregarina blattarum (gregarine)

3. FROG. ADULT.

Rectum. *Endamœba ranarum* (ameba)
Trichomonas augusta (flagellate)
Hexamita intestinalis (flagellate)
Opalina ranarum (ciliate)
Nyctotherus cordiformis (ciliate)
Balantidium sp. (ciliate)
Blood. *Trypanosoma rotatorium* (flagellate)
Lankesterella ranarum (hemosporidium)
Cytamœba bacterifera (hemosporidium)

4. FROG. TADPOLE.

Surface. *Trichodina pediculus* (ciliate)
Small intestine. *Giardia agilis* (flagellate)
Rectum. *Euglenamorpha hegneri* (flagellate)

5. LIZARD.

Intestine. *Trichomonas lacertæ* (flagellate)
Prowazekella lacertæ (flagellate)
Blood. *Karyolysus lacertarum* (hemosporidium)

6. DOMESTIC FOWL.

Cecum. *Endamœba gallinarum* (ameba)
Endolimax gregariniformis (ameba)

Trichomonas gallinarum (flagellate)
Chilomastix gallinarum (flagellate)
Eimeria tenella (coccidium)

7. TURKEY.

Intestine. *Histomonas meleagridis* (flagellate)
Eimeria meleagridis (coccidium)

8. PIGEON.

Crop. *Trichomonas columbæ* (flagellate)
Blood. *Hæmoproteus columbæ* (hemosporidium)

9. ENGLISH SPARROW.

Feces. *Isospora lacazii* (coccidium)
Blood. *Plasmodium cathemerium* (hemosporidium)
Spleen and liver. *Toxoplasma paddæ* (hemosporidium ?)

10. LABORATORY RAT.

Small intestine. *Giardia muris* (flagellate)
Hexamita muris (flagellate)
Retortamonas sp. (flagellate)
Cecum. *Endamœba muris* (ameba)
Trichomonas muris (flagellate)
Trichomonas parva (flagellate)
Chilomastix bettencourti (flagellate)
Feces. *Eimeria miyairii* (coccidium)
Blood. *Trypanosoma lewisi* (flagellate)

11. LABORATORY MOUSE.

Small intestine. *Giardia muris* (flagellate)
Hexamita muris (flagellate)
Cecum. *Endamœba muris* (ameba)
Trichomonas muris (flagellate)
Feces. *Cryptosporidium muris* (coccidium)
Muscles. *Sarcocystis muris* (sarcosporidian)

12. GUINEA-PIG.

Small intestine. *Giardia caviæ* (flagellate)
Cecum. *Endamœba coboyæ* (ameba)
Endolimax caviæ (ameba)
Trichomonas caviæ (flagellate)
Chilomastix intestinalis (flagellate)
Retortamonas caviæ (flagellate)
Balantidium caviæ (ciliate)
Feces. *Eimeria caviæ* (coccidium)

13. RABBIT.

Small intestine. *Giardia duodenalis* (flagellate)
Cecum. *Endamœba cuniculi* (ameba)
    Chilomastix cuniculi (flagellate)
    Retortamonas cuniculi (flagellate)
Feces. *Eimeria stiedæ* (coccidium)

14. CATTLE.

Stomach. *Endamœba bovis* (ameba)
    Trichomonas ruminantium (flagellate)
    Diplodinium ecaudatum (etc.) (ciliates)
Genital tract. *Trichomonas fœtus* (flagellate)

15. PIG.

Cecum. *Endamœba polecki* (ameba)
    Iodamœba suis (ameba)
    Trichomonas suis (flagellate)
    Balantidium coli (ciliate)

16. RHESUS MONKEY.

Mouth. *Endamœba gingivalis* (ameba)
Small intestine. *Giardia lamblia* (flagellate)
Cecum. *Endamœba histolytica* (ameba)
    Endamœba coli (ameba)
    Trichomonas hominis (flagellate)
    Balantidium sp. (ciliate)
Vagina. *Trichomonas vaginalis* (flagellate)

17. CHIMPANZEE.

Feces. *Balantidium coli* (ciliate)
    Troglodytella abrassarti (ciliate)

18. ANIMALS CONTAINING ONE OR SEVERAL SPECIES OF PARTICULAR INTEREST.

Hydra	*Trichodina pediculus*	(surface: ciliate)
Carolina locust	*Gregarina locustæ*	(intestine: gregarine)
Cricket (*Gryllus*)	*Gregarina oviceps*	(intestine: gregarine)
House fly	*Herpetomonas muscarum*	(intestine: flagellate)

Water strider	*Crithidia gerridis*	(intestine: flagellate)
Termites (wood-eating)	Intestinal flagellates	
Crimson-spotted newt (aquatic)	*Trypanosoma diemyctyli*	(blood: flagellate)
Duck	*Leucocytozoön anatis*	(blood: hemosporidium)
Heron	*Giardia ardeæ*	(flagellate: small intestine)
Field mouse	*Giardia microti*	(small intestine: flagellate)
Horse	Ciliates	(cecum and colon)

CHAPTER II

INTRODUCTION TO THE SARCODINA

I. *Classification*

As noted in the previous chapter the SARCODINA are characterized by the presence of pseudopodia. These are more or less temporary processes formed by the cytoplasm. They serve primarily for purposes of locomotion and for the capture and ingestion of food material. Some of the SARCODINA include in their life-cycle a flagellated stage. In the following table are listed the more important divisions into which the Class SARCODINA may be divided. Most of the parasitic species that are of particular interest with respect to man and his domesticated animals are included in a single family, the ENDAMŒBIDÆ.

Class SARCODINA. PROTOZOA with pseudopodia.

Subclass I. RHIZOPODA. SARCODINA with lobose or reticulose pseudopodia; no axial filaments in pseudopodia; creeping forms.
Order I. AMŒBINA. RHIZOPODA with lobose pseudopodia; skeleton absent; simple shell may be present.
Suborder I. GYMNAMŒBA. AMŒBINA without skeleton or shell.
Family I. AMŒBIDÆ. Free-living gymnamœbæ. Examples: *Amœba proteus, Pelomyxa palustris.*
Family 2. ENDAMŒBIDÆ. Parasitic in cavities or tissues. Examples: *Endamœba histolytica, Endolimax nana.*
Suborder 2. THECAMŒBA. AMŒBINA with shell. Examples: *Arcella vulgaris, Chlamydophrys stercorea.*
Order 2. FORAMINIFERA. RHIZOPODA with reticulose pseudopodia; with shell. Example: *Globigerina bulloides.*
Order 3. MYCETOZOA. RHIZOPODA with multinucleate plasmodium. Example: *Plasmodiophora brassicæ.*

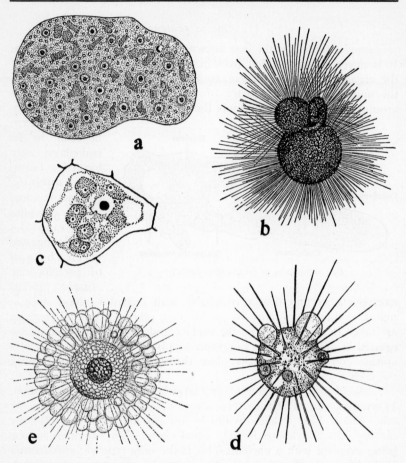

Fig. 5.—Types of Sarcodina. a. *Pelomyxa palustris,* a species with many nuclei. b. *Globigerina bulloides,* with globular chambers and long spines. c. *Plasmodiophora brassicae,* a mycetozoon; host cell containing several parasites. d. *Actinophrys sol.* e. *Thalassicolla nucleata.* (After various authors)

Subclass 2. ACTINOPODA. SARCODINA with radiating, unbranched pseudopodia; floating forms.

Order 1. HELIOZOA. ACTINOPODA with axial filament in pseudopodia. Example: *Actinophrys sol, Vampyrella lateritia.*

Order 2. RADIOLARIA. ACTINOPODA usually without axial filament; central capsule present. Example: *Thalassicola nucleata.*

II. *Amœba proteus*

Amœba proteus is the best known species in the Class SARCODINA. It is never a parasite, but lives in fresh water. A general view of the organism is shown in Fig. 6. This figure indicates the shape of the animal and the character of its pseudopodia. The clear area around the periphery represents the ectoplasm and the central granular area the en-

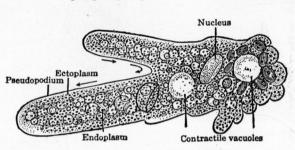

FIG. 6.—*Amœba proteus*. (After Leidy)

doplasm. In the endoplasm are located a biconcave nucleus, contractile vacuole, food bodies and crystals. Food is ingested with the aid of pseudopodia. *Amœba proteus* exercises a certain degree of choice with regard to food since it ingests certain types more frequently than others. The food particles are taken in at any point on the surface and undigested materials are egested at any point. The organism simply flows away from it. Excretion and respiration take place through the general surface of the body.

Amœba proteus reaches about 600 µ in length during locomotion. When this size is attained reproduction by binary division usually takes place. The nucleus divides by mitosis and then the cell-body divides into two approximately equal parts, each daughter amœba being supplied with a nucleus. This is the only type of reproduction in the life-cycle of *Amœba proteus* of which we are certain, although other types have been described.

Amebas move with the aid of pseudopodia. Many investigators have attempted to determine the method of ameboid movement. According to Mast, the central mass of protoplasm in *Amœba proteus* is a fluid, or sol, which he calls the plasmasol. Surrounding the plasmasol is a layer of more viscous protoplasm in the gel state, the plasmagel. Movement occurs as follows. The pseudopodia are temporary and may appear at any point. A pseudopodium is produced where the elastic strength of the plasmagel is weakest. A hyaline cap is formed and the plasmasol is forced into it by the contraction of the plasmagel at the opposite (temporary posterior) end, thus

extending the pseudopodium. The plasmagel solates at the posterior
end and this new plasmasol flows forward becoming a gel again just
back of the tip of the pseudopodium. Thus *Amœba* moves forward
in the direction of the pseudopodium as a result of the solation and
gelation of the endoplasm. The rate of locomotion depends in part
on the temperature; it increases to a maximum at 24° C., then decreases to 28° C., increases again to 30° C., and finally becomes zero
at 33° C. There is still much to be learned about ameboid movement,
but when the true explanation is found, "it will probably give a key
not only to the formation of pseudopodia but to the movement of
flagella, cilia, and even muscular contraction." (Mast.)

Amœba proteus responds to various stimuli, reacting positively to
some and negatively to others. In general it may be said that the
responses are such as to be of value to the individual, since reactions
are negative to such injurious agents as strong chemicals, heat and
mechanical impacts, but positive to beneficial agents.

III. *Parasitic Sarcodina in General*

Almost every large group in the Class SARCODINA includes species
of interest to parasitologists. The Order AMŒBINA contains, as
noted above, the Family ENDAMŒBIDÆ which includes most of the
important species of SARCODINA that live in man and lower animals.
These will be given special consideration in later chapters. In the
Family AMŒBIDÆ are a number of interesting so-called coprozoic
species belonging to the genera *Hartmannella, Vahlkampfia* and
Sappinia. These will be described in Chapter III.

The Suborder THECAMŒBA, besides many common fresh-water
species, includes a number of interesting coprozoic forms, especially
Chlamydophrys stercorea (Fig. 18, *i*).

The FORAMINIFERA are fresh-water and marine organisms. The
MYCETOZOA are terrestrial PROTOZOA living for the most part upon
moist leaves and decaying wood. One of the best known species in
this group is *Plasmodiophora brassicæ* which causes swellings on the
roots of cabbages and other plants.

Several parasites of somewhat doubtful systematic position may
be included in the Order HELIOZOA. *Vampyrella lateritia* and several
species of *Nuclearia,* for example, attack algæ.

The marine PROTOZOA of the Order RADIOLARIA are of interest
to parasitologists because many of them contain vegetable organisms
known as ZOÖXANTHELLÆ which apparently live with the PROTOZOA
in a state of symbiosis. Their yellow color gives the protozoön this
tinge when a large number of specimens are present.

CHAPTER III

AMŒBÆ LIVING IN MAN

I. *Generic and Specific Characteristics*

Although the number of genera of amœbæ living in man has not been definitely established most protozoölogists agree that there are at least four, namely, *Endamœba, Endolimax, Iodamœba* and *Dientamœba*. These genera may be distinguished from one another by the character of their nuclei.

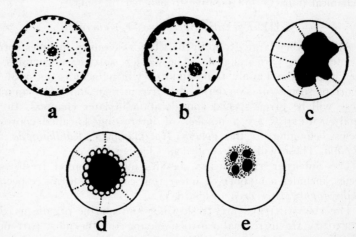

Fig. 7.—Diagrams of nuclei of various types of amebas that live in man. a. *Endamœba histolytica*. b. *E. coli*. c. *Endolimax nana*. d. *Iodamœba williamsi*. e. *Dientamœba fragilis*.

As indicated in Figure 7, the nucleus of *Endamœba* possesses a small, more or less central, karyosome and a layer of granules on the nuclear membrane.

The nucleus of *Endolimax* contains a large karyosome frequently irregular in shape and consisting of several portions attached to each other by strands; often linin fibers extend from the karyosome to the nuclear membrane. There is usually no visible layer of chromatin granules on the nuclear membrane.

46

The nucleus of *Iodamœba* likewise lacks the peripheral chromatin granules; the single large karyosome is surrounded by a layer of faintly staining globules. As in *Endolimax,* linin fibers may extend from the karyosome to the nuclear membrane.

The genus *Dientamœba* is characterized, as the name implies, by the presence of two nuclei in many of the specimens; the chromatin in these consists of granules, usually four in number, imbedded in a matrix of plastin; often one of the granules is larger than the others; this mass may be connected with the nuclear membrane by linin fibers.

The genus *Endamœba* is represented in man by three species. *Endamœba histolytica* lives primarily in the large intestine and secondarily in other parts of the body. The karyosome in the nucleus of this species is small and located in the center; the peripheral chromatin granules are delicate. *Endamœba coli* also lives in the large intestine; its nucleus has a larger karyosome eccentrically placed, and the chromatin granules on the nuclear membrane are coarse. The third species, *Endamœba gingivalis,* lives in the mouth. Its nucleus is not always spherical. The karyosome is usually subcentrally located and often can be seen to consist of several granules; and the peripheral chromatin may be irregularly distributed.

The other three genera contain one species each that live in man. These are *Endolimax nana, Iodamœba williamsi* and *Dientamœba fragilis.* All of them live in the large intestine. Species belonging to the genera *Endamœba, Endolimax* and *Iodamœba* have been reported from many of the lower animals; some of these will be described in Chapter IV.

II. *Incidence of Infection*

The amœbæ that live in man seem to be cosmopolitan in their distribution, but the percentage of individuals among the general population that are infected varies in different localities. In general it may be said that the incidence of infection is apt to be higher in the warmer regions than in the colder parts of the world and in the less well sanitated areas than in communities where effective sewerage systems exist. In the United States the following estimates have been made of the percentage of infection among the general population: *Endamœba histolytica,* 10 per cent, *Endamœba coli,* 50 per cent, *Endolimax nana,* 25 per cent, and *Iodamœba williamsi,* 10 per cent. Our knowledge of the incidence of infection with *Endamœba gingivalis* is less definite but probably about 50 per cent are infected. *Dientamœba fragilis* appears to be less common but in some localities

10 per cent of the inhabitants may be infected. Fortunately *Endamœba histolytica* is the only one of these species whose pathogenicity has definitely been established and even this species does not bring about a diseased condition except under favorable circumstances, most of those who are infected being carriers.

III. *Endamœba histolytica*

I. HISTORICAL

There is some doubt as to who first saw and described *Endamœba histolytica*. Lewis (1870) described an intestinal amœba from man in a report on cholera in India. A more careful study of this species (Cunningham, 1871) indicates that it was probably *Endamœba coli*. There is no doubt but that Loesch saw *Endamœba histolytica* in a young Russian peasant in 1873 (published in 1875). Loesch demonstrated the pathogenic nature of this organism by infecting a dog with it; dysentery developed in the dog and amœbæ were found in ulcers in its intestine. Koch (in Koch and Gaffky, 1887), first saw amœbæ in intestinal sections made from patients who had died of dysentery. This stimulated the investigations by Kartulis who in 1887 described amœbæ in liver abscess pus and was the first to find this parasite in amœbic abscesses of the brain (Kartulis, 1904). Osler (1890) was the first to report *Endamœba histolytica* in America. He found the organism in liver abscesses and this discovery led to the important work of Councilman and Lafleur (1891) on the pathology of amœbic dysentery and amœbic abscess of the liver.

For many years it was supposed that only one species of amœba lived in the human intestine, but Councilman and Lafleur (1891) suggested that there might be two species and this was demonstrated by Quincke and Roos in 1893. The exact status of the two organisms now known as *Endamœba histolytica* and *Endamœba coli* was not finally decided until 1913 when Walker and Sellards' experiments on human beings demonstrated beyond question that *Endamœba histolytica* is pathogenic and produces cysts with four nuclei, and *Endamœba coli* is non-pathogenic and produces cysts with eight nuclei. Since 1913 many investigators have added to our knowledge of *Endamœba histolytica*. The principal results of these investigations are presented in the following paragraphs.

2. LIFE-CYCLE

This species may live in the lumen of the bowel without access to the intestinal wall or may penetrate the latter. The active trophozoite divides by binary fission. In the human bowel, due to conditions still unknown, certain trophozoites may become smaller and lose their food inclusions; these are known as precystic forms. They become spherical and secrete a cyst wall about themselves and in this form pass out of the body in the feces. By two successive divisions the nuclei within the cyst increase from one to four. The infection of new hosts occurs by the ingestion of infective cysts which probably

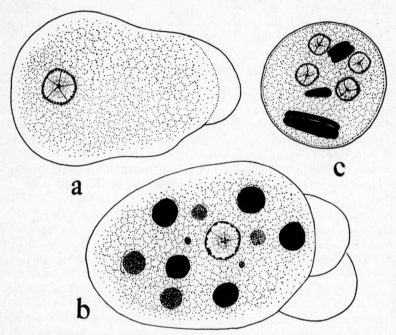

FIG. 8.—*Endamœba histolytica.* a. Type occurring within host tissue, without food inclusions. b. Type from intestine containing red blood cells. c. Cyst with four nuclei and two pairs of chromatoid bodies.

hatch in the small intestine. A quadrinucleate amœba emerges from the cyst and by nuclear and cell division produces eight amœbulæ. These pass on into the large intestine where they grow into adult trophozoites.

3. MORPHOLOGY

Trophozoite. The active, or trophozoite, stage of *E. histolytica* (Figure 8) varies greatly in size but is usually from 20 μ to 30 μ in diameter. The size variations are due principally to two factors (1) growth following binary division and (2) heritably diverse size races. The clear ectoplasm around the periphery of the body may be distinguished from the more granular endoplasm; and the pseudopodia, which are entirely of ectoplasm, are thin and blade-like and formed in an explosive manner. Within the cytoplasm are often food vacuoles containing red blood cells and a single nucleus, which, however, is rarely distinctly visible in living specimens. The nuclear structure is revealed in fixed and stained preparations. The nucleus is of the *Endamœba* type; it is from 4 μ to 7 μ in diameter; is "poor" in chromatin; and has a small, centrally located karyosome and a layer of fine chromatin granules on the nuclear membrane. The figure published by Dobell in 1919 has usually been accepted as that of a typical specimen. This has resulted in considerable confusion, since, although organisms occur containing a nucleus such as he has drawn, many specimens possess a nucleus with the several granules comprising the karyosome somewhat spread out and with the peripheral chromatin less regularly distributed. Reproduction of the trophozoite is by binary fission. The nuclear membrane remains intact throughout. The number of chromosomes according to Kofoid and Swezy (1922) is six (Fig. 4b); these divide in the metaphase and migrate to the poles in the anaphase. Then the nucleus constricts into two.

Precystic stage. Before encysting, *E. histolytica* loses its food inclusions; decreases in size; becomes sluggish; and rounds up. Elmassian in 1909 believed this stage to be a distinct species and gave to it the name *Entamœba minuta*. Frequently vacuoles containing glycogen and rod-like refractile (chromatoid) bodies appear before encystment occurs.

Cyst. A thin peripheral wall is secreted by the precystic organism, thus forming a spherical body, the cyst (Fig. 18c), which ranges from 5 μ to 20 μ in diameter. Different size races are indicated by differences in the size of the cysts. The mature cyst contains four nuclei, each of which appears like that of the trophozoite, but cysts with one, two and three nuclei are frequently passed. Often glycogen vacuoles and chromatoid bodies are present in young cysts, but these are usually absorbed later. The chromatoid bodies are characteristic in shape, being in the form of blunt rods, and are frequently present in pairs, the two members of which are approximately equal in size.

4. HOST-PARASITE RELATIONS

Incidence of infection. Many surveys have been carried out to determine the incidence of *E. histolytica* among human beings in various parts of the world. The results vary with the methods used and the experience of the investigators, but from them an estimate can be made of the number infected. Boeck and Stiles (1923) examined 13,043 specimens from 8,029 persons in the United States and noted 333 cases or 4.1 per cent of infection; Mathews and Smith (1919) report 2.97 per cent of 202 army recruits in England; Meleney (1930) found 17.3 per cent of 4,987 rural inhabitants in Tennessee; and Wenrich, Stabler and Arnett (1935) discovered 4.1 per cent of 1,060 college freshmen in Pennsylvania. The actual percentages were much higher than these figures since not all infections are revealed unless half-a-dozen or more examinations are made of each person. Andrews (1934) estimates that the study of single purged stools reveals at least 75 per cent of the protozoan species present but this method is seldom employed in surveys.

Epidemiology of transmission. The infection of new hosts, as noted above, is brought about by the ingestion of cysts. Cysts, when they are passed, may contain one, two, three or four nuclei. One patient may pass mostly uninucleate or binucleate cysts at one time and quadrinucleate cysts at another time; and cysts passed by different hosts may differ with respect to their nuclear number. It is generally believed that only the quadrinucleate cysts are infective, but Yorke and Adams (1927) have proved that cysts with one or two nuclei may continue to develop in culture media and Hegner, Johnson and Stabler have shown that immature cysts ripen in the small intestine after they have been swallowed by a monkey; such cysts may possibly become infective after they have been ingested by a host.

The successful infection of new hosts depends to a considerable extent upon the viability of cysts outside of the body. Moisture is necessary for long-continued existence since, although protected with a resistant wall, drying is soon fatal to them. The distribution of viable cysts in a dried condition is, therefore, impossible. Various tests have been used to determine the viability of cysts. The method most frequently used is the addition of eosin in a concentration of 1 : 1000. This is supposed to penetrate and stain dead cysts but not those that are alive. This method is not entirely satisfactory. It is now possible to cultivate *Endamœba histolytica* in artificial media and under proper conditions excystation occurs. In this way the viability of cysts can be determined without question. Perhaps the best method of proving viability is to use laboratory animals such as kittens; but this method is far from simple.

Cysts in nature remain in the feces in latrines until they die or are carried away by flies and other animals, or on the surface of the soil where they are destroyed by drying, are disseminated by animals or washed into the soil or into ponds and streams by the rain. The viability of cysts in raw and diluted feces and the probability of their dissemination by flies and other animals are thus subjects of public health importance.

It has been found that when cysts remain in moist feces they may live for several weeks. Dilution of the feces with water seems to be favorable for their continued existence. Cysts are able to withstand a wide range of temperatures, for example, Yorke and Adams (1926) were able to obtain cultures from cysts that had remained in raw feces at room temperature for nine days, and in water at 0° C. for seventeen days; and Dobell (1927) states that cysts may remain alive at room temperature for as long as 37 days but usually only a few days at 37° C. The pasteurization of milk probably raises the temperature to a high enough point (60° C.) for a sufficient time to destroy any cysts that may be present and of course bringing water to the boiling point accomplishes the same result. This appears to be the only known method of killing cysts in water. Various experiments have been reported with disinfectants; these indicate that cresol in a strength of 1 : 20 kills cysts almost instantly.

There is only one conceivable way in which new hosts can be infected and that is by the ingestion of viable cysts. It seems probable that cysts usually reach the mouth in contaminated food and drink, although they might also be carried there on soiled hands. Among the most important factors that bring about the dissemination of cysts are unsanitary conditions, the handling of food by infected persons, the common use of toilet, wash bowl, and towel and dissemination by insects and perhaps other animals. It has been shown that house-flies will ingest large numbers of cysts at a single meal and that these may be deposited on food or in drink in a living condition in the vomit or feces of the fly from five minutes to at least sixteen hours after feeding. Flies no doubt play a rôle in the dissemination of *Endamœba histolytica*. Other animals are probably less important. Ants and cockroaches are possible distributing agents. Several investigators have shown that rats and mice may become infected, but these animals probably play a minor rôle in transmission (Andrews and White, 1936).

As pointed out above, most hosts infected with *Endamœba histolytica* are carriers, that is, they are infected and are passing cysts but do not exhibit any symptoms of disease. Carriers are particularly dangerous since in them the infective cysts are formed, whereas patients suffering from acute amœbic dysentery pass only the noninfective trophozoites. It has been suggested that carriers among certain classes of people, such as food-handlers, be eliminated by treatment but this is at present impracticable.

An interesting fact regarding the epidemiology of amœbiasis is the greater number of acute cases that occur in the tropics as compared with the temperate regions. Three principal reasons have been offered to account for this: climate, lack of sanitation and the presence of more virulent strains. None of these, however, has been demonstrated. Epidemics of amœbiasis have been reported but are uncommon.

An important fact that has been brought out by studies on the transmission of protozoan cysts is that the host is entirely responsible for his own infection. The parasite remains passive while in the infective stage and can only reach the intestine of a new host by the activities of that host.

Parasitological and clinical periods. The prepatent period in infections in man with *Endamœba histolytica,* according to the work of Walker and Sellards (1913), ranges from one to forty-four days; that is, cysts were recovered from the stools of patients from one to forty-four days after they had swallowed gelatin capsules containing infective cysts. The prepatent period in most of these cases was four or five days. The patent period may last for years, the infected person becoming a carrier. Walker divided carriers into two types, contact carriers who have never exhibited symptoms and convalescent carriers who pass cysts after recovering from an attack of dysentery. Carriers frequently suffer relapses during which symptoms reappear. The incubation period in Walker's experiments ranged from twenty to ninety-five days. In cats, which are very susceptible to infection, the incubation period lasts about two weeks if cysts are injected *per os* but only about two days if rectal injections of trophozoites are given.

Distribution and localization within the host. Since the primary site of infection of *Endamœba histolytica* is the large intestine, cysts that are ingested by a host must pass through the stomach and small intestine. Cysts have no powers of locomotion, hence they are passively carried along in the stomach and intestinal contents. They may reach the large intestine within four hours. Where excystation occurs is not known. It is generally believed that this takes place in the small intestine. Cysts fed to monkeys were found to hatch in the small intestine (Hegner, Johnson and Stabler, 1932) but may possibly hatch in the large intestine also.

For many years it was thought that cysts did not develop outside of the body but that they require the stimuli furnished by digestive

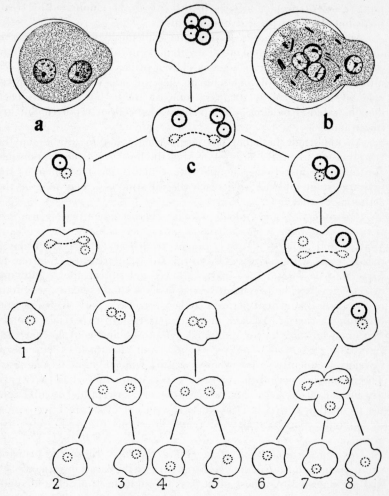

FIG. 9.—*Endamœba histolytica.* a. Binucleate cyst hatching. b. Quadrinucleate cyst hatching. c. Derivation of eight amebulæ from a quadrinucleate cyst after hatching. The darker nuclei are those contained in the cyst; the lighter nuclei are those derived from them. (a, b, after Hegner, Johnson and Stabler; c, after Dobell)

juices for excystation. We now know that cysts will develop from the uninuclear and binuclear stage to the quadrinuclear stage not only in culture media but also in raw feces (Hegner, Johnson and Stabler, 1932). Apparently moisture and a suitable temperature are the only factors necessary to bring about excystation. There seems to be some inhibiting substance, however, in the intestinal contents of the host that prevents the hatching of the cysts in the host in which the cysts are formed (Yorke and Adams, 1927). The evidence at present available indicates that a four-nucleated amœba emerges from the cyst and subsequently divides into four uninucleate amœbæ.

Excystation in *Endamœba histolytica* has been observed and described by several investigators. Immature cysts as well as mature cysts may excyst in the small intestine, at least under experimental conditions (Hegner, Johnson and Stabler, 1932; Tanabe, 1934). In every case the contents of the cysts emerge as a single organism. Then, as Dobell (1928) and Cleveland (1930) have shown with material grown in cultures, and Tanabe (1934) in cysts fed to rats, each quadrinucleate ameba produces eight amebulas by a complicated series of nuclear and cytoplasmic divisions. The accompanying diagram illustrates the usual sequence of events (Fig. 9).

Primary site of infection. The amœbæ that escape from the cysts and succeed in reaching the intestinal wall may establish themselves in the large intestine, which is the primary site of infection. No doubt many cysts and many excysted amœbæ are carried out of the body in the feces. Those parts of the intestine where stasis is first encountered are most frequently infected. This is indicated by the experimental work of Sellards and Theiler (1924) on kittens and by the results of post-mortem examinations on human beings. Clark (1924), for example, shows that in a total of 186 cases, ulcers were scattered throughout the colon in 113 cases (60.7 per cent), but in 63 cases (33.8 per cent) were limited to certain regions.

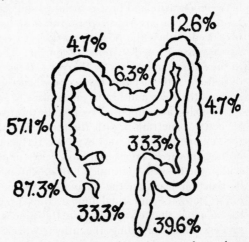

Fig. 10.—Appendix, colon and rectum of man showing the regional distribution of lesions in sixty-three cases of amœbic dysentery. (After Clark)

These regions, as indicated in Figure 10, are dependent portions where greatest stasis occurs, that is, the cecum, ascending colon, rectum, sigmoid and appendix.

Secondary sites of infection. Amœbæ may possibly migrate from the large intestine into the ileum but very few infections in the ileum have been reported. Amœbæ may also gain entrance to the blood stream by way of the ulcers in the intestinal wall and may be carried to various parts of the body. They may set up infections wherever favorable conditions exist. The most frequent secondary site of infection is the liver. In this organ they produce abscesses, most often in the right lobe, and sometimes so large that they contain over a gallon of pus. These abscesses may rupture into the lung. Amœbic abscesses occur in a large proportion of patients who die of amœbic dysentery. For example, Kartulis (1887) noted 55 per cent in 500 cases at autopsy, Craig (1911) records 33 per cent of seventy-eight cases and Clark (1924) reports 51 per cent of 186 cases. Abscesses of amœbic origin may also occur in the lung, brain and spleen. Certain investigators believe that *Endamœba histolytica* is responsible for various diseased conditions of obscure etiology.

Pathogenesis. Endamœba histolytica may behave as a tissue parasite and as such is always pathogenic to the host although, as noted above, very few persons who are infected exhibit symptoms but are in the carrier condition. Apparently in such cases a state of equilibrium between parasite and host is attained during which the injuries caused by the amœbæ are repaired by the host-tissue as rapidly as they are produced. When the host is not able to repair the lesions as rapidly as they are caused symptoms appear. The most common symptom of intestinal amœbiasis is diarrhea. This is frequently followed by dysentery. Other symptoms occur when the invasion of other organs, such as the liver and brain, takes place.

Amœbæ are supposed to invade the tissues of the intestinal wall by active penetration with their pseudopodia, or by dissolving away the cells with the aid of a cytolytic ferment which they secrete. They do not appear to ingest red blood cells or other tissue elements while within the tissues. Continued multiplication of the amœbæ and cellular destruction leads to the formation of an abscess which eventually bursts into the intestinal lumen, thus producing an ulcer. Some of the amœbæ that escape invade the mucosa near by and repeat the process, thus spreading the infected area. At the same time, those that remain in the ulcer continue the destruction of the tissues at the sides and bottom. Further pathological effects result from a continuation of this process. These tissue-invading amœbæ are large and never of the precystic type; the latter, as well as cysts, occur only in the lumen of the intestine.

Immunology. The evidence available indicates that an age immunity may exist in both man and lower animals to infections with

Endamœba histolytica. Young kittens, for example, are more susceptible and suffer a more acute attack than older animals. There is some
evidence also that some races are more resistant to infection than
others.

Several attempts have been made to perfect a complement fixation
test in amœbiasis. The most recent is that of Craig (1927, 1934).
Craig found cytolytic and complement binding substances in absolute
alcohol extracts of forty-eight-hour old cultures of *Endamœba
histolytica;* the complement fixation substance was apparently specific
for *Endamœba histolytica* since the blood sera of individuals infected
with other species of amœbæ gave negative reactions. Wagener
(1924) seems to have obtained some success in perfecting a precipitin
test in cats using antigen from scrapings of ulcerated areas of infected animals; and Scalas (1923) claims to have worked out an
intradermal reaction for man using antigens prepared from the fresh
feces of a case of acute dysentery.

Changes may take place in the aggressivity of the parasite as well
as in the resistance of the host, but apparently whether a host becomes a carrier or suffers an acute attack depends on the physiological
condition of the host and not on the virulence of the amœbæ. For
example, Walker and Sellards (1913) fed cysts from a convalescent
carrier to a fresh host who became a contact carrier; cysts from this
contact carrier when fed to a third person produced another contact
carrier; but cysts from this third case when fed to a fourth individual
brought about an attack of dysentery three weeks later. These facts
indicate that the fourth person in this series was less resistant rather
than that the virulence of the parasite changed.

Host-parasite adjustments. The presence of parasites in a host
without the appearance of symptoms is often spoken of as latency.
How long a carrier condition or period of latency may last is not
known, but it seems probable that an infection once established per-
sists for many years and possibly even throughout the life of the
host. Carriers, however, are liable to exhibit symptoms at any time;
such an occurrence in convalescent carriers is spoken of as a relapse.
Just what modifications in the host or parasite are responsible for
relapses is not known with certainty.

There are three principal points of view with regard to the character of the host-parasite relations during the carrier period. The
amœbæ may live as harmless commensals in the lumen of the intestine; amœbæ may attack the tissues of the intestinal wall but not
severely enough to bring about symptoms; or the amœbæ may, by
their invasion of the tissues, bring about what is known as chronic

amœbiasis with recognizable symptoms. Further study of this subject is necessary before a final conclusion is possible.

5. PREVENTION AND CONTROL

Amœbiasis is a preventible disease just as are bacillary dysentery, typhoid fever and similar diseases. Acute cases are not dangerous since no infective cysts are passed by them. Carriers, however, may pass as many as 300,000,000 cysts in a single day (Kofoid, 1923). The control of carriers and the transmitting agents, or the destruction of cysts after they are passed, are obvious methods of preventing the spread of amœbiasis. Individuals may be protected by preventing the contamination of their food and drink. In certain countries, such as China, where night-soil is used as fertilizer, vegetables and fruit should not be eaten until they have been immersed in water at 80° C. for ten seconds (Mills, Bartlett and Kessel, 1925). Community efforts for prevention and control should be directed primarily toward improvements in the water supply, milk supply and general sanitation. The effect of a change in the water supply is shown in statistics furnished by Clark (1924). Clark found in Panama, among 4,000 autopsies from 1905 to 1914, 170 cases of amœbiasis or 4.25 per cent. A better water supply was then furnished and during the period 1914 to 1923 among 2,800 autopsies only sixteen cases or 0.57 per cent of amœbiasis were reported. The epidemic of amœbiasis that occurred in Chicago in 1933 appears to have been due to the contamination of drinking water in two hotels by sewage containing cysts. Almost 1,000 cases and 58 deaths were traced to infections acquired in these hotels (Bundeson, 1935). A recent analysis of methods of treatment of amœbiasis is that published by Craig (1934).

6. HOST-PARASITE SPECIFICITY

Endamœba histolytica is a natural parasite of man. Spontaneous infections with this species have been reported in cats, dogs, rats and monkeys but these were probably brought about by the ingestion of cysts passed by man. Experimental infections have been obtained in monkeys, cats, dogs, rats, mice, guinea-pigs and rabbits. Monkeys seem to be infected in nature with an amœbæ which is apparently *Endamœba histolytica*. Kittens and puppies may be infected in the laboratory; older cats and dogs are more difficult to infect. Both these animals and monkeys have been found to suffer from amœbic liver abscess. Kessel (1923) was the first to successfully infect rats and mice. Baetjer and Sellards (1914) and Chatton (1917, 1918) are the only ones to report successful infections in guinea-pigs. Rabbits have been infected by Huber (1909) and Thomson (1926). Monkeys, dogs, rats and mice that are infected may pass cysts, but kittens undergo an acute infection without the passage of cysts and thus far no cysts have been observed in guinea-pigs and rabbits.

IV. *Endamœba coli*

1. HISTORICAL

As previously stated, *Endamœba coli* was first reported by Lewis in 1870 and more accurately described by Cunningham (1871). Accounts of it were later given by Grassi (1879), by Quincke and Roos (1893) and by Casagrandi and Barbagallo (1895, 1897). Schaudinn (1903) distinguished definitely between *Endamœba coli* and *Endamœba histolytica,* and recognized the former to be non-pathogenic and the latter pathogenic. Because a pathogenic organism is more interesting than a non-pathogenic species, more work has been done on *Endamœba histolytica* than on *Endamœba coli.*

2. LIFE-CYCLE

The life-cycle of *Endamœba coli* is similar to that of *Endamœba histolytica* except that the organism lives only in the lumen of the intestine and does not invade the tissues. The trophozoite may pass through the precystic stage and produce cysts in which, by three successive divisions, eight nuclei are formed. Cysts pass out of the body and bring about new infections if they are ingested by a susceptible host.

3. MORPHOLOGY

Trophozoites. The trophozoites of *Endamœba coli* (Figure 11) are never as abundant in a particular host as are the cysts of *Endamœba histolytica.* They live in the large intestine. In size they range from 18 μ to 40 μ, being usually from 20 μ to 30 μ in diameter; they are thus of about the same mass as *Endamœba histolytica.* The distinction between endoplasm and ectoplasm is not well marked. Pseudopodia are granular and not clear as in *Endamœba histolytica,* and are formed slowly rather than explosively as in the latter. Movement is sluggish. The nucleus, which is generally visible in the living animal, contains a rather large karyosome eccentrically placed and a thick layer of chromatin granules on the nuclear membrane. The food of *Endamœba coli* consists of organic material in the intestine, but red cells and tissue elements are not ingested. The trophozoite of *Endamœba coli* reproduces by binary fission.

Precystic stage. The precystic stage involves the casting out of food bodies and the assumption of a spherical shape. The precystic stage of *Endamœba coli* can be distinguished from that of *Endamœba histolytica* by the difference in the nuclear structure.

Cysts. The cysts of *Endamœba coli* (Figure 11) range from 10 μ to 30 μ or more in diameter. Size is a criterion that cannot be used with certainty to distinguish this species from *Endamœba histolytica,* but cysts less than 10 μ in diameter are usually those of *Endamœba histolytica,* whereas cysts more than 20 μ in diameter are usually

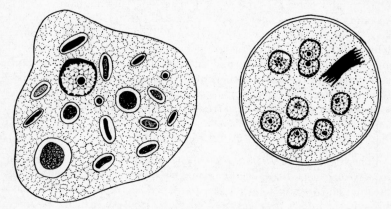

Fig. 11.—*Endamœba coli.* Trophozoite (at left) containing nucleus and food bodies. Cyst (at right) with eight nuclei and a mass of chromatoidal substance.

those of *Endamœba coli.* From one to eight nuclei ordinarily are present in the cysts, although as many as twenty have been reported. The normal mature cyst contains eight nuclei. Mitosis within the cyst (Figure 4a) has been described by Swezy (1922). It occurs within the nuclear membrane and the chromosome number is six. In young cysts, glycogen bodies occur; these are usually larger than similar bodies in *Endamœba histolytica.* Chromatoid bodies also occur in the cyst; these are splinter-like and often in bundles, and do not have blunt rounded ends as do those of *Endamœba histolytica.* They gradually disappear as the cysts increase in age.

4. HOST-PARASITE RELATIONS

The transmission of *Endamœba coli* from one host to another is no doubt brought about by the contamination of food or drink with feces containing cysts, and the factors that are responsible for the dissemination of the cysts are similar to those described for *Endamœba histolytica*. The cysts are carried through the stomach and into the small intestine, where they probably hatch, and thence into the large intestine. Excystation has been observed outside of the body (Yoshida, 1920; Hegner, 1927), but nothing is known of this process within the host. There is no good evidence that *Endamœba coli* invades the tissues, hence its host-parasite relations are very simple. At least 50 per cent of the general population appear to be infected with this species indicating the prevalence of the fecal contamination of human food and drink. Why *Endamœba coli* should be more successful than *Endamœba histolytica,* which infects only about 10 per cent of the general population, has not been determined.

5. HOST-PARASITE SPECIFICITY

That man is a good host for *Endamœba coli* was demonstrated by Walker and Sellards (1913) ; of twenty men who were fed cysts from five different hosts seventeen became infected; none of these exhibited symptoms. An amœba resembling *Endamœba coli,* and which may be identical with it, has been reported from monkeys. Kessel (1923) reported the infection of rats with *Endamœba coli* and the following year the experimental infection of monkeys (Kessel, 1924).

V. *Endamœba gingivalis*

1. HISTORICAL

This species appears to be the first entozoic amœba of any animal to be discovered, and the first amœba of man to be described. Gros (1849) reported amœbæ from the tartar of the teeth of man which must have been this species. It was reported by Steinberg (1862), by Grassi (1879) and by others at intervals up to the year 1915 when Smith and Barrett and Bass and Johns decided that this species is a tissue invader and the probable etiological agent of *pyorrhea alveolaris*. These publications brought the organism into great prominence and resulted in the stimulation of numerous investigations.

2. LIFE-CYCLE

So far as is known, *Endamœba gingivalis* occurs only as a trophozoite, no cyst ever having been found. Multiplication is by binary fission. There is probably no life outside the body of the host, the amœbæ being passed directly from one host to another.

3. MORPHOLOGY

The trophozoites of *Endamœba gingivalis* (Figure 12) range from 6 μ to 60 μ in diameter but are rarely over 20 μ. The clear ectoplasm is distinct from the granular endoplasm and locomotion is fairly active. Kofoid and Swezy (1924) describe a distinct pellicle. The nucleus is of the endamœba type, smaller than that of *Endamœba coli* and with a karyosome either centrally located or eccentric. The food vacuoles contain bacteria, leucocytes and the like; red cells have rarely been reported.

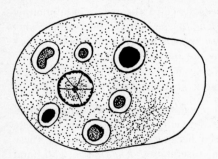

Fig. 12.—*Endamœba gingivalis* containing a nucleus and food bodies.

4. TRANSMISSION

The transmission of *Endamœba gingivalis* from host to host no doubt takes place in the trophozoite stage and plenty of opportunity is afforded for direct passage during kissing. It is thus easy to account for the high incidence of infection in the general population which probably averages at least 50 per cent. The absence of a cyst stage in an amœba that is transmitted by direct contact is worthy of note.

5. PATHOGENICITY

E. gingivalis lives in various places in the mouth, but especially in the tartar of the teeth and in the materia alba around them; it has been reported from many suppurative and inflamed conditions of the mouth and throat. That this species does not require access to the tissues is indicated by the fact that Lynch (1915) found them in the crevices between the false teeth of persons with healthy gums. Various new species have been described from abscesses in the jaw and tonsils, but these were probably all somewhat modified *E. gingivalis*. The presence of large numbers of these amœbæ in the lesions of *pyorrhea alveolaris* led Smith and Barrett (1915) and Bass and Johns (1915) to conclude that they are responsible for this disease, and on their recommendation emetin was widely used in its treatment. More recent studies indicate that the species is harmless. Its food consists principally of leucocytes and a few bacteria (Kofoid and Swezy, 1924). Smith and Barrett (1915) record the ingestion of red cells and Howitt (1926) finds that washed red cells of the guinea-pig are eaten by specimens in artificial cultures, but erythrocytes are probably very seldom devoured in nature. The colonization of the intestine by this species as a result of swallowing trophozoites seems impossible according to the work of Howitt (1926), who found that they were unable to withstand human gastric juice containing the normal amount of acid, and quickly exploded when subjected to human bile.

6. HOST-PARASITE SPECIFICITY

Amœbæ have been found in the mouths of certain lower animals. Goodrich and Moseley (1916) reported them from the dog and cat suffering from pyorrhea, and Nieschulz (1924) described what he considers a variety of the human species *E. gingivalis* var. *equi* from around the teeth of the horse. Monkeys are frequently infected with oral amœbæ. Thus Hegner and Chu (1930) found amœbæ in the mouths of 37 of 44 wild monkeys that they examined in the Philippine Islands. It remains to be determined whether these are specifically distinct from the form occurring in man. Hecker (1916) found it impossible to infect guinea-pigs with amœbæ from the human mouth and Drbohlav (1925) was equally unsuccessful with a kitten into the intestine of which he injected specimens grown in culture, and with a young dog into the gingivæ of which similar material was inoculated. Hinshaw (1928), however, reports the successful inoculation of dogs with *E. gingivalis* from man.

VI. *Endolimax nana*

I. HISTORICAL

Endolimax amœbæ were seen by various observers during the early years of this century but were not recognized as belonging to a separate genus until 1917 when Wenyon and O'Connor found them to be common inhabitants of human beings in Egypt. They have since been widely studied and are now known to be among the commonest of human amœbæ. Species have also been reported from the cecum of fowls, the large intestine of frogs, the colon of cockroaches, the cecum of rats and the large intestine of monkeys.

2. LIFE-CYCLE

The life-cycle of *Endolimax nana* resembles that of *Endamœba coli*. Trophozoites live in the lumen of the large intestine where they feed on organic material; precystic stages occur, which develop into cysts; these pass out of the body in the feces and bring about infections if ingested by susceptible hosts.

3. MORPHOLOGY

Trophozoite. This is a comparatively small species, the trophozoite (Fig. 13) measuring only 6 μ to 12 μ in diameter. It has clear, blunt pseudopodia but is usually sluggish. The food vacuoles contain bacteria and other food bodies. The nucleus possesses a membrane free from chromatin granules. Within it is a large conspicuous karyosome

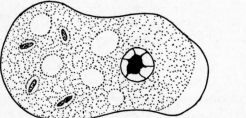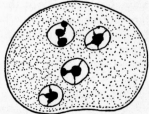

FIG. 13.—*Endolimax nana.* Trophozoite (at left) containing nucleus and food bodies. Cyst (at right) with four nuclei.

usually irregular in shape and sometimes divided into 2 or 3 parts. Linin fibrils connect the karyosome with the nuclear membrane.

Precystic stage. As in *E. histolytica* and *E. coli* the precystic stage loses its food bodies, but does not become much smaller than the adult trophozoite.

Cyst. The cysts are typically ovoidal, but sometimes are spherical or irregular in shape (Fig. 13). They are from 8 μ to 10 μ in length and about 6 μ in breadth. The fully developed cysts contain four nuclei but younger cysts with one, two or three nuclei occur. No chromatoid bodies are present but diffuse glycogen masses may occur from the precystic to the four-nucleate stage.

4. HOST-PARASITE RELATIONS

Endolimax nana is probably a harmless commensal living in the large intestine of man. Transmission no doubt occurs in the cyst stage and differs in no essential feature from that described for *Endamœba histolytica*. Excystation *in vitro* has been described by Hegner (1927) but has never been seen in the living animal. There is no evidence of pathogenicity. Kessel (1923) claims to have infected rats and monkeys (1924) by feeding them cysts from man.

That *Endolimax nana* is a common inhabitant of the human intestine is indicated by the reports of various surveys. The following are based mostly on a single examination of each person: Boeck and Stiles (1923), 13.2 per cent positive of 8,029 persons from various parts of the United States; Magath and Ward (1928), 13.3 per cent positive of 457 persons at the Mayo Clinic; Meleney, Bishop and Leathers (1932), 11.9 per cent positive of 20,237 persons in Tennessee; Wenrich, Stabler and Arnett (1935), 11.4 per cent positive of 1,060 freshmen college students. Other investigators report over 29 per cent of positives. The average among the general population, considering the number of positives missed on one examination, would probably reach 25 per cent or more.

Endolimax amœbæ from lower animals exhibit the characteristics of the genus but their specificity is largely based on the hosts in which they occur.

VII. *Iodamœba williamsi*

1. HISTORICAL

The genus *Iodamœba* was proposed by Dobell in 1919 for a species of human amœba that appears to have been described first by Prowazek in 1911 under the name *Entamœba williamsi*. There is still some question whether this amœba is the species Prowazek found at that time or the species he described in 1912 as *E. bütschlii*, hence both specific names occur in the literature. Cysts of an amœba were noted by Wenyon (1915, 1916) and others in human feces that contained huge masses of glycogen. Since these masses stained a deep mahogany color when tinted with iodine, the cysts were called iodine cysts until their relation to the trophozoites of *I. williamsi* was established.

2. LIFE-CYCLE

Iodamœba williamsi lives in the lumen of the large intestine of man. The trophozoites divide by binary fission; a precystic stage occurs; and most of the cysts are uninucleate.

3. MORPHOLOGY

Trophozoite: Unstained.—Ectoplasm and endoplasm are not easily distinguished except when ectoplasmic pseudopodia appear. Movement is slow and little progress results. Specimens range from 5 to 20 μ in diameter the average being from 9 to 14 μ. The nucleus is usually not visible in the living animal. Many food vacuoles may be present; these contain bacteria and intestinal debris but not red cells.

Trophozoite: Stained (Fig. 14).—The principal feature revealed by staining is the character of the nucleus. This is a large body with a distinct membrane. The karyosome is large and centrally located. When stained with hæmatoxylin and then properly decolorized the

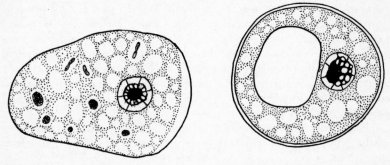

Fig. 14.—*Iodamœba williamsi.* Trophozoite (at left) containing nucleus and food bodies. Cyst (at right) with nucleus and glycogen body (clear).

central portion of the karyosome remains deeply stained but a peripheral layer of lightly stained bodies appears completely surrounding the central mass. Fibers may appear passing from the karyosome to the nuclear membrane. No chromatin occurs on the nuclear membrane.

Precystic Stage.—As in other species, the trophozoites loose their food bodies before encysting. Unlike other species they decrease very little in size.

Cyst: Unstained.—The cysts range from about 6 to 17 μ in diameter, averaging about 9 μ. They are often irregular in shape. Most of the cysts contain one or several glycogen masses. There is a well-defined cyst wall.

Cyst: Stained.—When stained with iodine the glycogen masses become very conspicuously colored; they appear as clear vacuoles after hæmatoxylin. The nucleus differs in structure from that of the trophozoite. The deeply staining portion of the karyosome is eccentric, sometimes lying against the nuclear membrane on one side, and the lightly staining granules become aggregated on the opposite side as shown in Fig. 14. Very few cysts contain more than one nucleus;

only 2 specimens with 2 nuclei were encountered by Taliaferro and Becker (1922) among 2000 cysts examined.

4. HOST-PARASITE RELATIONS

Iodamœba williamsi appears to be a harmless commensal feeding on bacteria and organic matter in the large intestine. The incidence of infection ranges probably from about 5 to 10 per cent. Boeck and Stiles (1923) report 5 per cent among 8,029 persons from all over the United States on the basis of a single examination; and Meleney, Bishop and Leathers (1932) report 4.1 per cent among 20,237 persons in Tennessee, also from one examination. The actual incidence of infection was probably 8 or 10 per cent. Wenrich (1937) noted *Iodamœba* in 26 of 1700 human beings and in 25 of 55 apes and monkeys examined. Transmission no doubt takes place in the cyst stage as in *E. histolytica, E. coli* and *Endolimax nana*. Smith (1927) has described excystation *in vitro* in guinea-pigs. Apparently moisture and a suitable temperature are the required stimuli; cysts in a weak saline solution on a slide under a cover-glass, when maintained at a temperature of 37° C. for about five hours, were seen to excyst on a number of occasions. When injected into the stomach of guinea-pigs, cysts are carried into the small intestine where they may excyst in the jejunum within a period of three hours. Kessel (1923) and Smith (1928) appear to have brought about infections in rats with cysts from man. It is possible that amœbæ belonging to this genus that have been reported from pigs, monkeys and other lower animals may belong to the same species as that from man. For example, *I. suis* from the intestine of the pig may really be *I. williamsi,* in which case the pig serves as a reservoir host of the human species.

VIII. *Dientamœba fragilis*

1. HISTORICAL

Only one species of the genus *Dientamœba* is known; this occurs in man and monkeys and was described by Jepps and Dobell (1918) as *Dientamœba fragilis* because of its apparent delicacy.

2. MORPHOLOGY

Trophozoite. This measures usually from 3.5 μ to 12 μ but may reach over 20 μ in diameter (Fig. 15). It is active, has clearly defined ectoplasm and endoplasm, and sends out leaflike, hyaline pseudopodia.

Two nuclei with the characteristics already described are usually present in more than 50 per cent of the specimens, hence the genus name *Dientamœba*. The food consists of bacteria and yeasts. *D.*

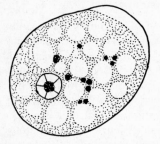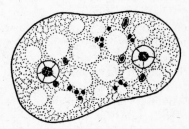

FIG. 15.—*Dientamœba fragilis.* Uninucleate trophozoite (at left); binucleate trophozoite (at right).

fragilis is not as fragile as at first supposed, but will live for a day or two in fecal material outside of the body.

Cyst. One observer has reported cysts but this has not been confirmed.

3. HOST-PARASITE RELATIONS

D. fragilis is more common than most protozoan surveys indicate; for example, Wenrich, Stabler and Arnett (1935) report it from 4.3 per cent of 1,060 freshmen college students on one examination. It appears to be as widely distributed geographically as other species of human amœbæ. Several investigators have reported intestinal disturbances associated with infections with *D. fragilis* (Hakansson, 1936; Wenrich, 1936, 1937) but its pathogenicity is still in doubt. Amœbæ indistinguishable from this species were found by Hegner and Chu (1930) in two of 44 wild monkeys (*Macacus philippinensis*) captured near Manila, Philippine Islands.

IX. *Doubtful Species of Amœbæ Reported from Man*

The six species of amœbæ described above are recognized as "good" species by practically all protozoölogists. Besides these, almost one hundred other species have been described as human parasites but have not become established as distinct species. Most of these doubtful forms have been described by persons who were careless in their work or knew very little about protozoölogy. Several stages in the life-cycle of a single species have sometimes been described as distinct species, and in some cases stages in the life-cycle of several species have been combined under one specific name. Four of these doubtful species have received more attention than any of the others; they are *Councilmania lafleuri* described by Kofoid and Swezy in 1921, *Caudamœba sinensis* described by Faust in 1923, *Karyamœbina falcata* described by Kofoid and Swezy in 1924 and *Endamœba dispar* named by Brumpt in 1925.

None of these species has been generally accepted by protozoölogists. *Councilmania lafleuri* is usually considered to represent stages in the life-cycle of *Endamœba coli*; *Caudamœba sinensis* may be an aberrant form of *E. histolytica* or a degenerating specimen of the flagellate, *Trichomonas hominis* such as Castellani (1905) named *Entamœba undulans*; and *Karyamœbina falcata* may have been named from degenerating trophozoites of *E. histolytica*. *Endamœba dispar* is supposed to be morphologically indistinguishable from *E. histolytica* but physiologically different; it is non-pathogenic and does not ingest red blood cells.

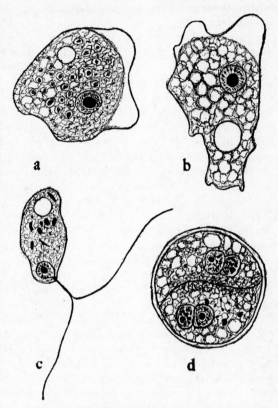

FIG. 16.—Coprozoic amœbæ.
a. *Hartmannella hyalina.* Trophozoite.
b. *Dimastigamœba gruberi.* Amœboid form.
c. *Dimastigamœba gruberi.* Flagellate form.
d. *Sappinia diploidea.* Trophozoite. (All after Dobell and O'Connor. x 2000)

X. *Coprozoic Amœbæ*

PROTOZOA that live in fecal material are said to be coprozoic. They are free-living species which either find their way into the feces after passage from the body, or else are swallowed in the cyst stage, pass through the alimentary canal unchanged and hatch after their escape from the body. Coprozoic PROTOZOA are of particular importance because they may be confused with parasite species, especially when stools are kept moist and warm for some hours before examination.

Hartmannella hyalina (Fig. 16) has frequently been cultivated from human feces (Musgrave and Clegg, 1904). It possesses a single contractile vacuole; and a cyst stage, but not a flagellated stage, occurs in its life-cycle. *Dimastigamœba gruberi* is another common coprozoic species that possesses a contractile vacuole; both cyst stage and a flagellate stage occur in its life-cycle (Wilson, 1916). *Sappinia diploidea* occurs commonly in the feces of lower animals and more rarely in those of man. It possesses a contractile vacuole and two nuclei. A cyst stage has been described consisting of two individuals within a single wall. The shelled rhizopod, *Chlamydophrys stercorea,* was reported by Schaudinn (1903) from human feces, but he probably confused this form with one of the parasitic amœbæ. *C. stercorea,* however, occurs commonly in the feces of frogs, pigs and horses. The trophozoite (Fig. 18, *i*) is surrounded by an egg-shapèd, transparent shell about 15 μ in length, through a pore in one end of which pseudopodia are extruded. Cysts occur in its life-cycle.

XI. *Methods of Obtaining and Preparing Amœbæ for Study*

I. COLLECTION OF MATERIAL

Fecal samples should be collected in clean, dry containers that are free from antiseptics. If possible they should be deposited directly into a container and not in a water-closet first. They should also be kept free from urine. The sigmoidoscope has been used by Paulson and Andrews (1927) for obtaining material directly from the intestine but this is not necessary under ordinary conditions.

Whenever possible the entire stool should be obtained. If this cannot be accomplished, then samples from several parts of the stool should be selected. The paraffin pasteboard containers commonly used for transporting ice-cream are well adapted for the collection of samples. Small pill boxes may be used for smaller samples and these may be sent by mail in ordinary cylindrical mailing cases. Feces obtained after a saline purge reveal a greater number of protozoan species than naturally-passed stools.

Fecal samples should be examined as soon as possible after they are passed, since the active trophozoites become quiescent when the material becomes cold and soon die. It is advisable to keep the feces warm either in a vacuum bottle or in a thermopack. A stool in a pasteboard container, if placed in a thermopack with several containers filled with water at body temperature, will remain warm for a considerable period. A warm stage is not necessary for a rapid examination. The cysts of intestinal amœbæ live for many days in fecal material, hence they may be looked for in older stools. Active amœbæ that appear in old stools are coprozoic species and not former inhabitants of the human intestine. Since the protozoa may be distributed irregularly in a stool, it is desirable whenever possible to stir up the entire sample in saline solution.

2. PREPARATION OF SMEARS

Living specimens. The amœbæ of man can be identified usually in the living condition. It is important, however, that fresh material be used for this purpose and that it be prepared in such a way as not to destroy the organisms. Amœbæ that are moving about, and cysts, can be detected with a 16 mm. objective and a number 10 ocular. After the organism is found the species can be determined with the 4 mm. objective. A simple method of preparing a smear is to take very small samples from various parts of the stool and emulsify them with a toothpick on a slide in 0.7 per cent saline solution. A number 1 cover-glass can be added and the material spread out beneath it until a very thin layer is formed. A frequent mistake is the use of too much material, thus forming such a thick smear that the protozoa cannot be distinguished. Organisms are often to be found in the mucus on the outside of formed stools, hence samples from both outside and inside should be made. The smear, of course, should never be allowed to dry since this quickly kills the amœbæ and modifies their shape so that they cannot be identified. The addition of neutral red or eosin 1 : 10,000 may aid in diagnosis since the débris is stained but not the cysts. The trophozoites are not killed by these dyes.

Dead specimens killed with iodine. The identification of cysts of amœbæ depends largely on the number and character of the nuclei they contain. Nuclei are often difficult to observe in living specimens, hence it is customary to add to the smear an iodine solution. A saturated solution of iodine in 5 per cent aqueous potassium iodide should be used. The amœbæ are killed by this solution and the number and much of the structure of the nuclei can then be determined; the presence or absence of glycogen and its mass and shape can also be observed.

Dead specimens killed with Schaudinn's solution and stained with iron-hæmatoxylin. In some cases it is impossible to determine with certainty the species present in anything but a fixed and stained smear. The best method of making such preparations is to spread a thin moist film on a slide or cover-glass, drop it before it has a chance to dry into Schaudinn's fixing solution and then stain it in iron-hæmatoxylin. The following is a short outline of the steps in the preparation and staining of smears by the Heidenhain iron-hæmatoxylin process.

1. A small bit of feces is smeared on a cover-glass with a glass rod so as to form a thin moist film.
2. Drop immediately face downward into warm (heated only to point where steam rises) Schaudinn's fluid which is composed of the following:

   Distilled water saturated with mercuric chloride (Hg_2Cl_2) 65 pts.
   95 per cent alcohol .... 33 pts.
   Glacial acetic acid .... 2 to 5 pts.
   The film will float on the surface at first. After a few seconds it can be completely immersed and left in the fluid for from 10 to 20 minutes.
3. Wash and harden by the following steps:
   a. Wash in 50 per cent alcohol for a few minutes.
   b. Transfer to 70 per cent to which has been added a few drops of alcoholic iodine solution (to remove sublimate) for at least 10 minutes.
   c. Harden in 95 per cent alcohol. When speed is essential this hardening may be shortened to a few minutes, but it is best to leave the film in the alcohol for an hour and even a few days does not injure it.
   d. Hydrate by successive immersions for a few minutes in 70 per cent and 50 per cent alcohol and distilled water.
4. Mordant by placing in a 2 per cent aqueous iron alum solution (ammonium-ferric sulphate) 30 minutes or longer (over night answers as well). While 30 minutes will suffice it is best to mordant for at least 2 hours.
5. Wash in distilled water for a few seconds.
6. Stain in 0.5 per cent aqueous hæmatoxylin solution. This should be made up several weeks previous to its use and allowed to "ripen." Several hours is sufficient for staining, but a longer time, viz., over night, is better.
7. Wash in distilled water.
8. Differentiate in 1-2 per cent aqueous iron-alum solution. This is by far the most difficult part of the process and can be done accurately only after practice. The overstained films are placed in the iron-alum solution and at intervals taken out, rinsed in distilled water and examined under the microscope. When each film is destained enough, it is washed in distilled water and then placed in running tap water for at least 20 minutes.

It is often an advantage to start the differentiation with 2 per cent iron-alum solution, and as the films become destained to dilute the solution to about 0.5 per cent so that the end point is reached more slowly.

9. Wash in distilled water.
10. Dehydrate by immersing successively for about five minutes each in 50 per cent, 70 per cent, 95 per cent and absolute alcohol (2 changes).
11. Clear by immersing in two changes of xylol (5 minutes each).
12. Mount by lowering the smear face-downward over a drop of Canada balsam on a slide and pressing it down gently.

Johnson (1935) has devised a modification of the above which, by the use of a 0.25% solution of iron alum for decolorizing, permits a time instead of visual control of the process. In abbreviated form the technique is as follows:

Minutes

1. Fix in hot Schaudinn's solution plus 5 to 10 per cent acetic acid 10
2. 95 per cent alcohol plus iodine (port wine color) 5
3. 70 per cent alcohol 5
4. Rinse in tap water 1–3
5. 4 per cent iron alum 15
6. Rinse in tap water 1–2
7. Stain (0.5 per cent aqueous hematoxylin) 10
8. Decolorize in 0.25 per cent iron alum 12
9. Wash in running water 3–30
10. Dehydrate, clear and mount

For *Dientamœba* use 15 to 20 per cent acetic acid for best results. Flagellates also require more acid. If slides are for diagnosis only, a short washing period is sufficient; but if intended for permanent record they should be washed at least thirty minutes. At no stage in the staining process should the smears be allowed to dry.

3. CONCENTRATION METHODS

Often the cysts of amœbæ are present in fecal material in such small numbers that they cannot be found in smears without undue effort. To obviate this difficulty concentration methods have been perfected. Some of these methods are so complicated that they are of use only to professional protozoölogists. A simple method of washing and sedimentation, however, that is valuable for concentrating cysts may be described here. Fecal material is thoroughly stirred up in water and strained through two layers of cheese-cloth into a tall cylindrical graduate containing about two liters of water.

This is allowed to settle for a few hours and then some of the material at the bottom is removed with a long pipette and smears made. In some cases it is desirable to repeat this process several times.

Simple centrifugation has been practiced on a large scale for survey diagnosis by Meleney (1932). The details are as follows:

About a gram of feces are placed in a 25 cc. test tube with 10 cc. of tap-water. The fecal material is broken up by shaking, and the suspension filtered through cotton into a 50 cc. centrifuge tube. Additional tap-water up to 40 cc. is then poured through the cotton to wash through any cysts which have been held in the cotton. The tube is then centrifuged at 1800 revolutions for one-half to one minute, the supernatant fluid poured off, and a portion of the fine sediment examined microscopically on a slide.

XII. *Methods of Cultivating Amœbæ*

I. FREE-LIVING AND COPROZOIC AMŒBÆ

These are easily cultivated on a medium of Musgrave and Clegg (1904) which consists of

Agar ....20.0 grams
Sodium chloride ....0.3-0.5 grams
Extract of beef ....0.3-0.5 grams
Distilled water ....1000 c.c.

This is rendered 1 per cent alkaline and made up in the same way as nutrient agar. It is poured into Petrie dishes and when congealed the material containing amœbæ is spread on the surface; the cultures must be kept moist and at a temperature of 20° C. to 25° C.

2. ENTOZOIC AMŒBÆ

Cutler (1918) appears to have been the first to cultivate an endamœba although no one has succeeded in repeating his work. An endamœba from the turtle, *E. barreti,* was cultivated by Barret and Smith (1924). Their medium consisted of 0.5 per cent sodium chloride solution, nine parts, and human blood serum, one part, and was kept at either room temperature or at 10° C. to 15° C.

A medium devised by Boeck and Drbohlav (1925) for the cultivation of *Endamœba histolytica* has been found to be very successful. This is known as the L.E.S. medium, inasmuch as it is made up of Locke's solution, egg, and human blood serum. The L.E.S. medium is prepared as follows:

"1. Four eggs were washed, brushed with alcohol and broken into a sterile flask containing glass beads. Fifty (50) cc. of Locke's physiological solution are then added and the mixture broken up by shaking.

2. Test tubes are then filled with a sufficient quantity to produce slants from about 1 to 1½ inches in length upon coagulation by heat.

3. These tubes are now slanted in an inspissator and heated (70° C.) until the egg mixture has solidified. They are then transferred to the autoclave and sterilized for 20 minutes at 15 pounds of pressure.

4. The tubes are now covered to a depth of 1 cm. above the egg slant with a mixture composed of 8 parts of sterile Locke's solution and 1 part of sterile inactivated human blood serum. They are then incubated to determine sterility.

5. The Locke solution is made up as follows:

Distilled water ....1000 cc.
NaCl ....9.0 grams
CaCl ....0.2 grams
KCl ....0.4 grams
NaHCO$_3$ ....2.2 grams
Glucose ....2.5 grams

The solution is sterilized, either in the Arnold or the autoclave, according to the ordinary methods." (Boeck and Drbohlav, 1925.)

A second medium devised by Boeck and Drbohlav is the L.E.A. mixture, which differs from the L.E.S. medium by the substitution of a 1 per cent solution of crystallized egg albumin for the human serum. The work of Boeck and Drbohlav was first confirmed by Andrews (1925) and later by many other investigators.

A number of modifications and simplifications of these media have been reported. The most simple are those of Craig (1926). His Locke-Serum medium is made up as follows:

Sodium chloride ....9.00 grams
Calcium chloride ....0.24 grams
Potassium chloride ....0.42 grams
Sodium bicarbonate ....0.20 grams
Dextrose ....2.50 grams
Distilled water ....1000 cc.

This solution is filtered, autoclaved at fifteen pounds pressure for fifteen minutes and allowed to cool. There is then added one part of inactivated human, horse or rabbit serum to each seven parts of the Locke solution used. After adding the blood serum the mixture is thoroughly shaken and filtered through a Mandler or Berkefeld filter. Later (Craig, 1926) two simpler media were devised; the Ringer-Serum medium is prepared by combining seven parts of a modified Ringer solution and one part of an inactivated human blood serum. The Ringer solution has the following formula:

Sodium chloride ....8.0 grams
Calcium chloride ....0.20 grams
Potassium chloride ....0.20 grams
Distilled water ....1000 cc.

Craig's Normal-Salt-Serum medium is the most simple of all but has given this investigator good results. This medium is prepared by adding one part of inactivated human blood serum to seven parts of normal salt solution (0.85). The salt solution is autoclaved at fifteen pounds pressure for fifteen minutes before adding the serum, and the mixture is filtered, tubed, and tested for sterility in the same manner as the Locke-Serum and Ringer-Serum media. These results demonstrate that sodium chloride is the only constituent necessary besides blood serum for the continued cultivation of *Endamœba histolytica*. Much has been learned regarding the life-cycle of *E. histolytica* by means of artificial cultures as may easily be judged from the investigations of Yorke and Adams (1926a, 1926b, 1927), Dobell and Laidlaw (1926) and Dobell (1927). Craig and St. John (1927) have shown that this method may even be used to determine the presence of *E. histolytica* in stools and that a larger percentage of positives may be determined in this way than by the smear method. Dobell (1927) also states that "A culture frequently supplies a more accurate test of the presence of amœbæ than a microscopic examination." It remains to be proved that this method can be employed successfully under field conditions.

Cleveland and Sanders (1930) devised the following medium for the cultivation of *Endamœba histolytica* and report that the organism grows far better in it than it does in its natural environment. The medium is made up as follows:

Slants of liver infusion agar are covered with fresh horse serum—saline (one part serum to six parts physiological saline) containing rice flour. The Liver Infusion Agar is prepared by the Digestive Ferments Company of Detroit, Michigan, and each pound contains in addition to the infusion from 500 grams of beef liver, 10 grams of peptone, 5 grams NaCl and 20 grams of agar.

The best results in making the liver infusion agar slants are obtained by using 30 grams per liter of distilled water instead of 55, the amount called for in the directions of the Digestive Ferments Company. This makes a softer slant and is not so rich. These slants are covered to the depth of the slant with fresh horse serum-saline (1-6) and a 3 mm. loop of sterile rice flour added.

In this medium *Endamœba histolytica* carries on its entire life-cycle. When a heavy inoculation is made, encystation begins within 18 to 24 hours after the inoculation and continues for 72 hours or more. As soon as the cysts reach the four nucleate stage and become mature, they excyst and the life-cycle continues.

Tsuchiya's (1934) medium consists of a nutrient broth prepared by dissolving 10 gms. of peptone, 3 gms. of meat extract, and 5 gms. of NaCl in 1000 cc. of *neutral* distilled water. This is tubed in 8 cc. quantities and autoclaved. Each tube is enriched by the addition of two 4 mm. loopfuls of a thoroughly triturated mixture of 2 parts of rice starch to one part of animal charcoal. The author emphasizes the fact that primary cultures are more likely to be successful if they are inoculated with washed material obtained by simple sedimentation or centrifugation of the stool. A modification of this technique suggested and recommended by Tsuchiya is to overlay an egg-slant with the broth and to add the starch-charcoal mixture.

XIII. *Pseudoparasites in Human Feces*

Besides coprozoic PROTOZOA, various objects in fecal material, such as vegetable organisms, human intestinal cells and mechanical artefacts may be mistaken for entozoic amœbæ. Various types of

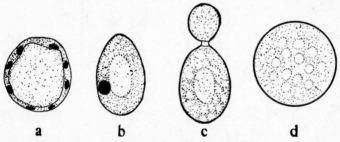

a   b   c   d

FIG. 17.—Vegetable organisms in human feces.
a. *Blastocystis hominis.*
b. Intestinal yeast.
c. Intestinal yeast, budding.
d. Intestinal mold. (All after Kofoid, Kornhauser and Swezy. x 2800)

vegetable organisms resemble amœbic cysts; the most common of these are *Blastocystis hominis,* intestinal yeasts and fecal molds (Figure 17). Dysenteric stools contain many bodies that may be mistaken for PROTOZOA, especially macrophage cells, and polymorpho-

TABLE I

DIFFERENTIAL DIAGNOSIS OF HUMAN INTESTINAL AMŒBÆ

	Stage and Condition	Endamœba histolytica	Endamœba coli	Endolimax nana	Iodamœba williamsi
Diameter	Trophozoite living	Usually 20 μ to 30 μ	Usually 20 μ to 30 μ	Usually 6 μ to 12 μ	Usually 9 μ to 14 μ
Locomotion ..	Trophozoite living	Active	Sluggish	Sluggish	Sluggish
Pseudopodia .	Trophozoite living	Blade-like, hyaline, explosive	Blunt, slowly formed	Blunt, slow, several	Blunt, slowly formed
Cytoplasm ...	Trophozoite living	Ectoplasm sharply differentiated	Ectoplasm not sharply differentiated	Ectoplasm not sharply differentiated	Ectoplasm not sharply differentiated
Nucleus	Trophozoite living	Faint or invisible	Visible	Faintly visible	Sometimes visible
Inclusions ...	Trophozoite living	Red blood cells, no bacteria	Bacteria and débris	Bacteria and débris	Bacteria and débris
Nucleus	Trophozoite, stained with iron-haematoxylin	4 μ to 7 μ; karyosome small, central; thin peripheral chromatin; membrane thin	4 μ to 8 μ; karyosome large, eccentric; heavy peripheral chromatin; membrane thick	1 μ to 3 μ; one large or several connected karyosomes; no peripheral chromatin	2 μ to 3 μ; one large central karyosome surrounded by refractile granules
Diameter	Cyst, living	5 μ to 20 μ	10 μ to 30 μ	8 μ to 10 μ by 6 μ	8 μ to 12 μ
Shape	Cyst, living	Spheroidal	Spheroidal	Ellipsoidal	Spheroidal or irregular
Nucleus	Cyst, living	Faint or invisible	Visible	Usually invisible	Faint or invisible
Glycogen	Cyst, stained with iodine	Present in young cysts; stains dark mahogany brown	Present in young cysts; usually larger than in E. histolytica	Sometimes present in young cysts	Almost always present and large
Nuclei	Cyst, stained with iron-haematoxylin	4, structure as in trophozoite	8, structure as in trophozoite	4, structure as in trophozoite	1, refractile granules at one side
Chromatoid bodies	Cyst, stained with iron-haematoxylin	Often present; rod-like with rounded ends	Sometimes present; like splinters of glass	None	None

nuclear leucocytes which may ingest red blood cells. Beginners often mistake such objects as air bubbles and oil globules for cysts of amœbæ, but one soon learns to recognize these as mechanical artefacts.

XIV. *Differential Diagnosis of Human Amœbæ*

Table I presents the principal features of the four common amœbæ that live in man in such a manner that they may easily be compared. The criteria of importance in identifying living trophozoites are size, speed of locomotion, character and method of formation of the pseudopodia, differentiation between ectoplasm and endoplasm, visibility of the nucleus and character of the inclusions. In trophozoites stained with iron-hæmatoxylin the nuclear structures are clearly exhibited; these are size, mass, number and location of the karyosomes, the presence or absence and thickness of the peripheral chromatin, if present, and the thickness of the nuclear membrane. Living cysts may be distinguished by their size, shape and visibility of the nuclei. Cysts stained with iodine show the number of nuclei and the presence or absence and characteristics of glycogen bodies, if present. Nuclear number and structure and chromatoid bodies are revealed in cysts stained with iron-hæmatoxylin.

CHAPTER IV

AMŒBÆ OF LOWER ANIMALS

I. *Amœbæ of Monkeys*

At least eleven species of amœbæ belonging to three genera have been described from monkeys. One of these, named *Endamœba nuttalli* by Castellani in 1908, resembles *Endamœba histolytica* so closely, both in the trophozoite and cyst stages, that many authorities believe them to belong to the same species. Another, named *Endamœba pitheci* by Prowazek in 1912, is structurally indistinguishable from *Endamœba coli* both in the trophozoite and cyst stages. It seems probable that seven of the other species named from monkeys belong to one or the other of these two species. Brug in 1921 described a species of *Iodamœba* from a monkey to which the name *Iodamœba kueneni* was given; this species may be the same as *Iodamœba williamsi* in man. The same investigator (Brug, 1923) described an *Endolimax* from a monkey for which he proposed the name *Endolimax cynomolgi;* this may be the same species as *Endolimax nana* in man. Amœbæ belonging to these various species have been reported from the gorilla, chimpanzee, orang-utan, baboon and a number of other species of monkeys from both the Old World and the New World. Most of the monkeys in which the amœbæ have been found were in captivity and it is possible that they may have become infected with human amœbæ. However, Hegner and Chu (1930) found as many protozoa in wild monkeys in the Philippine Islands as had previously been reported from captive animals. Of 44 monkeys examined, 37 (84 per cent) were found to be infected with amœbæ indistinguishable from *Endamœba gingivalis,* 22 (50 per cent) with *E. coli,* 10 (23 per cent) with *E. histolytica,* 22 (50 per cent) with *Endolimax nana,* and 2 (4.5 per cent) with *Dientamœba fragilis.* Apes and monkeys either in a wild state or in captivity are therefore excellent sources from which to obtain material for study. The histolytica-like amœba may produce in monkeys both amœbic dysentery and amœbic liver abscesses. As already noted, there is evidence that *E. histolytica, E. coli* and other species of amœbæ can be transferred from man to monkeys successfully (Kessel, 1924).

II. *Amœbæ of Domesticated Mammals and Birds*

Amœbæ have been found in practically all of the domesticated mammals and birds. Many of these have been considered specifically different from those described from man and have been given specific names. How many of these are actually distinct species remains to be determined. None of these species seem to be severely pathogenic but usually live the lives of harmless commensals in the mouth or intestine.

I. FOOD ANIMALS

Amœbæ were described from the stomach of cattle by Liebetanz (1905) and given the name *Endamœba bovis.* Nieschulz (1922) reported the finding of cysts in the feces of cattle but whether these belong to the same species or not is unknown. An amœba called *Endamœba intestinalis* was reported by Gedoelst (1911) from horses; this species has been found by Fantham (1920) in the colon and cecum of horses in South Africa as well as a second species, *Endamœba equi* (Fantham, 1921), which ingests red blood cells and is presumably pathogenic. Pigs harbor not only endamœbæ but also iodamœbæ. Amœbæ were discovered in the intestinal ulcers of pigs by Theobald Smith (1910); they were probably of the species named *Endamœba polecki* by Prowazek (1912). A second species of endamœba, *E. debliecki,* which is smaller than the first, has been described by Nieschulz (1924). An iodamœba was described by O'Connor (1920) from pigs in the Ellice Islands; to this the name *I. suis* was given. Several investigators have since found iodamœbæ in pigs in various parts of the world, including the United States (Hegner and Taliaferro, 1924). It is still to be determined whether the iodamœbæ of man and the pig belong to the same species. An extensive report on the protozoa of pigs has recently been published by Kessel (1928). An amœba named *Endamœba ovis* has been reported from sheep (Swellengrebel, 1914) and another, named *Endamœba capræ,* from goats (Fantham, 1923). Endamœbæ have been described from the mouth of the horse as *Endamœba gingivalis* var. *equi* (Nieschulz, 1924).

2. PETS

Household pets, such as cats and dogs, are frequently infected with amœbæ. Spontaneous amœbic dysentery in both dogs and cats has been reported by a number of investigators. The amœba concerned is probably *E. histolytica.* As noted above, experimental

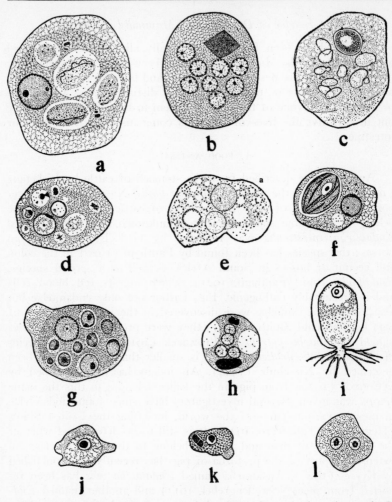

FIG. 18.—Some amœbæ of lower animals. a. *Endamœba muris*, from the rat. b. *E. muris*, cyst. c. *E. blattæ*, from the cockroach. d. *E. thomsoni*, from the cockroach. e. *E. testudinis*, from the tortoise. f. *E. minchini*, from the crane-fly larva. g. *E. ranarum*, from the frog. h. *E. ranarum*, cyst. i. *Chlamydophrys stercorea*, from the feces of frogs, horses, etc. j. *Endolimax blattarum*, from the cockroach. k. *Endolimax caviæ*, from the guinea-pig. l. *Dientamœba fragilis*, from the monkey. (a, b, d, f, g, h, j, k, after Wenrich, x 1500; c, from Kudo, x 400; d, from Kudo, x 665; i, from Wenyon, x 500; l, from Hegner and Chu, x 1500)

infections may be set up in both of these animals with *E. histolytica* from man. An amœba indistinguishable from *E. gingivalis* has also been reported from the dog (Goodrich and Moseley, 1916).

3. LABORATORY ANIMALS

Many rodents are susceptible to amœbic infections, An amœba of the *Endamœba coli* type, named *E. cuniculi,* has been found in rabbits (Brug, 1918). Guinea-pigs harbor a similar form named *E. cobayæ* (Walker, 1908). Cysts containing both four nuclei (Leger, 1918) and eight nuclei (Holmes, 1923) have been found in guinea-pigs. The amœbæ of rats and mice have been studied more carefully than those of other rodents. The commonest species, known as *E. muris,* is of the *E. coli* type, but amœbæ resembling *E. histolytica* have also been reported (Brug, 1919; Chiang, 1925). Andrews and White (1936) examined 2515 wild rats captured in the city of Baltimore and report the following numbers of infections with amœbæ; *E. histolytica* in 28 (1.1 per cent), *E. muris* in 262 (10.4 per cent), and *Endolimax nana* in 1. An endolimax indistinguishable from *E. nana* was reported by Chiang and given the name *E. ratti* because this investigator was unable to infect rats with *E. nana* from man.

4. BIRDS

Amœbæ have been described from the intestine of grouse, fowls and ducks. A species named *Endamœba lagopodis,* whose cysts contain four nuclei, was reported from grouse by Fantham (1910). Amœbæ with eight-nucleate cysts have been recovered from fowls (Hartmann, 1913; Tyzzer, 1920) and a species named *E. anatis* has been described from ducks in South Africa (Fantham, 1924). The cecum of the fowl is also the habitat of an endolimax. Tyzzer (1920) gave this form the name *Pygolimax gregariniformis,* but it no doubt belongs to the genus *Endolimax* (Hegner, 1926) and should be referred to as *Endolimax gregariniformis.*

Methods have been devised for finding amœbæ and other protozoa that may be present in the digestive tract of birds and other animals but are too few in number to be detected by smear examination. The culture method, which was found by Craig and St. John (1927) to be successful in the diagnosis of amœbæ in human feces, might also be of value if applied to lower animals. Of proven worth is the use of chicks a few days old. Fecal samples, when injected into chicks either *per os* or *per rectum,* very soon reach the ceca where certain protozoa, both amœbæ and flagellates, may increase very rapidly in number and become numerous enough within two or three days to be found without difficulty (Hegner, 1929).

III. *Amœbæ of Other Animals*

Many species of amœbæ have been described from other lower animals; a few of these, of particular interest because of the ease with which they may be obtained or of the nature of their hosts, may be mentioned here. *Endamœba ranarum,* which occurs in the intestine of certain frogs, is indistinguishable morphologically from *E. histolytica,* but attempts to infect tadpoles with histolytica cysts have failed (Dobell, 1918). After excystation, eight amœbulæ are formed just as in *E. histolytica* (Sanders, 1931). Tadpoles and young frogs appear to be more often infected than older animals. For example, Brandt (1936) reports *Endamœba ranarum* in 3.03 per cent of bullfrogs over 100 mm. long and in 13.2 per cent of bullfrogs less than 100 mm. long.

As noted in Chapter III (page 74), the first endamœba of a cold-blooded animal to be cultivated was *E. barreti* which occurs in the turtle (Barret and Smith, 1923; Taliaferro and Holmes, 1923). Amœbæ have been reported from the intestine of other reptiles, for example, snakes and lizards, and may even be pathogenic to these animals (Geiman and Ratcliffe, 1936). Species have also been described from the newt and from the intestine of fish. Many invertebrates also serve as hosts of endamœbæ. The vagina of the horse-leech is the habitat of *Endamœba aulastomi.* Various insects are infected, for example the larvæ of the crane fly by *E. minchini* (MacKinnon, 1914), the water-bug, *Belostoma,* by *E. belostomæ,* and the honey-bee by *E. apis.*

The amœba of the cockroach, *E. blattæ,* which is the type species of the genus *Endamœba* (Leidy, 1879) has been studied more than any other amœba that occurs in invertebrates. The trophozoite (Figure 18, *c*) is very large and may reach a diameter of 120 μ, being usually about 50 μ. The nucleus is large, often lemon-shaped, and possesses a very thick membrane. There is no central karyosome, the chromatin material being arranged in a broad peripheral zone of granules.

The most recent account of the life cycle of *Endamœba blattæ* is that by Morris (1935). The stages described are shown in the accompanying diagram (Fig. 19).

If we take the large adult amoeba (1) showing no indication of recent fission to be the zygotic adult form, this gives rise, by a series of mitotic fissions (2 to 8), to a number of smaller mononucleate animals, only slightly larger than the cysts, as shown in stage 9.

Within these the number of nuclei is increased, by further mitoses,

to an average of about sixteen; after which mitotic activity halts, the
nuclei become spherical, and take on an appearance more like those of
the cysts (10). A rest period appears to precede the actual secretion
of the cyst wall (11), which is followed immediately by another division
—possibly meiotic in nature. The segregation of the two cytoplasmic

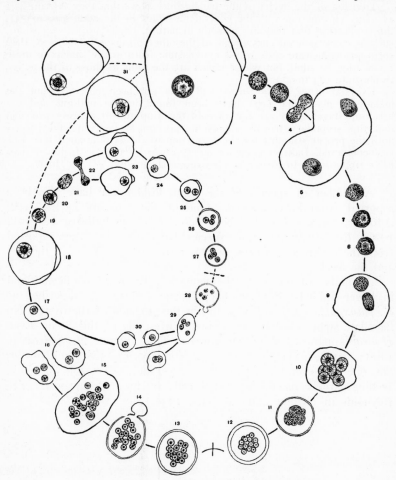

FIG. 19.—*Endamœba blattæ*. Life cycle. (After Morris)

phases completes the cyst formation, giving rise to the form capable of
infecting other roaches (12).

In the mid-gut of the second host the digestive juices modify the
appearance of the cyst (13), by what appears to be a change of perme-
ability, and soon after reaching the hind-gut excystation occurs (14).

Within the plasmodial metacystic amoeba (15) the nuclei undergo a gradual transformation which is completed during the break up of the former (16). The resultant amoebulae (17) grow to a size comparable to that of the smaller adults (18) and these trophozoites conform entirely with the descriptions of E. thomsoni (Lucas, 1927).

Division of the nuclei of the trophozoite shows that they contain half as many chromosomes as the equivalent stages in the adult (19 to 23), thus indicating that they are gametic in nature. Under proper conditions, such as cause general encystment of the other protozoa of the host, they form quadrinucleate cysts whose cytoplasmic features are similar to those formed by the adult, but whose nuclei are the same as those of the active trophozoite (24 to 27).

Excystation of these forms (28) has not been observed, but the metacystic plasmodia (29) have been found in the mid-gut and the break-up stages (30) are not rare in the hind-gut. It appears probable that this secondary trophozoite cycle may repeat itself indefinitely, or until the proper stimulus for the formation of the zygotic adult type (1) is encountered. Indirect evidence points toward syngamic fusion of two large trophozoites to form a single zygotic large adult (31). (Morris)

A number of species of the genus *Endolimax* have also been reported from lower animals. One of these occurs in the frog. Another, *E. reynoldsi,* has been described from a lizard (McFall, 1926). *Endolimax blattæ* is a species that has recently been reported from the cockroach (Lucas, 1927). Other species occur in the flea and the leech.

A number of species of the genus *Vahlkampfia* have been found in lower animals. For example, Hogue (1921) has described as *V. patuxent* a species that occurs in the stomach of the oyster. No flagellate stage could be found in the life-cycle of this form. Even *Hydra* is parasitized by an amœba. This species, *A. hydroxena* (Entz, 1912), is very large, ranging from 100 μ to 368 μ in diameter, has one or several contractile vacuoles and is ectozoic in habit, feeding largely on the epithelial cells of its hydroid host. (See Reynolds in Hegner and Andrews, 1930.)

CHAPTER V

INTRODUCTION TO THE MASTIGOPHORA

I. *Classification*

Although the presence of one or more flagella in the so-called adult stage is the most conspicuous characteristic of the MASTIGOPH-ORA, flagella are not always present, and certain SARCODINA have a flagellated stage in their life-cycle. With these reservations the statement that MASTIGOPHORA are PROTOZOA with flagella is correct. There are two primary types of MASTIGOPHORA, those belonging to the subclass PHYTOMASTIGINA being plant-like, and those in the subclass ZOÖMASTIGINA being animal-like. Comparatively few of the PHYTOMASTIGINA are parasitic, whereas large numbers of parasites occur among the ZOÖMASTIGINA. In the following classification certain families are listed under the order PROTOMONADIDA because most of the flagellates parasitic in man and animals belong to this order.

Class MASTIGOPHORA. PROTOZOA with flagella.

    Subclass 1. PHYTOMASTIGINA. Plant-like flagellates.

        Order 1. CHRYSOMONADIDA. Small, simple, with one or two flagella. Examples: *Chrysamœba radians, Chromulina flavicans.*

        Order 2. CRYPTOMONADIDA. Small, oval, with rigid periplast and two flagella. Examples: *Cryptomonas ovata, Chilomonas paramœcium.*

        Order 3. DINOFLAGELLIDA. Mostly marine, with two flagella, one in a groove. Examples: *Gymnodinium roseum, Oödinium parasiticum.*

        Order 4. EUGLENOIDIDA. One or two (rarely three) flagella; complex vacuole system. Examples: *Euglena viridis, Copromonas subtilis, Euglenamorpha hegneri.*

        Order 5. PHYTOMONADIDA. Mostly with thickened cuticle forming a lorica, with two flagella. Examples: *Volvox globator, Hæmatococcus pluvialis.*

    Subclass 2. ZOÖMASTIGINA. Animal-like flagellates.

        Order 1. PANTASTOMATIDA. One to many flagella, no cytostome, pseudopodia. Examples: *Mastigamœba volutans, Mastigina hylæ.*

Order 2. PROTOMONADIDA. One nucleus, few flagella.

Family 1. MONADIDÆ. Examples: *Oikomonas termo, Heteromita uncinata.*

Family 2. TRYPANOSOMIDÆ. Examples: *Leptomonas ctenocephali, Crithidia gerridis, Trypanosoma gambiense.*

Family 3. BODONIDÆ. Examples: *Bodo caudatus, Rhynchomonas nasuta.*

Family 4. PROWAZEKELLIDÆ. Example: *Prowazekella lacertæ.*

Family 5. EMBADOMONADIDÆ. Example: *Retortamonas (Embadomonas) intestinalis.*

Family 6. CHILOMASTIGIDÆ. Example: *Chilomastix mesnili.*

Family 7. CERCOMONADIDÆ. Examples: *Cercomonas longicauda, Enteromonas (Tricercomonas) hominis.*

Family 8. CRYPTOBIIDÆ. Example: *Cryptobia helicis.*

Family 9. TRICHOMONADIDÆ. Examples: *Trichomonas hominis, Polymastix melolonthæ.*

Family 10. DINENYMPHIDÆ. Examples: *Dinenympha gracilis.*

Order 3. HYPERMASTIGIDA. One nucleus, many flagella. Examples: *Lophomonas blattarum, Trichonympha agilis.*

Order 4. DIPLOMONADIDA. Two nuclei, body bilaterally symmetrical, flagella paired. Examples: *Giardia lamblia, Hexamita muris.*

Order 5. POLYMONADIDA. More than two nuclei, many flagella. Examples: *Calonympha grassii, Stephanonympha silvestrini.*

II. *Euglena*

Euglena is a very common plant-like flagellate that occurs in bodies of fresh water in which they are sometimes so numerous that they produce a greenish tinge. The body has a definite shape as indicated in Figure 20, the peripheral layer of ectoplasm being modified into a firm but flexible cuticle on which there are longitudinal spiral markings. A single flagellum arises at the anterior end from a depression, the cytostome. The cytostome leads into a short gullet which connects with a vacuole-like reservoir into which a number of small contractile vacuoles discharge their contents from time to time. It is supposed that excretory products are discharged from the body by way of the reservoir. Near the anterior end of the body is a reddish structure known as the stigma or eye-spot. A single nucleus lies near the center of the body. In the endoplasm are many chlorophyll-bearing bodies known as chromatophores; these give the animal its green color. Besides this, other inclusions consist of paramylum which is carbohydrate in nature.

Euglena probably obtains its nutriment by all three of the most common methods. With the aid of chlorophyll, sunlight and carbon dioxide it is able to manufacture food in the form of paramylum; this is a plant-like method of nutrition known as holophytic. There is good evidence that euglena also absorbs nutriment, in the form of decomposed organic material, through the general body wall, and is thus saprophytic. Recent observations indicate that in some cases euglena may actually ingest bacteria through the cytostome; if this is correct, holozoic nutrition may be added to the other two types.

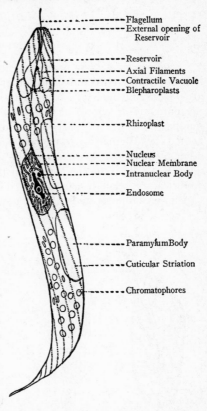

FIG. 20.—*Euglena spirogyra*, a plant-like flagellate (x 700). (After Ratcliffe)

Locomotion in euglena is effected by means of the flagellum, the organism swimming through the water in a spiral course. Euglena is also capable of movements, known as euglenoid movements, consisting of peristaltic waves, which pass over the animal from the anterior to the posterior end. Various external stimuli have effect on the movements of the organism, especially changes in the intensity and direction of the light.

Reproduction in euglena is principally by longitudinal division.

Under certain conditions the organisms may encyst, becoming spherical and secreting about themselves a thin cyst wall. They may emerge from the cyst without dividing or may undergo one or several divisions before the cysts hatch.

III. *Parasitic Mastigophora in General*

I. PARASITIC PLANT-LIKE FLAGELLATES

Euglena viridis has been presented as a representative of a plant-like flagellate. This and many other species of the PHYTOMASTIGINA are free-living in habit. Many of the plant-like flagellates, however, are parasitic or coprozoic. Of these several of the euglenoidida and dinoflagellida are of particular interest. A species of euglenoidida, named by Wenrich (1923) *Euglenamorpha hegneri,* differs from other members of this order in the possession of three flagella (Hegner, 1923). This species occurs in the intestine of tadpoles in North America. A related species was discovered by Brumpt and Lavier (1924) in tadpoles in Brazil. A new genus, *Hegneria,* was proposed

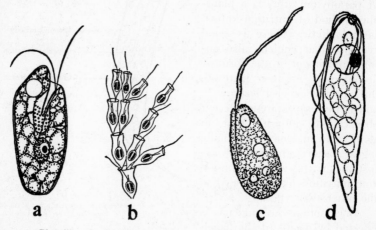

FIG. 21.—Plant-like flagellates. a. *Chilomonas paramecium.* b. *Dinobryon sertularia.* c. *Copromonas subtilis.* d. *Euglenamorpha hegneri.* (After various authors)

for this species, and the organism, which possesses seven flagella, named *Hegneria leptodactyli.* The genera *Euglenamorpha* and *Hegneria* were placed by Brumpt and Lavier in the family HEGNERELLIDÆ. Several species of the genus *Astasia* are parasitic, for example, *A. captiva* is endoparasitic in a flatworm and *A. mobilis* in the egg sacks and digestive tract of cyclops. It seems possible that the parasitic habit of such species as *Euglenamorpha hegneri* may have evolved as a result of the ingestion of free-living euglenoids by tadpoles and other aquatic animals or by their entrance through the rectum into the intestine.

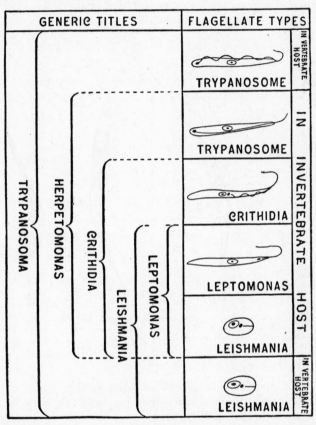

FIG. 22.—TRYPANOSOMIDÆ. Stages in the life-cycle of five genera in vertebrate and invertebrate hosts. (After Wenyon)

Large numbers of parasites occur among the dinoflagellates. The family BLASTODINIDÆ contains only parasitic species. Many types and degrees of parasitism are exhibited by members of this family (Chatton, 1920). Some are ectoparasitic, and others endoparasitic in tissues or cavities.

2. TRYPANOSOMIDÆ, EXCLUSIVE OF THE GENERA TRYPANOSOMA AND LEISHMANIA

The family TRYPANOSOMIDÆ contains a large number of hemo-flagellates and allied forms. Those belonging to the genera *Trypanosoma* and *Leishmania* are of particular importance to us since many of them are pathogenic to man and domesticated animals. These are

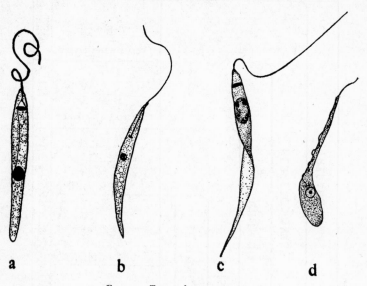

a   b   c   d

FIG. 23.—Types of TRYPANOSOMIDÆ.
a. *Herpetomonas muscæ-domesticæ* (x 2500). (After Swezy)
b. *Leptomonas ctenocephali* (x 2000). (After Shortt)
c. *Phytomonas elmassiani* (x 3000). (After Holmes)
d. *Crithidia gerridis*, with divided blepharoplast (x 2140). (After Becker)

treated in Chapter VI. The genera belonging to this family and some ·idea of the stages through which they pass and the hosts in which they live are indicated in Figure 22.

Members of the genus *Leptomonas* exist in the leishmania and leptomonas stages, which live only in invertebrate hosts, from one to another of which they are transmitted in the form of cysts that are passed in the feces.

Members of the genus *Crithidia* exist in three forms, leishmania, leptomonas and crithidia; they are limited to invertebrate hosts and transmitted by means of cysts that are passed in the feces.

Members of the genus *Herpetomonas* exist in four stages, leishmania, leptomonas, crithidia and trypanosome; occur only in invertebrate hosts; and are transmitted by cysts passed in the feces.

Members of the genus *Leishmania* exist in two stages, leishmania and leptomonas, but occur in both vertebrate and invertebrate hosts, one stage in the life-cycle probably being passed in each; methods of transmission in this genus are not well known.

Members of the genus *Trypanosoma* pass through all of the stages illustrated and may occur in both vertebrate and invertebrate hosts, passing from invertebrate to vertebrate or from vertebrate to invertebrate.

Members of the genus *Phytomonas* resemble leptomonads, but live both in plants and in invertebrates, the latter being the transmitting agent.

Leptomonas. The leptomonads are the simplest of all the types of TRYPANOSOMIDÆ and from them the other genera seem to have evolved. *Leptomonas ctenocephali* (Figure 23b), a species that lives in the intestine and malpighian tubules of the flea, has been studied extensively. It occurs only in the invertebrate host and in the two stages, leptomonas and leishmania. The leptomonas form is slender, often curved, and up to 18 μ in length; all gradations exist between this and leishmania forms no more than 3 μ in diameter. There is a nucleus, an anterior flagellum and a parabasal body; the latter is referred to by most English protozoölogists as a kinetoplast and by the French as a centrosome. The organism multiplies by binary fission and is transmitted in the leishmania stage which arises in the hind gut and is cyst-like. Laveran and Franchini (1913, and later papers) claim to have infected vertebrates with this and other flagellates from the intestine of insects. A number of investigators have attempted to repeat these experiments without success (Hoare, 1921; Glaser, 1922; Shortt, 1923; and Becker, 1923). These flagellates may be cultivated in the N. N. N. medium (Novy-MacNeal-Nicolle, see page 109). Tyzzer and Walker (1919) compared the growth of *Leptomonas ctenocephali* and *Leishmania donovani* in culture media and note various differences which indicate that these two forms do not belong to a single species.

Crithidia. The members of this genus are also exclusively parasites of invertebrates, especially insects; but crithidia that occur in certain insects may simply be a stage in the development of a trypanosome. The crithidia stage is long and slender; the blepharoplast is near and in front of the nucleus and an undulating membrane, along the edge of which the flagellum is attached, extends from the blepharoplast to the anterior end. *Crithidia gerridis* (Figure 23d) occurs in a large percentage of North American water striders, *Gerris remigis* (Becker, 1923). The organisms occur from the first stomach to the rectum; in the latter cysts and encysting forms may be found; multiplication is by binary fission. The detailed life history of another species, *Crithidia euryophthalmi,* has been worked out by McCulloch (1917, 1918). This species lives in the intestine of *Euryophthalmus convivus,* an hemipterous insect that feeds on sap. Infection is brought about by the contamination of food with infected feces.

Herpetomonas. *Herpetomonas muscæ-domesticæ* (Figure 23a) is a representative of the genus *Herpetomonas* that may be obtained from the intestine of house-flies. It differs from leptomonads in the presence of a trypanosome stage in the life-cycle. Transmission is brought about by the contamination of food by infected fecal material. Herpetomonads from various species of flies have been given different specific names, but the work of Becker (1923), who found that flagellates from any one of six species of naturally infected flies were capable of producing an infection in the other five species when inoculated *per os,* indicates that the forms occurring in these different species of flies are actually all one species.

Phytomonas. The phytomonads are usually referred in the literature to the genus *Herpetomonas,* but their presence in both plants and insects makes it worth while to place them in a separate genus. They occur in leptomonas and leishmania stages. They were discovered first in the latex of euphorbias (La Font, 1909) and later in milkweeds (Migone, 1916). *Phytomonas elmassiani* (Figure 23c) has been found in many of the milkweeds of Maryland (Holmes, 1925a) and as far north as the northern boundary of New Jersey and in Honduras and the Philippines (Hegner) and Haiti (Kunkel). It does not parasitize the entire plant but lives as an intracellular, but not an intracytoplasmic, parasite in certain latex cells. The hemipterous insect, *Oncopeltus fasciatus,* is the vector; the flagellates occur in the dorsal and anterior lobes of the trilobed salivary glands of this bug (Holmes, 1925b, 1925c). Strong (1924) believes he has demonstrated that certain lizards become infected from insects in which plant flagellates occur and that specimens from the lizard are capable of producing lesions following subcutaneous inoculation in the monkey. This work needs confirmation.

3. PARASITIC ANIMAL-LIKE FLAGELLATES

All of the orders of the ZOÖMASTIGINA and all of the families of the PROTOMONADIDA listed above contain parasitic species. A number of genera are reserved for more detailed consideration in Chapter VII, and only a few of the more interesting species are described here.

Histomonas meleagridis (Fig. 24, c). This is an organism about which much has been written. It was described as *Amœba meleagridis* by Theobald Smith in 1895, but recent investigations indicate that it

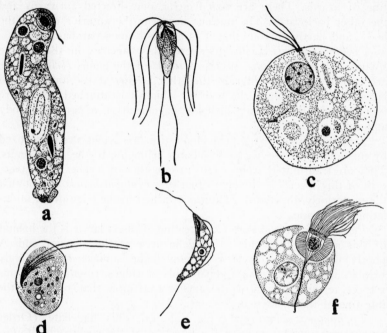

Fig. 24.—Animal-like flagellates. a. *Mastigina hylæ*, from large intestine of frog (x 515). b. *Hexamita muris*, from small intestine of mouse (x 2000). c. *Histomonas meleagridis*, from cecum of turkey (x 500). d. *Costia necatrix*, from skin of fish (x 1050). e. *Cryptobia helicis*, from reproductive organs of snail (*Helix*) (x 1900). f. *Lophomonas blattarum*, from colon of cockroach (x 1150). (a, after Becker; b, c, after Wenrich; d, after Maroff; e, after Bělař; f, after Kudo)

is a flagellate with one to four flagella that lives in the intestine of fowls and is able to invade the tissues (Tyzzer, 1924; Drbohlav, 1924). It is a pathogenic species and gives rise to what is known as blackhead in fowls and turkeys. It is transmitted by the fecal contamination of food and also in the eggs of a nematode worm (*Heterakis gallinæ*) that lives in the cecum of birds. Cultures have been prepared successfully with infected intestinal material (Tyzzer, 1934; De Volt, 1936) as well as with tissue from liver lesions (Bishop, 1937).

Costia necatrix (Fig. 24, d). This is a flagellate parasitic on the skin of fish. It possesses two flagella and a contractile vacuole. Longitudinal division takes place and a cyst stage occurs in the life-cycle. Young fish, to which the flagellates attach themselves by their flagella, may be killed by the attack.

Prowazekella lacertæ. Flagellates of this species live in the intestine of lizards. There are two flagella, one directed forwards and the other backwards. The nucleus lies near the anterior end of the body, and partly surrounding it is a conspicuous parabasal body.

Cryptobia helicis. Leidy discovered this flagellate in 1846 in the sexual organs of various species of snails of the genus *Helix*. There are two flagella, one anterior, the other arising at the anterior end but running back along the body to which it is attached. There are two blepharoplasts from which the flagella arise, a parabasal body and a nucleus.

Trypanoplasma borreli. The blood of fish is sometimes parasitized by this and other species of flagellates belonging to the same genus. They are transmitted from one fish to another by leeches. The structure of this species is similar to that of *Cryptobia helicis* except that the posteriorly directed flagellum is attached to the edge of an undulating membrane.

Polymastix melolonthæ. The intestine of insect larvæ is the habitat of this species. Two pairs of flagella arise at the anterior end. A poorly developed axostyle is present. The surface of the body exhibits more or less longitudinal folds or ridges, resembling in this respect certain species of the HYPERMASTIGIDA that occur in the intestine of the cockroach.

Lophomonas blattarum (Fig. 24, f). This flagellate (Order HYPERMASTIGIDA) occurs in the intestine of the cockroach. It possesses many flagella arranged in two tufts at the anterior end. There is a parabasal body associated with the nucleus, and an axostyle.

Hexamita muris. This species (Fig. 40, 2) is a representative of the order DIPLOMONADIDA. It occurs in the intestine of rats and mice, and possesses two nuclei, two groups of three anterior flagella and two posterior flagella which arise from axonemes. Cysts are formed in which nuclear division occurs. Transmission is no doubt by the ingestion of these cysts in contaminated food.

4. INTESTINAL FLAGELLATES OF TERMITES

Flagellate inhabitants of the intestine of termites are of special interest because of the number of species, the number of individuals in a single termite, their complexity, the large number of flagella possessed by many of them and the symbiotic relations between some of them and their hosts (Fig. 25). Species from at least eleven families and forty genera of flagellates have been reported from termites (Cleveland, 1923). Thanks to Cleveland's brilliant investigations (Cleveland, 1923, 1924, 1925a, b, c, d) we have been furnished with an excellent example of symbiotic relations between certain of these flagellates and their hosts. Cleveland proved that the flagellates ren-

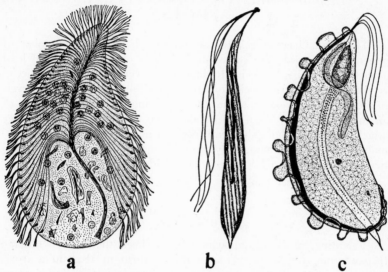

a   b   c

FIG. 25.—Flagellates of termites. a. *Snyderella tabogæ*, from *Lobitermes longicollis* (x 40). b. *Streblomastix strix*, from *Termopsis laticeps* (x 1200). c. *Trichomonas termitidis*. (a, b, after Kirby; c, after Wenrich)

der the cellulose (in wood) eaten by termites digestible by the insects and that without the aid of the flagellates the wood eaten is not digested and the termites starve to death. By starving the termite, *Termopsis nevadensis*, and subjecting it to oxygen under pressure, Cleveland (1925d) found that the insects live indefinitely when all four species of flagellates that inhabit this insect are removed except *Leidyopsis sphærica;* that they live from three to four weeks when all are removed except *Streblomastix strix* or when all four are removed; and that they live for about ten weeks when *Trichonympha campanula* and *Leidyopsis sphærica* are removed and *Trichomonas termopsidis* and *Streblomastix strix* remain. These results indicate that *Streblomastix* is of no value, that *Trichomonas* helps keep the insect alive for a few weeks and that *Trichonympha* alone is able to complete the necessary symbiotic relationship.

CHAPTER VI

HÆMOFLAGELLATES OF MAN AND LOWER ANIMALS

The term "hæmoflagellate" as here used, includes a number of genera of the PROTOMONADIDA, the members of which spend at least a part of their life-cycle in the blood of a vertebrate. Many species require two different species of hosts, spending part of the life-cycle in the blood of a vertebrate and the remaining part in the intestine of an insect. Many of them are of enormous importance because they attack and bring about the death of both man and domesticated animals. Two of the genera, *Trypanosoma* and *Leishmania,* are of particular significance and will now be considered in some detail.

I. *The Genus Trypanosoma*

I. HISTORICAL

Valentine, in Berne, appears to have been the first to observe trypanosomes in the blood, having seen them in 1841 in a trout, *Salmo fario.* Two years later Gruby (1843) established the genus *Trypanosoma* for an organism that he found in the blood of frogs (Figure 30a). The first trypanosomes of mammals were described from rats in India by Lewis (1879). Up to this time not much attention was paid to these blood-inhabiting PROTOZOA, but the genus *Trypanosoma* was brought into prominence the following year by Evans (1880) who discovered what is now known as *T. evansi* in horses and camels suffering from the disease known as surra. Fifteen years later Bruce (1895) discovered trypanosomes in horses and cattle in Africa that were suffering from the disease known as nagana. The first trypanosomes were seen in human blood by Forde in 1901 and recognized as such by Dutton in 1902. These organisms were next seen by Castellani (1903) in the cerebro-spinal fluid of a patient in Uganda who was suffering from sleeping sickness. This observation was confirmed and the relation between the trypanosomes and sleeping sickness demonstrated shortly afterward by Bruce and Nabarro (1903). These authors, and several others, established the fact that the transmitting agent of Gambian sleeping sickness is the tsetse fly, *Glossina palpalis*. In 1905 atoxyl was introduced by Thomas as a therapeutic agent in the treatment of trypanosomiasis. Since 1903 thousands of reports have been published as a result of investigations of trypanosomes. Trypanosomes occur in many species of lower animals, but not in man in the United States. They are responsible for Chagas' disease in man in South and Central America and in Mexico and for Gambian and Rhodesian sleeping sickness in Africa.

For methods of treating trypanosome diseases, the reader is referred to Manson's *Tropical Diseases* or some other book on tropical medicine.

2. MORPHOLOGY OF A TYPICAL TRYPANOSOME

Most of the trypanosomes are characterized by the possession of a more or less spindle-shaped body, a central nucleus, and a spherical or rod-shaped parabasal body, with which is closely associated a small blepharoplast, and a flagellum which arises from the

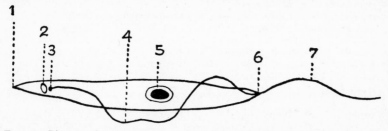

FIG. 26.—Diagram of a trypanosome. 1, Posterior end; 2, Parabasal body; 3, Blepharoplast; 4, Undulating membrane; 5, Nucleus; 6, Anterior end; 7, Flagellum.

blepharoplast and extends anteriorly. The protoplasm of the body unites with the flagellum to form the undulating membrane. The general arrangement of these organelles can be seen by an examination of Fig. 26.

3. IDENTIFICATION OF SPECIES

Specific distinctions of trypanosomes include the degree and type of motility, size and shape of the body, variations in the size and relative position of the nucleus and the kinetoplast, the degree of development of the undulating membrane and the anterior flagellum, variations in life-cycle, hosts involved, loci of colonization in hosts, pathogenicity, and immunological, serological and cultural reactions. In many instances a combination of characteristics, morphological and physiological, have been used to describe species, and many alleged species are so similar in appearance that it is virtually impossible to distinguish them by morphological criteria alone. For a more comprehensive discussion of this group, and for specific descriptions of trypanosomes, the first volume of Wenyon's "Protozoölogy" is recommended. The following list of species with their hosts contains representative forms.

Species	Vertebrate Host	Invertebrate Host	Disease Produced
T. gambiense	Man	Glossina palpalis	African sleeping sickness
T. cruzi	Man	Reduviidæ	Chagas' disease
T. brucei	Domesticated animals	Glossina spp.	Nagana
T. evansi	Domesticated animals	Tabanus spp.	Surra
T. lewisi	Rat	Rat flea	None
T. vespertilionis	Bat	Bed-bug	None
T. legeri	Ant-eater	?	?
T. prowazeki	Monkey	?	?
T. theileri	Cattle	Tabanus spp.	None
T. melophagium	Sheep	Sheep ked	None
T. paddæ	Birds	?	?
T. vitattæ	Soft tortoise	Leech	?
T. kochi	Crocodile	?	?
T. najæ	Cobra	?	?
T. rotatorium	Frog	Leech	Pathogenicity varies
T. rajae	Skate	Leech	?

4. LIFE-CYCLE OF TRYPANOSOMA LEWISI

Vertebrate host. One of the easiest trypanosomes to obtain for demonstration and study is *T. lewisi,* a species that occurs in wild rats and can readily be subinoculated into laboratory rats. It occurs in the blood of rats all over the world and appears to be non-pathogenic to these animals, since enormous numbers may be present without bringing about the appearance of symptoms. When trypanosomes are inoculated into a rat a prepatent period of from two to four days ensues during which no organisms can be found in the blood. Following this, multiplication stages may be found in the blood for from four to seven days. Multiplication ceases at the end of this period and all of the trypanosomes remain in what may be called the adult stage, until they die. This stage of adult infection ranges from seven to one hundred days. It has been shown by Taliaferro and by Coventry (1925) that a reaction product is built up by the rat which gradually inhibits reproduction. Not only is reproduction inhibited but at the end of about ten days after inoculation most of the trypanosomes are destroyed in the blood in some unknown way. The few that remain continue active for several weeks; finally all disappear and the rat is then immune to another infection for a considerable period, often during the rest of its life.

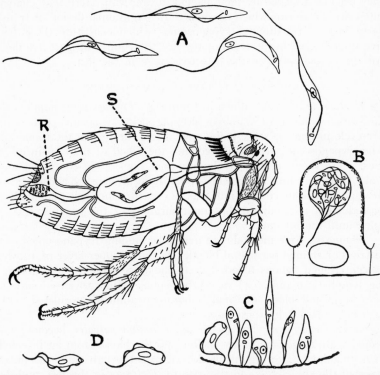

FIG. 27.—Diagram of *Trypanosoma lewisi* in the blood of the rat and in the flea. A. Trypanosomes as seen in the rat at late phase of infection. B. Intracellular phase of development in stomach. C. Attached flagellates in rectum; evolution of crithidia into metacyclic trypanosome form. D. Free metacyclic trypanosomes which bring about infection when ingested by rat. R. Rectal phase. S. Trypanosomes in stomach of flea. (After Wenyon)

Invertebrate hosts. Trypanosomes are transmitted from rat to rat by the rat-flea; not by the bite of the flea, but in the feces of the flea which are licked off its fur and swallowed by the rat or in the flea itself which is eaten by the rat. We owe to Minchin and Thomson (1915) a detailed account of the life-cycle of *T. lewisi* in the flea. This is shown in Figure 27. Trypanosomes are taken into the stomach of the flea when it sucks blood from an infected rat. They lose their infectivity, probably about one-half hour afterward. Some of them succeed in penetrating epithelial cells of the stomach wall where they undergo multiple fission and give rise to a number of daughter trypanosomes; these may reinfect epithelial cells and repeat the process or may be carried through the intestine into the rectum where they become attached by their flagella to the wall. Here they change into crithidial forms which reproduce by longitudinal fission or transform into short, stumpy trypanosomes which constitute the infective stage passed in the feces of the flea. It requires at least five days for the development of the infective stage in the flea.

5. LIFE-CYCLE OF TRYPANOSOMA GAMBIENSE

Vertebrate host. As shown in Figure 28, *Trypanosoma gambiense,* the causative agent of Gambian sleeping sickness, spends part of its life-cycle in man or some game animal and the rest in the tsetse fly. The trypanosomes are inoculated into the blood of man by infected flies. Here they multiply by longitudinal division in the blood and make their way into the cerebro-spinal fluid. When trypanosomes of this species are inoculated into rats, no reaction product that inhibits reproduction is produced, but multiplication of the organisms continue until the rat dies.

Diagnosis. Five methods are available; finding trypanosomes (1) in fresh or stained peripheral blood, (2) in the upper layer of 100 cc. of centrifuged venous blood, (3) in the juice obtained by puncturing lymphatic glands, (4) in cerebro-spinal fluid (advanced cases), or (5) in the blood of small laboratory animals inoculated with material obtained by these procedures.

Invertebrate host. The tsetse fly, *Glossina palpalis,* becomes infected with *T. gambiense* by sucking up the blood from an infected man or animal. The organisms do not pass through an intracellular stage in the stomach, as in the case of *T. lewisi* in the flea, and do not produce infective stages in the rectum, but migrate from the stomach into the salivary glands, where they pass through the crithidial stage and then transform into infective trypanosomes ready to be transmitted to another host when the fly bites.

6. HOST-PARASITE RELATIONS OF T. GAMBIENSE

Transmission. As stated above, *T. gambiense* is transmitted from man to man by the tsetse fly, *Glossina palpalis,* and perhaps by several other species of this genus. The flies do not become infected until about three weeks after they have ingested trypanosomes; then they

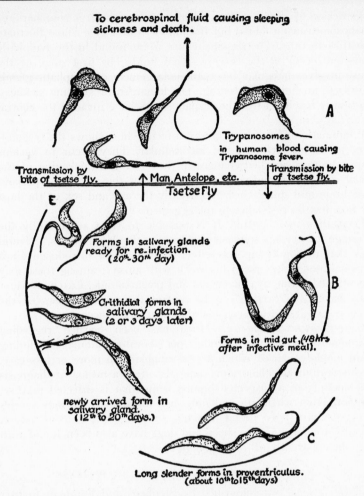

To cerebrospinal fluid causing sleeping sickness and death.

A

Trypanosomes in human blood causing Trypanosoma fever.

Transmission by bite of tsetse fly.

↑ Man, Antelope, etc.

Tsetse Fly

Transmission by bite of tsetse fly.

E

Forms in salivary glands ready for re-infection. (20ᵗʰ-30ᵗʰ day)

Crithidial forms in salivary glands (2 or 3 days later)

B

Forms in mid gut, (48 hrs after infective meal).

D

newly arrived form in salivary gland. (12ᵗʰ to 20ᵗʰ days.)

C

Long slender forms in proventriculus. (about 10ᵗʰ to 15ᵗʰ days)

FIG. 28.—*Trypanosoma gambiense*, life-cycle in man and tsetse fly (x 1500). (From Chandler. After Robertson)

are able to transfer infective stages from their salivary glands to the blood of man during the biting process. Transmission probably also occurs from animal reservoirs, such as antelope, to man through the agency of tsetse flies.

The course of the infection. It is difficult to determine the incubation period in man because, as a rule, the time of inoculation is not known; apparently, however, this period may range from two or three weeks to seven years. There are never large numbers of trypanosomes in the blood but the numbers in a given host fluctuate from time to time. The organisms are to be found in the lymphatic glands and occur in the cerebro-spinal fluid. The first stage of the disease involves irregular fever, the enlargement of lymphatic glands and spleen, anæmia and wasting. The lethargic, or sleeping sickness, condition is reached after the trypanosomes have invaded the central nervous system.

Examination of tissues from an infective host shows the trypanosomes to be intercellular, not intracellular. They occur in various organs, the most marked changes in these being a thickening of the arterial coat and round cell infiltration about the arteries, especially of the brain and spinal cord. Apparently the age and sex of the host have no effect on resistance to the organism.

Prevention and control. It is possible to treat successfully the first stage of trypanosomiasis but rarely the later stages. Several drugs that are more or less effective have been introduced since Thomas (1905) announced his work with atoxyl; among these may be mentioned antimony, Bayer 205 and tryparsamide. Extensive campaigns have been carried out to control the insect vectors or the animal reservoirs with a considerable degree of success.

Host-parasite specificity. Much has been learned regarding *T. gambiense* by means of studies on laboratory animals, including certain monkeys, all of which are inoculable with more or less ease. The susceptibility of laboratory animals offers a means of diagnosis since blood from a suspected human being that is infected may set up an infection when injected into such an animal. Various species of animals have been found infected with *T. gambiense* in nature, especially antelope. Cattle, sheep and dogs have also been found with infections apparently of *T. gambiense.*

7. HOST-PARASITE RELATIONS OF T. RHODESIENSE

T. rhodesiense was described by Stephens and Fantham (1910) as a separate species because of the presence in some specimens of a nucleus located posteriorly. About 5 to 6 per cent of the short forms of this species exhibit this condition. As the specific name indicates, this type of sleeping sickness occurs in the Rhodesian region of Africa. Several characteristics besides the appearance of specimens with posterior nuclei indicate differences between this species and *T. gambiense. T. rhodesiense* is more virulent both to man and to laboratory animals; it is more resistant to drugs, such as atoxyl; it differs in its serological reactions; and is transmitted by a different species of tsetse fly, namely, *Glossina morsitans*. The relations between *T. rhodesiense* in wild and laboratory animals are similar to those of *T. gambiense*. It seems probable that *T. rhodesiense* represents members of the species *T. brucei* that have become adapted to life in the human host.

8. THE LIFE-CYCLE
OF TRYPANOSOMA
CRUZI

Vertebrate host.
Trypanosoma cruzi (Figure 29) exists in the mammalian host more frequently as a tissue parasite, a leishmania, than in the trypanosome stage. Bugs of the species *Triatoma megista* are the insect vectors. The trypanosomes do not multiply in the blood of man but penetrate tissue cells, where they transform into the leishmania forms that multiply by fission. These leishmania forms may transform into trypanosomes and, when liberated into the blood, either penetrate other cells or are ingested by the insect host.

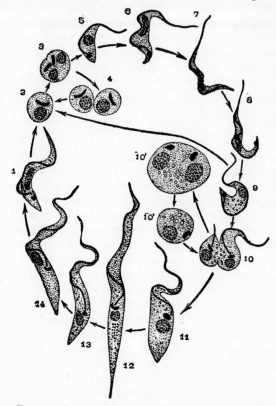

FIG. 29.—*Trypanosoma cruzi*, life-cycle in man, 2-9, and in the bug, 9-14 and 1. The infective trypanosomes from the rectum of the bug (1) become leishmanias in the tissue of man (2-4) or trypaniform stages in the blood of man (5-9). Stages taken into the digestive tract of the bug (9), divide (10), become crithidias (11, 12) and then infective trypanosomes (13, 14, 1). (After Brumpt)

Invertebrate host. In the stomach of the *Triatoma* the ingested trypanosomes change to the leishmania form and multiply by fission. They then transform to crithidias, which are carried into the intestine, where they multiply by fission and finally change into infective trypanosomes. It is probable that these infective trypanosomes find their way into the blood of a new host through wounds made by the bug in biting, near which the organisms have been deposited by the bug in its feces.

Diagnosis. This type of trypanosomes is not constantly present in the peripheral blood, hence diagnosis based upon the demonstration of trypaniform stages is uncertain. Chances of finding parasites are enhanced by inoculating small laboratory animals with the suspected blood, or by allowing insect vectors known to be free from the flagellate, to feed upon suspected individuals. These animals are subsequently examined for evidence of infection.

9. HOST-PARASITE RELATIONS OF T. CRUZI

T. cruzi was discovered in Brazil by Chagas (1909) in certain hemipterous insects of the genus *Triatoma* that inhabit the huts of the natives, where they find hiding places in cracks in the walls. Later, trypanosomes of this species were found in human beings. The transmitting agent is *Triatoma megista* and probably several other members of this genus. Several species of armadillos are infected in nature and serve as reservoirs. Monkeys and cats have also been found naturally infected, and infections may be set up by inoculating the organisms into many laboratory animals, including monkeys.

The disease due to the presence of *T. cruzi* is known as South American trypanosomiasis or Chagas' disease. It is acute in children under one year of age and chronic in older children and adults. The incubation period is from ten days to one month. The organisms are scanty in the blood but the disease can be diagnosed by inoculating laboratory animals. Invasion of the tissues by the parasites brings about fever, anemia and enlargement of lymph glands, the thyroid, liver and spleen. Degeneration of the invaded cells occurs and fibrous tissue is greatly increased. None of the drugs that are effective in cases of African sleeping sickness have any effect on *T. cruzi*. The best method of controlling this organism seems to be by attacking the transmitting agent.

10. TRYPANOSOMES OF LOWER ANIMALS

A large number of species of trypanosomes have been described from lower vertebrates and there are, probably, many others not yet discovered. All of those described may not be distinct species but there is no doubt but that the members of the genus are widely distributed, both as regards species of host and the geographical distribution of these hosts.

(1) TRYPANOSOMES OF MAMMALS. *Primates*. Trypanosomes have been discovered in many species of primates other than man and about a half dozen of these have been given specific names. Infections have been recorded in South American monkeys and marmosets, in African monkeys, chimpanzees and gorillas. Besides these natural

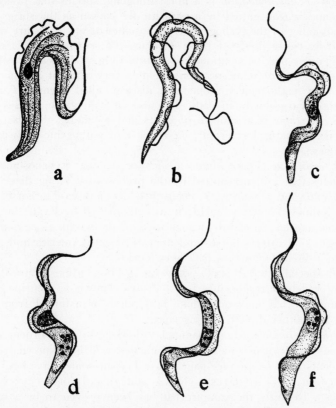

FIG. 30.—Trypanosomes of lower animals. a. *T. rotatorium*, from frog (x 1400). b. *T. diemyctyli*, from crimson-spotted newt (x 1600). c. *T. equinum*, from horse (x 2500). d. *T. brucei*, from domestic animals (x 2500). e. *T. evansi*, from domestic animals (x 2500). f. *T. equiperdum*, from horse (x 2500). (a, after Laveran and Mesnil; b, after Hegner; c-f, after Wenrich)

infections it has been found that monkeys may be infected in the laboratory by blood inoculation.

Ungulates. Cattle, horses, sheep, goats, antelope and other types of ungulates are infected by various species of trypanosomes in different parts of the world. As noted above, the game animals of

Africa serve as reservoirs for *T. gambiense* and *T. rhodesiense*. Some of the trypanosomes of ungulates are apparently non-pathogenic and others pathogenic. Of the non-pathogenic species two may be mentioned here. *T. theileri* occurs in cattle in South Africa and is probably transmitted by tabanid flies in which infective forms develop. *T. melophagium* is a non-pathogenic species that occurs in sheep and is transmitted by a parasitic fly known as the sheep ked.

A number of the pathogenic trypanosomes of ungulates are transmitted by tsetse flies. Of these *T. brucei, T. congolense, T. simiæ* and *T. vivax* may be mentioned. *T. brucei* (Fig. 30d) is a parasite of wild game and of domestic animals; it is very virulent and accordingly very pathogenic, producing a disease called nagana. *T. congolense* occurs chiefly in cattle but also in wild game, horses and sheep. *T. simiæ* is a parasite of goats and monkeys; the wart hog serves as a natural reservoir. *T. vivax* is a pathogenic parasite of antelopes.

T. evansi and *T. equinum* (Fig. 30c, e) are trypanosomes of ungulates that are transmitted by the proboscis of biting flies, such as *Tabanus* and *Stomoxys*. *T. evansi* produces a disease in horses and other animals known as surra; it was discovered by Evans in 1880 in India and has spread to various parts of the world. *T. equinum* is a species that infects horses and mules in South America and gives rise to a disease known as mal de caderas.

Of special interest is *T. equiperdum* (Fig. 30f), a parasite of horses which is responsible for a disease known as dourine; this trypanosome has no intermediate host but is transferred from one horse to another directly during coitus.

Other mammals. Many mammals belonging to other orders serve as hosts for trypanosomes. The commonest and best known species in rodents is *T. lewisi* (see page 100). Trypanosomes have been discovered in the CHIROPTERA (bats), and INSECTIVORA (moles and shrews). Recently the vampire bat has been proven to be a transmitting agent of *T. hippicum* in the horses of Panama (Dunn, 1932). Of the EDENTATA, the ant-eater is known to be infected by trypanosomes; the armadillo, as noted above, serves as a reservoir for *T. cruzi,* and the two-toed sloth serves as a host for a trypanosome-like hæmoflagellate known as *Endotrypanum schaudinni,* which lives inside of the red blood cells.

(2) BIRDS. Trypanosomes have been described from birds in various parts of the world. One of the best known is *T. paddæ* of the Java sparrow; this is a pathogenic species which can be transferred

to canaries and other birds. Another well known species is *T. noctuæ* of the little owl.

(3) REPTILES. Crocodiles, turtles, snakes and lizards all serve as hosts for trypanosomes. The land-inhabiting species are transmitted by blood-sucking arthropods and the water-inhabiting species by leeches.

(4) AMPHIBIA. The easiest trypanosomes to obtain in America are those of frogs, toads and salamanders. Frogs and toads are frequently infected by the type species of the genus, *T. rotatorium* (Figure 30a), and in some localities all specimens of the crimson spotted newt, *Diemyctylus viridescens,* are infected with *T. diemyctyli* (Figure 30b) (Hegner, 1921).

(5) FISH. Trypanosomes have also been described from fish. These likewise are probably transmitted by leeches. Both fresh-water and marine fish serve as hosts.

II. THE CULTIVATION OF TRYPANOSOMES

The first trypanosome to be cultivated in artificial media was *T. lewisi,* which was grown by Novy and MacNeal (1903) in a blood-agar mixture. A blood-agar medium suitable for cultivating *T. lewisi* is made up by adding 30 c.c. of 2 per cent bacteriological nutrient agar to 270 c.c. of 0.85 per cent sodium chloride solution; 10 c.c. of this mixture is placed in each test-tube, autoclaved at 120°C., then cooled at 50°C; to each is then added twenty drops of rabbit's blood and the tubes are finally ready for use after being incubated at 37°C. for twenty-four hours.

A medium widely used for growing trypanosomes is the Novy-MacNeal-Nicolle (N.N.N.) medium. This may be made up as follows: water, 900 c.c., agar, 14 grams, and NaCl, 6 grams, are mixed together during heating and a column three to four centimeters high placed in test-tubes while still hot. From 2 to 3 c.c. of sterile rabbit's blood is added to each test-tube when the agar has cooled to 50°C., mixed by revolving, and allowed to solidify in a sloped position. When incubated at 37°C. for twenty-four hours condensation liquid accumulates at the bottom of the tube; into this a small amount of infected blood or tissue is placed and the tubes incubated at from 22°C. to 25°C. Organisms may later be recovered from the liquid of condensation or from scrapings from the agar surface above the liquid. Sub-cultures should be made about every two weeks.

Many trypanosomes grown in culture media pass through stages resembling those that occur in the invertebrate host. For example, crithidia stages develop at the low temperatures; these may transform into the trypanosome stage if the temperature is increased and these may again change to the crithidia stage if the temperature is lowered. Cultivation in artificial media is of some value in diagnosis, since positive cultures are often obtained from patients in whom microscopic examination has failed to reveal the organisms. It has been found difficult to sub-culture *T. cruzi* and cultures of *T. gambiense* are not very successful, since this organism does not multiply to any great extent. *T. rotatorium,* when cultivated in blood-agar medium, rounds up, and each individual by binary division produces, after several days, a cluster of about 150 crithidia forms. This type of multiplication probably resembles what takes place in the intermediate host, the leech. *T. cruzi* has been cultivated successfully in tissue culture of embryonic heart muscle in which its development is the same with respect to both time and stages of its cycle as it is in the body of the living vertebrate host (Kofoid, Wood and McNeil, 1935).

II. *The Genus Leishmania*

I. HISTORICAL

Leishmania bodies (Figure 31) were first seen by Cunningham (1885), who described them as parasitic organisms, in the

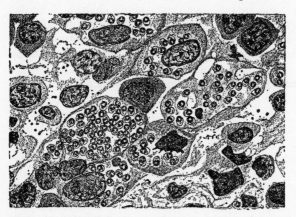

tissue of Delhi boil in India. He supposed them to be spores contained in amœbæ, the latter really being large macrophages. In 1903 both Leishman and Donovan described similar organisms from cases of dum-dum fever. Since then the leishmania stages have often been referred to

FIG. 31.—*Leishmania donovani.* Leishman-Donovan bodies in the spleen cells of an infected dog (x 1500). (After Brumpt)

as Leishman-Donovan bodies. Laveran and Mesnil (1903) supposed these bodies to be piroplasmas and Ross (1903), who believed them to be sporozoa, proposed the generic name *Leishmania* for them. The connection of *Leishmania donovani* to kala azar was discovered by

Bentley in 1904. Up to this time only the leishmania stage was known, but in 1904 Rogers discovered that when spleen pulp containing Leishman-Donovan bodies was placed in sodium citrate solution at a temperature of 22°, flagellates developed of the leptomonas type. The organism of oriental sore, first described by Cunningham (1885), was rediscovered by Wright (1903) in an Armenian child in Boston. This parasite is indistinguishable from that of kala azar but has a different life history and produces different lesions in the host. Its scientific name is *Leishmania tropica*. The flagellate stage of this species (Figure 32) was obtained in cultures by Nicolle in 1908. The leishmania parasite that occurs in so-called South American leishmaniasis is by some considered to be a separate species to which the scientific name *Leishmania brasiliensis* was given by Vianna in 1911. The type of leishmaniasis that occurs in the countries bordering the Mediterranean has been considered a separate disease for which Nicolle (1908) proposed the name infantile kala azar and for the organism of which he proposed the name *L. infantum*. The evidence now available indicates that kala azar and infantile kala azar are caused by the same parasite; Noguchi (1924) finds that *L. infantum* and *L. donovani* give the same serological reactions. Leishmanias occur in dogs and cats and have been reported from lizards and several other animals.

2. MORPHOLOGY OF LEISHMANIA

The flagellate stage of *L. donovani* is slender and spindle-shaped and about 10 or 12 μ in length. There is no undulating membrane. Near the center of the body is an oval nucleus and near the anterior end is a parabasal body and a blepharoplast. From these an axoneme extends forward giving rise to a free flagellum about as long as the body. The tissue-inhabiting stage is round or oval (Fig. 31) and measures from 1 to 5 μ in diameter. In it are visible a nucleus and a rod-shaped parabasal body and blepharoplast.

3. LEISHMANIA DONOVANI AND KALA AZAR

Geographical distribution. Kala azar occurs in various parts of Asia, including India, Ceylon, China, Russia, Turkestan and Asia Minor; in Africa, including Tunis, Tripoli, Algeria and Egypt; and in Europe, including Greece, Italy, Spain and Portugal.

Life-cycle. As indicated in the diagram on page 91, members of the genus *Leishmania* occur as leishmania bodies in vertebrate and invertebrate hosts and as leptomonads in invertebrate hosts. As a matter of fact, there is still some doubt regarding the invertebrate host of *L. donovani* although, as noted above, the leptomonad stages occur in culture media. The flagellate stage in the life-cycle, as revealed in cultures, has the characteristics of a leptomonad. The flagellates measure from 10 μ to 20 μ in length and from 1.5 μ to 4 μ in breadth. They reproduce by binary fission. All stages between the leishmania and leptomonas forms occur in cultures. The leishmania bodies (Figure 31) vary in size from 2 μ x 1 μ to 4.5 μ x 2.5 μ. They contain a spherical or slightly ovoidal nucleus near one side, a much smaller spherical or rod-shaped parabasal body and sometimes a thread-like prolongation from the parabasal body which is the rudiment of a flagellum. The leishmania bodies divide by binary fission.

Host-parasite relations. As noted above, the transmitting agent of *L. donovani* is supposed to be an invertebrate host in which the leptomonad form occurs, but this is not yet known with certainty. Bedbugs, flies, mosquitoes, lice, house-flies, ticks and sand-flies have all been accused of transmitting kala azar but none of them has yet been found guilty with certainty although species of the sand-fly, *Phlebotomus,* are probably the vectors. Within the human body leishmanias are intracellular; they are particularly numerous in the endothelial cells of the blood and lymph capillaries and in leukocytes; they have been described from practically all organs of the body but occur especially in the spleen, liver, bone marrow and lymph glands. This distribution of the parasites among the internal organs has suggested the name visceral leishmaniasis in contrast to cutaneous leishmaniasis which is due to *L. tropica.* The leishmania bodies are probably distributed throughout the body in the blood stream. They multiply within the cells until liberated into the blood stream by the rupture of the cell wall. They gain entrance to other cells probably by their own activity.

The incubation period of kala azar ranges from several weeks to several months, usually being difficult to determine because the time of entrance of the parasite is generally unknown. The principal symptoms produced are irregular fever, upon which quinine has no effect, enlargement of the spleen and liver, anemia and emaciation. Almost all untreated cases end in death. It seems probable that these symptoms result from the destruction of enormous numbers of cells, the disintegration products of which are liberated into the blood. Vianna in 1913 discovered tartar emetic to be effective in the treatment of South American leishmaniasis and this drug was later found to be effective also in the treatment of kala azar; most of the cases treated with this drug recover.

Cultivation and diagnosis. As noted above, Rogers (1904) succeeded in cultivating the organism of kala azar. Although the diagnosis of kala azar may be made by finding the parasite in material obtained by puncture of the spleen or in blood films stained with Romanowsky stains, the culture method is also valuable, since tubes of N. N. N. medium to which a few drops of blood are added, when incubated at 22°C. to 25°C., may reveal the parasites which may be too few in number to appear in ordinary smears.

Control. The control of kala azar may be effected in two ways, first by the treatment of all cases with drugs, and second by the removal of human beings from habitations where infection is present to new homes. It was found by Rogers (see Rogers, 1919) that a distance of three hundred yards is sufficient to prevent the spread of kala azar although the reasons for this result are not known.

4. LEISHMANIA TROPICA AND ORIENTAL SORE

Geographical distribution. The cutaneous leishmaniasis of the old world is commonly known as Oriental sore, although it is also called Delhi boil, Bagdad boil, Aleppo boil, and so on. Oriental sore is widely distributed in Asia; it occurs in North Africa and in Spain, Italy and Greece.

Life-cycle. The leishmania stage of Oriental sore occurs within the cells of the human host. Flagellate forms have also been reported from the sores. When leishmanias are grown in N. N. N. medium they transform into flagellates which multiply by binary fission (Figure 32). Both leishmania and leptomonos stages are indistinguishable from these stages in the life-cycle of *L. donovani.* The invertebrate hosts of *L. tropica* are supposed to be certain sand-flies of the genus *Phlebotomus* in which presumably the leptomonad stage occurs.

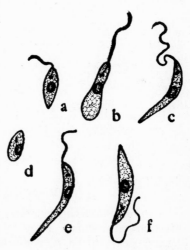

FIG. 32.—*Leishmania tropica.* Flagellate stages in culture medium (x 1480). (After Adler and Theodor)

Host-parasite relations. The organisms of Oriental sore can be transmitted from man to man by inoculation. The lesions in most cases are limited to the skin of the exposed parts of the body. One attack confers immunity. According

to Manson, this fact has led the Jews of Bagdad for many years to
inoculate their children in some unexposed part of the body to prevent the occurrence of scars on the face. The incubation period of
Oriental sore is usually about two months. The symptoms are slight;
a small red papule first appears; this increases in size and may give
rise to a shallow ulcer which finally dries leaving behind it a slightly
depressed scar. The leishmania bodies occur within leucocytes and
epithelial cells in the papules or ulcers. Smears or cultures may be
made from this material which reveal the organisms. For methods
of treatment, the reader is referred to Manson's *Tropical Diseases*
or some other book on tropical medicine.

5. LEISHMANIA BRASILIENSIS AND SOUTH AMERICAN LEISHMANIASIS

The fact that *L. brasiliensis* cannot be distinguished morphologically from *L. tropica* and that the lesions produced by these two
organisms are similar have led many to the conclusion that they both
belong to the same species. That there is a serological difference,
however, is indicated by the work of Noguchi (1924) who found
that the serum from a rabbit inoculated with *L. tropica* agglutinated
this organism but not *L. brasiliensis,* and that the serum from a
rabbit inoculated with *L. brasiliensis* agglutinated this species but not
L. tropica. South American leishmaniasis occurs principally in Brazil
and Peru. It has also been reported from several other South American countries and from Central America. The disease is known as
espundia, uta or forest yaws. The method of transmission of the
organism is unknown.

Recently the use of the viscerotome, by means of which liver
samples have been obtained from large numbers of dead persons
without the necessity of autopsy, has led to the discovery that leishmaniasis in South America is in many cases accompanied by visceral
lesions.

6. LEISHMANIAS OF LOWER ANIMALS

Natural and laboratory infections with human species. Natural
infections with human species of leishmanias are rare except in dogs.
What appears to be *L. donovani* has been reported from dogs in
various parts of Asia, Africa and Europe. The parasites in the dog
cannot be distinguished from those in man. The disease in dogs that
are naturally infected and that are inoculated with parasites from
man runs the same course. Canine leishmaniasis is similar in geographical distribution to human kala azar except in India. The only
other animal in which a natural infection with *L. donovani* has been

reported is one case of an infected cat. Both *L. tropica* and *L. brasiliensis* have been reported in dogs living in regions where these parasites are known to be present in man.

A number of laboratory animals are susceptible to infection with all three species of human leishmanias. Dogs are easily infected; monkeys, rats, mice and guinea-pigs are more refractory. The infections in these animals develop slowly and small numbers of parasites are produced. A small rodent that lives in North China, called the hamster, has been found by Smyly and Young (1924) to be especially susceptible to *L. donovani* and to bring about an extremely heavy infection. This animal may become very important as a host for carrying out laboratory experiments.

Other species of leishmanias in lower animals. A number of species of leishmanias have been described from lizards. The transmitting agents are probably insects that are eaten by these reptiles. A species known as *L. tarentolæ* occurs in the gecko in North Africa. Sand-flies, that are known to feed on the gecko, may be the transmitting agent. Other species have been reported from lizards of the genus *Anolis,* from the chameleon and from the Indian gecko, and flagellates of the leptomonas type have been reported by Strong (1924) in the intestine of Central American lizards.

CHAPTER VII

INTESTINAL FLAGELLATES OF MAN AND LOWER ANIMALS

I. *Classification and Diagnosis*

In this chapter will be considered the intestinal flagellates of man and certain of their allies in lower animals. Among these are species that live in the mouth or vagina and are hence not really intestinal flagellates; they are usually included in this category however. Five different genera and seven different species are represented among these flagellates that live in man. Three species of the genus *Trichomonas* (Figure 34) belong to the family TRICHOMONADIDÆ. *Chilomastix mesnili* (Figure 33) is a member of the family CHILO-MASTIGIDÆ. *Retortamonas (Embadomonas) intestinalis* (Figure 36) belongs to the family EMBADOMONADIDÆ. *Enteromonas (Tricerco-monas) hominis* (Figure 37) has been placed in the family CERCO-MONADIDÆ and *Giardia lamblia* (Figure 38) is a member of the order DIPLOMONADINA. Intestinal flagellates belonging to these genera, and perhaps in some cases even to the same species, as those just mentioned, have been reported from many types of domesticated and wild animals.

Flagellates of the genera *Trichomonas, Chilomastix* and *Giardia* are widespread among the general population. *Retortamonas intestinalis* and *Enteromonas hominis* appear to be so rare that the chances of encountering them are not good. It is possible to determine the genus of the three common types just mentioned in the living condition. Material from the mouth, vagina or intestine should be stirred up in a drop of normal saline solution, confined under a cover-glass and examined with a 16 mm. objective. If active flagellates are present they will be seen moving about in this medium. The trichomonads (Figure 35) possess anterior flagella which lash backward bringing about a jerky sort of progression. Along one side is an undulating membrane, which can easily be seen with the 4 mm. objective and is the most important structural feature of use in distinguishing this genus from the others in the living condition. The flagellates are rotated on their axis by means of this undulating membrane. At the posterior end of trichomonas extends out a slender rod known as the axostyle. The cell membrane of trichomonas is evidently very pliable because the shape of the organism changes frequently and pseudopodia-like projections are often extended.

Chilomastix (Figure 33) resembles trichomonas in appearance but the shape of the body does not change to any considerable extent. The body is frequently twisted along its longitudinal axis resulting in a peripheral spiral groove. It is propelled forward and spirally in a jerky manner by three anterior flagella. On one side near the anterior end is a large cytostome which can often be seen in the living animal. There is no undulating membrane and although an axostyle is absent there is frequently a spinelike projection at the posterior end that resembles the axostyle of trichomonas.

The conspicuous feature of living specimens of giardia (Figure 38) is the presence of a large sucking disc occupying the anterior ventral surface; the anterior dorsal surface of the body is correspondingly convex. Giardia does not possess an undulating membrane and the axostyles do not extend beyond the posterior end of the body. No changes in the shape of the body occur during locomotion except movements of the tail and very little progress results from the movements of the flagella.

II. *Chilomastix in Man*

1. LIFE-CYCLE

One species of the genus *Chilomastix,* known as *Chilomastix mesnili,* occurs in man. This form lives in the large intestine and is present in about 10 per cent of the general population in many parts of the world. Cysts are formed in the intestine, pass out in the feces and represent the stage that brings about infection in new hosts. The trophozoites multiply by binary fission and division has been reported within the cyst.

2. MORPHOLOGY

Trophozoite (Figure 33a). The living trophozoite of *Chilomastix mesnili* has been described above; its principal characteristics are presented in the table on page 118. The body is pear-shaped and ranges usually from 10 μ to 15 μ in length and from 3 μ to 4 μ in breadth. There are three anterior flagella and a fourth flagellum that is situated in the cytostome and directed posteriorly. The cytostome is almost half as long as the entire body; along either side of it is a

supporting fibril. Near the anterior end of the body is a large
spherical nucleus containing one or several blocks of chromatin and
on the outside of the nuclear membrane are located several blepharoplasts from which the flagella arise. The food of chilomastix consists

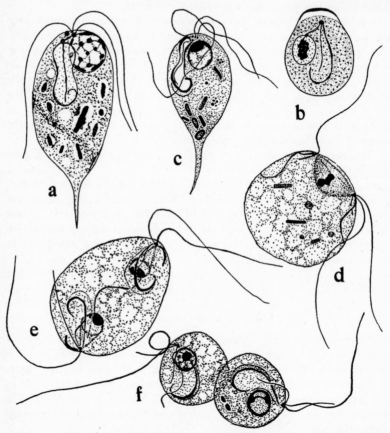

FIG. 33.—*Chilomastix*. a. Trophozoite of *C. mesnili*, from large intestine of man
(x 4000). b. Cyst of *C. mesnili* (x 4000). c. Trophozoite of *Chilomastix* from the intestine of a toad, *Bufo vulgaris*. d, e, f. *Chilomastix* from *Bufo vulgaris* grown in culture
showing three successive stages in division (x 2000). (a, b, after Hegner; c-f, after
Bishop)

largely of bacteria and the cytoplasm is usually so crowded with
food vacuoles that the structures just described are often obscured.

    Cysts. The cyst of chilomastix in the living condition is lemon-
shaped and usually from 7 μ to 9 μ in length and from 4 μ to 6 μ in
breadth. Practically no structure can be seen within the living cyst.

In specimens fixed in Schaudinn's solution and stained with iron-hæmatoxylin (Figure 33b) the wall of the cyst is seen to be thickened at the anterior end and separated slightly from the protoplasmic body within. Food bodies are extruded before encystment takes place, hence the nucleus and cytostomal structures are often more conspicuous in the cyst than in the trophozoite.

3. HOST-PARASITE RELATIONS

Chilomastix mesnili is transmitted from man to man in the cyst stage and infections are the result of the ingestion of contaminated food or drink. Cysts will live for months in water and apparently retain their infectivity (Boeck, 1921). They are probably often carried to food or drink by flies, since these insects readily ingest fecal material and the cysts may be deposited later in a viable condition (Root, 1921). A disease known as flagellate diarrhea has been attributed to the presence of *C. mesnili* because these flagellates have been found in persons suffering from diarrhea, in which no other causative organism could be discovered. It has not yet been definitely proved, however, that chilomastix is guilty.

III. *Chilomastix in Lower Animals*

Chilomastix occurs in many of the lower animals. It has been reported from the chimpanzee and orang-utan and several species of monkeys, from the rumen of the goat, the cecum of the rabbit, rat and guinea-pig, the cecum of the fowl, and from the intestine of the lizard, frog and fish. Separate specific names have been applied to these various types but whether they all represent "good" species is still to be determined. They resemble *Chilomastix mesnili* in general features.

Some of the species that may be encountered are as follows: rat, *C. bettencourti;* goat, *C. capræ;* rabbit, *C. cuniculi;* guinea-pig, *C. intestinalis;* fowl, *C. gallinarum;* frog, *C. caulleryi;* fish, *C. motellæ;* leech, *C. aulastomi.*

IV. *Trichomonas hominis*

1. LIFE-CYCLE

This species is known only in the trophozoite stage. It lives in the large intestine and probably is present in about 10 per cent of the general population in various parts of the world.

2. MORPHOLOGY

The most common trichomonad that lives in the human intestine possesses four interior flagella, but specimens with three or five are sometimes found. The offspring of these, when grown in culture, have the same number of flagella as their parents, that is, the number of flagella appears to be a constant characteristic. It has been proposed that these three types of intestinal trichomonads be considered as belonging to three different genera, in which case the type with four flagella retains the name *Trichomonas hominis,* that with three must be placed in the genus *Tritrichomonas* (Figure 35e) and the form with five in the genus *Pentatrichomonas.* These three types are considered in this book together under the name *Trichomonas hominis.*

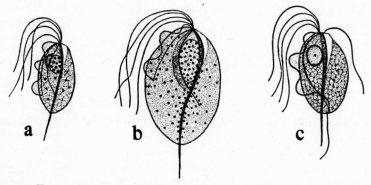

FIG. 34.—Human trichomonads. a. *Trichomonas elongata,* from the mouth. b. *T. vaginalis,* from the vagina. c. *T. hominis,* from the intestine (x 2000). (After Wenrich)

As indicated in the table on page 132, *Trichomonas hominis,* when fixed in Schaudinn's solution and stained with iron-hæmatoxylin, exhibits, besides the anterior flagella, a flagellum that is attached to the outer edge of the undulating membrane and becomes free at the posterior end of the body. On one side near the anterior end is a comma-shaped cytostome; a hyaline rod, the axostyle, passes through the center of the body longitudinally. Near the anterior end is a more or less spherical nucleus, several blepharoplasts from which the flagella arise and a chromatic basal rod which arises from a blepharoplast and extends posteriorly at the base of the undulating membrane. The body of *T. hominis* varies greatly in size but is usually from 8 μ to 15 μ in length and from 3 μ to 5 μ in breadth.

3. HOST-PARASITE RELATIONS

Since there is apparently no cyst stage in the life-cycle of *T. hominis,* this species must be transmitted from one person to another in the trophozoite form, and the only conceivable method of entrance to the host is in contaminated food or drink. It is obviously necessary, if this is correct, for the trophozoite to withstand the digestive juices in the stomach and to pass through the small intestine unharmed before an infection can be established in the large intestine. That this is probable has been shown in the case of rats, cats, guinea-pigs, and monkeys (Hegner, 1924, 1926, 1934; Brumpt, 1925; Wenrich and Yanoff, 1927) to which were fed trichomonads that were later recovered in a viable condition from the intestine.

The resistance of *T. hominis* to conditions outside of the body have recently been demonstrated by a series of experiments (Hegner, 1928). It was found that viable trichomonads could be recovered from the fecal material in which they passed out of the body eight days later, the fecal material in the meantime being kept at room temperature ($22°$C.), summer temperatures ($25°$C. and $31°$C.) and low temperature ($5°$C.). Viable trichomonads were also recovered at the end of seven days from fecal material deposited on garden soil. When fecal material is highly diluted with water, however, the osmotic pressure is so greatly changed that death occurs within a few hours, hence the danger of becoming infected through drinking water appears to be slight.

Experiments on the transmission of *T. hominis* by cockroaches and house-flies (Wenyon and O'Connor, 1917; Root, 1921; Hegner, 1928) indicate that there is little danger of trichomonads surviving ingestion by cockroaches, but that flies that ingest fecal material may deposit living trichomonas in their vomit or droppings at intervals of from twenty minutes to four hours after ingestion. It seems probable, therefore, that the house-fly plays an important rôle in the transmission of this flagellate.

The question of the pathogenicity of *Trichomonas hominis* has not yet been decided. This species has been accused of causing flagellate diarrhea and dysentery. The five-flagellate pentatrichomonas (Figure 34a) was reported from a number of diarrheic or dysenteric patients and hence considered particularly pathogenic, but cases have been described (Hegner, 1925) of persons infected with this form who had never exhibited any symptoms of diarrhea or dysentery. The habit of pentatrichomonas of ingesting red cells has also been advanced as evidence of pathogenicity, but recent experiments (Hegner,

1928) prove that many types of trichomonads ingest red cells and that these are accepted for food just as are bacteria and other food particles.

Intestinal trichomonads can be eliminated from both animals and man by treatment with an arsenical known as carbarsone (Hegner and Eskridge, 1935; Gabaldon, 1936).

V. *Trichomonas* (*buccalis*) *elongata*

1. LIFE-CYCLE

Trichomonas (*buccalis*) *elongata* is an inhabitant of the human mouth and apparently exists only in the trophozoite stage. It divides by binary longitudinal fission and multiple fission has also been reported (Ohira and Noguchi, 1917). No other stages in the life-cycle of this species have been observed.

2. MORPHOLOGY

The trophozoite of *T. elongata* (Figure 34a) varies in size usually from 12 μ to 16 μ in length and from 4 μ to 8 μ in breadth. There are four anterior flagella which often seem to arise in pairs from the trilobed blepharoplast. The undulating membrane extends posteriorly only about two-thirds the length of the body and the flagellum on its outer edge does not extend beyond the end of the membrane. The chromatic basal rod is inconspicuous. The axostyle is thread-like and stains deeply in iron-hæmatoxylin. A parabasal body has been described by Wenrich in specimens fixed in chromic or osmic acid. It is "biscuit-shaped," and located anterior to the level of the nucleus. In the center of it is a densely-staining chromatic fibril. A clear slit-like area, sometimes visible near the anterior end, is the cytostome. The nucleus is similar in position and structure to that of *T. hominis*.

3. HOST-PARASITE RELATIONS

Trichomonas elongata may be found in scrapings from the gingival space at the base of the teeth. They are not commonly found in smear preparations, but may be cultivated in serum-saline-citrate medium; the data obtained in this way indicate a high incidence of infection; probably 50 per cent of the general population carry this organism. Transmission, no doubt, usually occurs during kissing. A definite relation seems to exist between the presence of *T. elongata* and a diseased condition of the oral region (Hogue, 1926; Hinshaw,

1926) ; that is, more positive cases have been recorded from persons giving a history of pyorrhea, acute gingivitis or abscessed teeth than from those with normal mouths. The flagellate itself is probably not pathogenic but finds the diseased condition favorable for growth and multiplication.

VI. *Trichomonas vaginalis*

I. LIFE-CYCLE

This is the type species of the genus *Trichomonas*. It occurs only in the trophozoite stage. It is widespread among women and a high incidence of infection has been reported (Brumpt, 1913; Reuling, 1921; Hegner, 1925), from 5 per cent to 50 per cent being infected. A few cases of infection have been reported from the urinary tract of man (Dock, 1896; Hegner and Taliaferro, 1924; Katsunuma, 1924; Dastider, 1925; Lynch, 1930).

2. MORPHOLOGY

The length of *Trichomonas vaginalis* varies usually from 15 μ to 20 μ and the breadth from 6 μ to 18 μ. The four anterior flagella usually emerge from the body in pairs. The organism (Figure 34b) resembles the other trichomonads in structure but has a very short undulating membrane with a flagellum on its outer edge that does not extend beyond the side of the body. The chromatic basal rod is thin and the axostyle is likewise thin and stains deeply with iron-hæmatoxylin. Surrounding the axostyle are a number of spherical bodies that stain deeply with iron-hæmatoxylin. A sausage-shaped parabasal body has been observed in this species which extends past the posterior end of the nucleus sometimes for half the length of the body.

3. HOST-PARASITE RELATIONS

How *Trichomonas vaginalis* is transmitted from one host to another is unknown. Specimens could easily gain access to the urinary tract of man during coitus. Investigations on monkeys indicate that the intestinal and vaginal trichomonads may belong to the same species (Hegner, 1928). If this is true, then the vagina may become infected by contamination with the intestinal form. The pathogenicity of *T. vaginalis* is also uncertain. Flagellates of this species are reported to be present when the vaginal mucous membrane is in an abnormal condition and when the reaction of the vaginal mucus is acid. Treatment with sodium bicarbonate is therefore recommended by some physicians so as to change the vaginal contents to an alkaline condition. A pentavalent arsenical known as aldarsone has recently been advocated for the treatment of trichomonas vaginitis (Bland and Rakoff, 1936).

VII. *Trichomonas in Lower Animals*

Trichomonads seem to be distributed more widely among vertebrates than any other type of intestinal protozoa. They are present

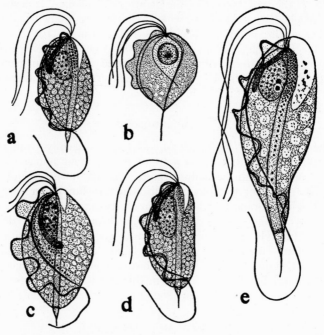

FIG. 35.—Trichomonads from lower animals. a. *Trichomonas* sp., from the intestine of the rhesus monkey. b. *T. columbæ*, from the crop of the pigeon. c. *T. muris*, from the cecum of the rat. d. *T. fœtus*, from the vagina of the cow. e. *T. augusta*, from the intestine of the frog (x 2000). (After Wenrich)

in almost every species of domesticated animal as well as in most of the wild animals that have been examined. One species that probably belongs to the genus *Trichomonas* has been reported from pond water (Bishop, 1935, 1936).

Most of the mammals closely associated with man appear to be infected with trichomonads; flagellates belonging to this genus are commonly present in the intestine of rats, mice, guinea-pigs, rabbits, dogs and cats. They have also been reported from the mouth of the dog, cat and monkey, from the genital tract of cattle and monkeys, from the stomach of the pig, the rumen of cattle, the cecum of fowls, the crop of pigeons and doves, the intestine of reptiles, amphibians and fish and from leeches, molluscs and termites. Trichomonads have been reported from the intestine of various species of monkeys and from the vagina of the rhesus monkey. *Macacus rhesus,* and the intestinal form from the latter has apparently been successfully transmitted to the vagina of the same species of monkey (Hegner, 1928). The species most easily obtained for study are *Tritrichomonas augusta* (Figure 35e), from the rectum of the frog, and *Tritrichomonas muris* (Figure 35c), from the cecum of the rat. Both of these organisms are more easily prepared for study than is *T. hominis* from man and exhibit the characteristics of the genus much more distinctly. Of special interest in connection with the trichomonads of lower animals is the fact that a cyst stage occurs in the life-cycle of certain species and that multiple fission as well as binary fission may occur. During multiple fission the two daughter flagellates do not separate following division and their offspring likewise remain together until a so-called somatella is formed consisting of eight merozoites. Eventually these merozoites separate one by one from the somatella. Some of the species described from lower animals are as follows:

Pig	*T. suis*	Lizard	*T. lacertæ*
Cattle	*T. ruminantium*	Tortoise	*T. brumpti*
Cattle	*T. fœtus*	Toad	*T. batrachorum*
Horse	*T. equi*	Frog	*T. augusta*
Cat	*T. felis*	Fish	*T. legeri*
Rat	*T. muris*	Termite	*T. termopsidis*
Guinea-pig	*T. caviæ*	Snail	*T. limacis*
Fowl	*T. gallinarum*	Leech	*T. sanguisugæ*
Pigeon	*T. columbæ*		

Among the more interesting species of trichomonads are *Tritrichomonas fecalis, Trichomonas columbæ* and *T. fœtus. Tritrichomonas fecalis* was isolated repeatedly by Cleveland (1928) from the stools of one person. The organism could not be found or cultivated until approximately four weeks after the stool had been passed. It grew luxuriantly in diluted feces and in serum-saline medium.

Trichomonas columbæ (Figure 35b) is a parasite associated with diseased conditions in pigeons and doves. Its primary site of infection is the digestive tract between the crop and the glandular stomach. Tissues are actually invaded and liquefied (Cauthen, 1936).

Trichomonas fœtus (Figure 35d) occurs in the genital tract of cattle and is held responsible for early abortion and other reproductive disabilities. Transmission is from infected bulls to cows, but Andrews and Miller (1936) have shown that virgin heifers may become infected by association with diseased cows.

VIII. *Retortamonas (Embadomonas) intestinalis*

This species was reported by Wenyon and O'Connor (1917) from two human cases in Egypt. It is apparently a rare species in man but has been found in widely separated regions. It probably lives in the

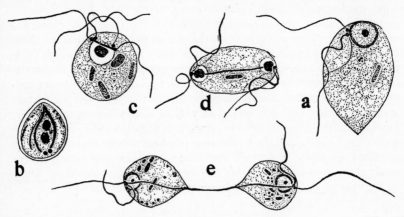

FIG. 36.—*Retortamonas (Embadomonas) intestinalis.* a. Trophozoite. b. Cyst. c, d, e. Stages in binary division (x 3000). (After Bishop)

large intestine. Both trophozoites and cysts occur (Figure 36) and infections may last for at least six weeks. The trophozoite is ovoidal and from 4 μ to 9 μ in length and 3 μ to 4 μ in breadth. It is characterized by the presence of two flagella, one extending out from the anterior end and the other, which is much thicker, arising from the large cytostome which is situated on one side and extends from near the anterior end to about the middle region of the body. Near the anterior end is a spherical nucleus containing a large karyosome. The cysts are pyriform in shape, 4 μ to 6 μ in length and 3 μ to 4 μ in breadth.

IX. *Retortamonas in Lower Animals*

Specimens belonging to this genus have been recorded from the larva of the crane fly, from a waterbug, frog and tortoise. Wenyon (1926) records specimens from the cecum of the guinea-pig and

wild rat morphologically identical with *R. intestinalis* in man. Specimens have been reported from several species of monkeys (Fonseca,
1917; Kessel, 1927); from the sheep and three-toed sloth (Hegner
and Schumaker, 1928); and from rabbits, various amphibians and
the cockroach. Whether these are all "good" species is still to be
determined.

X. *Enteromonas hominis*

The genus *Enteromonas* was founded by Fonseca (1915) for a
single species, *E. hominis*. It has been reported from North America
and various other coun-
tries but appears to be
comparatively rare. The
trophozoite (Figure 37)
is pear-shaped and has
the structure characteristic of the genus *Cerco-
monas,* but possessès
three anterior flagella
and a posterior flagellum
which is attached to the
flattened side of the or-
ganism. The length of
the trophozoite varies
from 4 μ to 10 μ and the

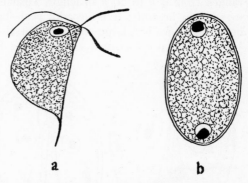

FIG. 37.—*Enteromonas hominis* from man. a.
Trophozoite. b. Cyst (x 4500). (After Wenyon and
O'Connor)

breadth from 3 μ to 6 μ. There is no cytostome. There is a large
anterior nucleus of the vesicular type. Reproduction is by longitudinal binary fission. The cysts of *E. hominis* are elongate oval, 6 μ to
8 μ in length and 3 μ to 4 μ in breadth, and when mature contain
four nuclei. Nothing is known regarding the relations of the organism to its human host. Considerable confusion has existed regarding
this species and one named *Tricercomonas intestinalis* by Wenyon
and O'Connor (1917). It seems probable that organisms that have
been found in man and in the guinea-pig and placed in the genus
Tricercomonas have either been specimens of *E. hominis* or of some
other species of flagellate.

XI. *Giardia lamblia*

I. LIFE-CYCLE

The species of giardia living in man possesses both trophozoite
and cyst stages in its life-cycle. The trophozoites divide by binary

fission and division also occurs within the cyst. The surveys of intestinal protozoa made in various parts of the world indicate that *Giardia lamblia* is present in about 12 per cent of the general population. Infection is brought about by the ingestion of cysts, which excyst in the small intestine and remain there; this is the section of the digestive tract where these flagellates are usually located.

2. MORPHOLOGY

Trophozoite (Figure 38). The trophozoite of *Giardia lamblia* ranges from 9 μ to 20 μ in length (usually 12 μ to 15 μ) and 5 μ to 10 μ in breadth; it is broadly pear-shaped and bilaterally symmetrical. There is a large anterior ventral sucking disc, as shown in Figure 38, two nuclei, two axostyles and four pairs of flagella. The "axostyles" are probably a pair of axonemes connecting the caudal flagella with the blepharoplasts. The two anterior lateral flagella arise from blepharoplasts at the anterior ends of the axostyles, pass forward through the cytoplasm, cross each other near the extreme anterior end, follow the edge of the body for a short distance and then emerge one on either side.

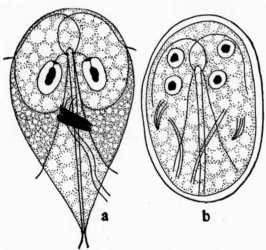

FIG. 38.—*Giardia lamblia* from man. a. Trophozoite (only the bases of the flagella are shown). b. Cyst (x 4000). (After Hegner)

The posterior lateral flagella have a similar origin but pass posteriorly along the edges of the lateral shields and emerge near the posterior end of the body. The caudal flagella extend out from the caudal ends of the axostyles, and the ventral flagella arise directly from the axostyles a short distance posterior to the nuclei. Between the two blepharoplasts is an arch-shaped fibril in the center of which is an interblepharoplastic granule. A rhizoplast connects each nucleus to the blepharoplast on its side of the body. Just posterior to the ventral sucking disc are a pair of "parabasal bodies" that are more or less intimately fused together; these resemble the chromatoid bodies of amœbæ. Basal granules are sometimes visible at the points where the anterior lateral and caudal flagella emerge from the body. The diamond-shaped region between the lateral shields is much thinner than the rest of the body. The ventral sucking disc is used by the organism to attach itself to epithelial cells of the intestine and no doubt helps it to maintain itself there against the action of peristalsis. While thus located, the ventral flagella are in active movement, thus creating a current which renews the medium and is probably valuable in bringing nutritive material to the flagellate. There is no cytostome, food substances being absorbed through the general surface of the body.

Cyst (Figure 38). The cyst of G. lamblia is ovoidal and varies from 8 μ to 14 μ in length and from 6 μ to 10 μ in breadth. Fibrils are visible in the living cyst. In cysts that are fixed in Schaudinn's solution and stained with iron-hæmatoxylin the axostyles and cytoplasmic portions of the anterior lateral and posterior lateral flagella are visible as well as groups of fibrils which probably are the remains of those that lie along the edge of the sucking disc and lateral shields in the trophozoite. There may be two, four, eight or sixteen nuclei within the cyst; these are spherical and are usually distributed, two near the anterior end, two near either end, four near the anterior end or four near either end. Excystation has been described (Hegner, 1927).

3. HOST-PARASITE RELATIONS

Transmission. As in other intestinal protozoa that have a cyst stage in their life-cycles, Giardia lamblia is transmitted from one human host to another by the contamination of food or drink by cysts. The work of Boeck (1921) indicates that these cysts may remain alive outside of the body for several months. They are unable, however, to withstand drying, hence their infectivity depends upon the continued presence of moisture.

Pathogenicity. The terms "lambliasis," "giardiasis" and "flagellate diarrhea" all refer to a pathogenic condition supposed to be brought about by G. lamblia. It is still to be proved, however, that this flagellate is responsible for the symptoms of diarrhea observed. It seems probable that the organisms find the diarrheic condition favorable for their growth and multiplication. Most of the persons infected with G. lamblia do not exhibit symptoms but must be considered carriers in whom the organisms multiply and produce cysts, the latter being passed by the host and responsible for the initiation of new infections. Cholecystitis or inflammation of the gall bladder has been attributed to these flagellates (see Hegner, 1927). Children appear to be more heavily infected with *G. lamblia* than do adults, a fact which indicates an age resistance to the organism.

XII. *Giardia in Lower Animals*

Species of the genus *Giardia* have been reported from a large number of lower animals including monkeys, lions, cats, dogs, sheep, cattle, goats, horses, rabbits, guinea-pigs, rats, mice, herons, lizards, tadpoles, fish and nematodes (Figure 39). These resemble *Giardia*

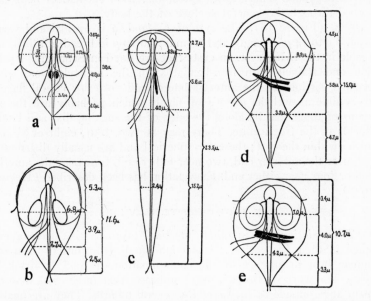

FIG. 39.—Giardias from lower animals. Diagrams drawn to scale to illustrate differences in size, shape, parabasal bodies, and other structural features (x 2600). (After Hegner)
a. *Giardia muris* from the rat.
b. *Giardia sp.* from the great blue heron.
c. *Giardia agilis* from the tadpole.
d. *Giardia duodenalis* from the rabbit.
e. *Giardia caviæ* from the guinea-pig.

lamblia in the general structure of both the trophozoite and cyst, but careful measurements indicate differences in body size and differences in the relative shape and size of various parts of the body. The number, size, shape and location of the parabasal bodies also differ in the organisms from different species of hosts. Because of these morphological differences many of these forms are considered to be distinct species. Apparently host-parasite specificity is very rigid among members of the genus *Giardia* since almost every host species is infected by a distinct species of the genus (Hegner, 1927). *Giardia muris* of the rat (Figure 40) is the species most easily obtained. Trophozoites occur in the small intestine of a considerable proportion of laboratory rats and mice. Encysting specimens may be found in

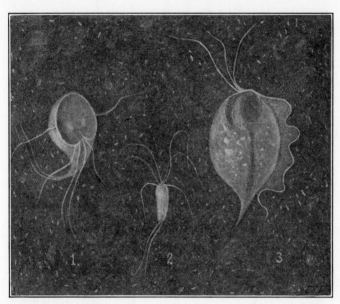

FIG. 40.—Flagellates from the intestine of the rat as seen when alive. (After Hegner)
1. *Giardia muris.*
2. *Hexamita muris.*
3. *Tritrichomonas muris.*

the small intestine and cysts may be recovered from the cecum or the feces. *G. muris* differs in only minor respects from *G. lamblia*. Another species that can easily be obtained, and is very distinctive in shape and structure, is *G. agilis* which occurs in the duodenum of tadpoles (Figure 39c). Some of the common species of *Giardia* are as follows:

Rabbit	*G. duodenalis*	Goat	*G. capræ*
Rat	*G. muris*	Horse	*G. equi*
Field mouse	*G. microti*	Cattle	*G. bovis*
Dog	*G. canis*	Heron	*G. ardeæ*
Cat	*G. cati*	Lizard	*G. varani*
Guinea-pig	*G. caviæ*	Tadpole	*G. agilis*

TABLE II

INTESTINAL FLAGELLATES OF MAN

		Trophozoite		Cyst	
	Structural Characteristics	Shape	Size	Shape	Size
1. *Chilomastix mesnili* (Wenyon, 1910)	3 free ant. flag.; 1 flag. in cytostome	Pear-shaped	10 μ-15 μ x 3 μ-4 μ	Lemon-shaped	7 μ-9 μ x 4 μ-6 μ
2. *Trichomonas hominis* (Davaine, 1860)	3, 4 or 5 free ant. flagella; 1 post. flag. on margin of undulating membrane; axostyle present	Pear-shaped	8 μ-15 μ x 3 μ-5 μ	Cysts unknown	
3. *Trichomonas vaginalis* (Donné, 1837)		Pear-shaped	15 μ-20 μ x 6 μ-18 μ	Cysts unknown	
4. *Trichomonas elongata* (Steinberg, 1862)		Pear-shaped	6 μ-12 μ x 4 μ-8 μ	Cysts unknown	
5. *Retortamonas intestinalis* (Wenyon and O'Connor, 1917)	2 ant. free flag. unequal in thickness; cytostome large	Ovoid	4 μ-9 μ x 3 μ-4 μ	Pyriform	4 μ-6 μ x 3 μ-4 μ
6. *Enteromonas hominis* (Fonseca, 1915)	3 ant. free flag.; one post. flag. on surface of body	Pear-shaped	4 μ-10 μ x 3 μ-6 μ	Elongate oval	6 μ-8 μ x 3 μ-4 μ
7. *Giardia lamblia* (Stilse, 1915)	Bilaterally symmetrical; anterior ventral sucking disc; 2 nuclei, 2 axostyles, 4 pairs of flagella	Pear-shaped	9 μ-20 μ x 5 μ-10 μ	Oval	8 μ-14 μ x 6 μ-10 μ

SPOROZOA IN GENERAL AND GREGARINES IN PARTICULAR

I. *Classification*

The groups of protozoa that are brought together in the class SPOROZOA have certain characteristics in common but are not necessarily closely related. They are combined in one class largely for the sake of convenience. Sporozoa are all parasitic. They are especially common among vertebrates and arthropods and less common among other invertebrates. They form spores at one stage in their life-cycle which usually serve to set up infections in new hosts. There are no locomotor organelles in the adult stage and food is absorbed through the general surface of the body. The following is a convenient arrangement of the groups in this class:

Class SPOROZOA. All species parasitic; locomotor organs absent, sexual reproduction results in the formation of sporozoites.

 Subclass 1. TELOSPORIDIA. Intracellular during part of the life-cycle; spore formation ends the life of the individual.

  Order 1. GREGARINIDA. Inhabitants of cavities (cœlozoic); schizogony usually omitted from life-cycle.

  Order 2. COCCIDIA. Typically inhabitants of epithelial cells (cytozoic); both schizogony and sporogony occur in a single host.

  Order 3. HÆMOSPORIDIA. Blood-inhabiting species (cytozoic) of vertebrates; schizogony in a vertebrate and sporogony in an invertebrate host; resistant spores usually absent.

 Subclass 2. CNIDOSPORIDIA. Usually multinucleate in adult stage; spore formation occurs during the life of the individual.

  Order 1. MYXOSPORIDIA. Adult, a large multinucleate plasmodium; spores large, with usually two polar capsules.

Order 2. MICROSPORIDIA. Spores small, with usually one polar capsule.
Subclass 3. ACNIDOSPORIDIA. Protozoa of doubtful affinities that produce simple spores.
Order 1. SARCOSPORIDIA. Spores in sac-like tubules in muscle cells of vertebrates.
Order 2. HAPLOSPORIDIA. Parasites of lower vertebrates and invertebrates. No polar capsules.

II. *Life-Cycles*

The life-cycles of the sporozoa are as a rule more complex than those of protozoa belonging to the other three classes. This is apparently the result of the fact that there is often an alternation of hosts, part of the life-cycle being passed in a vertebrate and part in an invertebrate. In a typical life-cycle two sorts of reproduction occur; schizogony, during which large numbers of offspring are produced asexually, and sporogony, which involves sexual phenomena and ends in the production of spores.

Various types of life-cycles will be described in this and the following chapters, hence it is not necessary to describe them here in detail. It may, however, be worth while to review briefly three typical but different life-cycles.

1. MONOCYSTIS

Certain gregarines of the genus *Monocystis* are parasitic in the seminal vesicles of the earthworm. The entire life-cycle (Figure 41) is passed in a single host. The trophozoite penetrates and grows at the expense of a group of sperm mother cells. There is no asexual reproduction of the trophozoite but two fully grown trophozoites conjugate and surround themselves with a double wall, thus forming a cyst; within, the organisms, which now may be considered gametocytes, produce large numbers of gametes; these copulate in pairs and form spores, the resistant wall of which is known as a sporocyst; within each spore eight spindle-shaped sporozoites arise; these represent the stage that infects new hosts.

2. ISOSPORA

Another type of life-cycle that includes asexual reproduction in the trophozoite stage may be illustrated by means of the coccidium of the cat and dog, *Isospora felis* (Figure 44). The sporozoites that

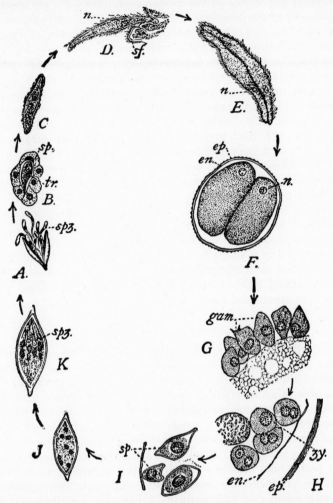

Fig. 41.—*Monocystis,* an acephaline gregarine parasitic in the seminal vesicles of the earthworm. A, the eight sporozoites (*spz.*) escaping from the sporocyst. B, a young trophozoite (*tr.*) among the sperm-mother cells (*sp.*) of the earthworm. C, a free individual with a few withered sperm cells adhering to it. D, a mature individual attached to the sperm-funnel (*sf.*) of the earthworm. E, two mature individuals joined side by side. F, two individuals have formed a cyst; *en.,* endocyst; *ep.,* epicyst; *n.,* nucleus. G, gametes (*gam.*) formed by one individual within the cyst. H, conjugation of gametes to form zygotes (*zy.*). I, zygotes (sporoblasts, *sp.*) that have secreted spore coats or sporocysts. J, a single spore in which the nucleus has divided, forming eight daughter nuclei. K, a fully developed spore containing eight sporozoites (*spz.*). (From Hegner. After Cuénot and Bourne)

escape from the spores in the intestine of the host (30) penetrate epithelial cells of the intestinal wall (1) and become trophozoites (2); each trophozoite is a schizont which produces a number of daughter merozoites asexually (3-8); this multiplicative process is known as schizogony. The merozoites may enter other epithelial cells (8 to 1) becoming trophozoites and pass through another period of asexual reproduction, or, after the penetration of epithelial cells, may produce merozoites which are gametocytes; these penetrate other epithelial cells (9) where they develop into macrogametocytes (19) or microgametocytes (11). Each gametocyte produces either one large macrogamete (22) or a large number of microgametes (18). One microgamete copulates with each macrogamete (23), a process that may be considered fertilization, thus producing a zygote. A wall forms about the zygote and the body is then known as an oöcyst (24). The protoplasm within divides to form two sporoblasts (28) each of which forms a sporocyst about itself thus becoming a spore (29). Within each spore four sporozoites develop (29). This life-cycle, which is passed in a single host, includes a period of asexual reproduction, known as schizogony, followed by sexual processes which lead to a second type of reproduction (sporogony) ending in the formation of spores and sporozoites.

3. MALARIA PARASITE

The third type of life-cycle, well illustrated by that of the malaria parasites (Figure 52), involves stages similar to those just described, but part of them are passed in a vertebrate host, for example man, and the rest in an invertebrate host, for example certain anopheline mosquitoes. Sporozoites inoculated into the blood by the mosquito penetrate red cells, becoming trophozoites; these are schizonts which produce merozoites by asexual reproduction. Some of the trophozoites become gametocytes; these do not undergo development in the human body, but, in the stomach of the mosquito, each macrogametocyte produces one macrogamete and each microgametocyte produces a number of microgametes. Copulation (fertilization) then occurs, an oöcyst is formed, and large numbers of sporozoites develop within it.

III. *Gregarines*

Gregarines are among the simplest of the sporozoa and are easily obtained for study, since they are common parasites in the digestive tract and body cavity of insects and earthworms. We may recognize two groups, the first known as the EUGREGARINIDA which do not

have a period of schizogony in their life-cycle, and the SCHIZOGRE-
GARINIDA which do.

1. ACEPHALINE GREGARINES

These are EUGREGARINIDA without an epimerite or "head." The
species of the genus *Monocystis,* the life-cycle of which was described
on page 134 (Figure 41), are common in the seminal vesicles of the
earthworm. If the seminal vesicles of the worm are dissected out,
large trophozoites and cysts containing spores may usually be found,
as well as other stages in the life-cycle.

Other interesting species of acephaline gregarines are *Cystobia
irregularis,* which lives in the blood vessel of the sea cucumber,
Holothuria nigra; Urospora sænuridis, an inhabitant of the seminal
vesicles and body cavity of the annelid worm, *Tubifex tubifex; Gonospora minchina,* which occurs in the cœlum of the annelid, *Arenicola
ecaudata;* and *Lankesteria culicis,* that parasitizes the gut of the
yellow-fever mosquito, *Ædes ægypti.*

2. CEPHALINE GREGARINES

These are especially abundant in insects and can be obtained
easily from the intestine of grasshoppers, cockroaches or meal-
worms. The sporozoites penetrate the epithelial cells of the intestinal
wall and the trophozoites which develop from them are at first intracellular; later the trophozoites break out of the epithelial cells to
which they are attached for a time by the head or epimerite (Figure
42a); this, the cephalont stage, consists of two parts, the posterior
deutomerite which contains the nucleus, and an anterior protomerite
and epimerite. When the cephalont becomes detached from the cell
it loses its epimerite and is then known as a sporont (Figure 42b).
The sporonts within the intestine unite end to end, a condition known
as syzygy (Figure 42c). Two sporonts conjugate and surround
themselves with a wall thus forming a cyst (Figure 42d); they are
gametocytes, each of which produces a large number of gametes.
The gametes copulate in pairs, thus becoming zygotes, and secrete
sporocysts and hence are spores (Figure 42e). Within each spore
eight sporozoites are produced. The sporozoites that are liberated
in the intestine of the hosts that have ingested the spores bring about
new infections.

Some of the common species of cephaline gregarines are as follows: *Gregarina blattarum* lives in the digestive tract of the cockroach, *G. locustæ* in that of the Carolina locust and *G. oviceps* in

that of crickets of the genus *Gryllus; Hirmocystis harpali* is an intestinal parasite of the beetle, *Harpalus pennsylvanicus erythropus; Leidyana erratica* inhabits the intestine of crickets, *Gryllus abbreviatus* and *G. pennsylvanicus; Acutispora macrocephala* occurs in the gut of a chilopod, *Lithobius forficatus;* and *Porospora portunidarum* is a very large species that lives in crabs (*Portunus*) and mollusks (*Cardium*).

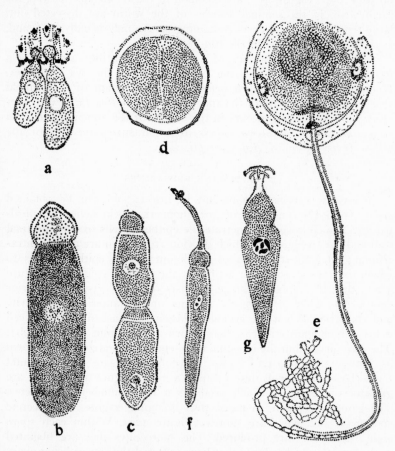

Fig. 42.—Cephaline gregarines of insects. (After Watson)

a. Trophozoites of *Leidyana erratica* attached to host cells of the cricket (x 245).
b. Adult sporont of *Leidyana erratica* (x 245).
c. Sporonts of *Gregarina blattarum* of the cockroach in syzygy.
d. Two sporonts of *Leidyana erratica* within a cyst (x 60).
e. Mature cyst of *Leidyana erratica* extruding a chain of spores (x 245).
f. *Stylocephalus longicollis* of the church-yard beetle.
g. *Ancyrophora uncinata* of the water-beetle.

3. SCHIZOGREGARINES

These are principally intestinal parasites of arthropods and annelid worms. As noted above, asexual reproduction, or schizogony, occurs in the life-cycle of the members of this group. Sometimes several types of schizonts occur in the life-cycle of a single species. Considerable variation exists in the various life-cycles in the method of formation of gametes and spores. *Schizocystis gregarinoides* lives in the gut of fly larvæ of the genus *Ceratopogon; Ophryocystis mesnili* occurs in the mealworm, *Tenebrio molitor;* and *Caulleryella pipientis* parasitizes the gut of *Culex pipiens*.

CHAPTER IX

COCCIDIA

I. General Characteristics

The coccidia are sporozoa whose life-cycle includes both schizogony and sporogony and is passed in a single host. They are parasitic in vertebrates, myriapods, mollusks, insects, annelids and flatworms. The life-cycle of *Isospora felis* (Figure 44) that occurs in the cat and the dog has already been described (page 134). The life-cycles of other species resemble this but differ in certain respects. For example, the oöcysts of the genus *Eimeria* contain four spores, each with two sporozoites (Figure 43d); a species known as *Caryotropha mesnili,* that lives in the body cavity of an annelid, has about twenty spores in its oöcysts, each of which produces twelve sporozoites; *Cyclospora caryolytica,* which parasitizes the nuclei of the intestinal epithelium of the mole, produces oöcysts in which two spores are formed each with two sporozoites; and other variations occur in the different species. The hæmogregarines represent a suborder of the Coccidia. Three common genera are *Hæmogregarina, Hepatozoön* and *Karyolysus.* In these an intermediate host is required for transmission.

II. Coccidia in Man

A number of species of coccidia have been reported from man but only one of these, *Isospora hominis,* has been definitely established as a human parasite. Several coccidia reported by Dobell (1919) as new species from man, namely, *Eimeria wenyoni* and *E. oxyspora* (Figure 43d) and a third species, named by Dobell (1921) *E. snijdersi,* have since been proved by Thomson and Robertson (1926a, 1926b) to be parasites of fish, the oöcysts of which had been eaten by the human host, had passed through the intestine and been found in the feces.

I. MORPHOLOGY AND LIFE-CYCLE OF ISOSPORA HOMINIS

This species is known only in the oöcyst stage (Figure 43a, b). The oöcysts which pass out in the feces of the host measure from 25 μ to 33 μ in length and from 12.5 μ to 16 μ in breadth. Their

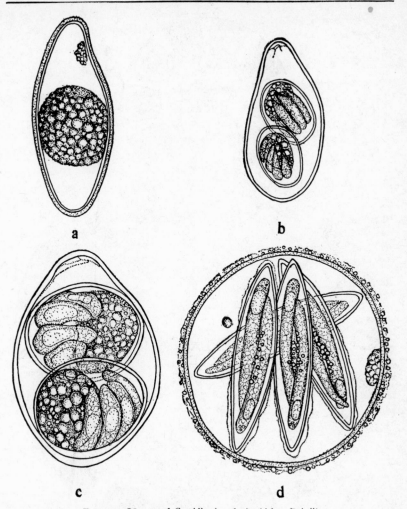

FIG. 43.—Oöcysts of Coccidia (x 1600). (After Dobell)

a. *Isospora hominis* of man, before spore formation.
b. *Isospora hominis* of man, containing two spores each with four sporozoites and a residuum.
c. *Isospora bigemina* of the cat.
d. *Eimeria sardinæ* (= *E. oxyspora*) of fish.

protoplasmic contents are usually in the form of a ball when they emerge in the feces. During the life outside of the body of the host the nucleus divides and the protoplasm separates into two uninucleate sporoblasts. Each sporoblast secretes two walls (sporocysts) about

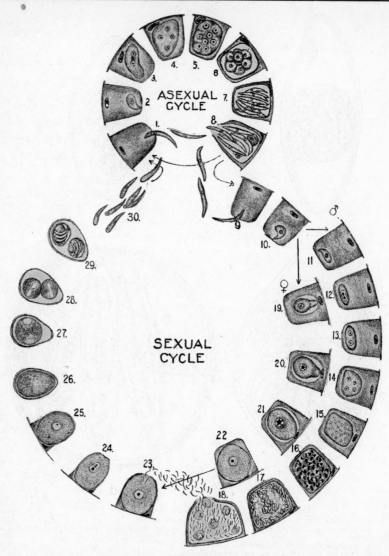

Fig. 44.—*Isospora felis,* life-cycle. (From Hegner. After Andrews) Stages 26, 27, 28 and 29 are oöcysts which pass out of the body with the feces; in each oöcyst two sporoblasts are formed (28) and in each sporoblast four sporozoites (29). When ingested by a susceptible animal the sporozoites escape from the oöcyst (30), enter epithelial cells (1) where they undergo schizogony (2-8). The merozoites produced may repeat the asexual cycle (8 to 1 to 8) or initiate the sexual cycle (9-25). In the latter, female cells (♀) or macrogametes (19-22) and male cells (♂) or microgametes (11-18) develop. Fertilization (23) is followed by the formation of the oöcyst (24-26).

itself thus becoming a spore. Within each spore four uninucleate sausage-shaped sporozoites are formed. Part of the protoplasm is not included in the sporozoite but remains behind as a residue; such a residue also occurs in certain other coccidia. The asexual cycle and sexual phenomena are not known in *Isospora hominis,* but are probably similar to those of *Isospora felis* in the cat, which are illustrated in Figure 44 and described on pages 134-136.

2. HOST-PARASITE RELATIONS OF ISOSPORA HOMINIS

Human coccidiosis is apparently rare, only about two hundred cases having been reported. The reasons for this low incidence are not known with certainty, but it is probable that cases are frequently overlooked because the cysts do not appear in the feces until the symptoms have disappeared. Also, only a small number of oöcysts are passed by the human host. It is even possible that *I. hominis* may be a natural parasite of some lower animal and only occasionally infects man.

The oöcysts of coccidia are very resistant to factors in the external environment. Haughwout (1921), for example, exposed oöcysts of *I. hominis* in the sporoblast stage to the sun for three hours every day for a week and found that at the end of this period some of them developed sporozoites when water was added. The oöcysts thus probably remain viable for long periods outside of the body and have excellent opportunities for being ingested by man in contaminated food or drink. The sporozoites probably escape from the spore and excyst in the small intestine, and immediately penetrate the epithelial cells; they are thus always pathogenic although probably large numbers must be ingested before symptoms are brought about. The stages within the human body are probably similar to those of *I. felis* in cats and dogs (see Figure 44).

The best account of a human infection with *Isospora hominis* is that of Connal (1922). Six days after swallowing oöcysts the patient suffered from diarrhea; oöcysts appeared in the feces twenty-two days after the diarrhea began and were present daily for the succeeding thirteen days. Coccidial infections are of particular interest because, as in this case, the incubation period (six days) is shorter than the prepatent period (twenty-eight days), whereas in most other pathogenic protozoa of man the prepatent period is shorter than the incubation period.

III. *Coccidia in Lower Animals*

The coccidia most easily obtained for study are those in the rabbit, *Eimeria stiedæ* (Figure 45a, c, d). Oöcysts of this species may be found in the feces of a large proportion of these animals. They are in an unsegmented stage when passed but segmentation may be

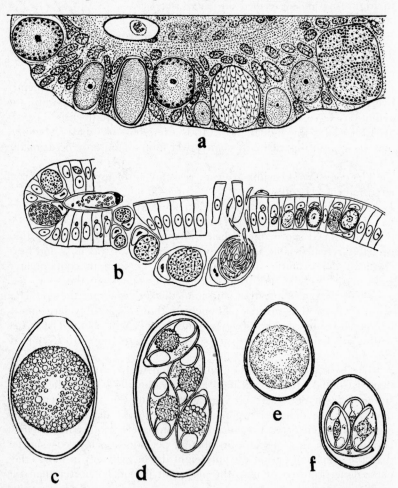

FIG. 45.—*Eimeria* of lower animals. a. *E. stiedæ:* various stages in life-cycle in epithelial cells of bile duct of rabbit (x 700). b. *E. tenella:* various stages in life-cycle in cecum of fowl. c. *E. stiedæ:* unsegmented oöcyst from rabbit. d. *E. stiedæ:* segmented oöcyst. e. *E. miyiarii:* unsegmented oöcyst from rat. f. *E. miyiarii:* segmented oöcyst. (a, after Wenrich; b, after Tyzzer; c, d, after Perard; e, f, after Becker. c-f, x 1130.)

observed if the material is placed in a 5 per cent aqueous solution of potassium bichromate to inhibit the growth of bacteria. Segmentation into sporoblasts and the formation of sporozoites takes place in about three days.

Eimerias of other species (Figure 45) occur in various species of mammals, birds, reptiles, amphibia and fish. All of these are pathogenic if their life-cycles are similar to that of *E. stiedæ* in the rabbit, but most of them do not injure the host very severely. *E. stiedæ* frequently brings about the death of rabbits, however, and *E. zürnii* is the cause of diarrhea in cattle, especially in Switzerland, Sweden and Denmark. The eimeria in birds, *E. tenella,* is likewise lethal under certain conditions, especially when epidemics occur among young chickens.

Coccidia of the genus *Isospora* also occur in vertebrates of all classes. Cats and dogs are commonly infected with *I. felis* and *I. rivolta.* Other species occur in birds and cold-blooded vertebrates.

The genera of the common coccidia are distinguished by the number of sporocysts and sporozoites present in the mature oöcysts. Species differ in size, shape, color, surface markings, presence or absence of oöcystic or sporocystic residues, pathogenicity, localization in the host, course of infection and species of host. Some of the species that live in familiar animals are as follows:

Cat and dog	*Isospora felis*	Rabbit	*E. stiedæ*
Cat	*Eimeria felina*	Rat	*E. miyiarii*
Dog	*E. canis*	Pig	*E. debliecki*
Guinea-pig	*E. caviæ*	Fowl	*E. tenella*
Mouse	*E. falciformis*	Turkey	*E. meleagridis*
Cattle	*E. zürnii*	Sparrow	*Isospora lacazii*

IV. *Hæmogregarines*

The hæmogregarines are unpigmented parasites that occur in both red and white cells in the peripheral blood of vertebrates. The species most easily obtained for study occur in the blood of frogs.

I. HEPATOZOÖN MURIS

An excellent account of this species has been provided by Miller (1908). As shown in Figure 46, schizogony (4-8) occurs in the rat and sexual phenomena and sporogony (9-21) in a mite (*Lelaps echidninus*) which feeds on the blood of the rat. When infected mites are eaten by a rat, sporozoites escape from the spores (22), penetrate the intestinal villi (1-2), enter the blood stream (3) and

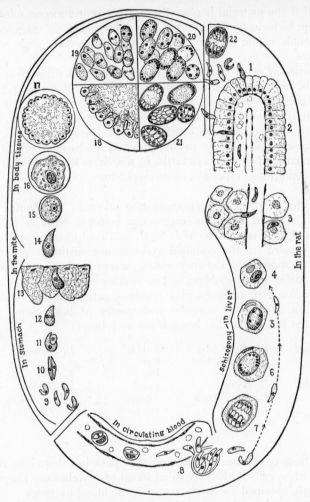

FIG. 46.—*Hepatozoön muris*. Stages in the life-cycle in the rat and the mite. (After Miller)

are carried to the liver, where they enter the liver cells (3). During schizogony within these cells (4-8) from twelve to twenty merozoites are produced. These may likewise enter liver cells and undergo schizogony or may break out into the blood stream (8), penetrate mononuclear leucocytes and develop into gametocytes. If these gametocytes are sucked up into the stomach of a mite they copulate in pairs, one member of the pair becoming a large macrogamete and the other a smaller microgamete (9-11). The zygote thus formed becomes an oökinete (12) which makes its way through the intestinal wall into the body cavity (13-14) and forms an oöcyst in the tissue of the body (15-16). The oöcyst increases in size and from fifty to 100 sporoblasts are formed (17-18), each of which secretes a sporocyst and becomes a spore (19). About sixteen sporozoites are formed in each spore (20-22).

2. HÆMOGREGARINA

Hæmogregarina occur in many aquatic vertebrates (Figure 47). The life-cycle of *Hæmogregarina stepanowi* has been worked out in detail (Reichenow, 1910). It is a parasite of the European turtle,

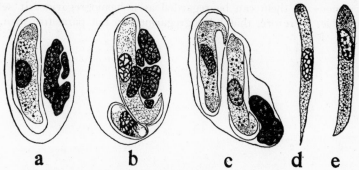

a   b   c   d   e

FIG. 47.—Hæmogregarines of frogs. a, b, c, within red cells; d, e, free in the blood stream (x 1400). (After Kudo)

Emys orbicularis and is transmitted from turtle to turtle by a leech, *Placobdella catenigera*. Sporozoites introduced by a leech invade red blood corpuscles of the turtle in which they become vermicules; these eventually segment into from 13 to 24 merozoites. Multiplication by asexual reproduction continues in the vertebrate and gameto-cytes are also formed. These, when ingested by a leech, undergo maturation and fertilization in the intestine. In the zygote, or oöcyst, thus formed, 8 sporozoites develop. They break out, make their way into the dorsal blood vessel and are carried into the proboscis of the leech, where they probably enter the proboscis-sheath from which they are transferred to the blood of any turtle attacked by the leech.

3. KARYOLYSUS

The species in this genus are parasites of reptiles. Often they have a karyolytic action on the nucleus of the cells of the host caus-ing it to fragment, hence the genus name. The life-cycle is best known in *K. lacertarum* which lives in the wall lizard, *Lacerta muralis,* and is transmitted by a mite, *Liponyssus saurarum.* Schizogony occurs in the endothelial cells of the vertebrate and gametocytes develop in the red blood corpuscles. These undergo maturation and fertilization in the mite and sporozoites are produced in the oöcyst that develops from the zygote thus formed.

4. "HÆMOGREGARINES" OF MAN

At least five species of "hæmogregarines" have been described from the blood of man. Wenyon (1923, 1926) has critically examined the evidence on which these species are based and concludes that none of them can be regarded as a hæmogregarine. It seems probable, therefore, that hæmogregarines do not parasitize man.

CHAPTER X

HÆMOSPORIDIA EXCLUSIVE OF MALARIAL PARASITES

The hæmosporidia, as the name implies, are sporozoa that live in the blood. They penetrate the blood cells of vertebrates where they pass through schizogony and go through part of their life-cycle in invertebrate hosts where sporogony occurs. The most important species are the malarial parasites of man; a consideration of these will be deferred until the next chapter.

Three families with five genera and a number of doubtful species are considered here.

Family 1. PLASMODIDÆ. Schizogony occurs in the peripheral blood of vertebrates. Genus *Plasmodium.*

Family 2. HÆMOPROTEIDÆ. Gametocytes only occur in the peripheral blood; schizogony takes place somewhere else. Genus *Hæmoproteus.*

Family 3. BABESIDÆ. Minute parasites in erythrocytes. Genera *Babesia* and *Theileria.*

I. *The Genus Hæmoproteus*

The members of this genus live in the endothelial cells of the blood vessels or in the red blood cells of vertebrates. The gametocytes (Figure 48) within the red blood cells are halter-shaped and hence are often known as halteridia. Pigment granules are produced by trophozoites in the red blood cells. It was in *Hæmoproteus* that MacCallum (1898) discovered the formation of microgametes and fertilization which led to the solution of the "exflagellation" phenomena noted by previous investigators in malarial parasites of man.

The best known species of this genus is *H. columbæ,* a parasite of the common pigeon that has been reported from various parts of the world. The life-cycle of this species includes asexual reproduction in the endothelial cells of the blood vessels of the pigeon's lungs and other organs. The trophozoites in the endothelial cells grow to large size, become multinucleate and then segment into large numbers of merozoites. These penetrate red blood cells where they develop into male or female gametocytes. When infected red cells are taken into the stomach of the hippoboscid fly, *Pseudolynchia maura,* the micro-

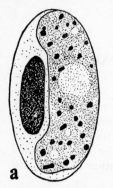 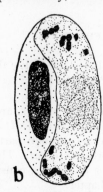

gametocytes continue their development producing a number of filamentous microgametes which ferti- lize the macrogametes that have developed, one from e a c h macrogametocyte. The zygote thus formed becomes a motile vermicu- lous oökinete; this pene- trates the wall of the midgut where pigmented oöcysts are formed (Adie, 1915, 1924). Large num- bers of sporozoites arise within the oöcysts; they

FIG. 48.—*Hæmoproteus columbæ,* in red blood cells of the pigeon. a. Macrogametocyte. b. Microgameto- cyte (x 3900). (After Roudabush and Coatney)

eventually escape and some of them reach the salivary glands where they are ready to be inoculated into the blood of any pigeon that chances to be bitten by the infected fly. This life-cycle, which requires ten to twelve days in the fly, resembles that of malarial parasites. Halteridia occur in a number of other species of birds, and in local- ities where flies of the genus *Pseudolynchia* are absent, hence in these cases the invertebrate transmitting host must belong to some other genus.

Coatney (1936) lists 45 species of *Hæmoproteus* that have been described from birds and reptiles. About 600 species of birds have been found to be infected and about 22 species of reptiles.

Very little is known, however, regarding the life-cycle and trans- mitting agents of these species.

II. *The Genus Leucocytozoön*

The leucocytozoa are parasites of birds, in which they occur in red cells. The characteristic appearance of the gametocytes is that of an oval body in a spindle-shaped cell (Figure 49). Filamentous microgametes develop from the microgametocytes and fertilize the macrogametes; the zygote thus formed becomes an oökinete. Schizog- ony apparently occurs in mononuclear cells in the internal organs or in the plasma and is probably similar to this process in hæmo- proteus. Skidmore (1932) was able to transmit *Leucocytozoön smithi* from infected turkeys to clean turkeys by means of flies of the species

Simulium occidentale which were fed on infected turkeys, then ground up in sterile physiological salt solution, and injected intravenously and subcutaneously into non-infected poults. *Leucocytozoon anatis* is a species that infects both wild and domestic ducks in which it causes serious juvenile losses. Gametocytes which are present in the red blood cells are ingested by the female of the blood-sucking black fly, *Simulium venustum*. Gametogenesis, fertilization and oökinete formation take place in the stomach of the fly. Sporozoites develop in oöcysts on the outer wall of this organ. Merozoites develop into schizonts in the lungs, liver, spleen and kidneys of ducks which have been bitten by infected flies.

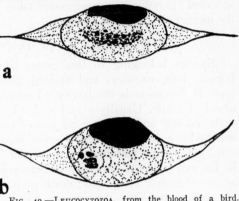

FIG. 49.—LEUCOCYTOZOA, from the blood of a bird. a. Microgametocyte. b. Macrogametocyte. (After Wenyon)

The earliest gametocytes are to be found in the blood cells on the seventh day following the fly bites. On the tenth day the first mature gametocytes are found. Death of a bird may occur at this time but it usually takes place on the twelfth day unless recovery occurs in the meantime. The time required for the different stages in the sexual cycle of the parasite in the fly has not been determined. Observations indicate that it may take place in as short a time as five days. This would allow fifteen days for the entire life-cycle in both the vertebrate and the invertebrate host. There is evidence that all of the merozoites which enter blood cells are capable of developing into gametocytes and that trophozoites do not occur. (O'Roke, 1931.)

A catalog and host-index of the genus *Leucocytozoön* recently published by Coatney (1937) contains the names of 68 species of parasites, all from bird hosts.

III. *Babesidæ (Piroplasmidæ)*

The members of this group parasitize the red blood cells of mammals and are non-pigmented. They reproduce in the red cells by division, usually into two, but sometimes into four daughter parasites. One species, *Babesia (Piroplasma) bigemina,* which causes

Texas fever, or red water fever, in cattle, is of peculiar historical importance because this was the first protozoön whose transmission from host to host was demonstrated to be due to an arthropod; Smith and Kilborne (1893) not only proved that *B. bigemina* is transmitted by ticks of the genus *Margaropus* (*Boöphilus*) but that so-called "hereditary" transmission takes place through the egg from the mother tick to its offspring.

I. THE GENUS BABESIA (PIROPLASMA)

Species belonging to this genus occur in cattle, sheep, goats, horses, dogs, monkeys and various game animals of the ungulate type. *B. bigemina* is the largest of several species that occur in the blood of cattle. Usually a pair of pear-shaped organisms appear in each red cell and as many as 50 per cent of the red cells may be infected in a diseased animal. Reproduction takes place within the red cell by a sort of budding process. Some of the organisms contained in the red cells are probably gametocytes. Infected animals exhibit acute or chronic symptoms; death may occur in a week or ten days or gradual recovery may ensue. Fever, anemia, jaundice and the excretion of urine colored red by the excretion of hæmoglobin by the kidneys are characteristic symptoms. Cattle that recover still carry the parasites in their blood for long periods.

Babesia canis, which is responsible for malignant jaundice in dogs, has been more carefully studied than the other species. It has been reported from many parts of the world including Florida (Eaton, 1934; Sanders, 1937). The parasites resemble *B. bigemina* in appearance; they are about 5 μ long and contain a nucleus from which extends a filament of fine granules and a vacuole. When division occurs, the filament becomes bifurcated at the end; then two bud-like processes appear into which the filaments extend; a vacuole arises in each bud; then the nucleus divides and finally the cell body divides and two pear-shaped daughter cells result. A flagellate form in the blood of dogs has been described.

The cycle in the tick (*Rhipicephalus sanguineus*) has been described by Christophers (1907) and by Shortt (1936) but not all of the stages that occur and their sequence are known with certainty.

The life-cycle of *B. bigemina* in the tick, *Margaropus annulatus,* is illustrated in Figure 50 and described by Dennis (1932) as follows.

When blood which is infected with *B. bigemina* is taken into the gut of the tick, many of the intracorpuscular parasites are soon freed. Certain of these normal-appearing parasites become transformed into gametes through growth and slight structural modification. The gam-

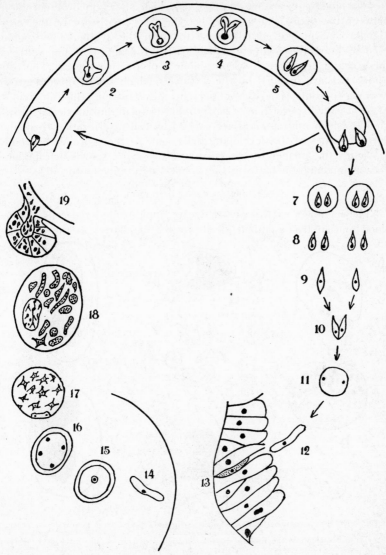

FIG. 50.—Diagram of the life-cycle of *Babesia bigemina*. 1-6, cycle of binary division in the red blood cells of cattle. 7, infected red cells as ingested by tick. 8, trophozoites free in gut of tick. 9, vermicule-like isogametes. 10, union of gametes in a pair. 11, fusion of gametes. 12, motile oökinete. 13, 14, oökinete passes through wall of gut (13) into ovum (14). 15, sporont. 16, 17, formation of sporoblasts. 18, sporokinetes in cell destined to form part of salivary acinus. 19, sporozoites resulting from fragmentation of sporokinetes, in acinus of salivary gland of larval tick, ready to be transferred to a new host. (After Dennis)

etes are motile vermicule-like bodies which show no differentiation between the sexes. The gametes become associated in pairs, the individuals of which eventually fuse to form the zygote. The zygote becomes a motile oökinete which passes through the thin wall of the gut and penetrates the contiguous reproductive organs. The ova of the tick are invaded by the oökinetes which round up and grow to form sporonts. The sporont secretes a cyst within which it divides to form naked sporoblasts. The sporoblasts form multinucleate sporokinetes which migrate, and are carried by cell proliferation throughout the tissues of the developing tick; some of the sporokinetes come to occupy the anlagen of the salivary glands. The sporokinete undergoes fragmentation to form the minute infectious sporozoites.

2. THE GENUS THEILERIA

The members of this genus live in unpigmented red cells in the blood and in the endothelial cells of the capillaries in the internal

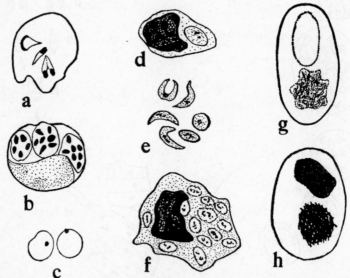

FIG. 51.—HÆMOSPORIDIA. a. *Theileria parva*, in red blood cell of a calf. b. *T. parva*, in a lymphocyte of a calf. c. *Anaplasma marginale*, in red blood cells of an ox. d, e, f. *Toxoplasma paddæ*, from the English sparrow: d, in leucocyte from bone marrow; e, spores from the liver; f, in leucocyte from liver. g, h. *Cytamœba bacterifera*, in red blood cells of the frog: g, as it appears in the living cells; h, after staining. (a, b, after Cowdry and Danks; c, after Theiler; d, e, f, after Herman; g, h, after Hegner)

organs. They occur in cattle, the best known species being *Theileria parva* (Figure 51a, b) and have been reported from sheep and goats but appear to be rare in these animals.

Theileria parva causes a disease in cattle, known as East Coast fever, that occurs in Africa and to a lesser extent in Asia. The anemia, jaundice and hæmoglobinuria, characteristic of infections with *B. bigemina,* are absent in this disease; furthermore, cattle that have recovered from infections with *B. bigemina* are not immune to *T. parva.* From 80 per cent to 90 per cent of the red cells may be parasitized in infected animals. The organisms are mostly oval or rod-shaped. Schizogony, which occurs in the endothelial cells of capillaries in the lymphatic glands, spleen and other organs, results in the production of large numbers of minute merozoites which break out of the parasitized cells and either penetrate other endothelial cells and repeat the schizogonic cycle or else parasitize red cells. When an animal recovers, the organisms completely disappear from the body. *T. parva* is transmitted by ticks of the genus *Rhipicephalus.* The cycle in the tick appears to be similar to that of *B. canis* in its intermediate host.

IV. *Doubtful Species of Hæmosporidia*

A large number of bodies resembling protozoa have been described from the blood of man and lower animals and included in this group. Their exact nature still remains to be determined. Three genera may be mentioned here: *Toxoplasma, Cytamœba* and *Anaplasma.*

I. TOXOPLASMA

This genus was proposed (Nicolle and Manceaux, 1909) for a parasite discovered in a North African rodent. The organism is crescent shaped and from 4 μ to 6 μ in length (Figure 51d, e, f). Reproduction is by longitudinal binary division and schizogony has also been described. Bodies supposed to represent species belonging to this genus have been reported in various species of mammals and birds and one species, *T. pyrogenes* (Castellani, 1914), has been reported from the blood and spleen of man. The exact status of these bodies is yet to be determined. Recently toxoplasmas have been reported from North American birds by Manwell and Herman (1935), and the latter (Herman, 1937) suggests that the avian forms all belong to one species, *T. paddæ,* and the mammalian forms to another species, *T. gondi.*

2. CYTAMŒBA

The name *Cytamœba bacterifera* was applied by Labbé (1894) to bodies that occur in the red blood cells of European frogs. Similar bodies occur in the red blood cells of *Rana clamitans* and *R. cates-beiana* of North America (Hegner, 1921). They are located at one end of the red cell and, in freshly drawn blood, exhibit amœboid changes in shape (Figure 51g, h). After a few minutes they become spherical. Within them are many rod-shaped, actively moving bodies named *Bacillus krusei* by Laveran (1899). The nature and systematic position of these bodies are doubtful.

3. ANAPLASMA

Theiler (1910) applied the name *Anaplasma marginale* (Figure 51c) to minute spherical bodies that appear near the margin of the red cells of cattle suffering from infection with *Babesia bigemina* and considered them to be protozoa consisting entirely of chromatin. Similar bodies have been noted in the red blood cells of other animals.

Anaplasma occurs in cattle in scattered areas over the United States. It may be transmitted by several species of ticks, including *Boöphilus annulatus, Rhipicephalus sanguineus, Dermacentor variabilis, D. andersoni* and *Ixodes scapularis* (Rees, 1934), as well as mechanically by biting flies, such as *Tabanus æquales, Chrysops sequax* and *Stomoxys calcitrans.*

CHAPTER XI

MALARIAL PARASITES OF MAN

I. *Introduction*

The three species of malarial parasites that live in man belong to the genus *Plasmodium* and to the family PLASMODIDÆ. Besides these, there are a number of other species belonging to the same genus and family that parasitize species of mammals, birds and lizards. The morphology and life-cycles of all of the different species of plasmodia are similar. There is an asexual cycle in a vertebrate host and a sexual cycle in an invertebrate vector. Malaria is the most important disease of man due to an animal parasite. It is the most important of all diseases in many tropical and semitropical countries. It must be eradicated from these localities before they can be developed, hence the economic phases of malariology are of particular interest.

II. *The Discovery of the Malarial Parasites in Man and Mosquito*

Many theories were proposed to account for the symptoms that accompany malaria before the real etiological agent was discovered by Laveran in Algeria in 1880. At the time Laveran made his discovery the attention of scientific men was largely directed toward the so-called *Bacillus malariæ* which Klebs and Tomassi-Crudeli had announced as the causative organism of malaria. Thus, although the real parasite was described in 1880, it was not until 1885 that students in general accepted Laveran's work. In that year March'afava and Celli gave the name *Plasmodium malariæ* to the organism of quartan malaria. The species name *vivax* was given to the tertian parasite by Grassi and Feletti in 1890 and that of *falciparum* to the estivo-autumnal parasite by Welch in 1897. Golgi, who distinguished the different types of malarial parasites, described in 1885 and 1886 the asexual cycle of the quartan parasite in the blood of man and later the asexual cycle of the tertian parasite. Golgi also realized the significance of the presence of crescents in the blood and recognized the third type of malaria due to *Plasmodium falciparum*.

The discovery of the sexual cycle of malarial parasites in mosquitoes was due to the prediction by Sir Patrick Manson (1894) that malaria would be found to be transmitted by mosquitoes and to the investigations of Sir Ronald Ross. Ross did his work in India. He observed in 1895 the formation of gametes from crescents in the stomach of the mosquito, a process then known as exflagellation, the significance of which was not realized until 1897 when MacCallum proved it to be a maturation process followed by the fertilization of female gametes. Oöcysts were found by Ross in 1897 in the stomach of a mosquito that had fed on infected human blood. In the following year Ross (1898) worked out the whole life-cycle of the organism of bird malaria in culex mosquitoes. Circumstances over which he had no control prevented Ross from completing the stages of the sexual cycle of human malarial organisms in mosquitoes; this was done by Grassi, Bignami and Bastianelli (1898) in the same year, but after Ross's results on bird malaria had been published. These Italians succeeded in infecting three men by allowing infected mosquitoes to bite them, and Manson in 1900 infected a man in London by means of mosquitoes imported from Italy, thus finally demonstrating the rôle of the mosquito as the transmitting agent of malaria.

III. *The Asexual Cycle of the Malarial Parasites in Man*

I. PLASMODIUM VIVAX

The three species of human malarial organisms differ in their life-cycles in minor details only. For this reason a rather full account of the tertian parasite, *Plasmodium vivax,* will be presented, followed by briefer descriptions indicating the differences between this and the other two species.

Sporozoite. The stage in the asexual cycle that is inoculated into human beings by the bite of an infected mosquito is a sporozoite. This is spindle-shaped, 10 μ to 12 μ in length and 1 μ to 2 μ in breadth, and contains an oval nucleus (Figure 52, *1*). The sporozoites apparently penetrate the red blood corpuscles by means of boring movements (Figure 53a, b, c). Several thousand of them are probably inoculated during the bite of a mosquito but many of these are no doubt destroyed by phagocytes.

Trophozoite. Within the red cell the organism changes into an amœboid hyaline body known as a trophozoite (Figure 52, *2*). This throws out pseudopodia actively, hence the specific name *vivax.* The trophozoite grows at the expense of the cytoplasm in the corpuscle

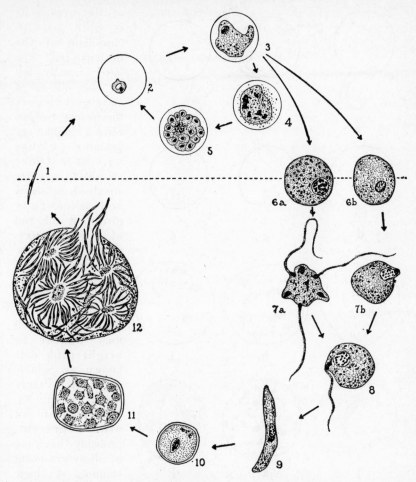

FIG. 52.—Life-cycle of the tertian malarial parasite, *Plasmodium vivax*. The stages above the dotted line occur in the peripheral blood of man, whereas those below are found only in the mosquito. 1, Sporozoite. 2, Trophozoite, in red cell. 3, Full-grown schizont. 4, Schizont with chromatin in several masses. 5, Segmentation stage. 6a, Male gametocyte. 6b, Female gametocyte. 7a. Exflagellation of male gametocyte—formation of microgametes. 7b, Female gametocyte extruding chromatin from nucleus. 8, Fertilization of macrogamete by microgamete. 9, Oökinete. 10, Young oöcyst. 11, Oöcyst with many nuclei. 12, Ripe oöcyst discharging sporozoites. (After Hegner and Cort)

and as it becomes larger the infected cell increases in size (Figure 54, A*2*). Pigment granules, which represent the by-products of the digestion of hæmoglobin, appear within the parasite in about six to eight hours. When stained by the Romanowsky method the cytoplasm

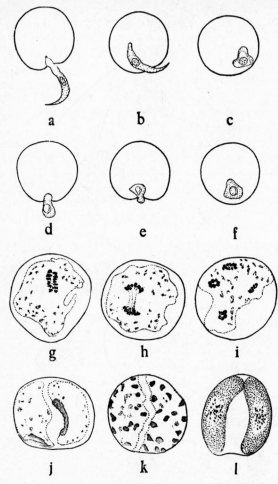

of the trophozoite is blue and the chromatin of the nucleus red. The latter usually lies at one side of a vacuole which gives the young trophozoite a ringlike appearance (Figure 54, A1). Older trophozoites are amœboid in shape and when fully grown at the end of forty hours, practically fill the enlarged red cell (Figure 53, g). Degeneration spots in the protoplasm of the parasitized cell may appear as bright pink dots known as Schüffner's dots (Figure 52, 4; Figure 54, A2); these are not always present, probably because of idiosyncrasies in staining. A single red cell may be parasitized by more than one trophozoite, especially when large numbers are present (Figure 53j, k, l).

FIG. 53.—Malarial parasites of man. (a-i, after Schaudinn; j, k, after Thomson and Woodcock; l, after Manson-Bahr)

   a, b, c. Sporozoite penetrating a red cell.
   d, e, f. Trophozoite penetrating a red cell.
   g, h, i. Schizont undergoing nuclear division.
   j. Two macrogametocytes in a single red cell.
   k. Two schizonts, ready to segment, in a single red cell.
   l. Two gametocytes (crescents) in a single red cell.

Schizogony. A trophozoite may become a sexual stage (gametocyte) or an asexual stage (schizont). The full-grown schizont is 8 μ to 10 μ in diameter (Figure 52, 3; 54, A2). Its nucleus, by successive divisions (Figure 53g, h, i), produces from fifteen to twenty-four daughter nuclei. Each daughter nucleus with a portion of the cytoplasm is then cut off as a minute cell known as a merozoite, and the pigment granules become aggregated near the center of the schizont (Figure 52, 5; Figure 54, A3). Then the infected red cell breaks down, liberating the merozoites, pigment granules and the remains of the red cell into the blood stream. It is possible that toxins elaborated by the parasite are also liberated at this time and are partly responsible for the symptoms of chills and fever.

The liberated merozoites penetrate fresh red corpuscles (Figure 53e, f, g) and repeat the asexual cycle, which requires a period of forty-eight hours. In the case of *P. vivax*, young red cells are usually invaded. The pigment granules are engulfed by leukocytes and carried to the internal organs, especially the spleen, liver and brain. Asexual reproduction continues as long as a host is parasitized, and, when a sufficient number of parasites are present, a number estimated by Ross (1911) as 150,000,000, symptoms are exhibited by the patient.

Whether the trophozoite is within or attached to the outside of the red blood corpuscle is a problem that has been under discussion for many years. Most observers believe that the parasite penetrates and lives within the red cell, but a few believe that the parasite is attached to the outside. The work of Ratcliffe (1927) involving the fixation and sectioning of infected blood of both man and bird seems to prove conclusively that the malarial organism is intracellular and not extracellular.

The penetration of a single red cell (Figure 53j, k, l) by two or more parasites is not as common in the case of *Plasmodium vivax* as in that of *P. falciparum* where it occurs so frequently as to be of diagnostic value. Double or triple infections with *P. vivax* are also frequent; that is, two or three groups of parasites may live in a single host at the same time, undergoing schizogony on different days and thus bringing on symptoms at more frequent intervals than usual.

Gametocytes. Some of the parasites that penetrate the red blood cells do not undergo schizogony, but develop into sexual stages known as gametocytes (Figure 52, 6a, 6b; Figure 54, A4). These are unable to develop into gametes in the body of the vertebrate host, but degenerate in time if they are not sucked up into the stomach of a mosquito. Gametocytes usually appear in the blood after several generations of merozoites have been produced. They may be distinguished from schizonts, and macrogametocytes and microgametocytes may be separated on the basis of morphology. The macro-

gametocytes are from 13 μ to 16 μ in diameter; the cytoplasm stains
a dark blue; the chromatin consists of a small compact mass excen-
trically placed and the pigment consists of long rods. The microgametocytes are 9 μ to 11 μ in diameter; the cytoplasm stains light blue;
the chromatin consists of a large diffuse mass centrally located; and
the pigment is in small rods.

2. PLASMODIUM MALARIÆ

The asexual cycle of *Plasmodium malariæ*, the organism of
quartan malaria, differs from that of *P. vivax* in the following
respects. The entire period from the penetration of the red cell to
the liberation of merozoites is seventy-two instead of forty-eight
hours. The infected red cell is approximately normal in size and no
degeneration spots such as Schüffner's dots appear (Figure 54, B).
The schizont is small and so frequently quadrilateral in shape as to
be of diagnostic importance (Figure 54, B2). Pigment occurs within
the organism in the form of large irregular granules. The merozoites
number from six to twelve; they are often arranged in a single
rosette with the pigment granules in the center (Figure 54, B3). The
gametocytes are similar in appearance to those of *P. vivax* but much
smaller (Figure 54, B4). As in *P. vivax,* one red cell may contain
several parasites, but this is comparatively rare. Also one host may
be infected with two or more groups of parasites, due to inoculation
by mosquitoes on different days; hence clinical symptoms may appear
at shorter intervals than seventy-two hours. Apparently there is no
antagonism between groups of parasites belonging to the same species or to different species, since a single host may be infected with
P. vivax and *P. malariæ* at the same time.

3. PLASMODIUM FALCIPARUM

P. falciparum, the organism of estivo-autumnal malaria, has an
asexual cycle of from twenty-four to forty-eight hours. It is believed
by some (Craig, 1921) that two distinct varieties of *P. falciparum*
exist differing in the length of the asexual cycle. The size of red
cells infected with *P. falciparum* is approximately normal (Figure
54, C). Spots known as Maurer's dots, which stain a brick red, may
be present in the cytoplasm of the infected cells (Figure 54, C2).
The schizont is small and more or less circular in outline. The pigment granules are smaller than those of *P. malariæ* and irregular in
shape. Schizogony occurs almost entirely in the capillaries of internal
organs and segmenting parasites are not numerous in the peripheral
blood. From eight to ten or more merozoites are produced by a single

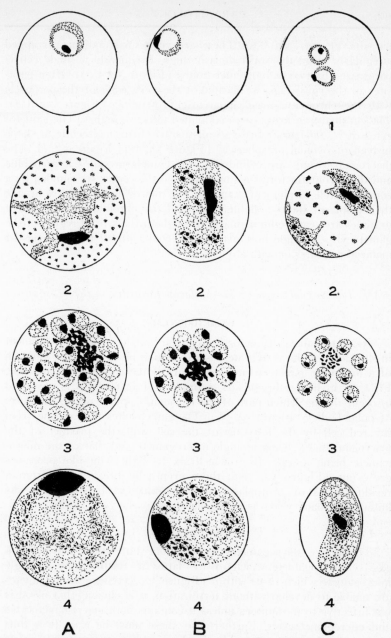

FIG. 54.—Four stages in the life-cycle of each of the three malarial parasites of man illustrating characteristics of diagnostic importance. (After Hegner and Cort)
A. *Plasmodium vivax.* 1, Ring stage; 2, schizont; 3, segmenter; 4, gametocyte.
B. *P. malariæ.* 1, Ring stage; 2, schizont; 3, segmenter; 4, gametocyte.
C. *P. falciparum.* 1, Ring stage; 2, schizont; 3, segmenter; 4, gametocyte.

parasite (Figure 54, C3). These are very small and are arranged irregularly or in the form of two rings. Frequently a single cell is parasitized by two or more merozoites (Figure 54, C2). Often parasites in the ring stage are located at the very edge of the corpuscle with the chromatin mass apparently protruding (Figure 54, C2). The chromatin in many cases is divided into two bodies. The gametocytes of *P. falciparum* are very distinctive, being crescentic in shape instead of ovoidal or spherical (Figure 54, C4; Figure 53, *l*). The macrogametocytes are cylindrical; the cytoplasm stains a deep blue and the chromatin forms a single mass in the center surrounded by a compact circle of pigment granules. The microgametocytes are broad; the cytoplasm stains a lighter blue and the chromatin and pigment granules are scattered irregularly throughout the central region of the gametocyte. A single host may be infected with all three species of malarial parasites or with any two of them.

IV. *The Sexual Cycle of the Malarial Parasites in the Mosquito*

1. GAMETOGENESIS

As stated above, gametocytes cannot complete their development in the blood of the vertebrate host. In drawn blood or in the stomach of a mosquito gamete formation occurs if the gametocytes are ripe. First, as in higher organisms, a process of maturation is supposed to occur during which part of the chromatin is cast out in the form of polar bodies (Figure 52, 7b). The gametocytes then escape from the red cell by the bursting of the cell wall, the product of the macrogametocyte being a single macrogamete and that of the microgamete being a body from which six to eight whip-like processes grow out (Figure 52, 7a); these eventually break away from a residual mass of protoplasm as microgametes. This process was known for many years as exflagellation.

2. FERTILIZATION

The active microgametes swim about until they encounter a passive macrogamete. Each of the latter is fertilized by a single microgamete which fuses with it (Figure 52, 8). Since macrogametes are unable to develop without fertilization, it is obvious that blood is not infective to mosquitoes unless it contains both macrogametocytes and microgametocytes. Furthermore, these must be ripe. It is thus evident that hosts in whose blood only one type of gametocyte exists are not dangerous as reservoirs of infection. Cases are on record of such hosts. As is pointed out in Section III of this book, only a comparatively few species of mosquitoes of the genus *Anopheles* are capable of transmitting malaria. Huff (1927) has shown that fertilization occurs in mosquitoes that do not transmit malaria but that the later stages of the sexual cycle do not occur.

3. SPOROGONY

The zygote, which results from the fusion of a microgamete with a macrogamete, soon becomes elongated and active and is then known as an oökinete or vermicule (Figure 52, *9*). The oökinete makes its way to the stomach wall by gliding movements resembling those of gregarines, penetrates the tissues and becomes located between the outer epithelial layer and the muscular layers of the stomach wall. Here it becomes a spherical oöcyst (Figure 52, *10*). The period from the ingestion by the mosquito to the oöcyst stage occupies about forty hours. The oöcyst obtains nutrition from the tissue in which it lies and grows from an original size of from 12 μ to 14 μ in diameter to 50 μ to 60 μ in diameter. There may be as many as five hundred oöcysts in the stomach wall of a single mosquito.

The nucleus of the fully grown oöcyst produces by successive divisions from twenty to thirty daughter nuclei; then vacuoles appear which eventually become connected in such a way as to divide the cytoplasm into irregular masses (Figure 52, *11*). Projections grow out from these masses which become spindle shaped and in each of which is a nucleus; thus the sporozoites are developed (Figure 52, *12*). It requires four or five days for the fully grown oöcyst to produce sporozoites. From several hundred to as many as ten thousand sporozoites may develop within a single oöcyst.

Eventually the oöcyst bursts and the sporozoites are liberated into the body cavity. They are carried about in the blood stream to all parts of the body, many of them finding their way into the salivary glands where they lie ready to be injected into the next man or animal bitten by the mosquito.

The sexual cycles of the three species of malarial parasites of man are similar in most respects. Different species of mosquitoes, however, differ with regard to their susceptibility to infection with the different species of parasites. The parasites differ also in the length of the period from the time gametocytes are ingested by the mosquito to the liberation of the sporozoite. The optimum temperature for the development of the three species within the mosquito also differs. For example, *Plasmodium vivax* passes through its sexual cycle in eight or nine days at 25° C. to 30° C., *P. malariæ* in from eighteen to twenty-one days at 22° C., and *P. falciparum* in ten to twelve days at 30° C.

V. *Host-Parasite Relations*

1. TRANSMISSION

The malarial parasites of man are transmitted in nature only by certain species of mosquitoes belonging to the genus *Anopheles* (see Section III). Apparently lower animals, with the possible exception of certain monkeys, cannot be infected with human malarial parasites (Bass, 1922), hence there are no animal reservoirs of these organisms, and mosquitoes can only become infected by ingesting blood from parasitized human beings.

2. PARASITOLOGICAL AND CLINICAL PERIODS

The prepatent period in a malarial infection depends on the method of study. Ross (1911) has estimated that if 150,000,000 parasites are present in an average human being it would require from ten to fifteen minutes to find a specimen in a thin film. If one thousand sporozoites are inoculated by a mosquito, and ten merozoites from each segmenting schizont succeed in infecting fresh red cells at the end of each asexual cycle, it would require twelve days to produce as many as 150,000,000 parasites; twelve days may thus be considered the length of the prepatent period, although this period obviously would be shorter if a larger number of sporozoites were inoculated by a mosquito, and longer in the case of *P. malariæ* than in *P. vivax* because the asexual cycle in *P. malariæ* occupies a greater length of time. The length of the patent period varies greatly depending on many factors, including the physiological condition of the host and whether or not treatment is given. Usually parasites eventually become so few in number that they are very difficult to find during the subpatent period, but the host is subject to other patent periods at intervals which correspond to periods of relapse. A host once infected may remain infected for many years.

The incubation period of tertian malaria is from fourteen to eighteen days, of quartan malaria from eighteen to twenty-one days, and of estivo-autumnal malaria from nine to twelve days. As noted above, symptoms appear when about 150,000,000 parasites are present and continue for periods that vary in length in different individuals. If the patient recovers with or without the aid of a therapeutic agent, a latent period ensues to be followed frequently by one or more periods of relapse.

TABLE III.

Differential Diagnosis of Human Malarial Parasites (Stained Preparations)

Species	Plasmodium vivax	Plasmodium malariæ	Plasmodium falciparum
Type of Fever	Tertian (benign tertian)	Quartan	Malignant tertian (Estivo-Autumnal, Subtertian)
Length of asexual cycle in man	48 hours	72 hours	24-48 hours
Size of infected cell	Greater than normal	Approximately normal	Approximately normal
Dots in infected cell	Schüffner's dots	None	Maurer's dots
Shape of schizont	Circular in outline	Quadrilateral	Circular
Size of schizont	Large	Intermediate	Small
Size and shape of pigment granules	Short rods	Large, irregular	Smaller, irregular
Number of merozoites	15 to 24	6 to 12	8 to 10 or more
Arrangement of merozoites	Two rings or irregular	One ring, a rosette	Two rings or irregular
Shape of gametocytes	Ovoidal or spherical	Ovoidal or spherical	Crescentic

3. DISTRIBUTION AND LOCALIZATION WITHIN THE HOST

The malarial organisms are primarily intracellular parasites although they are free in the blood in the sperozoite and merozoite stages, and in the body of the mosquito during part of the sexual cycle. They are distributed throughout the human body in the blood stream and are as abundant in the blood vessels of the internal organs as in those of the peripheral circulation. *P. falciparum* is peculiar in that the segmenting stages are, for some unknown reason, retained in the internal organs. They are especially abundant in the spleen, liver, brain, bone marrow and placenta.

4. SYMPTOMS

One of the most conspicuous characteristics of malaria is its periodicity. The most prominent symptoms are chills and fever occurring every twenty-four, forty-eight, or seventy-two hours, depending on the species. The typical paroxysm consists of a chill, during which the skin is cold, the pulse weak and the lips blue, a rise in temperature accompanied by hot, dry skin, flushed face, strong pulse and thirst, and a decrease in temperature which is the sweating stage, and ends in apparent recovery. After a series of attacks with high temperature, the temperature at each attack becomes lower until symptoms cease.

5. PATHOLOGY

Three of the primary characteristics of malaria are pathological in nature. These are the deposition of pigment in the tissues, enlargement of the spleen and anemia. The last named condition is due to the destruction of red blood cells during schizogony and possibly to the reproduction by the parasites of a hæmolytic agent. There is a reduction in hæmoglobin corresponding to the reduction in number of the red cells. The pigment granules, which escape when the parasitized red cells break down, are engulfed by leucocytes and distributed throughout the body, but especially to the spleen, liver, brain and bone marrow. This pigment occurs in no other disease. The enlargement of the spleen in human beings infected with malarial organisms is a characteristic of diagnostic value since the disease and its severity may often be judged by the extent of this enlargement. The swelling is due to distention with blood as a result of lowered vascular tone. The spleen filters out pigment and the remains of infected red cells. The liver also commonly becomes enlarged during an attack of malaria. In infections with *P. falciparum* there is a mechanical mass-ing of parasites and pigment in the capillaries of the cerebrum and other organs.

6. IMMUNITY

Immunity to malaria may apparently be acquired by frequent infection and reinfection. In highly malarious countries children become infected and exhibit symptoms but those who survive and reach the age of about ten years, although still infected, do not exhibit symptoms. Immunity of this type can also be established in adults by frequent inoculation with blood containing *P. vivax,* the degree of immunity acquired varying directly with the number of inoculations and the strain of parasite used. Results of this sort have been obtained in experiments on the effects of malaria on patients suffering from general paralysis.

In both bird malaria and human malaria the strain of parasite used is of the greatest importance, since in some cases as long as parasites of a certain strain are present in a host, that host cannot be reinfected with the same strain, but a superinfection may be secured with another strain belonging to the same species.

Apparently the destruction of parasites within the host is due largely to the phagocytes, known as macrophages, that live on the walls of the blood-vessels of the internal organs. The spleen seems to be especially important since if this organ is removed from a monkey that has acquired immunity, an attack of malaria develops at once. An instructive discusion of this subject is furnished by Hackett (1937).

7. LATENCY, RELAPSE AND THE CARRIER CONDITION

Latency. We may distinguish two types of latency in malarial infections, primary latency, which is often simply an extended period of incubation, and secondary latency, which represents the periods between relapses. The period of primary latency may extend over months or even years, the parasites, because of lack of virulence or a natural resistance of the host, being unable to increase in numbers sufficiently to bring about symptoms. During periods of secondary latency, a few parasites remain in the body, where they continue to reproduce asexually, but appear to be destroyed in large numbers by the resistance of the host. Both types of latency may end as a result of a change in climate or exposure to cold, inebriation and other factors that tend to lower resistance. In some cases infected persons show slight symptoms but are able to be about; they are said to be suffering from ambulatory malaria.

Relapse. As indicated in the diagram (page 13) latent periods are ordinarily followed by periods of relapse. Relapses occur in all three types of human malaria, often in from one to three weeks after the end of the primary attack. Over half of the patients suffering from quartan malaria experience relapses, slightly less than half of the patients suffering from tertian malaria and about one fourth of those with estivo-autumnal malaria. Longer periods of latency, sometimes called recurrences, are characteristic later in the course of the disease. These range from a few months to a year or more.

There are a number of theories to account for relapse but the one that seems to be correct is that asexual reproduction occurs during the latent periods at the same rate as during the incubation period and period of symptoms, but that the resistance of the host is sufficient to destroy most of the parasites but not all of them. Relapse is of great importance in the control of malaria since in many regions mosquitoes do not remain infected throughout the winter season but become reinfected in the spring from persons suffering from relapse who have large numbers of gametocytes in their blood. If all of the parasites could be eliminated from the human host there would be no reservoir from which the mosquito could become infected and malaria would, therefore, cease to exist in certain localities.

Carriers. Two types of carriers may be recognized among human beings infected with malaria. Potential carriers are those in whose blood parasites occur in such small numbers as to be non-infective to mosquitoes. Active carriers, on the other hand, have a sufficient number of ripe gametocytes of both sexes to bring about infection in mosquitoes. The number of carriers in a malaria district is indicated by the figures obtained by Bass (1919), who found in Bolivar County, Mississippi, during 1916 to 1917, 6,664, out of 31,459 persons examined, to be infected. About 45 per cent of those infected had no symptoms when examined and had had no symptoms during the previous year. A carrier in whose blood there are few gametocytes is not as infective to mosquitoes as one containing large numbers of gametocytes.

VI. *Treatment, Prevention and Control*

I. TREATMENT

Several therapeutic agents are of importance in the treatment of malaria. The best known of these is quinine, which is derived from the bark of a tree, and the curative powers of which were discovered by the Indians of Peru and became known to the Spaniards about 1600. Quinine may be administered by mouth, by intravenous injection or by intramuscular injection. It is quickly absorbed into the blood but its method of destroying the malarial parasites is not known with certainty; it may kill the parasite directly or act through the body of the host.

The second therapeutic agent, known as plasmochin, was derived from quinoline and tested on birds infected with malaria. This drug is especially effective against benign tertian and quartian infections but not so destructive to *P. falciparum*. It is especially active against gametocytes which are destroyed long before the schizonts are affected. Plasmochin is rather toxic, hence it is often given in combination with quinine.

More recently a third drug, known as atebrin, has been synthesized which is now being used as a therapeutic agent. It attacks particularly the schizonts of all three species of human parasites. The student is referred to recent books and journals for methods of administratio.

2. PREVENTION AND CONTROL

Malaria depends for its existence on the presence of (1) certain species of mosquitoes and (2) human gametocyte carriers. Individuals may protect themselves from infection by screening the houses in which they sleep or in other ways preventing infected mosquitoes from biting them. Prophylactic doses of quinine, plasmochin or atebrin may prevent the appearance of symptoms even if parasites are inoculated by mosquitoes. Communities may be protected either by antimosquito measures (see Section III), or by the elimination of human carriers. The latter involves attacks on the parasite in the body of the host. The use of quinine, plasmochin and atebrin has not been very successful in sterilizing carriers.

There are many difficulties involved in the sterilization of malaria carriers. Our methods of detecting the carrier condition are not entirely satisfactory; carriers when once detected are not always willing to take the proper treatment, and no treatment has yet been devised that will eliminate all of the parasites from the body with certainty. What is neded more than anything else is a therapeutic agent that will destroy *all* of the parasites in the human host and thus prevent the carrier condition.

VII. *Therapeutic Malaria*

No account of the malarial parasites of man would be complete without at least a brief statement of their use in therapeutics. Wagner von Jauregg of Vienna, in 1887, suggested the use of malaria for treating general paralysis, but it was not until 1917 that he actually inoculated nine patients suffering from this disease with blood containing *Plasmodium vivax*. The favorable results obtained led to further inoculations in 1919. Since then many hospitals in various parts of the world have introduced malaria treatment with considerable success. The patient is infected and allowed to pass through from five to twelve febrile attacks. He is then treated with a drug. Many new facts regarding malaria in man have been secured as a result of the study of therapeutic malaria, since the exact time when the patient becomes infected can be controlled and various other factors determined.

VIII. *Methods of Obtaining and Preparing Malarial Parasites for Study*

I. LIVING SPECIMENS

If fresh blood from a patient suffering from malaria is placed under a cover-glass and examined at once with a compound microscope the parasites can be seen within the red cells. The older stages can be detected because of the presence of pigment granules, which are reddish brown in color, are actively motile in *P. vivax*, slightly motile in *P. malariæ*, and feebly motile in *P. falciparum*. Living trophozoites can be seen to throw out pseudopodia, those of *P. vivax* and *P. falciparum* being more actively amœboid than those of *P. malariæ*. If blood containing considerable numbers of gametocytes is examined under a cover-glass the formation of microgametes may occur within a few minutes, followed by the process of fertilization and the change of the spherical zygote into a vermicular oökinete.

2. CULTIVATION

Malarial organisms were first cultivated *in vitro* by Bass (1911) and Bass and Johns (1912). Blood containing malarial organisms was defibrinated and 0.1 c.c. of a 50 per cent solution of dextrose added to each 10 c.c. of blood. The mixture was placed in test-tubes and incubated at 40° C. Subcultures were made by centrifuging the cultures so as to throw the red cells to the bottom, thus freeing them from the leucocytes, and transferring the red cells to fresh culture tubes. Three asexual generations were obtained in this way by Bass and Johns. More refined methods of cultivation have been described by Row (1917) and Sinton (1922) but very little has been added to our knowledge of malaria by this means.

3. STAINED SPECIMENS

Malarial organisms are usually studied in blood films dried on slides and stained with Romanowsky stain. Films are of two types, thin and thick. Thin films are made as follows: the ear lobe or end of the finger is punctured with a Hagedorn needle and a drop of blood obtained one half inch from the end of a slide. Another slide is at once applied to this drop and drawn along, thus spreading the blood out into a thin film. This is then allowed to dry. If Wright's or Leishman's stain is used the film is covered with a few drops of stain and one minute later double the volume of distilled water is added; five minutes later this is washed off and the film is dried in the air. The cytoplasm of the parasite is stained blue and the chromatin red by this method. The pigment remains unstained. If Giemsa's stain is used the film is fixed in absolute methyl alcohol for five minutes; washed gently; and then one part of Giemsa plus ten parts of distilled water added for ten minutes. When washed and dried the parasites are stained as in Wright's or Leishman's stains.

Thick films are of value especially in detecting the presence of parasites, but the species of parasite is more difficult to determine than in thin films. Four drops of blood are obtained near the center of a slide and spread over an area of about one half of a square inch. When dried it is decolorized in 95 per cent alcohol, plus 2 per cent HCl for thirty minutes; washed for a few minutes and then stained with Wright's stain as described above. This method concentrates the parasites in a small area and hence a shorter length of time is required to find a specimen.

CHAPTER XII

MALARIAL PARASITES OF LOWER ANIMALS

I. *Malarial Parasites of Monkeys*

Malarial parasites were first detected in monkeys by Koch in 1898 and named *Plasmodium kochi* by Laveran in 1899. Since then at least seven more new specific names have been applied to malarial organisms reported from monkeys. Among the species of monkeys found to be infected are the chimpanzee, gorilla and orang-utan, several other species of Old World monkeys and several species of New World monkeys. Of particular interest is the fact that parasites resembling the three species that occur in man have been found in the chimpanzee and gorilla (Reichenow, 1917, 1920). Attempts have been made to determine whether these are identical with the human species, with conflicting results. For example, Mesnil and Roubaud (1920) claim to have infected one of two chimpanzees by the intravenous inoculation of human blood containing *P. vivax*. These investigators failed to infect a chimpanzee by means of bites of *Anopheles* mosquitoes infected with *Plasmodium falciparum*. Failure to infect a young chimpanzee with human blood containing *P. falciparum* has been reported by Blacklock and Adler (1924). The same authors in 1922 also failed to infect two human beings and an Anopheles mosquito with blood from an infected chimpanzee.

Recently a species of malaria has been discovered in monkeys that will live in human beings and is even being used for the treatment of general paralysis. This is *P. knowlesi* from the Malayan monkey, *Macacus irus*. For experimental studies *P. knowlesi* is very valuable. It occurs in *Macacus irus* in nature in Malaya and Java and produces a mild infection in this species of monkey. However, when transferred to *Macacus rhesus* a serious infection is induced which invariably ends fatally if treatment is not administered. *Macacus irus* is also infected in nature with another species of parasite, *P. inui*, which produced a mild infection in both *Macacus irus* and *M. rhesus* (Knowles and Das Gupta, 1934). No cross-immunity exists between these two species of malarial parasites.

ASEXUAL CYCLE

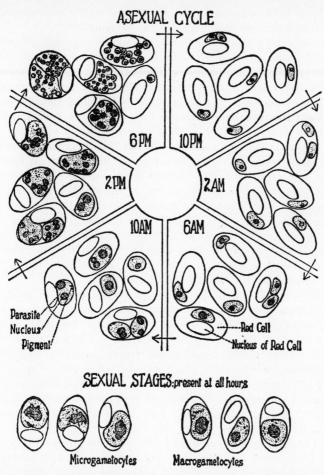

6 PM | 10 PM
2 PM | 2 AM
10 AM | 6 AM

Parasite
Nucleus
Pigment

----Red Cell
Nucleus of Red Cell

SEXUAL STAGES: present at all hours

Microgametocytes   Macrogametocytes

FIG. 55.—Diagrams representing the cycle of reproduction in bird malaria showing changes in size and variability. The outlines of the asexual stages (x 1500) of the parasites within the red cells, showing nuclei and pigment granules, were made at four-hour intervals during a consecutive period of twenty-four hours. Below are shown outlines of three microgametocytes and three macrogametocytes, which occur in small numbers at all hours throughout the infection. (After Taliaferro)

II. *Malarial Parasites of Birds*

That malarial parasites exist in birds has been known since 1890 (Grassi and Feletti). The name *Plasmodium præcox* has usually been applied to the organism, but other specific names for parasites that have been found in various species of birds in different parts of the world have been suggested, and Hartman (1927) and others have demonstrated that about ten species are recognizable.

The malarial parasites of birds are of considerable interest because they were used by Ross in working out the sexual cycle of malarial parasites in mosquitoes. They are also of great value for purposes of teaching and investigation since they can be transmitted easily from wild birds to captive canaries by blood inoculation, and when the latter are once infected they appear to remain infected throughout their lives. The method of procedure is to prick a vein in the leg and suck up a drop of blood into a syringe containing normal saline solution. This is then injected into the breast muscle or leg vein of a fresh bird. The average length of the prepatent period is about five days. The period of rise in the number of parasites is also about five days when from ten to 5,000 parasites per 10,000 red cells are present. Then a rapid fall in the number of parasites occurs and no more can be found in the blood except after long search. That the birds remain infected is evident from the fact that they suffer relapses, much as human beings do, and also by the fact that blood from the birds is infective to fresh birds.

It has been shown that the rate of reproduction of avian plasmodia in birds does not vary during the patent and subpatent periods and subsequent periods of relapse. It has also been demonstrated that the length of the asexual cycle (Figure 55) in a common species (*P. cathemerium*) that was obtained from a sparrow and that has been maintained in canaries for a number of years, is twenty-four hours (Taliaferro, L. G., 1925). During this period this strain must have passed through several thousand generations without the intervention of sexual reproduction and in a comparatively constant medium, the blood stream (Hegner, 1926).

Bird malaria is furthermore of value for the study of therapeutic agents. Drugs such as plasmochin and atebrin were first found to be effective against the plasmodia of birds and later of man (Roehl, 1926; Hegner and Manwell, 1927). Efforts to discover a better, more abundant and cheaper therapeutic agent than quinine are being made in various laboratories with the aid of birds infected with plasmodia.

Recently attention has been called to the peculiar relation that exists between old and young red cells and the parasites of bird malaria (Hegner and Hewitt, 1938). In certain species, when segmentation occurs in the bird, over 90 per cent of the merozoites invade young red cells. Why they do this is unknown. The effects of this phenomenon on the course of malaria infections, on relapses, geographical distribution, etc. are now being actively investigated.

III. *Malarial Parasites of Other Animals*

Malarial parasites have been described from domestic fowls and from a number of species of mammals and lizards and many new specific names have been proposed for them. Comparatively little, however, is known regarding their life-cycles in either the vertebrate or invertebrate host. Among the larger mammals in which malarial parasites have been noted are the goat and buffalo. Bats seem to be particularly susceptible to infection, several species having been named from these animals. Among other hosts in which plasmodia have been reported are the jumping rat and the squirrel.

Among the blood-inhabiting protozoa of lizards are a number of species that parasitize the red blood cells and resemble malarial parasites in their asexual cycle and in the production of gameto-cytes. The transmitting agent is unknown. Infected lizards have been reported from Africa and South America and a number of different specific names have been applied to the organisms discovered.

CHAPTER XIII

CNIDOSPORIDIA

The CNIDOSPORIDIA are not as well known as the TELOSPORIDIA, probably because many of them are extremely small and difficult to study, and comparatively few are to be found in man and domesticated animals. The two orders, the MYXOSPORIDIA and MICROSPORIDIA, are placed together under the heading CNIDOSPORIDIA because their spores are provided with one or more polar capsules.

I. *Myxosporidia*

The conspicuous characteristics of this order are: (1) the trophozoite is a multinucleate plasmodium with pseudopodia as locomotor

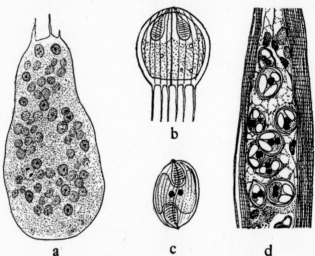

FIG. 56.—MYXOSPORIDIA.

a. *Chloromyxum leydigi*. Plasmodium from gall-bladder of dogfish, *Squalus acanthias*, showing spiky pseudopodia and nuclei (x 1600). (After Dunkerly)
b. *Mitraspora cyprini*. Fresh spore from kidney of carp, *Cyprinus carpio* (x 2000). (After Kudo)
c. *Myxidium oviforme*. Spore from gall-bladder of cod, *Gadus callarias* (x 1600). (From Kudo, after Parisi)
d. *Myxobolus orbiculatus*. Spores in muscle fibers of Gilbert's minnow, *Notropis gilberti* (x 900). (After Kudo)

organs (Figure 56a) and (2) the spores are comparatively large and contain usually two polar capsules (Figure 56b, c; Figure 57a). Myxosporidia are parasites of cold blooded animals, principally fish. Kudo (1919) listed 237 species of which 223 parasitize fish, eight amphibia, four reptiles, one insects and one annelids. Tissues, especially muscle and integument, and bodily cavities, such as the gall-bladder, urinary bladder and kidney tubules, are invaded by the organisms.

The trophozoite is at first a uninucleate amœbula which grows as a result of absorption of nutriment from the host through the general body surface. Its nucleus divides again and again as growth proceeds until the large multinucleate plasmodial stage is attained. Division of the trophozoite

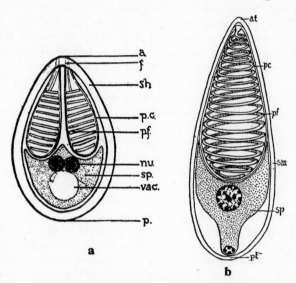

FIG. 57.—Diagrams showing the structure of neosporidian spores. (After Kudo)

a. Myxosporidian spore. *a.*, anterior end; *f.*, foramen of polar capsule; *nu.*, nuclei of sporoplasm; *p.*, posterior end; *p.c.*, polar capsule; *p.f.*, coiled polar filament; *sh.*, shell; *sp.*, sporoplasm; *vac.*, iodinophilous vacuole.

b. Microsporidian spore. *at.*, anterior end; *pc.*, polar capsule; *pf.*, polar filament; *sm.*, spore wall; *sp.*, sporoplasm.

(plasmotomy) may occur, but spore formation is the principal method of multiplication.

Spore formation occurs during the life of the individual, and the spores thus formed are liberated from time to time. The spore. is of great importance as an aid in determining the fact that the organism is a myxosporidium and the species to which it belongs, since the spores are very complicated in structure and differ widely from one another. The structure of a spore is shown in Figure 56. There is a resistant sporocyst consisting of two valves within which, at the posterior end, is a cytoplasmic body consisting of sporoplasm with a vacuole, probably glycogenous in nature, and two nuclei, and, at the anterior end, two polar capsules within each of which is a coiled, and probably hollow, filament.

The infection of new hosts is brought about by the ingestion of spores, the polar filaments of which are extruded through an opening in the anterior end when stimulated by the digestive juices, and attach the rest of the spore to the intestinal epithelium. The sporocyst then opens and the sporoplasm creeps out in the form of an amœbula. The two nuclei in the sporoplasm fuse into one. The amœbula then penetrates the intestinal wall and is carried in the blood stream or lymph to the primary site of infection. Frequently infections are severe and bring about the death of the host.

An idea of the host distribution and localization of MYXOSPORIDIA is indicated by the following selected species. *Leptotheca ohlmacheri* lives in the uriniferous tubules of frogs and toads; *Wardia ovinocua* parasitizes the ovary of the fish, *Lepomis humilis;* *Chloromyxum leydiga* occurs in the gall-bladder of the elasmobranchs, *Raja* and *Torpedo; Sphærospora polymorpha* inhabits the urinary bladder of the fish, *Opsaus tau; Unicapsula muscularis* invades the muscles and is responsible for "wormy" halibut on the Pacific coast of North America; *Myxidium lieberkühni* is a widely distributed species that lives in various species of the fish *Lucius; Myxosoma catostomi* is a muscle and connective tissue parasite of the sucker, *Catostomus commersonii; Lentospora cerebralis* is the agent of "twist-disease" in salmonoid fishes, due to the invasion of the cartilage and perichondrium; *Agarella gracilis* parasitizes the testis of the South American lung-fish, *Lepidosiren paradoxa; Myxobolus notatus* produces tumors in the subdermal connective tissue of the blunt-nosed minnow, *Pimephales notatus;* and *Henneguya psorospermica* forms cysts in the gills of the fish, *Lucius* and *Perca.*

II. *Microsporidia*

The MICROSPORIDIA are characterized by the presence of spores that are extremely small and possess usually only one polar capsule. Kudo (1924) records 178 species living in 222 different host species of which 149 are arthropods; the rest belong to other groups of invertebrates and to the cold-blooded vertebrates. Among the invertebrate hosts are included three species of sporozoa and one ciliate. Certain of the microsporidia are of great economic importance because they bring about the death of animals of value to man. For example, the species *Nosema bombycis* causes a chronic disease in silkworms known as pébrine. This species is generally distributed throughout the tissues of the host, including the eggs developing in the ovary. These eggs are deposited by the silkworm moth and the larvæ that hatch from them are thus infected by the so-called "hereditary" transmission. Pasteur was able to control silkworm disease, which once threatened to destroy the silk industry of France, by eliminating infected eggs which he was able to recognize with the aid of a microscope. Another important species economi-

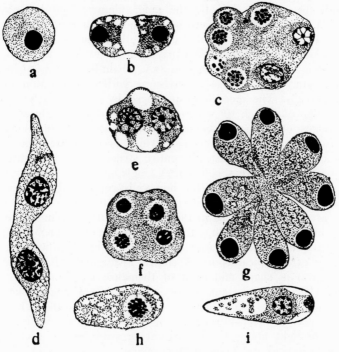

Fig. 58.—*Thelohania magna*, a microsporidium parasitic in the larva of the mosquito, *Culex pipiens*. Stages in the life-cycle (x 2360). (After Kudo)
a. Young schizont. b. Binary division. c. Multiple division. d. Binary division of the second type. e, f, g. Stages in formation of sporoblasts. h. Sporoblast. i. Young spore.

cally is *Nosema apis* which causes nosema disease in honey-bees. Infection is brought about by the ingestion of spores and is limited to the digestive tract. Other species of MICROSPORIDIA are to a certain degree beneficial because they attack harmful insects, for example, the larvæ of several species of anopheline mosquitoes that are carriers of human malaria may be infected (Hesse, 1904; Kudo, 1921, 1924). Infections with microsporidia have also been reported in the larvæ of black flies belonging to the genus *Simulium*. Many other species of insects, some of which are obnoxious, serve as hosts of microsporidia.

The life-cycle of a microsporidium is in general as follows. Spores are ingested by the host. As a result of the action of the digestive juices the polar filament is extruded and attaches the rest of the spore to the intestinal epithelium. After the filament becomes detached the cytoplasm (sporoplasm) within the spore creeps out through the opening left by the polar filament and becomes an amœbula. By means of pseudopodia the amœbula penetrates the epithelial wall and begins intracellular development. The trophozoite, or schizont (Figure 58a), may multiply by binary fission (b), by budding or by multiple fission (c). Chain-like forms are sometimes produced by successive divisions without separation of the daughter cells. The merozoites produced by schizogony eventually become sporonts each of which transforms into a single spore, or the nucleus of the sporont may undergo successive divisions into two, four, eight or more, each of which becomes the center of a cell known as a sporoblast, the entire structure being known as a pansporoblast (Figure 58e, f, g). A single spore (i) develops from each sporoblast (h). When the host cells rupture, the spores pass into the lumen of the intestine and out of the body in the feces. There are many variations in the life-cycles of different species.

As in the MYXOSPORIDIA, the spore of the MICROSPORIDIA is of particular importance because of its value in classification. The structure of a typical spore is shown in Figure 57b. Spores are usually oval in shape and most of them are from 3 μ to 8 μ in length. There is a resistant sporocyst containing a single polar capsule and a mass of sporoplasm in which are two nuclei. The polar filament may be fifty times the length of the spore; its extrusion can be brought about by mechanical pressure or by acetic acid, hydrochloric acid and iodine water.

III. Sarcosporidia and Haplosporidia

These two orders are placed in the Subclass ACNIDOSPORIDIA although their position among the protozoa is still uncertain as is even their protozoan nature. They differ from the CNIDOSPORIDIA in the production of spores that do not contain polar capsules.

SARCOSPORIDIA. These are parasites of vertebrates, being especially common in sheep, cattle and horses. They occur in reptiles and birds as well as mammals. The life-cycle of the sarcosporidium of rats and mice, *Sarcocystic muris,* is the best known. Spores ingested by mice hatch in the intestine, and liberate amœbulæ that penetrate the cells of the intestinal epithelium; here the trophozoites grow and multiply by schizogony. Apparently the merozoites migrate to the muscles where they become located in the fibers; here growth results in a multinucleate plasmodium which divides by plasmotomy. In the course of time the masses of parasites form long, slender, cylindrical bodies with pointed ends, known as "Miescher's tubes" (Figure 59a), within which immense numbers of sickle shaped spores (Rainey's corpuscles) measuring from 10 μ to 15 μ in length are formed.

Very little is known regarding the method of transmission of SARCOSPOR-IDIA. Mice become infected if they are fed on tissue containing spores (Smith, 1901). Mice have also been infected by feeding them tissue of sheep containing *Sarcocystis tenella* (Erdmann, 1910). The mouse parasite, *S. muris,* is capable of infecting guinea-pigs (Negri, 1908; Darling, 1910). Half a dozen cases of sarcosporidiosis have

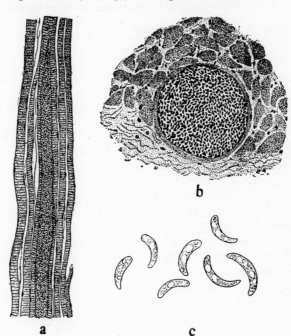

FIG. 59.—SARCOSPORIDIA.
a. Longitudinal section of Miescher's tube in muscle fibers of man (x 300). (After Baraban and St. Remy)
b. Transverse section of Miescher's tube in muscle fibers of man (x 300). (After Baraban and St. Remy)
c. *Sarcocystis muris.* Spores from the mouse. (After Koch)

been reported from man, the organisms usually being found at autopsy in heart muscle, laryngeal muscle, biceps or tongue (Figure 59a, b).

Darling has suggested that the SARCOSPORIDIA occurring in vertebrates are "sidetracked varieties of parasites of invertebrate animals." In most cases no serious results are brought about by the

infection, although *S. muris,* which spreads throughout the entire
body, brings about death in mice, and death sometimes also occurs in
sheep as a result of heavy infections. A toxic substance called sarcocystin, which is lethal to rabbits, was discovered by Pfeiffer (1891)
in SARCOSPORIDIA. The death of infected hosts may be due to this
toxin.

All of the known SARCOSPORIDIA are included in the genus *Sarcocystis.* Specific differentiation is not certain but the following names
have been proposed for organisms found in the different hosts named.

Man	*S. lindemani*	Cattle	*S. hirsuta*
Monkey	*S. kortei*	Horse	*S. bertrami*
Rat and mouse	*S. muris*	Pig	*S. miescheriana*
Sheep	*S. tenella*	Fowl	*S. horvathi*
Rabbit	*S. leporum*	Duck	*S. rileyi*

HAPLOSPORIDIA parasitize invertebrates and lower vertebrates.
The spores resemble superficially those of the MICROSPORIDIA, but
have no polar capsule nor filament. Some of the species that have
been described are as follows: *Haplosporidium nemertis* invades the
connective tissue of the flatworm, *Lineus bilineatus; Urosporidium
fuliginosum* lives in the body cavity of the polychete annelid, *Syllis
gracilis; Bertramia asperospora* inhabits the body cavity of many
common rotifers; *Ichthyosporidium giganteum* forms "cysts" in the
muscles, connective tissue or gills of the fish *Crenilabrus melops* and
C. ocellatus; and *Cœlosporidium periplanetæ* is a common and widespread parasite in the Malpighian tubules of various species of cockroaches.

CHAPTER XIV

PARASITIC INFUSORIA OF LOWER ANIMALS

I. *General Characteristics and Classification*

The INFUSORIA are characterized by the possession of cilia during a part or whole of their life-cycle. In most of them also the nuclear material is separated into a large macronucleus and a smaller micronucleus. Certain species belonging to the family OPALINIDÆ possess only one type of nucleus. The cilia of INFUSORIA cover the entire surface of the body in some species but are limited to certain areas in others. They are sometimes fused into spine-like processes, known as cirri, or side by side into membranelles. Most species ingest solid particles of food by means of a cytostome which leads into a cytopharynx, but a number of species, which are usually grouped together and called ASTOMATA, lack a mouth opening and absorb nutriment through the general surface of the body. The area surrounding the cytostome is known as the peristome; the arrangement of the cilia in this region differs in different groups and aids in classification. In some species there is an anal aperture, usually at the posterior end of the body, known as the cytopyge, and in certain of the OPALINIDÆ an excretory system with an external pore. One group of INFUSORIA, the SUCTORIA, possess cilia only in the young stages, the adults being provided with sucking tentacles.

Most of the INFUSORIA are free-living in fresh water or the sea. Many of them, however, are ectoparasites or endoparasites of man and other vertebrates and invertebrates. The INFUSORIA may conveniently be separated into two subclasses, the CILIATA and the SUCTORIA or ACINETARIA. The CILIATA may further be subdivided into four orders as follows.

Subclass I. CILIATA. Cilia in both young and adult stages.

Order I. HOLOTRICHIDA. Cilia usually covering the entire body and of approximately equal length. Examples: *Opalina, Isotricha.*

185

Order 2. HETEROTRICHIDA. Cilia of large size or fused into membranelles forming a spiral zone leading to the mouth. Examples: *Balantidium, Nyctotherus.*

Order 3. HYPOTRICHIDA. Body flattened dorso-ventrally; cirri on ventral surface. Examples: *Oxytricha, Kerona.*

Order 4. PERITRICHIDA. Cilia forming an adoral ciliated spiral and usually absent from the rest of the body; often sedentary in habit. Examples: *Vorticella, Trichodina.*

Subclass 2. SUCTORIA (ACINETARIA). Cilia in young stage but absent in adult stage; tentacles in adult stage; sedentary in habit. Examples: *Ophryodendron, Sphæro-phrya.*

II. *Nyctotherus cordiformis*

This species has been selected as a type of the ciliates by means of which the characteristics of this group may be illustrated. Species belonging to the genus *Nyctotherus* occur in various species of frogs and toads, in arthropods and in other types of hosts. *N. cordiformis* (Figure 60) occurs commonly in the rectum of frogs and tadpoles. It ranges from 60 μ to 120 μ in length. The body is entirely covered by parallel rows of cilia. On one side, near the anterior end, is a peristome supplied with long adoral cilia. This leads to a cytostome near the center of the body which opens into a long curved cytopharynx. A row of plates of fused cilia extends from the peristome into the cytopharynx. The macronucleus, which lies near the center of the body, is kidney-shaped and the small macronucleus lies on its concave side. Near the posterior end is a single contractile vacuole and at the posterior end a cytopyge.

The life cycle of the *Nyctotherus cordiformis* that lives in a frog (*Hyla versicolor*) as reported by Wichterman (1937) is illustrated in diagrammatic form in Figure 60. The stages shown are as follows:

A cyst (1) is swallowed by a young tadpole. The organism inside the cyst emerges (2) in the intestine of the host. The protozoön feeds on intestinal contents and grows (3). Ordinary binary fission follows (4) which may recur from time to time until the host is about to undergo metamorphosis. At this time smaller individuals are formed to produce the preconjugants (5). It is only these preconjugants that can take part in the sexual process. The preconjugants come together along their adhesive oral surfaces and fuse in pairs as conjugants (6, 7, 8, 9, 10). During conjugation, the macronucleus of each *Nyctotherus* undergoes fragmentation while the micronucleus of each passes through three pre-

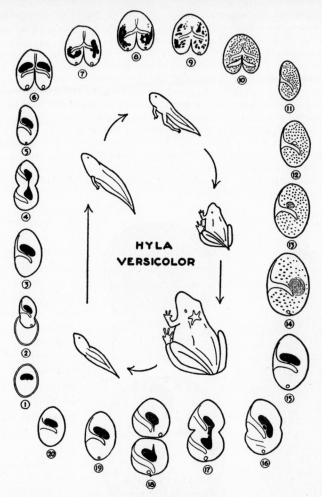

Fig. 60.—Diagram of the life-cycle of *Nyctotherus cordiformis* from the rectum of the frog. (After Wichterman)

gamic divisions leading to the formation of the stationary and migratory pronuclei (10). The migratory pronuclei are exchanged and proceed to fuse with their respective stationary pronuclei forming the amphinucleus. While the animals are fused in the conjugation process, the old ingestatory structures of each dedifferentiates, while an entirely new set of ingestatory structures differentiates posterior to the old set (10). The conjugants now separate (11) and the amphinucleus divides once to form two nuclear products (12), one destined to become the micronucleus of the reorganized *Nyctotherus* while the other body, the macronuclear anlage, undergoes a transformation involving the formation of a "spireme ball" or skein of chromatin. Exconjugants (11, 12, 13, 14) are found nearly exclusively in the recently transformed host. The macronuclear anlage grows in size while there is also a proportionate increase in size of the ciliate's body. The spireme-like macronuclear anlage (14) then transforms into a granular body which ascends to the anterior part of the animal coming to rest in the usual position of the macronucleus (15). The fragments of the old macronucleus are absorbed in the cytoplasm so that the animal assumes a form resembling the vegetative *Nyctotherus* except that it is larger in size. There are again, repeated divisions by binary fission (16, 17, 18). Some ciliates then encyst along with a dedifferentiation of structures (20) and a thick cyst wall is secreted (1). The cyst is then passed out the anus of the frog thus completing the life cycle of *Nyctotherus cordiformis*.

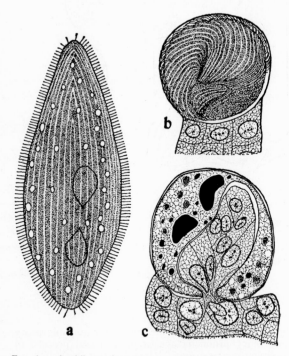

Another species of *Nyctotherus* that may easily be obtained for study is *N. ovalis* which occurs in the intestine of cockroaches and mole crickets. Other species have been reported from myriapods, termites and fish.

III. *Ectoparasitic Ciliates*

Among the ciliates are a number that live on the outside of aquatic animals. These represent all degrees of parasitism; some species attach themselves to an-

Fig. 61.—*Amphileptus branchiarum*, a holotrichous ectoparasite on the gills of tadpoles (x 550). (After Wenrich)
a. Free-swimming specimen showing cilia, surface striations, contractile vacuoles, and two nuclei.
b. Rounded-up specimen showing attaching membrane, cilia, and surface striations.
c. Specimen in optical section showing tissue of host being engulfed.

other animal and are carried about with no further effort on their part; others move about on the surface of the host and may migrate from one host to another, and a few invade the tissues of the host and may be considered pathogenic.

I. AMPHILEPTUS

An example of an ectoparasitic holotrich is *Amphileptus branchiarum* (Figure 61). This species is parasitic on the gills of frog tadpoles (Wenrich, 1924). There may be from one to almost two hundred on the gills on each side of a tadpole. They are usually

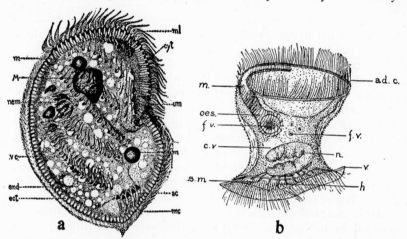

a   b

FIG. 62.—a. *Kerona pediculus*, a hypotrichous ectoparasite on *Hydra. ac.*, anal cirri; *cyt.*, cytostome; *ect.*, ectoplasm; *end.*, endoplasm; *m.*, micronucleus; *M.*, macronucleus; *mc.*, marginal cirri; *ml.*, membranelles; *nem.*, nematocyst; *vc.*, ventral cirri; *um.*, undulating membrane. (After Uhlenmeyer)
b. *Trichodina pediculus*, a peritrichous ectoparasite on *Hydra. ad.c.*, adoral cilia; *c.v.*, contractile vacuole; *f.v.*, food vacuole; *h.*, hooks; *m.*, mouth; *n.*, macronucleus; *oes.*, œsophagus; *s.m.*, striated membrane; *v.*, velum. (After Clark)

surrounded by the cuticular membrane of the gill epithelium. The ciliate, which measures about 61 μ in diameter, is spherical in this stage and actively rotates within the capsule thus formed (Figure 61b). It severs and engulfs tissues surrounding it (Figure 61c). Binary fission and conjugation take place within the capsules. When outside of the capsules the ciliate is free-swimming, about 122 μ in length and flattened dorso-ventrally (Figure 61a).

2. KERONA

Kerona pediculus (Figure 62a) is a parasitic hypotrich which lives on the fresh-water cœlenterate *Hydra*. It prefers *H. fusca* and

H. vulgaris to *H. viridis* (Uhlenmeyer, 1922). *K. pediculus* is modified for its mode of life; its anterior and lateral edges are flexible and fit closely to the host as the ciliate glides about on the surface. When detached from the host, it is free-swimming, but dies if it cannot find another suitable host, thus showing it to be an obligatory parasite. Living cells of the host are ingested by this parasite. Hydras thus attacked do not thrive and are eventually destroyed, but if they are freed from the parasites they again become vigorous.

3. TRICHODINA

Among the ectozoic peritrichs are several interesting species belonging to the genus *Trichodina*. *T. pediculus* (Figure 62b) lives on the outside of hydras, on the gills of certain salamanders and fish (Mueller, 1937) and on the skin of tadpoles. The posterior end of the organism is modified as an organ of attachment by means of a flap-like velum and teeth-like structures. *T. pediculus* appears to be an obligatory parasite since it dies when removed from the gills of its host (Fulton, 1923) but is not pathogenic since it feeds on particles in the surrounding medium and not on the tissues of the host. Cross-infection from the gills of the salamander to *Hydra* has been successfully accomplished. Another species of the genus *Trichodina*, *T. urinicola*, has been described from the urinary bladder of salamanders, fish and toads (Fulton, 1923). This differs from *T. pediculus* in both morphology and habit. It is suggested that this species changed its habitat from outside of the body to the urinary bladder and that this has been accompanied by changes in structure. *T. okajimæ* lives in the urinary bladder of Japanese salamanders. Trichodinas and keronas are sometimes associated on the same host. Clark (1866) says "At times the *Hydra* seems to be strangely knotted, and ungainly in outline, when upon close examination, we ascertain that it is crowded with a swarm of Keronas, upon several of whose convex backs, 1, 2, or 3 Trichodinas are seated, enjoying the pleasure of locomotion without the effort of producing it."

IV. *The Family Opalinidæ*

This is an interesting group of INFUSORIA that are very common in the rectum of frogs, toads and tadpoles. With the exception of one species, which occurs in a marine fish (*Box boops*), all of the approximately 150 species of opalinas live in the intestine of Amphibia. There are four genera (Figure 63), namely *Protoopalina* (a), with a cylindrical binucleate form, *Zelleriella* (b), with a flattened binucleate form, *Cepedea* (c), with a cylindrical multinucleate form, and *Opalina* (d), with a flattened multinucleate form. These are all characterized by a covering of cilia of equal length arranged

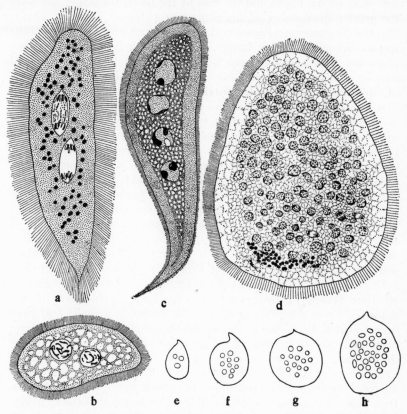

Fig. 63.—OPALINIDÆ. Examples of the four genera and a series of larval stages. (a-d from Metcalf, b and c after Bezzenberger; e-h, after Hegner and Wu)

a. *Protoopalina rhinodermatos.* A cylindrical form with two nuclei in the anaphase of mitosis (x 550).

b. *Zelleriella macronucleata.* A flattened form with two nuclei in the prophase of mitosis (x 500).

c. *Cepedea lanceolata.* A cylindrical form with four nuclei (x 900).

d. *Opalina ranarum.* A flattened form with many nuclei (x 250).

e. *Opalina larvarum.* Four stages in the growth of the young showing how the nuclei increase in numbers as the body increases in size (x 175).

in parallel rows, by the absence of a cytostome and by the presence of only one type of nucleus. An interesting characteristic of the OPALINIDÆ is the fact that in many species the nuclei come to rest in some stage of mitosis. The number of nuclei in the individuals

of various species ranges from two to several thousand. A study
of the growth of young opalinas of the species *O. larvarum* (Figure
63e-h) indicates that there is a definite relation between the number
and mass of the nuclei and the size of the body, the larger the body
the greater the number of nuclei present (Hegner and Wu, 1921).

Opalina ranarum (Figure 63d) is the commonest and best known
species belonging to this family. When alive it is opalescent in appearance. Some specimens reach a length of about a millimeter and
may be seen with the naked eye. The body contains a large number
of spherical nuclei evenly distributed throughout the cytoplasm.
Many small spindle-shaped bodies of unknown character are present
in the endoplasm. Reproduction is by binary division during most
of the year, but in the spring rapid division results in the production
of many small individuals which encyst and pass out in the feces
of the frog. These cysts, which are 30 μ to 70 μ in diameter, when
ingested by tadpoles, hatch in the rectum and give rise either to
macrogametocytes or microgametocytes. The gametocytes, which contain from three to six nuclei, divide into uninucleate macrogametes
or microgametes. These conjugate forming zygotes from each of
which a young opalina develops. *Opalina ranarum* may be kept alive
outside of the body of the frog for as long as three days in Locke's
solution (Larson, Van Epps and Brooks, 1925) and apparently has
been cultivated in Pütter's fluid (Tyler, 1926). Species belonging to
all four genera of OPALINIDÆ are frequently parasitized by en-
damebas. From 2 to 100 per cent of the ciliates in a single host have
been found to be infected. The endamœbas occur also in the opalinid
cysts and may be transmitted from adult frogs to tadpoles within
these cysts. Apparently the parasites do not injure the opalinids
although there may be over one hundred of them in a single ciliate.
Infected opalinids have been found in various widely separated countries indicating a world-wide distribution (Chen and Stabler, 1936).

V. *Ciliates of Mosquito Larvæ*

Ciliates have been reported from a number of insects among
which are the larvæ of mosquitoes (Figure 68f). A few words about
these are included here because mosquitoes are so important that
any organisms that parasitize them are of particular interest. A
species to which the name *Lambornella stegomyiæ* was given was
discovered by Lamborn (1921) in the Malay States, parasitic in
larvæ of the mosquito *Aedes* (*Stegomyia*) *scutellaris*. The ciliates
were present in the gills, body cavity, head and antennæ and 157
specimens were counted in a moderately filled gill. The larvæ appar-

ently were killed by the parasites which escaped when the gills ruptured shortly before death. Reproduction by fission was noted and cysts were observed attached to one of the larvæ (Keilin, 1921). Infection was probably by mouth.

Another species of ciliate was found by MacArthur (1922) in the body cavity of twenty-eight of eighty-seven larvæ and pupæ of *Theobaldia annulata* that were caught near Liverpool, England. All of the infected specimens were killed by the parasites; some larvæ contained as many as a thousand ciliates. Wenyon (1926) considers this species to be *Glaucoma pyriformis*.

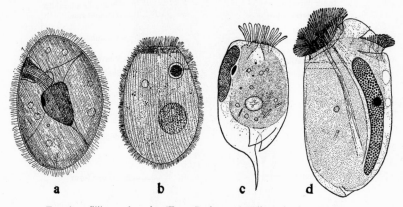

FIG. 64.—Ciliates of cattle. (From Becker and Talbott; b after Schuberg)
a. *Isotricha intestinalis* (x 500).
b. *Bütschlia parva* (x 850).
c. *Entodinium caudatum* (x 500).
d. *Diplodinium hegneri* (x 250).

VI. *Entozoic Ciliates of Cattle*

A number of different species of mammals harbor ciliates in their digestic tract. According to Buisson (1923) the types of mammals in which they occur, the number of species of hosts of each type and the number of species of ciliates are as follows:

	Species of Hosts	*Species of Ciliates*
Ungulates	11	128
Rodents	5	18
Primates	6	3
Hyracoidea	2	4
Proboscidea	1	1
	25	154

It is worthy of note that most of these ciliates occur in ungulates and rodents, which are herbivorous animals, and none occur in carnivorous animals. A number of other species have been described since Buisson made this compilation.

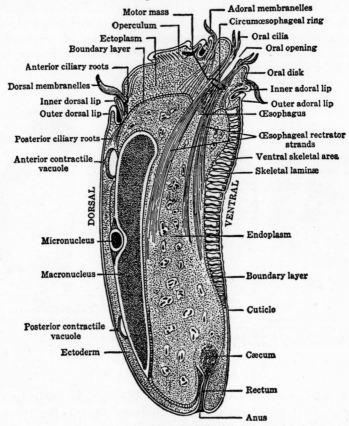

Fig. 65.—*Diplodinium ecaudatum*. A ciliate from cattle showing complicated structure. (After Sharp)

The first and second stomachs of cattle, that is the rumen and reticulum, are highly infected with protozoa, mostly ciliates. In this habitat two species of amœbæ, five species of flagellates and thirty-nine species and varieties of ciliates have been reported (Becker and Talbott, 1927). These belong principally to the genera *Isotricha* (Figure 64a), *Bütschlia* (b), *Entodinium* (c), and *Diplodinium* (d). The medium in the rumen and reticulum is neutral, or slightly acid or alkaline, and in the abomasum it is so strongly acid that, although cysts may pass through without injury, trophozoites are killed and digested. From two to sixteen or more species of ciliates may be present in the stomach of one animal. They feed on bacteria, other protozoa and fragments of the hosts' food. They are obligatory parasites since they die quickly if removed from their habitat. Their exact relations to the host are not known; some or all of them may be commensals or may assist in the digestion of the cellulose in the host's food and thus be symbiotic.

Among the ciliates of cattle are many species of great complexity. It is considered worth while to illustrate one of these here because protozoa are often erroneously considered to be simple organisms. The structure of *Diplodinium ecaudatum* is shown in Figure 65 and sufficiently described in the legend of this figure. Of particular interest is the so-called neuromotor apparatus consisting of a central motorium which is connected with nerve rings and fibrils that make up a complicated system.

VII. *Ciliates of Monkeys*

Ciliates have been reported from various species of primates other than man. One species, *Balantidium coli,* which is supposed to be the same as *B. coli* in man, has been reported from the chimpanzee, orang-utan, baboon and several other species of both Old World and New World monkeys. A species named *Balantidium aragãoi* has been reported from *Cebus caraya* in Brazil (Cunha and Muñiz, 1927) ; this may, however, also be *B. coli.* Several species of the genus *Troglodytella,* a genus that does not occur in man, have been reported from the chimpanzee and gorilla (Figure 66). One species, named *T. abrassarti,* was reported from a sick chimpanzee in the Belgian Congo (Brumpt and Joyeux, 1912). A supposed variety, named *T. abrassarti* var. *accuminata,* has been reported from a chimpanzee in Kamerun, and another species, named *T. gorillæ,* from a gorilla in the same locality (Reichenow, 1920).

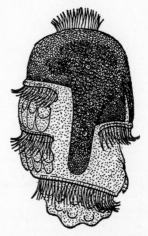

Fig. 66.—*Troglodytella gorillæ.* A ciliate from the intestine of the gorilla (x 250). (After Reichenow)

Chimpanzees that are kept in captivity in the United States are commonly infected with troglody-

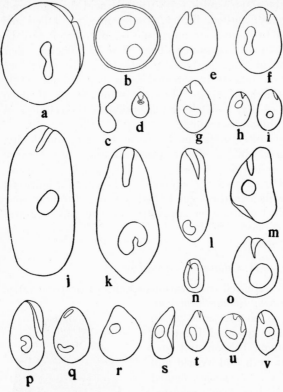

FIG. 67.—*Balantidium.* Outline drawings showing the shape and relative size of the body and nucleus of various species. a. *B. simile,* from *Macacus rhesus.* b. *B. simile,* cyst with 2 macronuclei. c. *B. simile,* macronucleus of trophozoite. d. *B. rhesum* from *M. rhesus.* e. *B. aragaoi* from *Cebus caraya.* f. *Balantidium* from the sheep. g. *B. coli* var. *bovis* from cattle. h. *B. piscicola* from *Piarectus brachypomus.* i. *B. granulosum* from *Salvelinus fontinalis.* j. *B. testudinis* from *Testudo græca.* k. *B. helenæ* from *Rana tigrina,* etc. l. *B. elongatum* from *R. tigrina,* etc. m. *B. blattarum* from *Blatta americana.* n. *B. orchestium* from *Orchestia* and *Talorchestia.* o. *B. luciensis* from *Orchestia littorea.* p. *B. duodeni* from *Rann tigrina,* etc. q. *B. entozoön* from *R. esculenta.* r. *B. falciformis* from *R. palustris.* s. *B. knowlesii* from *Culicoides perigrinus.* t. *B. amydalli* from *Bufo macrotis.* u. *B. bicavata* from *Bufo melanostictus.* v. *B. ovatum* from *Blatta americana.* (From Hegner)

tellas (Swezey, 1934; Hegner and Eskridge, 1934).

VIII. *The Genus Balantidium*

This genus deserves special emphasis because a species, *B. coli,* that is sometimes pathogenic to man, may apparently live in other primates and in pigs. The body is large, shaped as illustrated in Figure 3 (page 28), and covered uniformly with cilia. There is a peristome, at the posterior end of which is a cytostome, and a short cytopharynx, and a cytopyge near the posterior end.

Balantidium in pigs. Balantidia that occur in the intestine of pigs have long been considered to belong to the same species as that in man. A second species of *Balantidium, B. suis,* was described from pigs by McDonald (1922). This species has a more pointed posterior end and the greatest diameter is at or anterior to the center; whereas *B. coli* is rounded at the posterior end and the greatest diameter is posterior to the center. *B. suis* is approximately the same length as *B. coli* but not so broad, the average length of both species being 86 μ, but the breadth of *B. coli* is 66 μ and that of *B. suis* is 43 μ. The cytostome of *B. suis* is not almost terminal as in *B. coli* but is located about one-fifth of the length of the body posterior to the anterior end. The macronucleus of *B. suis* is rod or sausage-shaped, at least one-half of the length of the entire animal and about one-fourth as broad as long; whereas the macronucleus of *B. coli* is bean-shaped, about one-third of the length of the entire animal and about one-half as broad as long.

Balantidium in chimpanzee, pig and guinea-pig. An investigation of conjugation in balantidia (Nelson, 1934, Figure 71) has revealed a difference of a fundamental nature between the species that live in the chimpanzee and pig and in the guinea-pig. In the former two, during the reorganization of the nuclei after conjugation, the new macronucleus is formed by the fusion of two nuclei (placentæ); whereas in the balantidia of the guinea-pig, the macronucleus arises from a single nucleus (placenta). Thus, although the balantidia that live in these different types of mammals appear to be indistinguishable externally, they differ in nuclear reorganization following conjugation, and, at present, can be distinguished only at this stage in their life-cycle. The balantidia of man seem to resemble those of the chimpanzee and pig in their nuclear phenomena.

Cross-infection experiments with balantidia of mammals. The cross-infection experiments with balantidia reported in the literature have been summarized by Andrews (1932) in the accompanying table, positive results being indicated by a plus sign.

Source	Animal Into Which Inoculated					
	Monkey	Pig	Cat	Rabbit	Guinea-Pig	Rat
Man	+	+	+		+	+
Monkey		+				
Pig	+			+	+	+
Guinea-Pig						+

Andrews was unable to infect monkey, rabbit, cat, dog and lamb with human balantidia; monkey with pig balantidia; and monkey and rabbit with guinea-pig balantidia. He succeeded in infecting pig, guinea-pig and rat with human balantidia; pig with monkey balantidia; rabbit, guinea-pig and rat with pig balantidia; and rat with guinea-pig balantidia. It is important in evaluating the results of cross-infection experiments to know how long the parasite persisted in the "foreign" host since it is often possible for a parasite to live in

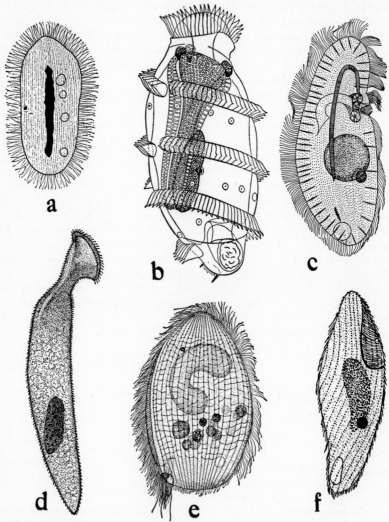

FIG. 68.—Some ciliates from lower animals. a. *Anoplophrya marylandensis*, from the earthworm. b. *Polydinium mysoreum*, from the elephant. c. *Lechriopyla mystax*, from the sea urchin. d. *Sieboldiellina planariarum*, from *Planaria*. e. *Ancistruma mytili*, from the clam. f. *Turchiniella culicis*, from the mosquito. (a, after Conklin; b, after Kofoid; c, after Lynch; d, after Bishop; e, after Kidder; f, after Grassé and Boissezon)

an unfamiliar environment for a short time and even to multiply there but to disappear within a few days. One may thus distinguish between a refractory host and a condition of weak host-parasite specificity.

Species of balantidia in lower animals. Balantidia have been described from many lower animals (Figure 67). A recent review of the genus (Hegner, 1934) indicates that about 30 species have been reported from almost that number of hosts. These hosts include besides man and various other species of primates, the pig, opossum, guinea-pig, sheep, cattle, ostrich, turtle, frogs and toads, fish, crustaceans, insects and snails.

IX.   *Other Ciliates of Lower Animals*

Many lower animals not previously mentioned are parasitized by ciliates (Figure 68). They are known to occur in the intestine of earthworms and aquatic annelids, in the gastrovascular cavity of medusæ, in the digestive system of flatworms (*Planaria*), in the blood vessel and cœlom of fresh-water CRUSTACEA, in the liver and uterus of mollusks, and in the gonads of echinoderms. No doubt large numbers of species that have never been reported live in or on the bodies of both invertebrates and lower vertebrates in this country.

One species of particular interest because it is pathogenic and may actually kill its host is the ectoparasite of fish known as *Ichthyophthirius multifiliis.* This species is parasitic in the skin and often occurs in aquaria. In the vegetative stage it is about 800 μ in diameter and lives in a cavity in the epidermis of the fish. When it escapes from this cavity it sinks to the bottom where it usually becomes encysted and undergoes 8 successive divisions resulting in the production of 256 minute uninucleated ciliates. The sexual phenomena that take place within the cyst are not accurately known, but the ciliates, when they break out, attack new fish hosts into whose skin they bore their way and develop to their full size.

X.   *Parasitic Suctoria*

Various types of parasitism are exhibited by the SUCTORIA (Figure 69) ; among these are ectoparasites that attach themselves to more or less definite species of aquatic animals, and endoparasites which live within other hosts. *Trichophrya salparum* lives on the surface of tunicates, such as *Molgula manhattensis; Dendrosomides paguri* attaches itself to hermit crabs, *Eupagurus excavatus* and *E. cuanensis; Ophryodendron porcellanum* lives on certain CRUSTACEA, especially *Porcellana platycheles; Sphærophrya stentoris* parasitizes free-living ciliates, such as *Stentor* and *Bursaria; Tokophrya cyclopum* fastens itself to *Cyclops, Diaptomus, Gammarus,* and other

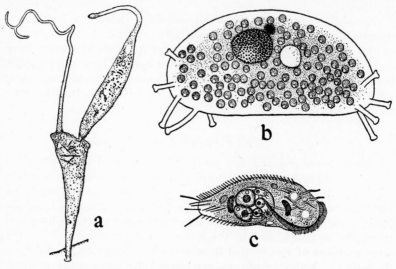

FIG. 69.—Some SUCTORIA from lower animals. a. *Ophryodendron prenanti,* from the surface of a nemertine worm. b. *Allantosoma intestinalis,* from the horse. c. *Sphærophrya* sp., inside of the body of a ciliate. (a, after Duboscq; b, after Hsiung; c, after Stein)

ENTOMOSTRACA; and *Endosphæra engelmanni* lives within the body of *Trichodina pediculus, Didinium nasutum,* vorticellas, and other protozoa. Collin (1912) has provided us with a magnificent monograph on the parasitic SUCTORIA.

CHAPTER XV

PARASITIC CILIATES OF MAN

I. *Balantidium coli*

The only species belonging to the class INFUSORIA that is known with certainty to be parasitic in man is the ciliate *Balantidium coli* (Figure 3, page 28).

1. LIFE-CYCLE

The trophozoite of *Balantidium coli* lives in the large intestine where it reproduces by transverse binary fission. Single organisms may encyst and pass out of the body in the feces; these represent the infective stage which brings about the transmission of the species to new hosts. The conjugation of two organisms occasionally occurs, followed by nuclear reorganization and binary fission.

2. MORPHOLOGY

Trophozoite (Figure 3). *Balantidium coli* is oval in shape, somewhat narrow and pointed at the anterior end and broader and rounded at the posterior end. The peristome, which is located near the anterior end, makes it possible to distinguish the ventral from the dorsal surface. *B. coli* is very large compared with other human protozoa and varies greatly in size; it ranges from 30 μ to 200 μ or more in length and from 20 μ to 70 μ in breadth, the usual range in size being from 50 μ to 70 μ long by 40 μ to 60 μ wide. The average length is 86 μ and the average breadth 66 μ and the ratio of length over breadth is 1.3. The entire body of the trophozoite is covered with cilia, which are arranged in parallel longitudinal rows in a somewhat spiral course; they are 4 μ to 6 μ in length on the general body surface and 8 μ to 12 μ in length on the adoral zone which surrounds the peristome. The cilia lie in the grooves between the ectoplasmic ridges and each cilium arises from a basal granule. The peristome is a slit-like depression on the ventral surface at the anterior end, at the bottom of which is the cytostome leading into the cytopharynx. A nonciliated oral plug in the peristome may completely close the cytostome (McDonald, 1922). At the posterior end is a rectal vacuole into which excretory materials are collected and from which they are forced out through a cytopyge. The body of *B. coli* is covered by a pellicle that is thrown up into parallel longitudinal ridges. Just beneath the pellicle is a layer of clear ectoplasm and within this is the more fluid granular endoplasm.

Within the body of *B. coli* are a macronucleus, a micronucleus, two contractile vacuoles and a number of food vacuoles. The macronucleus is large and kidney-shaped. It lies usually near the center of the body in a more or less oblique position. Chromosome-like masses of chromatin, constant in number (five to ten), have been observed in the macronuclei of balantidia from several species of hosts in addition to what appear to be minute chromatin granules scattered throughout the nuclear substance (Hegner and Holmes, 1923); the significance of these chromosome-like masses is not known. The micronucleus is small, subspherical in shape and lies against the macronucleus or in a depression in it. The two contractile vacuoles are located near the periphery of the body, one close to the posterior end and the other just anterior to the middle of the body; they expel excretory material in solution to the outside when they contract. The number of food vacuoles in the body depends on the state of nutrition of the organism. Food particles, such as starch grains, bacteria, red and white blood cells and organic débris, are driven by the adoral cilia through the cytostome and into the cytopharynx at the end of which the food vacuoles are formed. These food vacuoles are carried about in the endoplasm by a cytoplasmic movement known as cyclosis. Within them digestion is accomplished by enzymes secreted by the surrounding cytoplasm. The digested material passes out and is assimilated and the undigested particles are extruded through the cytopyge. A neuromotor apparatus has been described by McDonald (1922) in *B. coli*. It consists of a motorium, which is supposed to serve as a coördinating center, and a large number of fibrils which play a part in the swimming and feeding movements of the organism.

The trophozoite of *B. coli* reproduces by transverse binary fission (Figure 71, 1-2). The macronucleus apparently divides by amitosis; it becomes dumb-bell shaped and then the two approximately equal parts separate, one passing to either end of the body. The micronucleus undergoes a sort of intranuclear mitosis; one daughter micronucleus passes to each end of the body. Then a constriction appears at the center of the organism and the body is divided into two approximately equal parts; the cytostome of the parent is continued in the anterior daughter and a new cytostome arises at the anterior end of the posterior daughter cell. Rapid binary division sometimes results in "nests" of very small specimens within the tissues of infected hosts; these have been described as groups of spores (Walker, 1909) but sporulation probably does not take place in this species.

Cyst. The stimulus that initiates the process of encystment is not known. The ciliate secretes about itself a wall consisting of a thick outer layer and a thinner inner layer. These cysts, which are spherical or ovoid, measure from 50 μ to 60 μ in diameter (Figure 70). At first the organism moves about actively inside the cyst wall but eventually becomes quiescent and degeneration of the cilia then occurs. Encystment appears to be more frequent in the pig than in man.

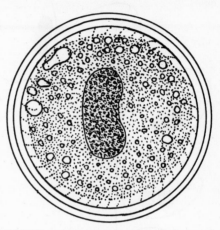

Fig. 70.—Cyst of *Balantidium coli,* from man. (After Andrews)

3. CONJUGATION

The best account of conjugation in *Balantidium coli* is that furnished by Nelson (1934) for balantidia obtained from the chimpanzee (Figure 71). The process of conjugation in this organism is similar to that of ciliates in general as far as the maturation divisions and the production and exchange of the pro-nuclei are concerned. Two maturation divisions of the micronucleus result in four nuclei of which three degenerate. The fourth divides again to produce the stationary and the migratory pronuclei. The migratory nuclei are exchanged and proceed to fuse with the stationary nuclei at which time the conjugants separate. After separation, the process most nearly resembles that in *Collinella* and *Nicollella* as described by Chatton and Perard (1921). The fusion nucleus divides to form one small nucleus and one large nucleus. The large nucleus undergoes a second division resulting in two equal nuclei. These are the placentæ destined to become the macronucleus. To do this, however, they go through a process of development until they resemble the vegetative nucleus in chromatin make-up at which time they fuse to form the

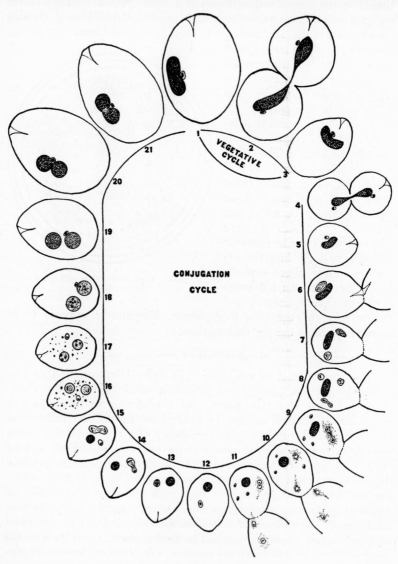

FIG. 71.—Stages in the conjugation cycle of *Balantidium coli*, from the chimpanzee. (After Nelson)

single kidney-shaped macronucleus. The small nucleus resulting from the first metagamic division undergoes slight changes and becomes the micronucleus (Figure 71).

4. HOST-PARASITE RELATIONS

Transmission. As is the case with other intestinal protozoa, *B. coli* is transferred from one host to another in the cyst stage (Figure 70), and it is the host that brings about its own infection, since the cyst is incapable of movement. The ingestion of food or drink contaminated by fecal material containing cysts is the probable method of infection. Trophozoites may possibly also be infective since they may live at room temperature for as long as ten days (Rees, 1927)

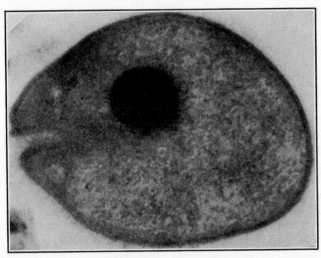

FIG. 72.—*Balantidium coli.* Photograph of a specimen within the intestinal wall of a human host. (From the Army Medical Museum)

and, at least in small animals (guinea-pigs), they are capable of passing unharmed through the stomach and small intestine and of reaching the cecum, which is the primary site of infection (Hegner, 1926). Cysts are more resistant than trophozoites; they will live at room temperature for several weeks if kept in a moist condition. It is generally supposed that human beings become infected by ingesting balantidia from pigs, since cysts appear to be rare in man; and a large percentage of human cases can be traced, more or less definitely, to pigs. Direct infection of man with cysts of *B. coli* from the pig has been attempted but with negative results (Grassi, 1888).

Pathogenesis. Where excystation occurs and the factors involved are not known. The primary site of infection is the large intestine, although cases have been reported of balantidia in the ileum (Reis, 1923). Apparently the excysted organisms are able to live and reproduce within the intestinal lumen without access to the tissues of the host; such organisms are non-pathogenic and the host is a carrier. In some cases, however, the organisms attack the intestinal wall and thus become pathogenic (Figure 72). Walker (1913) believes that the ciliates bore their way mechanically into the tissues of the intestinal wall thus causing irritation resulting in hyperæmia of the mucosa. The host tissues appear to be dissolved by ferments secreted by the parasites and used as food. Ulcers are formed and clinical symptoms appear, varying in severity from diarrhea to dysentery. The disease produced is known as balantidiasis, balantidial dysentery or ciliate dysentery.

5. CULTIVATION

Living balantidia may be obtained for study at any abattoir where pigs are slaughtered. McDonald (1922) found 68 per cent of 200 pigs infected, the parasites being most numerous in the cecum and first three or four feet of the colon. Barret and Yarbrough (1921) were the first to cultivate *Balantidium coli* in artificial medium; this consisted of sixteen parts of 0.5 per cent salt solution plus one part of inactivated human blood serum. Feces containing balantidia were inoculated at the bottom of tubes and incubated at 37° C. Maximum growth occurred in from forty-eight to seventy-two hours and subcultures were made every second day. Rees (1927) has confirmed this work although he used a modified Ringer's solution instead of 0.5 NaCl and substituted with success Loeffler's dehydrated blood serum for the human blood serum. A pure culture was obtained by picking out single individuals with a micropipette and inoculating them into test-tubes containing the medium. Cultures of the balantidia from the guinea-pig were also obtained by Rees and cysts occasionally appeared in these cultures. Other methods of cultivation have been described by Tanabe and Komada (1932), Atchley (1935), and Nelson (1937).

II. *Doubtful Ciliates of Man*

A number of ciliates have been reported from man by various investigators but none of them has as yet been established as a regular inhabitant of the human digestive tract. Among these are species belonging to the genera *Balantidium, Nyctotherus, Chilodon, Uronema* and *Colpoda*. It seems probable that all of these are poorly fixed specimens of *B. coli,* or coprozoic ciliates that have accidentally found their way into fecal material after it was passed or had passed through the digestive tract in the cyst stage and excysted in the stool. *B. minutum* was reported by Schaudinn (1899) and has been recorded by several investigators since then. Several varieties of this so-called species and of *B. coli* have been described from Italy, Germany, Honduras and Albania. A species named *Nyctotherus faba* was also described by Schaudinn (1899) from the same patient in whom *B. minutum* occurred. Several other species belonging to this genus have been reported from man. The free-living ciliate, *Chilodon uncinatus,* has been reported from human feces on several occasions. The species described from human feces as *Uronema caudatum* by Martini (1910) and *Colpoda cucullus* by Schultz (1899) are no doubt also free-living ciliates living under coprozoic conditions.

Section II

HELMINTHOLOGY

BY

DONALD L. AUGUSTINE

CHAPTER XVI

INTRODUCTION TO THE HELMINTHS

I. *General Classification*

The parasitic worms belong to a group of animals known as the helminths. This group was regarded by early zoölogists, Cuvier and others, as a single united division, not only biologically apart from other animals but systematically apart as well. On account of the great variety in the different types included in this division, the group is no longer regarded a systematic one. The association of its members is now looked upon as being only biological and the term "helminth" is used to specify certain lowly worms which lead parasitic lives.

Systematically, the helminths are represented in two different phyla, (1) PLATYHELMINTHES or flatworms, and (2) NEMATHELMINTHES or threadworms. Within these phyla the helminths are placed under five groups which usually rank as classes, namely, TREMATODA or flukes, and CESTOIDEA or tapeworms under the phylum PLATYHELMINTHES, and NEMATODA or threadworms, GORDIACEA or hair worms and ACANTHOCEPHALA or proboscis worms under the phylum NEMATHELMINTHES. While the GORDIACEA and ACANTHOCEPHALA have been classed by most writers as allies of NEMATODA they have little else in common with the nematodes except a general form of body and the parasitic habit. Some authorities have referred the GORDIACEA to the phylum NEMATOMORPHA, while others have regarded them as degenerate annelids. The proboscis worms have been placed under a separate phylum (ACANTHOCEPHALA) by some workers and others have pointed out possible relationships with the tapeworms for them. The GORDIACEA and ACANTHOCEPHALA are therefore of uncertain systemic position and until the morphology and embryology of these groups are better known, their affinities must remain problematical.

Phylum PLATYHELMINTHES Gegenbauer, 1859. METAZOA; triploblastic; bilaterally symmetrical; with bodies leaf-shaped or band-shaped; mostly hermaphroditic; without body cavity; alimentary canal incomplete or entirely lacking.

Class 1. TURBELLARIA Ehrenberg, 1831. PLATYHELMINTHES with bodies cylindrical to spindle-shaped; with ciliated ectoderm; with digestive system; development direct; with free-living habit.

Class 2. TREMATODA Rudolphi, 1808. PLATYHELMINTHES; unsegmented bodies oval or leaf-shaped; ciliated ectoderm present only in larval stage; with digestive system; living as ectoparasites or endoparasites; mostly hermaphroditic; with development by metamorphosis or alternation of generation; almost all, in the adult stage, parasites of vertebrates.

Class 3. CESTOIDEA Rudolphi, 1808. PLATYHELMINTHES; ribbon-shaped or band-shaped; mostly segmented; without mouth or alimentary canal; hermaphroditic; adults almost exclusively parasitic in alimentary canal of vertebrates.

Phylum NEMATHELMINTHES Vogt (Carus, 1863). METAZOA; triploblastic; bilaterally symmetrical; with elongated, cylindrical, unsegmented bodies; without cilia or appendages arranged on a regularly segmental plan, sexes usually separate; with body cavity in which organs float.

Class 1. NEMATODA Rudolphi, 1808, Diesing, 1861. NEMATHELMINTHES with bodies usually spindle-shaped, tapering at both ends rather than cylindrical; body cavity not lined by epithelium; alimentary canal usually complete; free-living and parasitic forms.

I. APPENDIX TO NEMATHELMINTHES

GORDIACEA von Siebold, 1848. NEMATHELMINTHES with bodies generally uniformly cylindrical with blunt, rounded ends; body cavity lined by epithelium; alimentary canal atrophied in sexually mature worms; parasitic in larval stage; adults free in bodies of fresh water.

ACANTHOCEPHALA Rudolphi, 1808. NEMATHELMINTHES with bodies tapering posteriorly; no trace of alimentary canal at any stage of development; with a proboscis; both larval and adult stages parasitic.

II. *Distribution and Incidence*

The helminths are world-wide in their distribution, and their incidence among the lower vertebrates is higher than in man. The presence of parasitic worms among the lower vertebrates is quite general. In man, however, their occurrence is apt to be greater in the tropical and subtropical countries where the climate and habits of the people are more favorable for their dissemination. Infection with a single species in such an environment may occur in 98 per cent of a given population and often several species may occur in a single host. It is a common occurrence to find hookworms, ascarids and whipworms in the same person. Often the number of different species of helminths in a single host is astonishingly high. In many instances, only a few parasites of a given species may be present in an infected host, or again, the number may be very large. Infections with 1000 hookworms, *Necator americanus,* are not uncommon. Pinworms also occur often in very great numbers. Perhaps the largest number of worms recorded from a single person is that reported by Sambuc and Baujean (1913). These authors obtained 21,000 liver flukes, *Clonorchis sinensis,* at autopsy from a patient in Indo-China. Some of the helminths are parasites of a single host species while others are common parasites of a more or less wide range of animals. For example, the pinworm, *Enterobius vermicularis,* is a parasite only of man, while the intestinal fluke, *Schistosoma japonicum,* not only infects man, but also occurs in cattle, horses, cats, dogs, swine and rodents under natural conditions.

The adult stages of helminths are more or less restricted to a single organ or system of organs of their hosts, occurring mainly in the intestines or certain portions of the alimentary tract, or in the liver, the lungs or the connective tissue. Hence, the derivation of their common names, such as the eye worm, the seat worm, the lung fluke, the liver fluke, the blood fluke and the like. Certain larval stages are not restricted, however, to a single organ and may have considerable range in their habitats for development. *Cysticercus cellulosæ,* the larval stage of the pork tapeworm of man, infects the intermuscular connective tissue, the brain and eye and has been found in many other localities. The hydatids of *Echinococcus* develop in the liver, lungs, kidneys, spleen, omentum, heart, brain and various muscles. On the other hand, the larvæ of *Trichinella spiralis* can develop to encystment only in the striated muscles of the host.

FACTORS DETERMINING DISTRIBUTION AND INCIDENCE

The type of life-cycle of a given species of the parasitic worms determines to a great extent its geographical distribution and incidence. In the majority of cases the parasitic stage alternates with a longer or shorter non-parasitic period. The development may be direct from host to host, or it may be exceedingly complicated involving both an alternation of generations and an alternation of hosts. The commonest and most widely distributed species of the helminths are those which have no intermediate host, with little or no development in the free stages, and infect a new host with ova which have escaped in the feces of the previous host. Thus the nematodes, *Ascaris lumbricoides, Trichuris trichiura* and *Enterobius vermicularis*, and the tapeworm, *Hymenolepis nana*, have become cosmopolitan in their distribution. The helminths which have a longer non-parasitic stage with larvæ developing in the soil are limited in their distribution to the warmer countries where the temperature and other factors are most favorable for their development and existence. The parasitic worms having intermediate hosts are necessarily limited in their distribution to the distribution of these hosts. The FILARIIDÆ are transmitted only by the bites of certain blood-sucking insects, and are therefore limited to the distribution of their specific intermediate hosts. It is probably for this reason that the eye worm of man, *Loa loa*, has not become established beyond the western coast of Africa, the habitat of its essential hosts, the mango flies, *Chrysops dimidiatus* and *Chrysops silacea*. On the other hand, there are several helminths, including the tapeworms *Tænia saginata* and *Tænia solium* of man, whose intermediate hosts are cosmopolitan. In such cases we may expect to find the parasite to be also cosmopolitan, providing certain habits of the host are favorable for their transmission. Many of the parasitic worms require certain food habits for their entrance into their final hosts. *Tænia saginata* and *Tænia solium* are introduced into their final hosts through the eating of infected raw or insufficiently cooked beef or pork respectively, and the fish tapeworm, *Diphyllobothrium latum,* and the liver fluke, *Clonorchis sinensis,* by the eating of infected raw or insufficiently cooked fish. *Trichinella spiralis* depends for its spread upon the eating of raw or undercooked pork containing the infective cysts of this parasite. Thus, the distribution of these helminths is limited to those countries, or certain districts within a given country or city, where raw meats or insufficiently cooked meats are eaten.

III. *Effects Produced by Helminths on the Host*

The relation of some of the helminths to disease is not always definite, while in other cases the pathogenicity is well established. In many helminth infections where clinical symptoms are manifest, the worms occur in relatively large numbers and the infection is of fairly long standing. On the whole, the onset of clinical manifestations due to the presence of parasitic worms is usually of a gradually increasing scale of severity rather than a rapid onset as in the case of infectious bacterial diseases. This is due to the fact that, as a rule, there is no multiplication of helminths within the host. Heavy infection is the result of frequent exposures to the infective stage. There are, however, some exceptions, particularly in the case of infection with *Trichinella spiralis,* whose progeny remain within the host harboring the adult. In this case the clinical symptoms may appear within a relatively few hours after the ingestion of the infective cysts of the worm, and the different stages in the course of the disease may be correlated with the different stages in the development of the parasite.

There is great variation in the susceptibility of different individuals to the attack of helminths. The worms may produce marked clinical symptoms in certain individuals while in others, equally parasitized, the infection may be entirely unnoticed. Marked clinical symptoms are most frequently met with in undernourished or otherwise weakened individuals.

The injuries produced by helminths depend on several factors, such as the size of the parasite, its mode of life, its habits within the host, the number present and the organs or tissues occupied. In general, the presence of helminths may injure the host in one or more of the following ways:

ROBBING OR STARVING THE HOST

All of the helminths derive their food from the host. The amount of injury to the host through the loss of such nourishment depends largely on the size of the parasite and on the number present. The amount of food taken directly from a host heavily parasitized with large tapeworms, or ascarids, is obviously considerable.

Hookworms are known to be voracious and extravagant feeders. Their food consists mainly of blood and lymph. It has been estimated, from direct observations, that one hundred dog hookworms remove about eighty-four cc. of blood from their host in twenty-four hours. Only an infinitesimal portion of this amount is used as food by the parasite.

WOUNDING THE HOST

Parasitic worms may wound the host either through their feeding habits or by boring through the tissues of the host during their migrations. Hookworms feed from the intestinal mucosa of their hosts, tearing it loose with their powerful teeth. Danger may arise from bacterial invasion through these wounds resulting in ulceration. *Ascaris lumbricoides* is frequently known to migrate out of its normal habitat, the small intestine, and in so doing may penetrate through the intestinal wall and cause a fatal peritonitis due to bacteria which are carried with it. Adult ascarids have been found to have penetrated practically every organ of the body. In such instances the danger to the host is not limited to the wandering action of the worm alone but to the invasion of bacteria as well.

The wounding action of the helminths is not restricted to the presence of adult worms, but is also met with in some larval stages. The infective larvæ of the hookworms, and of *Strongyloides stercoralis* among the nematodes, and the cercariæ of the blood flukes gain entrance to their hosts by actively penetrating the skin. In so entering their hosts, they produce an inflammation or dermatitis at their port of entry. Here again, complications due to secondary bacterial infections often arise and pustulation or extensive ulceration may follow. A number of larval nematodes have extensive courses of migration within the body of the host before the adult stage is reached. The larvæ of the hookworms and *Ascaris,* after their entrance into the portal system, pass through the liver and eventually to the lungs, where they break through the capillaries to the air spaces on their way up the trachea to the esophagus and thence into the intestines. Should the number of worms be large the hemorrhage may be considerable and the resultant inflammation so great that generalized pneumonia is likely to occur. The danger from the wounding action of the helminths then does not lie entirely in the wound itself; for, through the wound, they may bring about, or prepare the ground for a serious, superimposed infection by pathogenic bacteria.

MECHANICAL IRRITATION

Hyperplasia and overgrowth of specialized tissue are often the result of irritation from the presence of certain helminths. Metaplastic lesions have been attributed to *Paragonimus* in the lung and to *Schistosoma hæmatobium* in the urinary bladder. Liver flukes cause intense proliferation of the biliary epithelium and are believed to be a cause of cancerous growths. Malignant tumors have been traced to larvæ of the cat tapeworm, *Tænia tæniæformis,* in the liver of rats and to the nematode *Gongylonema neoplasticum* in the stomach of rats. There are many examples of helminths associated with the formation of neoplasms. The exact relationship is not clear. It is probable that certain individuals are particularly susceptible to such growths and that irritation by the worm stimulates rather than causes their development.

MECHANICAL OBSTRUCTION

Mechanical obstructions are often caused by the helminths. *Ascaris lumbricoides,* the common intestinal roundworm of man, frequently is the cause of intestinal obstruction and obstruction of the bile and pancreatic ducts. The majority of such cases occur in persons with heavy infections, from 60 to 5,000 worms, but equally serious complications have been noted repeatedly from infections with less than 10 worms. *Wuchereria bancrofti* produces stasis of the lymph which in time gives rise to lymphangitis, lymph scrotum and elephantiasis. Larval tapeworms, particularly hydatid cysts, produce obstruction by compression as they increase slowly in size. Liver flukes may completely block the bile ducts causing retention of bile and jaundice; and indirectly may produce angioma-like tumors through interference with the circulation.

TOXIC EFFECTS

Numerous toxic and nervous disorders have been attributed to helminth infections. Many individuals are susceptible to the toxic action of the secretions or body fluid of ascarids. Persons, particularly parasitologists and students of parasitology handling and dissecting fresh specimens, frequently carry the body fluid of the worm to the skin of the face or neck or to the eyes, which often produces a more or less severe reaction and conjunctivitis. General systemic reactions with urticaria over the entire body, swelling of face and eyes, rapid heart action and marked changes in the leucocyte count of the blood have been observed in certain cases exposed to very minute quantities of this fluid. The belief is general that heavy helminth infections may result in stunting the growth of the host. This is particularly evident in barnyard fowls, puppies and domesticated animals. It is doubtful, however, if any of the helminths produce true toxins. Their normal secretions and excretions which contain foreign proteins must be passed into the body of the host. These substances may be toxic and stimulate a reaction, which in many instances is demonstrable by serologic tests, such as the complement fixation, precipitin and intradermal reactions, now used in the diagnosis of certain helminth diseases.

IMMUNITY

There is no essential difference between bacterial and helminth immunity. Three more or less closely related phenomena are principally involved, generally termed "natural resistance," "age resistance" and "acquired resistance."

Natural resistance is a constitutional peculiarity which renders the host unsuitable for the complete development and establishment of certain parasites. As a rule, animals are naturally resistant in varying degrees to the helminths of physiologically unrelated animals. This protection is not always absolute, however, and is influenced markedly by diet. It has been shown repeatedly that animals raised on diets deficient in vitamin A have a lowered resistance to helminth infections. It has also been found that hosts which are highly insusceptible to their helminth infections lose their resistance when kept for a prolonged period on an inadequate diet. Resistance is spontaneously reëstablished, however, upon return to a proper regimen. The ascarids of man and of the pig are morphologically identical but represent two distinct varieties, the one developing only in man and the other in swine. However, it has been observed that the variety from man will develop in the pig when vitamin A is withheld from the diet.

A natural resistance is acquired with age and occurs in the absence of previous infection. In general, young animals are more susceptible to helminth infection than adults. Young pups are highly susceptible to infections with ascarids and hookworms, but old dogs show that the majority of these worms develop in the pups when the infection is given to the mother during gestation. Age resistance is not a constant feature in all hosts. Apparently man is always susceptible to the hookworms *Ancylostoma duodenale* and *Necator americanus*.

Studies on acquired resistance to helminths are of relatively recent date. It appears to develop most frequently in those infections which provoke severe tissue reactions or which cause extensive tissue damage. It has been shown that dogs are for a time susceptible to infection with *Strongyloides stercoralis,* but this period of susceptibility is of short duration and is promptly followed by a definite and specific resistance against this parasite. A single infection with *Trichinella spiralis* also protects to some extent against a later infection. Acquired resistance has also been established by injecting subcutaneously, intramuscularly and intraperitoneally products of helminths into susceptible hosts. In most cases acquired resistance appears to be limited and of short duration.

CHAPTER XVII

CLASS TREMATODA

I. *Characteristics of the Class*

All of the trematodes show marked modifications from their free-living relatives, the TURBELLARIA. There is an extreme development in the organs of attachment and reproduction and reduction or loss in the sensory apparatus, organs of locomotion or other structures usually present in free-living flatworms. This simplicity of structure of the TREMATODA is not a primitive simplicity but is the sign of specialization as a consequence of the development of the parasitic habit. Material for a general study of trematode morphology, movements, etc. may be readily obtained from the lungs of frogs which are usually infected with flukes of the genus *Ostiolum* (Figure 73) and of the genus *Hæmatolœchus*. These flukes are more or less transparent and the principal structures can be readily determined in the living organism. Detailed studies on the histology and the relation of the various organs may be made from toto mounts and serial sections (Figure 74).

EXTERNAL ANATOMY

The trematodes usually present a flattened, leaf-shaped or tongue-shaped body, or they may be barrel-shaped, conical, or attenuated (Figure 75). Most forms are small, ranging from about 1 mm. to 2 cm. or 3 cm. in length. Suckers, which may or may not be equipped with spines or hooks, are always present and vary in size and position according to the species. The ventral surface is marked by the opening of the genital pore which is usually located near the anterior border of the ventral sucker, the acetabulum. The anterior end is indicated by the oral opening which is surrounded by a sucker, the oral sucker. The excretory pore in endoparasitic forms is usually located at the posterior tip of the body; and a fourth external opening, microscopic in size, may also be present, located usually on the mid-dorsal surface. This pore is the opening of a small canal, Laurer's canal, which connects with the female reproductive system.

In ectoparasitic trematodes, the excretory system opens right and left at the anterior end of the dorsal surface.

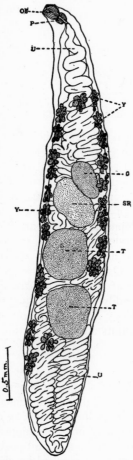

FIG. 73.—*Ostiolum medio-plexus*, dorsal view. *o.*, ovary; *os.*, oral sucker; *p.*, pharynx; *sr.*, seminal receptacle; *t.*, testis; *u.*, uterus; *v.*, vitellaria. (After Cort)

INTEGUMENT

Unlike the TURBELLARIA, the adult trematodes have no epithelium. The body is covered by a non-cellular, homogeneous layer, the cuticula, which is frequently supplied with spines (Figure 74). The cuticula is secreted by special cells which lie embedded in the underlying tissue.

MUSCULAR SYSTEM

Three distinct layers of muscles lie almost directly under the cuticula. These muscles consist of the outer circular muscles, a middle, thin layer of diagonal muscles and a third, or innermost layer of longitudinal muscles. These three sets of muscles make up what is termed the dermo-muscular sac and are used in producing alterations in the form of the body. Dorso-ventral muscles traverse the body from one surface to the other. The fibers of this set of muscles possess diverging brush-like ends which are attached to the inner surface of the cuticula. The suckers are muscular organs of attachment and are provided with special sets of muscles of equatorial, radial and meridional fibers. These muscles, particularly the radial fibers, are well developed and form powerful sucking, cupshaped discs by which the parasite fastens itself to its host.

PARENCHYMA

All the space between the muscles and the various systems is filled with a peculiar connective tissue consisting of a network of fibers which enclose spaces filled with fluid and contain many nuclei (Figure 74). This tissue is called parenchyma and is a mesenchyme.

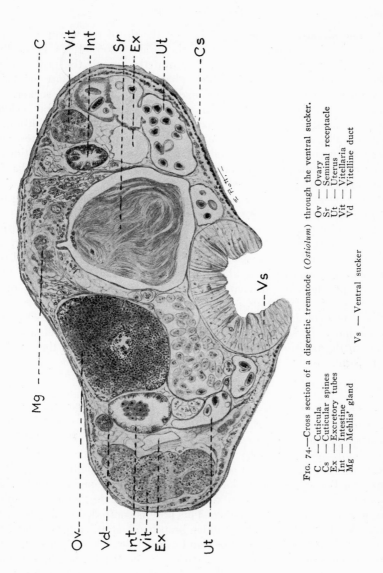

Fig. 74.—Cross section of a digenetic trematode (*Ostiolum*) through the ventral sucker.

C — Cuticula
Cs — Cuticular spines
Ex — Excretory tubes
Int — Intestine
Mg — Mehlis' gland

Ov — Ovary
Sr — Seminal receptacle
Ut — Uterus
Vit — Vitellaria
Vd — Vitelline duct

Vs — Ventral sucker

It is a characteristic of all the flatworms. There is no body cavity.

DIGESTIVE SYSTEM

The digestive system commences at the tip of the worm with the mouth, which is surrounded by the oral sucker. It is generally terminal or slightly sub-terminal. From the mouth the oral cavity leads backward into a muscular pharynx which is more or less globular and is usually smaller in diameter than the oral sucker. A short pre-pharynx may appear in some cases between the oral sucker and the muscular pharynx. Usually a very short, thin tube with muscular walls, the esophagus, connects the pharynx with the intestine. These structures of the so-called "foregut" are lined by a continuation of the cuticula surrounding the body. Unicellular, salivary glands are present and are located above the esophagus. These glands discharge by means of long ducts into the pharynx and the esophagus. The esophagus opens into the intestine which generally consists of two blind crura running backward and which vary in length according to the species. The intestinal crura are lined with tall cylindrical epithelium and have a weakly developed muscular layer composed of longitudinal and circular fibers. In species with no anal opening the waste products are discharged from the intestine through the oral opening which functions as both mouth and anus. The food of trematodes may consist of mucus, epithelial cells, intestinal contents of the host, blood, or secretions from the mucosa of the bile ducts, according to the position of the worm within the host and to the species of worm.

EXCRETORY SYSTEM

The excretory system of the trematodes is a definite tubular apparatus, symmetrically developed, and consists of the following parts: (1) a bladder, (2) collecting tubes, (3) capillaries, extensions of the flame cells, and (4) numerous, scattered flame cells (Figure 76). The bladder of endoparasitic forms usually occupies the median line of the posterior quarter of the body and opens to the exterior by a small pore at the posterior extremity, somewhat sub-terminal on the ventral surface. This pore is controlled by a sphincter muscle. The tubes of the bladder branch off at its anterior portion into the small collecting tubes and further branch off into smaller tubes which unite with the capillaries of the flame cells. The flame cell is a relatively large, hollow cell with a tuft of cilia projecting into the cavity toward the capillary (Figure 76). This tuft of cilia

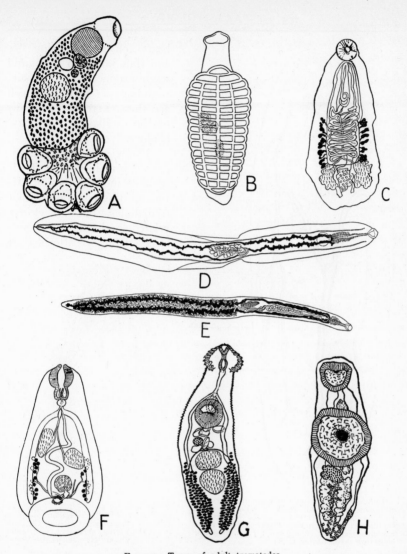

Fig. 75.—Types of adult trematodes.

A. *Polystoma megacotyle*. Mouth cavity of turtles. (After Stunkard)
B. *Aspidogaster conchicola*. Pericardial and renal cavities of fresh water mussels. (Redrawn from Stafford, internal structures omitted)
C. *Notocotylus quinqueserialis*. Cecum of American Muskrat. (Redrawn from Baker and Laughlin)
D. *Schistosomatium douthitti*. Male. Mesenteric veins of North American meadow mice. (After Price)
E. *Schistosomatium douthitti*. Female. (After Price)
F. *Diplodiscus temperatus*. Rectum of frogs. (After Krull and Price)
G. *Stephanoprora gilberti*. Intestine of water birds. (After Ward)
H. *Gorgodera minima*. Bladder of frogs. (After Cort)
(Figs. A, G and H reprinted by permission from *Fresh Water Biology* by Ward and Whipple, published by John Wiley & Sons, Inc.)

223

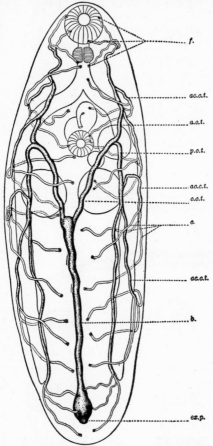

beats constantly during life and thus takes up the liquid waste products from the surrounding parenchyma which are then excreted by means of the capillaries, tubes and bladder.

Flame cells characteristically appear in groups. Their number and distribution differ in different families of trematodes, but all closely related species have the same basic excretory pattern. Cort

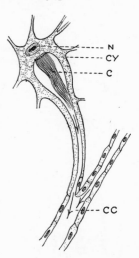

Fig. 76a.—Excretory system of *Margeana californiensis. ac.c.t.*, accessory collecting tube; *a.c.t.*, anterior collecting tube; *b.*, bladder; *c.*, capillaries; *c.c.t.*, common collecting tube; *ex.p.*, excretory pore; *f.*, flame cells; *p.c.t.*, posterior collecting tube. (After Cort)

Fig. 76b.—Diagram of a flame cell. C, cilia; CC, collecting capillary; CY, cytoplasm; N, nucleus.

(1917), Faust (1919) and Sewell (1922) and others have shown the importance of the excretory system as a basis for the establishment of a natural system of classification of TREMATODA. According to La Rue (1926), all trematodes of the subclass DIGENEA may be placed in two groups on the basis of the excretory pattern in the miracidium. In one group the miracidium has but a single flame cell on each side of its body, and is termed a "1" pattern, while in the other group the miracidium has two such flame cells on each side, a "1 + 1" pattern. In the larval stages succeeding the miracidium the flame cell number and arrangement undergo progressive modification. The number and distribution of the groups of flame cells in cercariæ have suggested family relationships.

LYMPH SYSTEM

Studies on the vascular or lymph system of trematodes have been confined almost wholly to monostomes and amphistomes. Looss was the first to recognize this system as an independent unit. More recent contributions are those of Stunkard (1929) and Willey (1930). The system consists of from 2 to 4 pairs of main channels which course along each branch of the intestine and which end blindly in oral and acetabular sinuses. It is intimately associated by complex ramifications with the intestinal crura throughout their length. The most active portions of the body, the testes, ovaries and genital suckers, receive the richest supply of lymph. The lymph is forced throughout the system as the worm elongates and contracts its body. The system obviously functions in the transfer of soluble nutrient substances from the intestine to the peripheral portions and probably, in some degree, in respiration, although respiration of most endoparasitic trematodes must be largely anærobic.

NERVOUS SYSTEM

The nervous system usually consists of a pair of cerebral ganglia situated to the right and left of and above the pharynx. These ganglia are connected with each other by a commissure dorsal to the pharynx, and from each ganglion three anterior and three posterior longitudinal nerves arise. The six nerves running backward are connected by numerous transverse commissures. Two of these six nerves are ventral, two dorsal and two lateral. Organs of special sense are lacking in adult endoparasitic forms but may be present in a few ectoparasitic forms and in the free-swimming stages of endoparasitic forms.

REPRODUCTIVE SYSTEMS

Most trematodes are true hermaphrodites, and contain complete organs of both sexes. A few, the SCHISTOSOMATIDÆ, are unisexual. The reproductive system is extremely developed, often exceedingly complicated, and the most conspicuous part of the worm. The sexual organs usually lie within the central field which is limited by the two intestinal crura.

The male genital system consists of two testes, their ducts and an organ for copulation (Figure 77). The testes are usually located in the posterior half of the body within the central field. They may lie side by side or one in front of the other and may be spherical, globular, lobed, branched or ramified, according to the species. From each testis a vas efferens originates and passes anteriorly to form,

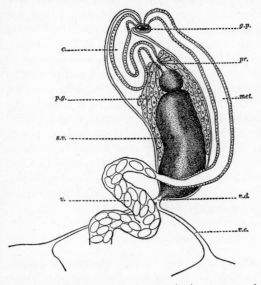

sooner or later, the vas deferens which passes into the so-called "cirrus sac." The cirrus sac envelopes three sections, (1) a dilated portion, the seminal vesicle, (2) the median section of unicellular prostate glands, and (3) the terminal muscular portion, the cirrus, which functions as the male organ of copulation. When functioning the cirrus may be protruded through the male genital pore, through the common genital atrium and into the female system by the

FIG. 77.—End ducts of the reproductive systems of *Margeana californiensis; c.,* cirrus; *g.p.,* genital pore; *met.,* metraterm; *p.g.,* prostate glands; *pr.,* prostate region; *s.v.,* seminal vesicle; *v.d.,* vas deferens; *v.e.,* vas efferens; *u.,* uterus. (After Cort)

evagination of its lumen during the contractions of the muscular walls of the cirrus sac.

The female genital apparatus consists of a single ovary, its oviduct, a seminal receptacle, two vitelline or yolk glands with their ducts, Mehlis' gland, and uterus (Figure 78). In many of the endoparasitic trematodes the female system is equipped with an additional canal, Laurer's canal, which leaves the oviduct near its union with the duct from the seminal receptacle and passes forward, opening on the dorsal surface of the body. In ectoparasitic forms, a similar canal, vitelline-intestinal canal, is found, but it leads to the intestine and not to the exterior. The ovary usually lies anterior to the testes.

It is smaller than the testes and may also vary in form according to the species. It is thin-walled, vesicular in structure and contains un-fertilized ova in different stages of development. The oviduct is usually very short and is soon joined by Laurer's canal and the duct from the seminal receptacle. The function of Laurer's canal is not well understood. Its main purpose may be for an escape of excess amounts of sperm and yolk material. The seminal receptacle is a thin-walled sac-like organ and its function is the storage of the

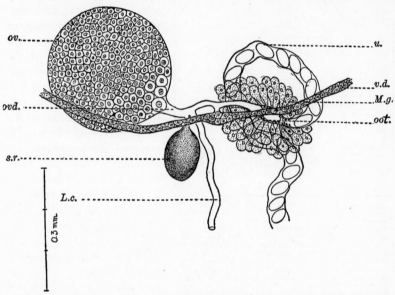

Fig. 78.—Connections of the ducts of the female reproductive system of *Margeana californiensis;* *L.c.,* Laurer's canal; *M.g.,* Mehlis' gland; *oot.,* oötype; *ov.,* ovary; *ovd.,* oviduct; *sr.,* seminal receptacle; *u.* uterus; *v.d.,* vitelline duct. (After Cort)

spermatozoa. Two yolk glands (vitellaria) are situated usually within the middle third of the body along each lateral field. These glands occur in grape-like bunches and are connected with each other by longitudinal excretory ducts which are connected with transverse ducts where they unite to form a common vitelline duct. The trans-verse ducts ·are ventral to the intestinal crura and usually pass somewhat below the ovary. At the union of the two transverse vitelline ducts a dilatation may occur which serves as a vitelline reservoir. The common vitelline duct joins the oviduct near the entrance of the duct from the seminal receptacle. Slightly beyond the point where the common vitelline duct joins the oviduct the tube

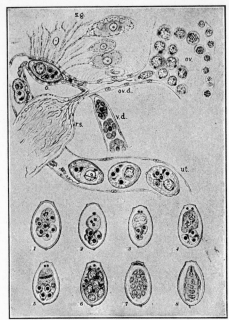

Fig. 79.—The development and fertilization of the egg in *Collyriclum faba* from the European sparrow. The cells are drawn to scale, but other structures are foreshortened and brought into one plane; *ov.*, ovary, with small, primitive ova at the periphery to the right; passing to left successive stages of development are shown—the rearrangement of the chromatin in chromosomes, the increase in the size of the ova, and the appearance of an extranuclear body, or attraction sphere, with the return of the nucleus to the resting state; *ov.d.*, oviduct in which the ova are mingled with the spermatozoa which pass from *r.s.*, receptaculum seminis; *v.d.*, vitelline duct filled with yolk cells with globules of granular material, which is liberated from these cells as they pass out of the duct; *s.g.*, Mehlis' gland—shown only in part—with secreting cells, showing cytoplasmic granules which are distributed along slender processes, extending to the oötype; *o.*, oötype, showing a peripheral membrane, enclosing a fertilized ovum, with spermatozoön coiled around the nucleus, and four yolk cells, from which the stored material has been utilized in the formation of the shell; *ut.*, the first portion of the uterus, containing several eggs, in which the yolk material has not yet been wholly incorporated into the shell. Masses of excess yolk and occasional spermatozoa are also shown. 1-8, successive stages in the development of the egg. 8, egg containing fully developed miracidium as it leaves the parent worm. (After Tyzzer)

may become considerably widened into a muscular portion known as the "oötype." The oötype is in turn surrounded by a number of unicellular glands (Mehlis' gland) which probably secrete a liquid in which the ova are suspended. The beginning of the uterus follows the oötype. The uterus of the adult endoparasitic trematodes is very long and follows an exceedingly tortuous course between the intestinal crura. It usually contains an enormous accumulation of ova and these more or less completely obscure all other organs. The terminal portion of the uterus usually lies beside the cirrus sac and discharges into the common genital atrium, which in turn opens to the exterior through the common genital spore. The very terminal portion of the uterus is often modified, and is known as the metraterm. It serves as a vagina.

FERTILIZATION

Both cross and self-fertilization are possible with the trematodes, although it is believed that self-fertilization is the commoner occurrence, especially among the endoparasitic forms. In both, the cirrus is the organ of copulation. Cross fertilization via Laurer's canal is possible and probably occurs from time to time. The spermatozoa, which are structurally similar to those of other animals, on entering the metraterm of the female system travel all the length of the uterus until they reach the seminal receptacle, in which they become stored up in great quantities. The ova, produced in the ovary, pass down the oviduct and become fertilized by the spermatozoa as they pass by the opening of the duct of the seminal receptacle. Yolk globules liberated from yolk cells in the vitelline ducts are poured into the oviduct. The fertilized ovum, together with a more or less constant number of yolk globules, passes into the oötype and there becomes enclosed in a shell. The shape of the egg is largely determined by the oötype which contracts energetically and serves more or less as a mold. Most trematode ova have operculated shells and may possess a characteristic knob or abbreviated spine which represents a slight projection of shell material into the oviduct. The shell is probably derived from the fusing together of liberated yolk globules, while the glands surrounding the oötype probably secrete a liquid in which the ova are suspended, serving more or less as a lubricant. The completed ovum is pushed forward into the uterus followed by other ova until the uterus is completely filled. Their escape to the exterior is via the metraterm into the common genital atrium and thence to the outside through the common genital pore. The endoparasitic trematodes produce immense numbers of ova which is an adaptation to the parasitic habit, and which counterbalances the loss incurred by the species in its transfer to new hosts. This early development is illustrated in Figure 79.

LARVAL DEVELOPMENT

All the ectoparasitic trematodes have a simple and direct manner of development. A ciliated larva develops within the ovum, which, upon hatching, swims about in the water until it attaches itself to its host where it feeds and grows directly into the adult stage. The endoparasitic forms, on the other hand, may have an extremely complicated life-cycle, involving both an alternation of generations and an alternation of hosts. There is multiplication by the production of fertilized ova by the adult worm in its final host, and by asexual generations which develop when the fluke is harbored by its first intermediate host. The germ cell cycle of endoparasitic trematodes has been a subject of much study and debate for more than a century. Hypotheses offered to explain their remarkable development in the snail host include metagenesis, heterogeny, pædogenesis, extended metamorphosis, germinal lineage, germinal lineage through poly-

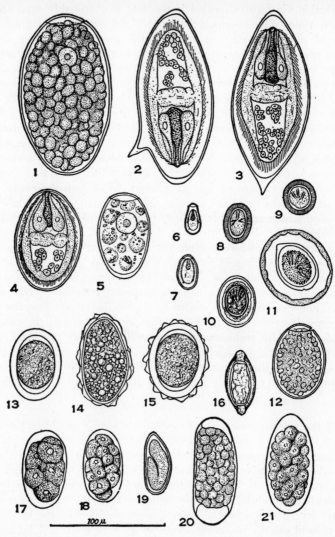

FIG. 80.—Eggs of the most important helminths of man. 1, *Fasciolopsis buski.* 2, *Schistosoma mansoni.* 3, *Schistosoma hæmatobium.* 4, *Schistosoma japonicum.* 5, *Paragonimus westermanii.* 6, *Clonorchis sinensis.* 7, *Metagonimus yokogawai.* 8, *Tænia saginata.* 9, *Tænia solium.* 10, *Hymenolepis nana.* 11, *Hymenolepis diminuta.* 12, *Diphyllobothrium latum.* 13, *Ascaris lumbricoides* (egg without outer coating). 14, *Ascaris lumbricoides* (abnormal egg). 15, *Ascaris lumbricoides.* 16, *Trichuris trichiura.* 17 and 18, Hookworm eggs. 19, *Enterobius vermicularis.* 20, *Heterodera radicicola* (*Oxyuris incognita*). 21, *Trichostrongylus orientalis.* (From Hegner, Cort, and Root, *Outlines of Medical Zoölogy*)

embryony and, finally, sexual reproduction. The more recent contributions on the generation have been made by Brooks (1930), Woodhead (1931), Anderson (1935) and Chen (1937).

The ova of many endoparasitic forms are completely developed at the time they reach the external world, while others may show no advancement whatever (Figure 80, 1-7). The ovum upon falling in fresh water may directly hatch or complete its embryological development, as the case may be. The embryo within the egg shell sooner or later escapes as a ciliated larva and swims about in search of a new host, a mollusc, which serves as its intermediate host. This larva is called the miracidium and may possess all the following structures: (1) a ciliated ectoderm with spine; (2) an elementary digestive organ; (3) secretory gland; (4) a collection of germinal cells attached to the body wall or lying freely within the body; (5) an excretory system; and (6) a nervous system (Figure 81). The miracidium is not a feeding stage. Its function is merely to carry the infection to the snail host, and unless it finds this host within a few hours, it dies. The miracidium usually enters its host by directly penetrating through the soft tissues and in so doing becomes denuded of its ciliated ectoderm. It then becomes an irregular, sac-like, extremely simple organism termed the sporocyst (Figure 82).

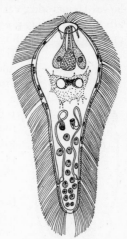

FIG. 81.—Miracidium of a digenetic trematode.

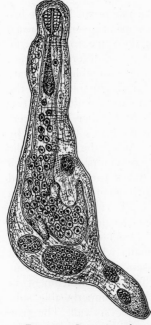

FIG. 82.—Sporocyst of a digenetic trematode containing a redia and developing germ cells.

The sporocyst possesses a body cavity which serves as a brood pouch for the developing daughter embryos. The daughter embryos grow to maturity and escape from the mother sporocyst by the rupture of the wall, and, in turn, produce young probably by parthenogenesis. This generation may also consist of simple organisms, sporocysts, which by a similar process give rise to larval trematodes, cercariæ; or they may consist of organisms, which are termed rediæ, possessing a rhabdocœle intestine with pharynx, an oral sucker and a birth pore (Figure 83). A granddaughter generation follows which may consist of cercariæ or another generation of rediæ which in turn gives rise to a generation of cercariæ. The cercariæ are a still more differentiated organism than the rediæ, showing both oral and ventral suckers, mouth, pharynx and bifurcated intestine, excretory system, specialized glands and a caudal appendage by which it propels itself through the water (Figure 84).

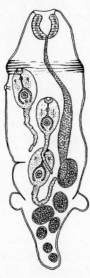

FIG. 83.—Redia of a digenetic trematode containing cercariæ and developing germ cells.

The cercariæ leave the molluscan host. It has been observed that they escape at given times each day. These times remain the same for a specific kind of cercaria, but differ for different species. Their function is to reach a suitable vertebrate host, the definitive host, for the completion of the life-cycle of the species to the adult stage. Entrance is gained into this host either by the cercariæ actively penetrating the host's tissues or by being taken in with the food of the host. In the first case, the cercariæ are equipped with well developed secretory apparatus for attacking and penetrating the tissues of the mammalian host. In the second case, the cercariæ may become encysted on vegetables which serve as food for the definitive host, or they may penetrate into a lower vertebrate (fish) or an anthropod (crayfish, crabs, or the like) or a mollusc (snail) which become food for the definitive host. Such cercariæ possess special cystogenous glands which not only secrete substances for their attachment to infective agents, vegetables, and so on, but also impermeable substances which surround the cercariæ, the true cyst wall. The true cyst wall protects the cercariæ against unfavorable conditions of the environment and against the acid medium of the stomach of the vertebrate host. The encysted stage of trematodes is generally termed the metacercaria (Figure 85). It is also known as the adolescaria. In every case, the cercaria, free or encysted, according to the species, is the only stage which is infective to the final, vertebrate host.

By placing snails from fresh-water ponds and streams into small glass receptacles and examining them closely with the unaided eye or a hand glass, small, white, exceedingly active organisms may be seen escaping from the snail. These are cercariæ. They may be collected with a pipette for microscopical study. The cercariæ, as well as other developing larval stages within the body of the snail, may also be obtained for study by cutting or crushing the shell so as to remove the body onto a glass slide for microscopic examination. If larval trematodes are present, some are almost invariably loosened from the infected part of the snail during this operation and may be found scattered around the snail in the water. The liver, or digestive gland, is apt to be the organ which is most heavily infected and may contain sporocysts, rediæ, cercariæ and

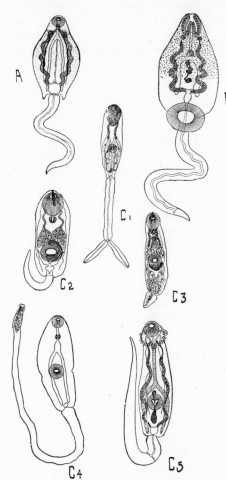

FIG. 84.—Examples of North American cercariæ: A, Monostome cercaria, *C. urbanensis.* B, Amphistome cercaria, *C. inhabilis.* C(1-5), Distome cercariæ; C1, Furcocercous, *C, douthitti;* C2, Xiphidiocercaria, *C, isocotylea;* C3, Microcercous, *C. trigonura;* C4, Gymnocephalous, *C, megalura;* C5, Echinostome, *C. trivolvis.* (After Cort)

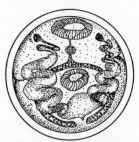

FIG. 85.—Encysted cercaria (metacercaria) of a digenetic trematode.

even metacercariæ. These may be studied in the living condition or killed in a sublimate fixing fluid and stained with hæmatoxylin.

A careful study of the cercariæ will show that they possess both (1) "adult characters" such as suckers, digestive and excretory systems, which foreshadow adult structure, and (2) "larval characters" which are merely temporary structures, the tail, stylet, cystogenous and cephalic glands, which are not carried over into adult life, but are developed only to meet the requirements of larval conditions. Types of cercariæ from North American molluscs are shown in Figure 84.

II. *Collection and Preservation of Trematodes*

Adult trematodes are commonly present in the intestine, liver, lungs and veins. Larval forms are less restricted in location and may be found in the body cavity, on various organs and within the muscles.

Small trematodes are best killed by Looss' shaking method. The specimens are shaken vigorously for a few minutes in a small amount of physiological salt solution. The killing solution, acetic-sublimate, is then poured on cold. After from four to eight hours in this solution, they are washed in 50 per cent alcohol for one-half hour, then in 70 per cent alcohol, tinged straw-color with iodine, for at least one hour. The specimens are then washed several times in 70 per cent alcohol until the color of iodine is entirely removed, after which they may be preserved in 80 per cent alcohol plus 5 per cent glycerine.

Large trematodes are best killed by pouring hot killing solution over them while they are flattened between slides.

The most satisfactory stains for trematodes are Delafield's hæmatoxylin and borax-carmine. Very dilute solutions should be used. The specimens should remain in the stain for several hours or overnight, and then rapidly destained in 70 per cent alcohol plus 2 per cent HCl. After dehydration the specimens may be cleared in carboxylol and mounted in Canada balsam or damar. Serial sections may be made of specimens stained *in toto,* or staining may be done after sectioning. The usual paraffin method is satisfactory.

Operculate trematode eggs are best preserved in 10 per cent formalin. Non-operculate eggs (SCHISTOSOMATA) should be first concentrated and then killed in hot 70 per cent alcohol plus 5 per cent glycerine. The alcohol should be allowed to evaporate slowly. Permanent mounts of eggs may be made by placing a small amount of the sediment in warm glycerine jelly on a slide and sealing the preparation with Noyer's lanoline cement.

III. *Classification of Trematodes*

The class TREMATODA is divided into three large subclasses, (1) MONOGENEA v. Beneden, 1858, (2) ASPIDOGASTREA Faust and Tang, 1936 and (3) DIGENEA v. Beneden, 1858. The monogenetic trematodes are mostly ectoparasites on aquatic vertebrates. They have powerfully developed posterior organs for attachment, carrying hooks and anchors (Figure 75A). In most forms the development is probably direct. The larva upon hatching is ciliated, but otherwise closely resembles the adult. After a free-swimming period, the larva attaches itself to its host, the cilia disappear and it grows, without metamorphosis, into the final stage. Development by true polyembryony has been noted in one species, *Gyrodactylus elegans* (Kathariner, 1904), a common parasite on the skin and gills of many fresh-water fishes; and an alternation of generations has been discovered in the life-cycle of *Polystoma integerrimum,* a parasite on the gills of tadpoles and in the rectum of frogs (Gallien, 1933). The aspidogastrid trematodes, the ASPIDOGASTREA, are parasites of cold-blooded animals including gasteropods, bivalves, crustaceans, fishes and turtles. They have a powerful ventral sucking organ. It is never supplied with anchors or hooks. It is usually in the form of a large sucking disc distinctly set off from the body and subdivided into numerous sucking alveoli (Figure 75B) or it may consist of a single series of small disconnected suckers. As far as is known, the life-cycle is simple and direct. The larva upon hatching possesses the fundamental characteristics of the adult and develops directly into the final stage, either in the same host or in another individual of the same or a different species. The members of the subclass DIGENEA are all endoparasites. They have a development through a complex series of stages involving an alternation of hosts, one of which is always a mollusc, and also an alternation of generations. All the trematodes parasitic in man, as well as those of economic importance in the lower vertebrates, belong to the subclass DIGENEA.

The older systems of classification of trematodes have been based largely upon the comparative anatomy of preserved adult worms. The arrangement of the reproductive organs has been used in making generic groups and in combining these into families. The orders and suborders have been based almost exclusively upon the external structure, such as the number, position and character of the organs of attachment. It has been shown by several workers that the organs of fixation are adaptive characters which have developed in connection with the parasitic habit. They are, therefore, cenogenetic structures and do not indicate genetic relationship. Cort (1917) in a study of the homologies of the excretory systems of five different forked-tailed cercariæ, which then represented three separate groups and two distinct families, discovered that the flame cell pattern in all five cercariæ was practically identical. This suggested a basis for the establishment of a natural system of classification. From this study and that of later workers, it is now evident that the excretory system is the only system of trematode anatomy which indicates genetic relationship. La Rue (1926) reorganized the classification of the digenetic trematodes on the basis of the fundamental flame cell arrangements in the miracidium. A main part of the classification given here is that proposed by La Rue. The classification cannot be considered complete because our knowledge of the life-cycles of many species and even of groups are not complete. By necessity, it includes groups established upon external anatomy and upon the flame cell pattern. Future study of the excretory systems of species and families will undoubtedly break up some of the now existing divisions. The student is referred to the following publications for detailed systems of trematode classification: Odhner, 1912; Ward, 1918; Gamble, 1922; Braun, 1925; Stiles and Hassall, 1926; Poche, 1926; Fuhrmann, 1928; Pearse, 1936; Price, 1937, and Dubois, 1938.

Class TREMATODA Rudolphi, 1808. PLATYHELMINTHES; living as ecto-parasites or endoparasites; cilia present only in larval stage; alimentary canal present; adult stage usually parasitic in vertebrates.

Subclass I. MONOGENEA v. Beneden, 1858. TREMATODA; usually ectoparasites; posterior organs of attachment extremely developed, always with chitinous anchors and hooks; uterus short, usually containing a single egg; development simple, direct. Parasites of fishes, turtles and amphibians.

Order 1. MONOPISTHOCOTYLEA Odhner, 1912. MONOGENEA; posterior organ of attachment single; vagina unpaired; no genito-intestinal canal; ectoparasite on skin and gills of fishes. Example, *Gyrodactylus elegans* v. Nordmann, 1832, on fresh water fishes, often cause of serious epidemic among young fishes at hatcheries and wild waters.

Order 2. POLYOPISTHOCOTYLEA Odhner, 1912. MONOGENEA; posterior organ of attachment multiple (two or many parted) ; vagina double; genito-intestinal canal present. Parasites of amphibians, turtles and fishes. Example, *Polystoma integerrimum* Zeller, 1872, on the gills of tadpoles and in the bladder of frogs, and *Sphyranura aligorchis* Alvey, 1936, on *Necturus maculosus.*

Subclass II. ASPIDOGASTREA Faust and Tang, 1936; TREMATODA; endoparasites; oral sucker absent or poorly developed; ventral sucking organ a powerful adhesive disc, frequently divided into series of sucking cups; intestine a simple blind sac; development probably direct; flame-cell pattern of larva "1 + 1 + 1"; parasitic on or in the soft parts of molluscs or in the intestinal canal of cold-blooded vertebrates. Example, *Aspidogaster conchicola* v. Baer, 1826.

Subclass III. DIGENEA v. Beneden, 1858; TREMATODA; endoparasites; organs of attachment consisting of one or two suckers of which the anterior is always single and median; without chitinous anchors and hooks; uterus long containing great masses of ova; flame cell pattern "1" or "1 + 1"; development by metamorphosis and alternation of hosts; all trematodes parasitic in man fall within this group.

Order 1. PROSOSTOMATA Odhner, 1905. DIGENEA; cercarial stage with unforked tail; adults hermaphroditic; mouth at or near anterior tip of body and usually surrounded by an oral sucker; a second sucker, if present, behind oral sucker, on ventral surface or at posterior end. Flame cell arrangement of miracidium is "1."

Order 2. STRIGEATOIDEA La Rue, 1926. DIGENEA, cercarial form with forked tail, with or without pharynx; flame cell arrangement or cercariæ reducible to a 1 + 1 pattern. Adults monoecious or dioecius, parasitic in intestinal tract of vertebrates or in the blood stream.

CHAPTER XVIII

THE DIGENETIC TREMATODES

Order *Prosostomata* Odhner, 1905

This order consists of three main groups, (1) MONOSTOMATA Zeder, 1800; (2) DISTOMATA Zeder, 1800; and (3) AMPHISTOMATA Bojanus, 1817, which rank as suborders. The MONOSTOMATA are fairly frequent parasites of birds and reptiles and occasionally have been encountered in mammals. Most of the trematodes of man as well as most of those of economic importance in lower animals belong to the DISTOMATA and AMPHISTOMATA.

I. Suborder MONOSTOMATA Zeder, 1800

The monostomes are particularly frequent in domestic and wild water fowl. As the name implies, they never possess more than one sucker, the oral sucker. The eggs of the commoner species carry long filaments at both poles. Some workers have looked upon the monostomes as isolated members of other groups that have lost all suckers except that surrounding the mouth, and that they should be classified in various families from which they originated. The monostomes are generally recognized as consisting of two families, (1) CYCLOCŒLIDÆ Kossack, 1911 and NOTOCOTYLIDÆ Lühe, 1909.

The CYCLOCŒLIDÆ are relatively large monostomes, varying from 5 mm. to 21 mm. in length. They lack a definite oral sucker. The intestinal crura may be simple, but in many species small ceca occur along the inner margins. They are also joined, thus forming a continuous arc at the posterior end of the body. The eggs do not have polar filaments. *Typhlocœlum cucumerinum* (Rudolphi, 1809) occurs in the esophagus, trachea, air sacs and thoracic cavity of domestic and wild ducks of Brazil, and *Tracheophilus cymbius* (Diesing, 1850) similarly occurs in European ducks. These parasites cause suffocation and even death to the host when occurring in large numbers. In their development the sporocyst stage is lacking. Upon hatching, the miracidium contains a fully developed redia. Within the snail host, species of *Planorbis* and *Lymnæa,* the redia gives rise to daughter rediæ in which cercariæ develop. The cercariæ are tailless and they encyst within the snail in which they develop. Ducks become infected by eating snails containing the encysted cercariæ.

The NOTOCOTYLIDÆ are small monostomes with three or five rows or groups of unicellular glands on the ventral surface. The uterus forms more or less regular transverse coils extending from the ovary to the posterior end of the cirrus sac. The eggs bear long polar filaments. They are intestinal parasites of aquatic birds and mammals. *Notocotylus quinqueserialis* Baker and Laughlin, 1911 (Figure 75c), and *Catatropis filamentis* Baker, 1915, occur in muskrats of North America. *Notocotylus attenuatus* (Rudolphi, 1809) (Figure 86) and *Catatropis verrucosa* (Frölich, 1789) occur in the cecum of water fowl. *Paramonostomum parvum* Stunkard and Dunihue, 1931, occurs in North

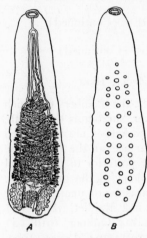

FIG. 86.—*Notocotylus attenuatus.* A, Adult, showing arrangement of internal structures; B, Adult, showing the grouping of the ventral glands. (Redrawn from L. and U. Szidat)

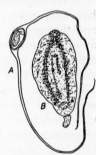

FIG. 87.—*Notocotylus attenuatus.* A, egg; B, cercaria. (Redrawn from Joyeux)

American ducks. According to Joyeux (1922), the sporocyst of *Notocotylus* contains two rediæ. The cercariæ (Figure 87) developing from these rediæ encyst within the snail host, *Planorbis rotundatus.* The final host becomes infected by eating snails containing the encysted cercariæ. These parasites are usually considered quite harmless to their hosts.

CHAPTER XIX

THE DIGENETIC TREMATODES (Continued)

Order Prosostomata Odhner, 1905 (Continued)

II. Suborder DISTOMATA Zeder, 1800

This suborder consists of several families, the members of which have two suckers. One sucker, the oral sucker, surrounds the mouth, and the second, the acetabulum or ventral sucker, is always located at or above the mid-area of the ventral surface of the body. The reproductive organs lie completely or largely posterior to the ventral sucker. Most of the trematodes of man belong to the DISTOMATA. The following families contain important parasites of man, domestic animals or lower vertebrates, (1) FASCIOLIDÆ Railliet, 1895, (2) OPISTHORCHIIDÆ Lühe, 1901, (3) DICROCŒLIIDÆ Odhner, 1910, (4) PLAGIORCHIIDÆ Lühe, 1901, (5) ECHINOSTOMATIDÆ Looss, 1902, (6) HETEROPHYIDÆ Odhner, 1914 and (7) TROGLOTREMATIDÆ Odhner, 1914.

I. Family FASCIOLIDÆ

These trematodes have fairly large, flattened, leaf-shaped bodies and usually a spiny cuticula. The ventral sucker is prominent and is located close to the oral sucker. The testes and ovary are greatly branched. The vitellaria are strongly developed. The uterus is usually short and lies anterior to the ovary. They are, for the most part, parasites in the bile ducts of sheep and cattle. One species, *Fasciolopsis buski* Lankester, 1857, is an important intestinal parasite of man.

1. *Fasciolopsis buski* (Lankester, 1857)

HISTORICAL

Fasciolopsis buski (Figures 88 and 89) was discovered by Dr. Busk in 1843 in the duodenum of a Lascar (East Indian) sailor who died in the Seamen's Hospital in London. Lankester, in 1857, described this parasite and named it *Distoma buskii*. Apparently Dr. Busk objected to this designation and the specimen was redescribed

in 1860 by Cobbold who gave it the name *Distoma crassum*. This
name, however, could not stand as it was already preoccupied for
another species of trematode; and further, according to the rules of
zoölogical nomenclature, the original specific designation had to be
accepted. In 1899 Looss carefully worked out the morphology of
this parasite and created the genus *Fasciolopsis* to which it was
assigned. Several species of *Fasciolopsis* have since been described
from man under the names of *Fasciolopsis rathouisi, F. fülleborni,*
and *F. goddardi,* but Goddard (1919) brings conclusive evidence that

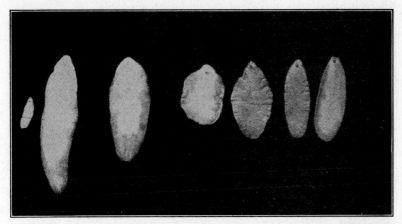

Fɪɢ. 88.—*Fasciolopsis buski.* Varieties of the fluke from man. Natural size. (After
Goddard)

they are all the same. Brown described in 1917 *Fasciolopsis spinifera*
from China, basing the specific differences on the presence of cuticular spines. Barlow (1925) has now shown that this specific division
is invalid, as it was based on differences which had been produced
by different ways in which the parasites had been recovered from
the patients and by the treatment they had undergone in various
preservative solutions. Brown's specific division is, therefore, un-
warranted and the conclusion can be drawn that there is but one
species of *Fasciolopsis* in man, i.e., *Fasciolopsis buski* (Lankester).

DISTRIBUTION AND FREQUENCY

Fasciolopsis buski is widely spread, having been reported from
many parts of China, as far north as the Yangtze Valley and as far
west as Chengtu and Suifu in Szechuen province and throughout the
southern provinces. It has also been reported from Russia, India,

Assam, Straits Settlements, Siam, Sumatra and Borneo. It occurs to the greatest extent in China, and there the most heavily infected endemic center is the Shaohsing area, a district of about 1,600 square miles containing between a million and a million and a half people. So prevalent is this parasite in this area that it is considered one of the principal causes of a severe illness and of a great loss of life. This area was recognized as an endemic center of fasciolopsiasis as early as 1893, and is apparently the only endemic center of this parasite in man in China and probably the only place in the world where it affords an important public health problem.

DESCRIPTION OF THE ADULT

Fasciolopsis buski is the largest trematode parasitic in man and may attain a length of 75 mm. and a width of 15 mm. The size of the parasites varies greatly, however, in different patients. It has

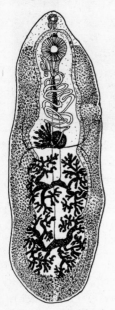

FIG. 89.—*Fasciolopsis buski*. Ventral view.

been observed that flukes from very poor people are smaller than those from patients of better financial status, indicating that the parasites thrive better on a more varied fare than the poor people provide them. Also where the infection is massive the parasites usually are smaller in size than where the infection consists of a few worms only. The largest flukes usually come from light infections. The average length is about 30 mm., average width about 12 mm. and average thickness about 2 mm. In the living condition the worms may be flesh-colored or the color of normal fresh blood, elongated, oval in outline and narrower anteriorly than posteriorly. The cuticula is covered with small, backward pointing spines arranged in transverse rows; these are most numerous about the acetabulum. The oral sucker is subterminal on the ventral side and is about 0.5 mm. in diameter. The acetabulum lies posterior and close to the oral sucker; it is from two to three times as large as the oral sucker, and has a pear-shaped opening. The prepharynx leads into the pharynx and there is practically no esophagus. The intestinal crura branch off almost directly from the pharynx and pass to the posterior extremity with two characteristic curves, one at the anterior border of the anterior testis, the other between the testes.

The testes occupy the posterior half of the body within the central field and lie one behind the other. They are dichotomously branched and their ducts unite in the middle portion of the anterior half of the body to form a seminal vesicle which passes forward as a convoluted tube within the cirrus sac which opens into the genital atrium, the pore of which opens immediately anterior to the acetabulum on the ventral surface.

The ovary is also branched and is situated in the middle of the body on the right of the median line. Mehlis' gland is well developed and is placed immediately to the left of the ovary. The vitellaria extend from the acetabulum along the lateral fields to the posterior tip of the body where they meet. The acini are very small. The uterus lies entirely anterior to the ovary and testes and is relatively short in comparison with that structure in many other trematodes. The eggs are usually very numerous in the feces from persons harboring the infection and even in very light infections it is almost impossible to overlook them by simple methods of examination. They average 138 μ in length and 83 μ in breadth and show no development when found in freshly passed feces (Figure 90). They are predominately oval in outline, brown in color, and are closed by a very delicate operculum.

LIFE-CYCLE

Fasciolopsis buski lives normally in the small intestine and to some extent in the stomach of man and pig. Dogs, monkeys and rabbits can be infected, but the worms do not develop to maturity in these animals (Young, 1936).

The development of *Fasciolopsis buski* closely parallels that of *Fasciola hepatica,* the sheep liver fluke, which has served for so many years as a classical illustration of the development of digenetic trematodes. Nakagawa (1921) worked out the life history of *Fasciolopsis buski* from pigs in Formosa, and Barlow (1925) followed the development in detail from human material in the Shaohsing area, China.

The ova when passed are in the one or two-celled stage and are surrounded by from twenty to forty yolk globules which disappear as the ovum develops. At the opercular end of the egg is a mucoid plug which probably acts as a protection against too early loosening of the operculum by the secretion of the miracidium.

The rate of development among a given lot of ova is uneven, some may show little or no advancement while in others the miracidia may be escaping from the shells. Usually at least twenty-two days are required for the miracidium to mature at optimum temperature, from 80° to 90° F. The fully developed miracidium within the shell is covered with a ciliated ectoderm composed of five tiers of six plates to the tier. There is present a well defined, pigmented eyespot and two flame cells. The miracidium also possesses a primitive digestive tract, a cul de sac, the mouth of which is patent. At the time of the escape of the miracidium from the shell the operculum opens following the dissolution of the mucoid plug by secretions of the miracidium and the miracidium swims away seeking a suitable host. The span of life of the free-swimming miracidium is limited to only a few hours unless it reaches and successfully enters its snail host, *Planorbis schmackeri* or *Segmentina nitedellus*.

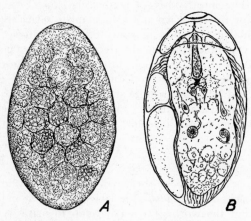

FIG. 90.—*Fasciolopsis buski*. A. Freshly passed egg. B. Egg containing fully developed miracidium. (After Barlow)

The miracidium may enter the snail hosts either through the respiratory orifice and then into the respiratory chamber where they enter directly into the body of the snail through the epithelial lining of the chamber, or they may actively penetrate any projecting surface of the snail. During the intrusion of its body into the tissues of the snail, the ectodermal plates become lost and the miracidium becomes the sporocyst. The development of the mother rediæ within the sporocyst is rapid. They emerge in about nine days and migrate up to the ovotestis of the snail. These mother rediæ produce daughter rediæ and the daughter rediæ in turn give rise to cercariæ. The cercariæ begin to emerge from the daughter rediæ in about twenty-five to thirty days after the infection of the snail by the miracidium, and, after leaving the daughter rediæ, they remain in the liver region for some time to mature before their migration down the lymph spaces to an exit from the snail.

The cercaria of *Fasciolopsis* has a straight, slender tail. There are two groups of well developed cystogenous glands, which later take part in the formation of the cyst. One set, the round-celled glands, secretes the material for the outer cyst wall and lies dorsally, and the other set, the rhabdoidal glands, secretes the material for the inner cyst wall. The free-swimming stage is brief and occupies only time enough for the cercaria to reach a plant where it attaches itself with its mouth and ventral suckers and begins to encyst. The outer cyst wall is formed first. This wall is well adapted to its purpose of acting as a simple supportive case for the cyst. It is extremely friable and easily detached from the plant. The inner cyst wall, however, is thick and tough. It is resistant even to hydrochloric acid, but is soluble in the intestinal juices. The cysts are more or less spherical; the outer cyst wall averages about $216\,\mu \times 187\,\mu$, while the inner cyst wall averages $148\,\mu \times 138\,\mu$.

Barlow found that the snails, from which the cercariæ have escaped, usually feed on caltrop and water nuts (*Trapa natans* and *Eliochairs tuberosa*), which vegetables are used as food by the human population of the endemic areas. The crops are fertilized with human feces and are raised in field-enclosed ponds. The ova of the parasite are thus directly introduced into the habitat of the snail host and the relationship between the snail and the plant brings the encystment of the cercaria to the place where it is most efficacious for the parasite and most dangerous for man.

These water nuts and caltrops are brought into the Chinese markets from the middle of July to the end of September for sale as fresh nuts. After September until the next spring they are sold as dry or stored nuts. As drying quicky kills the metacercariæ, it is only the fresh nuts that are of any danger. The danger of infection in the market is greatly enhanced because the vendor constantly sprinkles the caltrops with a brush dipped into unboiled canal water. Most of the caltrops are eaten raw at the time of purchasing, while those eaten in the fields are taken directly from the water where they grow just below the surface of the water on flesh root stalks. They are peeled with the teeth, during which process the outer cyst wall becomes ruptured and the cyst is deposited into the mouth and passes on to the duodenum. Here the inner cyst wall is dissolved away and the immature worm attaches itself to the mucosa of the upper intestine and rapidly grows into the adult stage. Barlow has found as many as 200 cysts of *Fasciolopsis buski* on a single caltrop. It is not surprising therefore that exceedingly heavy infections often occur in man in the endemic area.

SYMPTOMS

Intestinal trematodes, especially when occurring in large numbers, are known to cause abdominal discomfort, nausea, tenderness below the right costal margin, diarrhea, anemia, and edema. Large numbers, however, are not always necessary to give rise to noticeable symptoms, for many patients harboring but one or two worms often show appreciable disease.

Goddard (1919) recognizes three stages in fasciolopsiasis: (a) A period of latency in which there may be no marked symptoms but probably some asthenia and mild anemia. Barlow refers to this period as one of growth or development extending from the infection to a size sufficient to produce an amount of toxin which would cause apparent injury, and looks upon the onset of the clinical manifestations as occurring in a gradually increasing scale of severity, due to the growth of the parasites which develop to maturity without intermission. (b) A period of several months of diarrhea with abdominal pain. There is no jaundice and no blood in the stool. Diarrhea, according to Barlow, is not a constant symptom and may alternate with periods of constipation. (c) A period of edema in which the anemia is increased and the edema becomes more distressing. The edema may appear within twenty days of infection in case the patient is small or undernourished and the infection is massive. In fatal cases there is a marked edema with ascites and an extensive anasarca. Death, when it occurs, is apparently due to exhaustion. According to Barlow (1925) the apparent anemia is largely due to viewing the blood stream through an overlying edema. The edema does not involve the lungs and probably not the chest cavity even in advanced cases.

TREATMENT

Beta naphthol and carbon tetrachloride have been used with success in expelling intestinal flukes. Barlow finds carbon tetrachloride the most efficacious anthelmintic in the treatment of fasciolopsiasis.

The measures for prevention and control of fasciolopsiasis are, as in most cases of endemic helminth disease, simple in theory and exceedingly difficult to carry out in actual practice. They involve the changing of age-old customs, laws and religions of people who are, as a rule, ignorant, suspicious, more or less indifferent and superstitious. The control of human fasciolopsiasis is however hopeful, because it seriously affects only the people of a relatively small, limited area, the life history of the parasite is thoroughly understood, and the diagnosis of infected individuals is easily made from the ova, which are large and occur in large numbers, even in very light infections. A number of efficient and cheap drugs are also known which readily expel the adults from the host. Free clinics within the endemic area together with educational propaganda have resulted in noticeable improvement clinically.

Time-honored customs within the endemic area are, however, particularly favorable for the propagation of the life-cycle of *Fasciolopsis buski*. Fresh human excrement, urine and feces, is used for the fertilization of the caltrop crop. The farmers row their boats to the towns, buy the fresh night-soil at the door from housewives who have a few days' accumulation stored in large wooden pails. These boat-loads of fresh feces-urine are taken directly to their fields, diluted well with water and then applied, untreated, to the fields. There are also those who run public conveniences for a livelihood, placing them along the traveled roads for the use of the passing public. The fertilizer from such sources is more likely to be infected because these conveniences are patronized largely by persons afflicted with some intestinal disease, which makes it impossible for them to wait until they get home where they might defecate in their own receptacle thereby retaining possession of a saleable article. The farmer who buys from such sources thus brings the infection to his fields and it is he and his family who are often most heavily infected.

The free-living stages of *Fasciolopsis* as well as the snail hosts are sensitive, non-resistant organisms and are easily destroyed by several methods. The ova of the parasite are quickly killed in unslaked lime, even in dilutions of 1 : 1000. This dilution is also effective against the free-swimming stages and the snail hosts. The ova may also be destroyed by storing the night-soil, drying the feces, or exposing it to natural enemies, freezing and heating. Storage of the feces is perhaps the most desirable method and is the method used by farmers who can afford it. Fresh feces are used for fertilizer largely by the poorer farmers.

11. *Fasciola hepatica* Linnæus, 1758

Fasciola hepatica is the cause of a serious disease in sheep known as "liver rot." Its presence in man, although not infrequent and sometimes fatal, is regarded as incidental, and the common or characteristic hosts are sheep and cattle. This species is usually found in the biliary canals and the ducts of the liver and may occur as wandering parasites in the lungs and elsewhere.

F. hepatica is cosmopolitan in distribution and occurs where low, wet pastures and the presence of suitable snails make it possible for it to exist. In the United States, it occurs especially along rivers and tributary streams of the Atlantic and Pacific coasts and of the Gulf of Mexico. The states in which this fluke is most prevalent are Washington, Oregon, California, Texas, Arkansas, Louisiana, Alabama and Florida. Human infections have been reported from Venezuela, Chile, Argentina, Cuba, Puerto Rico, Algeria, France, Armenia, Italy and Turkestan.

MORPHOLOGY

Fasciola hepatica (Figure 91) is flattened, heart-shaped in outline and measures from 20 mm. to 30 mm. long and from 8 mm. to 13 mm. in breadth and possesses a cephalic cone from 4 mm. to 5 mm.

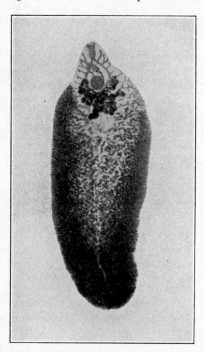

in length which is sharply differentiated from the body by a shoulder on each side. When in the living condition, it is brownish in color but becomes grayish when killed and kept in preservatives. The suckers are hemispherical and placed near to each other and are of about the same size. The pharynx is well developed and leads into the intestinal crura through the short esophagus. The intestinal crura extend to the caudal pole and are provided with numerous diverticula radiating outwards. The testes are greatly ramified and occupy the greater portion of the posterior part of the body, with the exception of the lateral and posterior borders. The ovary is also ramified and is situated lateral of the median line and in front of the transverse vitelline duct. The vitellaria are profusely developed and extend from the base of the

FIG. 91.—*Fasciola hepatica.* (Copyright by General Biological Supply House, Chicago)

cephalic cone to the extreme caudal pole, occupying nearly the entire posterior tip of the body. The uterus lies in front of the ovary and is short in comparison to the rest of the body; a cirrus sac is present and the genital pore is median, half-way between the oral sucker and acetabulum. The ova are yellowish brown, operculated, with development after oviposition and measure from 130 μ to 145 μ in length by 70 μ to 90 μ in breadth.

LIFE-CYCLE

The life-cycle of *Fasciola hepatica* closely parallels that of the large intestinal fluke of man, *Fasciolopsis buski*. The miracidium hatches from the egg in about three weeks after oviposition and finds its way into fresh water snails, especially species of the genera *Galba,* Lymnæa and Fossaria, where the cercariæ develop. The cercariæ upon their escape from the snail host swim to the surface of the water and there encyst, the encysted forms then float freely on the surface film of water. The cercariæ may also attach themselves to a submerged blade of grass or aquatic vegetation for encystment. When these cysts are swallowed by sheep, or other suitable host animals, when drinking or with grass, the young flukes escape from their cyst wall in the small intestine, penetrate through the wall of the intestine and enter the liver from its surface. They wander about in the liver a month or more before settling down in the bile ducts, where they mature. Young specimens that enter the blood stream may develop in unusual locations and may produce prenatal infection.

III. *Fascioloides magna* (Bassi, 1875)

Fascioloides magna is commonly known as the "large American liver fluke." It closely resembles *Fasciola hepatica* in structure except that it does not have a separate anterior portion or cephalic cone and the anterior end is bluntly rounded. The body is very large and may attain a length of 10 cm. It was first discovered in an European zoölogical garden in the wapiti elk. Its original home appears to be North America and it occurs in the liver and lungs of cattle, sheep and goats. In the United States it is most prevalent near the Gulf of Mexico, especially in Arkansas and along the coast and river valleys of Texas. It also occurs along the west coast in both the United States and Canada and has also been found in Colorado, Wisconsin and New York. *F. magna* occurs in the liver and lungs, commonly lying in cysts which contain one to several flukes and a quantity of dark-colored fluid filled with ova and débris. In cattle the parasites are completely encapsulated and further development is prevented. They seem to do but little damage aside from rendering the livers unfit for use as food. In sheep, however, a few worms may produce severe clinical symptoms (Swales, 1936). The life history of this parasite closely parallels that of *Fasciola hepatica.* The larval stages develop in the snail *Pseudosuccinea columella.* Development is completed in about two months.

IV. *Fascioliasis*

The pathology of fascioliasis in sheep is similar to that of Clonorchis infections in man (page 263). Necrosis of the liver parenchyma, hypertrophy of the biliary ducts with development of fibrous adventitia around them, and portal cirrhosis are characteristic lesions. The most prominent symptoms are severe anemia, marked weakness and emaciation. In heavy infections the skin is dry and the wool drops out in patches. The diagnosis is established upon finding the eggs of the parasite in the feces. Pure carbon tetrachloride is the preferred drug for sheep but it should not be given to cattle. Oleoresin of Aspidium is recommended for the latter.

Syrians and others who eat fresh, raw sheep livers are often troubled with adult flukes, accidentally ingested with the liver, attaching themselves to the pharyngeal mucosa. The flukes engorge themselves upon the tissues and tissue juices, and cause severe irritation and an edematous congestion of the throat. The condition is usually temporary but may persist for a week and death may result from asphyxiation.

PREVENTION

Wet pastures should be avoided and swampy areas should be drained, filled in or fenced off. When the infection is present in the flock, treatment should be given to infected animals at the beginning of winter, after the danger of fresh infection is past. Safe drinking supplies should be provided for the animals, as the infective cysts may be free, floating in infected marsh lands as well as on vegetation. Copper sulphate in proportions of one part in from 500,000 to 2,000,000 parts of water is known to destroy the snail hosts within forty-eight hours, but does not kill the eggs of the parasite nor those of the snail. It is therefore necessary to repeat this treatment of ponds in from two to three months. This solution is not injurious to the higher plants and animals or for bathing, drinking or irrigation, but may injure some species of fish, especially the young. Both slaked and unslaked lime in water also destroy the snail host.

II. Family OPISTHORCHIIDÆ

The members of the family OPISTHORCHIIDÆ are very transparent, small to medium in size, with the body tapering anteriorly. The oral and ventral suckers are close together and are very weakly developed. The testes are near the posterior end, one behind the other, and are either lobed or branched. There is no cirrus sac. These parasites occur in the bile ducts of mammals and birds. The second intermediate host is a fresh-water fish.

1. *Clonorchis sinensis* (Cobbold, 1875)

HISTORICAL

Clonorchis sinensis Cobbold was described by McConnell in 1875 from material obtained at autopsy of a Chinese carpenter living in Calcutta. The liver on this port-mortem examination was found to be greatly enlarged and tense with much distention of the bile ducts. On sectioning the liver, small worms escaped with the bile fluid and were believed by McConnell to be the cause of the pathological condition of the liver. Cobbold (1875) recognized that the fluke described by McConnell was a new species and gave it the name *Distoma sinense*. In 1877 MacGregor (1878) found the same trematode in several Chinese at Port Louis, Mauritius, and erroneously attributed a form of paralytic disease to its presence. In 1878 McConnell reported another case in a Chinese cook in Calcutta and suggested the possibility that the infection came from eating insufficiently cooked fish. It was also noted that all cases had been Chinese. In 1883 Kiyono, Nakahama, Yamagata and Suga published an account of the liver fluke in Japan. Baelz stated that these parasites were quite frequent in Japan, and recognized two species, separated principally on size differences. The smaller one he regarded as of pathological significance and named *Distoma hepatis endemicum perniciosum,* while the larger type was thought harmless and was designated as *Distoma hepatis innocuum.* Baelz found he had confused the clinical picture of the disease produced by this worm with that of schistosomiasis and later changed his views and came to look upon the two species as one and the same. Blanchard in 1895 created the genus *Opisthorchis* in which he placed the species *Distoma sinensis* Cobbold. It remained in that genus until 1907 when Looss established the genus *Clonorchis* for the Oriental liver fluke.

Looss concluded that there are two distinct species. The larger, which is the type found in China, was called *Clonorchis sinensis* Cobbold, and was believed to be harmless, and the smaller species, named *C. endemicus,* found mostly in Japan and in French Indo-China, was believed to be pathogenic. Verdun and Bruyant (1908) also made an extensive study of the species question in *Clonorchis* and concluded that while there were two distinct types, the differences were not sufficient to class them as distinct species and therefore established two varieties *Clonorchis sinensis major* and *Clonorchis sinensis minor*. Kobayashi (1917) by experimental methods and Ch'en Pang (1923) employing morphological comparisons proved that the differences found by earlier writers were individual variations and that there is only one species which should be referred to as *Clonorchis sinensis* Cobbold.

Saito (1898) was the first to study the viable ova and living miracidia, and Kobayashi (1911-1917) discovered the second intermediate host (various species of fresh-water fish) and was able to produce experimentally the adults from the encysted cercariæ found in the fish. Muto in 1918 found the cercaria of *C. sinensis* in a fresh-water snail, *Parafossarulus striatulus* var. *japonicus*. Faust and Khaw (1927) made an extensive study on the biology and epidemiology of *Clonorchis* infection in China.

DISTRIBUTION AND FREQUENCY

Clonorchis sinensis is a characteristic parasite of man and is frequently found in fish-eating mammals of the Orient including the countries adjacent to the China and Yellow Seas, namely Japan, Korea, China, Formosa and French Indo-China. The infection appears to be limited to the distribution of the snail host, *Parafossarulus striatulus* and its close relatives. In man it has been reported frequently from countries outside of the Orient, including the United States, but in all such cases the infection has been among Chinese or Japanese who originally came from endemic districts of China or Japan. There are no authentic records of the spread of this parasite into new regions by immigration. In Japan the liver fluke is clinically important only in the Okayama district, although it is more or less distributed throughout the mainland as well as in Shikoku and Kyushu. In Korea the infection is common only in the southern part of the peninsula. In China the most important infection with *Clonorchis* in man is in the Kwantung Province, Southeastern China, where the greater part of the infection is acquired through the eating of infected, raw, fresh-water fish. Occasionally native infections of *Clonorchis* in man are encountered in Central China but in North China the native population is free from this parasite. The most heavily infected area of French Indo-China, and probably of the entire endemic region, is found in the delta of the Red River. The persons most commonly infected are the native boatmen and soldiers. In children the infection usually is slight, but increases from fifteen years to old age, being highest after fifty years of age.

The number of individuals of *Clonorchis* in an infected host may be very great. Twenty-one thousand worms were obtained by Sambuc and Beaujean (1913) from a human case in Indo-China. Persons harboring more than 1,000 worms are not uncommon, but the average runs usually less than 100. Among the lower animals with natural infections, the number of clonorchids may also be very high.

The incidence of *Clonorchis sinensis* in field cats and dogs is high throughout endemic centers of China. Chen (1934) found about 44 per cent of the dogs and about 80 per cent of the cats of the Canton area, and about 59 per cent of the cats of the Foochow area infected. Other fish-eating mammals, badger, mink, marten, etc., may also harbor this parasite under natural conditions. However, cats and dogs are the most important reservoir hosts.

POSITION IN THE FINAL HOST

Clonorchis sinensis normally inhabits the bile passages of its host. It migrates to the more distal portions of the bile tracts when still immature and there grows to maturity. Apparently there is but little or no migration from this position during its adult life. The worms are usually found free in the cavity of the ducts, or crowded into the small bile capillaries, where they are bathed in the bile fluid. They have also been obtained from the gall bladder at autopsies of experimental animals under anesthesia. One lobe of the host's liver may sometimes be heavily infected (the left lobe) while the remainder of the organ will be relatively free from the infection. Post-mortem shows the common duct frequently blocked with worms which may also be found in the duodenum and the pancreatic duct, especially in heavy infections. It cannot, however, remain alive for any length of time in the alimentary tract since it is rapidly digested by the intestinal fluids.

The food of the adult flukes is believed to be the secretion from the mucosa of the bile ducts.

LONGEVITY OF ADULT IN THE BILE PASSAGES

No direct observations have been made on the longevity of the adult worm within the bile passages. Watson (1918) records an infection in a Chinese in Panama which was believed to exist for twenty years without reinfection, and Moore (1921) reports other cases with infections believed to be of from five to twenty years duration. Faust and Khaw (1927) have observed the infection in Chinese University students from Southern endemic centers who had lived continuously for several years in Peiping where raw fish is not eaten by man. Several of them had remained infected for a period of five years of abstinence. It seems probable, therefore, that after an infection with *Clonorchis sinensis* is once established, it may last from five to twenty years or more.

MORPHOLOGY OF THE ADULT FLUKE

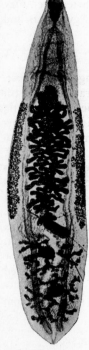

FIG. 92.—*Clonorchis sinensis*. (Copyright by General Biological Supply House, Chicago)

These trematodes (Figure 92) when alive are opalescent gray, but if allowed to die *in situ* preceding autopsy they become discolored through the absorption of the bile pigment and take on a deep brown color. They are mostly transparent and are very flabby, due to the weakly developed musculature. The body has a more or less rounded, tapering posterior end. The anterior end is more acute, terminating bluntly with the anterior sucker.

Marked differences have been recorded in sizes of *Clonorchis sinensis* which led Looss and others to believe this to be an important criterion of species in this genus. That size is not a species characteristic has been shown by a number of authors on this subject. Faust and Khaw (1927) have observed that (1) a few clonorchids in the bile passages of a large animal (man) have plenty of room to attain their full growth, and that the flukes obtained at autopsies of human cases are usually large; (2) that if a large number of these flukes live in the bile ducts of the same host, they crowd one another so that they do not usually attain such a size; and (3) large numbers of such flukes in the bile passages of small animals were usually small in size. In one experimental infection (cat) these authors obtained at autopsy eleven mature worms, one of which measured nearly twice the length of the other ten. The ten smaller ones were obtained from the distal bile capillaries of the left lobe, while the large worm was recovered from the proximal bile passage. The following table gives Faust and Khaw's measurements of over one hundred specimens of *C. sinensis* obtained from three human autopsies.

AVERAGE SIZE MEASUREMENTS OF CLONORCHIS FROM HUMAN AUTOPSIES

Case No.	Source	Worms Obtained	Worms Measured	Length in mm.	Breadth in mm.
I	Korea	93	93	12.1-20.1	3.4-4.6
2	South China	100	50	11.5-18.0	3.6-4.0
3	Hongkong	505	25	13.0-16.1	2.8-3.5

The normal egg of *Clonorchis sinensis* is a yellowish-brown color, oval in shape, resembling an old-fashioned carbon-filament, electric light bulb, and has an average size of 29 μ in length and 17 μ in breadth. The embryo is fully developed at the time the ova are expelled from the host. The operculum is located at the narrower pole and is vaulted, and so inserted within the rim of the shell that its contour usually does not follow that of the rest of the shell. The shoulders at the opercular rim are prominent and form a characteris-

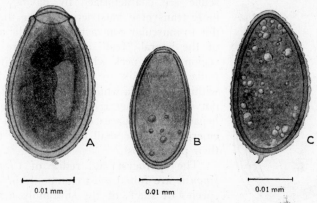

FIG. 93.—Eggs of *Clonorchis sinensis*. A, Normal egg; B, Incomplete egg; C, Anomalous egg. (After Yumoto)

tic for the diagnosis of *Clonorchis*. The shell shows on its surface an arabesque, polygonal pattern which is produced apparently by irregular thickness of its outer layer (Yumoto, 1936). Abnormal eggs may be encountered frequently. Of these Yumoto recognizes two main groups, (a) *anomalous* eggs, having neither miracidium nor operculum, and (b) *incomplete* eggs without miracidium but with operculum (Figure 93). The appearance of anomalous eggs takes place continuously during the life of the parasite, but incomplete eggs are characteristic of young or old worms, or during anthelmintic treatment.

LIFE-CYCLE

The ova of *Clonorchis* are deposited by the adult worms in the
biliary passages of the host and from there they pass to the intestinal tract, after being stored up in the gall bladder. To the present
day the exact method by which the snail host becomes infected with
Clonorchis is not definitely known. Experimental evidence, however,
indicates that the miracidia do not hatch in the open and actively
penetrate the snail host, as in the case of other flukes we have mentioned, but that the unhatched ova are taken passively with food into
the snail's digestive tract, and after hatching, the miracidia penetrate through the intestine into the vascular spaces and become
sporocysts. Here the sporocyst becomes an elongated structure, which
contains a number of young rediæ. These rediæ break out of the
thin-walled sporocyst and escape into the vascular sinuses. These

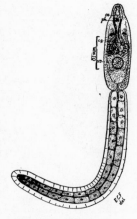

rediæ are characterized by having one or
more transverse constrictions along the body,
due to muscular contractions, and the absence
of the lateral "feet" and birth pore in the
region of the neck which is typical of many
rediæ. From six to eight cercariæ develop
within each redia which, upon maturity, break
out of the mother rediæ into the free inter-
hepatic lymph spaces of the host and finally
emerge from the snail into the water to seek
their piscine host.

The sporocyst and rediæ of *Clonorchis
sinensis* are found most commonly in various
species of snails of the subfamily BITHYNI-
INÆ. *Parafossarulus striatulus, P. striatulus*
var. *japonicus,* and *Bithynia fuchsiana* being
the more important hosts.

FIG. 94.—Cercaria of
Clonorchis sinensis; os., oral
sucker; *cg.,* cephalic secretory gland; *vs.,* acetabulum.
(After Faust)

The mature, free-swimming cercaria of
Clonorchis sinensis (Figure 94), when re-
laxed, measures from 250 μ to 275 μ in length by 60 μ to 90 μ in
breadth. The tail is long, 650 μ to 750 μ, with more or less truncated
tip. On either side of the tail, the integument is drawn out into
transparent alæ which run parallel to the tail margins. Six pairs of
unicellular, cephalic glands occupy the center of the body. The ducts
of these glands pass forward and end in hollow, attenuated boring
spines on either side of the oral aperture. These glands secrete a
substance which is histolytic and which aids the cercaria in its inva-

sion into the flesh of fresh-water fish, the second intermediate host. The cercariæ attach themselves to the body of the fish, and, after a shallow penetration into the tissues, encyst in this host, which may later become food of the final host. The encystment may take place in the musculature of the fish or on the underside of the scales or on the skin. Encystment usually occurs only after the cercaria has used up its histolytic secretions in its endeavor to gain a foothold in the tissues of the fish. The tail is cast off and the true cyst capsule is formed rapidly from the cystogenous granules

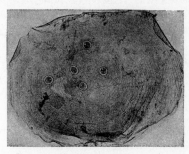

FIG. 95.—Encysted metacercaria on the under side of fish scale of *Hermiculter kneri*, a second intermediate host. Magnified. (Photograph from Faust)

which apparently absorb large quantities of water. The cystogenous fluid is exuded from the tissues of the larva and quickly forms into a comparatively thin, hyaline capsule. The cercariæ which encyst within the muscles of the fish possess an additional outer fibrous covering which is formed by the reaction of the host tissues. The mature cyst is elliptical in outline, measuring in the largest specimens 135 μ to 145 μ by 90 μ to 100 μ. The long axis of the cyst when it is embedded in the muscle lies parallel to the muscle fibers. When the cysts are located under the scales of the fish they are somewhat compressed and discoidal in shape (Figures 95 and 96).

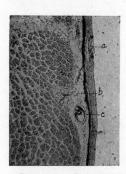

FIG. 96.—Section through superficial layers of *Culter brevicauda*, showing (a) the point of entrance of the cercaria into the subintegumentary layer; (b) strands of connective tissue with small round-cell accumulations in the region through which the larva has passed, and (c) the metacercaria recently encysted. (Photograph from Faust and Khaw)

More than thirty species of fresh-water fishes are known to harbor the cysts of *Clonorchis sinensis*. Of these *Pseudorasbora parva* is most commonly involved. It has a wide distribution and is often eaten raw, in vinegar or in soy sauce. Other hosts, *Crassius auratus, Ctenopharyn-godon idellus, Hypothalmichthys nobilis* and *Labeo jordani,* are especially prized for food in South China. The cysts occur most frequently in the flesh but many are found also in the head, under the dermal layers, in the gills, fins and scales and eye cavities (Kawai and Yumoto, 1936).

The encysted cercariæ can withstand high temperature. Kobáyashi (1917) found that they were killed if the flesh containing the cysts was roasted or boiled for fifteen minutes or kept in water at 100° C. for fifteen minutes. Faust and Khaw (1927) found that infected fish heated at 80° C. for one hour still harbored viable cysts. These observations show that infections can arise even from eating apparently "well-cooked" fish.

METHODS OF ENTRANCE INTO FINAL HOST

Three ways by which man may become infected with *Clonorchis* have been described by various writers: (1) by ingesting water containing living cysts which have been discharged or fallen from fish, (2) by handling the fish in the catching and preparation as food during which the cysts are transferred to the mouth and swallowed and (3) by eating raw or imperfectly cooked fish containing the *Clonorchis* cysts. While the first two methods are possible, it is probable that they occur but seldom under natural conditions. It is evident that the chief source of infection is by the direct ingestion of fish containing the cysts when served raw or only partially cooked.

DEVELOPMENT IN THE FINAL HOST

Upon ingestion of the cysts by the final host, the fibrous outer cyst wall, if present, is first digested away by the gastric juice and the encysted larva passes into the duodenum where the true cyst wall is ruptured, largely by the activity of the larva within, and the free form travels into the bile ducts where it grows to maturity. By the sixteenth day after ingestion of the cysts, some of the worms may be sexually mature and producing ova. Usually, however, it is not until the twentieth or twenty-fifth day or later that the majority reach sexual maturity.

PREVENTION AND CONTROL OF CLONORCHIASIS IN MAN

As in the endemic districts of fasciolopsiasis, age-old customs of the people are particularly favorable for the propagation of the *Clonorchis* life-cycle. This is especially true in South China where fish are raised for sale and are fed fresh, fecal wastes. Fish from these "culture" ponds constitute the principal food of the country population and are sold not only in the larger towns in the immediate vicinity but are also shipped alive in large numbers to outside markets.

The chief methods which have been suggested to effect the control of clonorchiasis in man are: (1) the disinfection of feces; (2) the eradication of the snail host; (3) educational propaganda regarding the danger of consuming raw fish; (4) legislation prohibiting raw fish, or permitting only salt-water forms to be consumed raw; and (5) therapeutic prophylaxis.

Ammonium sulphate ($[NH_4]_2SO_4$) has been recommended as a practical ovicide against *Clonorchis*. One part of a 0.7 per cent solution to ten parts of feces kills the larva within the egg in one-half hour's time. Ammonium sulphate is more desirable than other chemicals tested as *Clonorchis* ovicides in that it is also a well-proved chemical fertilizer and has been in use in China in the mulberry districts for a considerable period. Eradication of the snail host, *Parafossarulus striatulus* and related species is difficult, if not impossible. These snails are usually found only in the muck at the bottom of the fish ponds and any chemical applied to the water to destroy them would probably never reach them. Chemicals which would kill the snails would also kill the fish crop. The snails show marked ability to withstand desiccation and are not killed during the draining of the ponds. Control efforts against the snail host in clonorchiasis are held to be impracticable. The most effective and feasible method of attack against this infection is the attempt by education to prevent the eating of raw or partly cooked fresh-water fish.

Therapeutic measures against clonorchiasis are at present of doubtful value. Antimony and arsenic compounds have given some encouraging results. Gentian violet administered per os has been found effective against *Clonorchis* in laboratory animals by Faust and Khaw (1926) but has not been tested sufficiently to determine its efficacy in human infections. Measures should be taken to prevent cats and dogs feeding as scavengers at fish markets.

II. *Less Frequent Opisthorchiids of Man and Lower Animals*

Opisthorchis felineus (Rivolta, 1884) is a normal parasite of the cat, dog, fox and pig. It commonly occurs in man of the Ob Basin region in Siberia and in East Prussia. The normal habitat of the adult is in the bile ducts; it has also been found in the intestine and in the pancreatic ducts.

The adult form (Figure 97) is usually from 8 mm. to 11 mm. in length and 1.5 mm. to 2 mm. in breadth. The cuticula is smooth. The suckers are of about equal size and are separated from each other by one-fifth to one-sixth of the length of the body. Morphologically this species is quite similar to *Clonorchis sinensis* but the testes are lobed instead of branched as in *Clonorchis*. The eggs are small, light to dark yellowish-brown in color, with a sharply defined operculum at the more pointed pole, 30 μ long by 12 μ broad and contain a ciliated miracidium at oviposition.

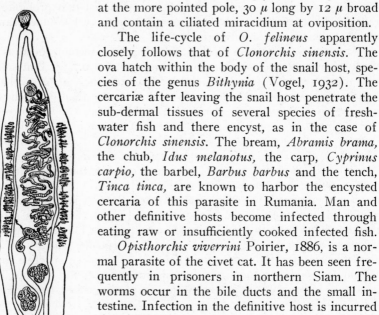

The life-cycle of *O. felineus* apparently closely follows that of *Clonorchis sinensis*. The ova hatch within the body of the snail host, species of the genus *Bithynia* (Vogel, 1932). The cercariæ after leaving the snail host penetrate the sub-dermal tissues of several species of fresh-water fish and there encyst, as in the case of *Clonorchis sinensis*. The bream, *Abramis brama*, the chub, *Idus melanotus*, the carp, *Cyprinus carpio*, the barbel, *Barbus barbus* and the tench, *Tinca tinca*, are known to harbor the encysted cercaria of this parasite in Rumania. Man and other definitive hosts become infected through eating raw or insufficiently cooked infected fish.

Opisthorchis viverrini Poirier, 1886, is a normal parasite of the civet cat. It has been seen frequently in prisoners in northern Siam. The worms occur in the bile ducts and the small intestine. Infection in the definitive host is incurred through eating raw fish.

Amphimerus noverca Braun, 1903, has been reported twice from man in Calcutta, India. It occurs commonly in the pariah dogs of that country and its presence in man is but incidental. Another species of this genus, *A. pseudofelineus* Ward, 1901, appears to be fairly common in cats and coyotes in central United States.

FIG. 97.—*Opisthorchis felineus*. (Redrawn from Stiles and Hassall)

Parametorchis complexus (Stiles and Hassall, 1894) and *P. noveboracensis* (Hung, 1926) have been described from the liver of domestic cats of New York.

III. Family DICROCŒLIIDÆ

The members of this family are small, elongated trematodes with poorly developed musculature and transparent bodies. The acetabulum is near the anterior end. The intestinal cæca are simple and do not extend to the posterior end. The excretory bladder is simple and tubular, reaching anteriorly to the center of the body. The ovary is posterior to the testes which lie posterior to the acetabulum. The genital pore is median, between the two suckers, near the fork of the intestine. Laurer's canal and a small seminal receptacle are present. The vitellaria are well developed and occupy the mid-region of the body, lateral to the intestinal crura. The uterus is long and occupies most of the space behind the ovary. The eggs are numerous, thick-shelled and deep brown in color. They are liver parasites of ruminants, swine, rodents, birds and man. Only one species, *Dicrocœlium dendriticum* (Rudolphi, 1819) is of clinical and economic importance.

1. *Dicrocœlium dendriticum* (Rudolphi, 1819)

Dicrocœlium dendritium (Figure 98) is a cosmopolitan liver fluke of sheep and other herbivores and has been observed in swine and wild rabbits. It is very common in Europe and occurs also in Algeria, Egypt, Siberia, Turkestan and North and South America. Its occurrence in man is incidental, but it has been encountered in several cases in Syria and the Lebanon, Rumania, Turkestan and Europe. It is characterized by a rather slender, elongate, flat body with more or less pointed ends. It is 8 mm. to 10 mm. in length and 1.5 mm. to 2.5 mm. in breadth. The acetabulum is usually more highly developed than the oral sucker. The cuticula is smooth. The pharynx passes into a moderately long esophagus and the intestinal crura are long and without branches. The genital pore is median and immediately anterior to the acetabulum. The testes are compact, nearly tandem to diagonal and lie directly posterior to the acetabulum. The ovary is median and lies immediately posterior to the testes. A seminal receptacle and Laurer's canal are present. The vitellaria are moderately developed and are lateral to the intestinal crura. The uterine loops are numerous, transverse and posterior to the ovary. The ova are of a deep brown color, operculated and slightly flattened on one side. They vary in size from 36 μ to 45 μ by 22 μ to 30 μ.

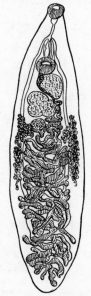

FIG. 98.—*Dicrocoelium dendriticum.* (Redrawn from Braun)

The life cycle of *Dicrocœlium dendriticum* is not completely known. The egg contains a fully developed miracidium which hatches only after being ingested by several species of land snails, *Helicella candidula, H. itala, Cochlicella acuta* and *Zebrina detrita,* in which hosts the cercaria develops. The manner in which the final host becomes infected remains unsolved. It is believed by Vogel (1929) and others that a second intermediate host is necessary to complete development, but Cameron (1931) reports having infected sheep by feeding them snails previously fed eggs of the parasite and known to harbor cercariæ.

Other species are *Dicrocœlium hospes* Looss, 1907, from the gall-bladder of cattle of the Sudan, and *D. macrostomum* Odhner, 1911, from the gall-bladder and bile ducts of guinea-fowl in Egypt. The life-cycles are not known.

IV. Diseases Due to Liver Flukes

A small number of flukes in the liver of the host usually give rise to no appreciable disorder and probably the majority of individuals harboring these parasites might be classed as carriers. When large numbers occur, however, they produce definite injury to the host. They may form a mechanical obstruction of the bile ducts so that jaundice results or they may exert a pressure on certain veins causing ascites or enlargement of the spleen. The pancreatic ducts may also be obstructed. The excretions and secretions of the parasites and substances derived from the bodies of dead worms probably produce disorders far more serious than those caused by mechanical means. These apparently are the cause of the severe anemia in long standing infections with *Clonorchis sinensis* and "aqueous cachexia" in sheep

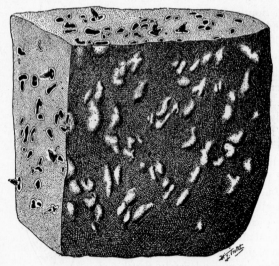

FIG. 99.—Human liver infected with *Clonorchis sinensis.*
(From Brumpt's *Précis de Parasitologie*)

infected with *Fasciola hepatica* and *Dicrocœlium dendriticum*. Bacterial infections and ulcers are frequent in the liver in fascioliasis.

PATHOLOGY

At autopsy the liver of the infected host may be somewhat hypertrophied and on its surface are white blebs which represent the projections of distended bile ducts (Figure 99). Upon sectioning, numerous cavities with thickened sclerotic walls are found which are

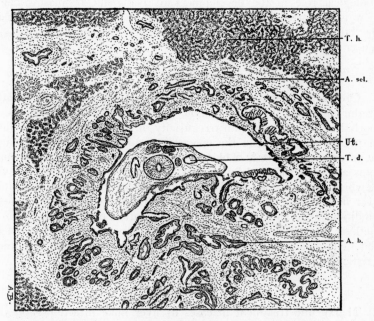

Fig. 100.—Lesions produced in the human liver by *Clonorchis sinensis*. T.h., liver tissue; A.scl., sclerotic tissue; Ut., uterus of the parasite; T.d., intestine of the parasite; A.b., biliary adenoma-like tissue. (From Brumpt's *Précis de Parasitologie*)

often filled with flukes and a brownish amorphous material containing thousands of ova, polymorphonuclear leucocytes and lymphoid cells. The walls of these cavities are the larger, hypertrophied bile ducts. Microscopic study of stained liver sections show an intense proliferation of the biliary epithelium producing an adenoma-like tissue. The connective and muscular tissues of the bile duct undergo intense hypertrophy followed by sclerosis which constantly increases in extent until in long standing infections it may involve several canals and produce a sclerotic area of considerable size (Figure 100). In this zone there is considerable infiltration of lymphoid cells and eosinophiles. The hepatic parenchyma, encroached on by the hypertrophied bile ducts, is poorly nourished and becomes atrophied. Through interference with the circulation, vascular areas resembling angioma may appear. In *Fasciola hepatica* infections marked destruction of the biliary epithelium and large ulcers may occur. It is believed by numerous investigators, Askanazy (1904), Joest (1919), Hoeppli (1933 a and b) and others, that liver flukes may play an etiological rôle in the development of malignant neoplasms. This view is supported by both histological evidence (marked changes in the biliary epithelium) and by the higher frequency of primary cancer in endemic areas.

SYMPTOMS

Ordinarily light or moderate infections with liver flukes usually produce no clinical manifestations. In clonorchiasis there may be a morbid sense of hunger, an irregularity of the bowels and a feeling of pressure and pain in the epigastrium and right hypochondrium. In severe cases there is a bloody diarrhea and icterus. These symptoms are soon followed by anemia, emaciation, ascites and cachexia to which the individual finally succumbs. Sheep in the early stages of liver fluke disease are likely to put on fat and seemingly improve in condition, apparently a result of a stimulation of the functions of the liver. The general course of the disease is very chronic and irregular. The diagnosis may be established readily upon finding characteristic ova in the feces of the host.

TREATMENT

Therapeutic treatment in cases of liver fluke infections appears thus far of doubtful value. Brug (1921) has, however, reported improvement in patients treated with tartar emetic and Shattuck (1924) found the stools of infected Chinese patients free from *Clonorchis* ova one month after treatment with antimony and arsenic compounds. Faust (1937) recommends the use of gentian violet and antimony salts against clonorchiasis and opisthorchiasis. Erhardt (1932) reports unsatisfactory results with gentian violet in opisthorchiasis, but found fuadin administered subcutaneously gave excellent results. Montgomerie (1926) reported exceptionally favorable results with carbon tetrachloride against *Fasciola hepatica* in sheep. This drug is, however, apparently ineffective against *Dicrocœlium dendriticum.* When carbon tetrachloride is employed treatment should be repeated after about five weeks, as immature worms are unaffected by it.

V. Family PLAGIORCHIIDÆ

These distomes are relatively small with oval and strongly flattened bodies. The cuticula usually bears small spines. A pharynx and esophagus are present, the intestinal crura are simple and variable in length. The excretory bladder is typically Y-shaped with the median stem dividing into two short branches behind the well developed Mehlis' gland. The genital pore is usually immediately anterior to the acetabulum. The cirrus sac is well developed, containing the cirrus, vesicle and prostate. The ovary is situated on the posterior margin of the acetabulum, generally to the right. The testes are usually oblique and close behind the ovary. The vitellaria are well developed and extend in vary-

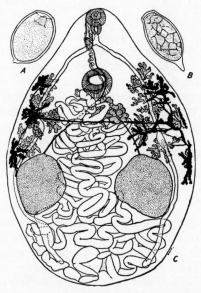

ing degrees along the lateral margins of the body. The uterus usually fills the posterior part of the body. The eggs are numerous, small and thin-shelled. Adults are principally parasitic in the intestinal tract or lungs of frogs, reptiles, birds, and occasionally mammals; metacercaria in insects. Examples, *Ostiolum medioplexus* (Stafford, 1902) in lungs of frogs and *Prosthogonimus macrorchis* (Macy, 1934), in the *bursa Fabricii* and lower intestine of poultry and wild fowl.

1. *Prosthogonimus macrorchis* Macy, 1934

The genus *Prosthogonimus* is world-wide in distribution. Its several species are, without doubt, the most pathogenic trematodes

A. Mature egg, showing normal spine.
B. Segmenting egg, showing abnormal spine.
C. Adult.

of poultry, frequently causing sharp decline in egg production, the laying of soft-shelled eggs, broken eggs and fatal peritonitis. *P. macrorchis* (Figure 101) is the prevalent species in North America, occurring frequently in the Great Lakes region. The adult worm occurs naturally in chickens and ducks. Experimental infection has been obtained in crows and sparrows (Macy, 1934). The adult worm is about 7 mm. in length and 5 mm. in width. The body is pyriform with the cuticula heavily spined in the anterior region. It is of a deep flesh color when alive. The ventral sucker is at least a half larger than the oral sucker. The testes are large, spherical to ovate and entire, and are located opposite each other in the third fourth of the body length and posterior to the ovary. The vitellaria are prominent and appear in snow-white clusters extending from the level of the ventral sucker to, but not posterior to the testes. The ovary is much lobed and lies posterior to the ventral sucker and slightly to the right of the body axis. The uterus is well developed, filled with eggs, and its coils appear blackish in contrast to the lighter shades of the body proper. The eggs are about 28 μ long by 16 μ wide and bear a small spine at the posterior pole.

LIFE-CYCLE

The cercaria of *P. macrorchis* develops in the common snail, *Amnicola limosa porata.* After leaving the snail host, the cercaria swims about, and if drawn into the rectal respiratory chamber of a suitable dragonfly nymph, particularly species of the genera *Leucorrhinia, Tetragoneuria* and *Epicordulia,* it migrates into the muscles of the nymph increases in size, and later encysts in the body cavity. When the infected nymph or adult dragonfly is eaten by a suitable avian host, the young trematode is liberated in the intestine. It then makes its way down the intestine to the cloaca and then to the *bursa Fabricii* or the oviduct where it grows to maturity in about one week.

PATHOLOGY AND SYMPTOMS

Prosthogonimus macrorchis causes marked irritation of the oviduct. The inflamed oviduct readily performs retroperistaltic movements. Broken eggs and bacteria are thus introduced into the body cavity where they frequently cause fatal peritonitis. A parasite is often included in the hen's egg.

Infected hens are usually inactive and show a marked tendency to sit on the nest. There is a sharp decline in egg production and frequent laying of soft-shelled eggs. The feathers about the cloacal region become encrusted with discharges from the oviducts. In advanced cases the abdomen is discolored and pendulous and the legs are held apart in walking. Diagnosis is made upon finding the characteristic ova by fecal examination. Carbon tetrachloride is recommended for removing the parasites. The disease may be prevented by keeping hens fenced away from lake shores, the natural habitat of the dragonfly, intermediate host of the parasite.

II. *Ostiolum medioplexus*

This distome (Figures 73, 74) and several other species of this genus and of the genus *Hæmatolæchus* are common parasites in the lungs of frogs. *O. medioplexus* is, perhaps, the commonest of lung flukes of *Rana pipiens,* which frog is used the world over for biological study. It is an elongate, slender fluke measuring about 7 mm. long and about 1 mm. in width at the region of the anterior testes. The body is fairly transparent. The darker internal structures give the worm a somewhat mottled appearance.

The acetabulum is very small and is located in front of the first third of the body length. The pharynx is prominent and leads into a short esophagus. The intestinal crura extend to the posterior end of the body. They are generally red from the ingested blood of the host. The testes are unlobed, round or oval, with squarish corners. They are slightly oblique. The cirrus sac is long and encloses the seminal vesicle, prostate and cirrus. The ovary is elongate oval. It lies a short distance back of the ventral sucker, either to one side or other of the body, with its long axis diagonal to the body axis of the worm and its anterior end toward the midline of the body. The seminal receptacle is larger than the ovary. It lies in the midline posterior to the ovary and overlaps the ovary for about half its length. The vitellaria are prominent and extend about half way between the anterior tip and the ovary to the region back of the posterior testes. Laurer's canal is absent. The folds of the uterus occupy the posterior portion of the body and the central field about the generative organs. The uterus is filled with eggs in varying stages of development. The eggs, when discharged, measure about 0.0255 mm. long and 0.015 mm. wide and contain a fully developed miracidium. The histology of this trematode in cross section at the level of the acetabulum is shown in Figure 74.

LIFE-CYCLE

The cercaria of *Ostiolum medioplexus* develops from sporocysts in *Planorbula armigera*. The dragonfly, *Sympetrum obtrusum,* is the second intermediate host which becomes infected during its aquatic life. The cercariæ after their escape from the snail host swim about in the water and, if carried into the rectal respiratory chamber of the dragonfly nymph by means of respiratory currents, penetrate the tissues of the bronchial basket and there encyst. Frogs become infected by eating adult dragonflies harboring metacercariæ. The student is referred to Krull (1930-34) and Ingles (1933) for detailed accounts of life-cycles of several North American frog trematodes.

VI. Family ECHINOSTOMATIDÆ

These trematodes are more or less elongate worms with a reniform collar surrounding the oral sucker on its dorsal and ventral margins. This collar bears either a single or double row of strong spines. The cuticula bears scales or spines. The esophagus is relatively long and bifurcates immediately above the acetabulum. The intestinal crura extend to the posterior portion of the body. The genital pore lies between the anterior margin of the acetabulum and the bifurcation of the esophagus. The testes are entirely or somewhat lobed, usually tandem, and located in the posterior half of the body. A cirrus sac is present. The ovary is anterior to the testes and usually median in position. There is no seminal receptacle. The vitellaria are well developed and occupy the lower two-thirds of the lateral fields and extend somewhat into the central field behind the testes. The uterus is relatively short and occupies the central field between the ovary and the acetabulum. The eggs are relatively large with thin shells. The adults are, for the greater part, intestinal parasites of birds and mammals, rarely of man, and usually appear to be of no particular pathogenic importance. Examples, *Echinostoma ilocanum* (Garrison, 1908) in man, dogs and rats, *E. revolutum* (Fröhlich, 1802) in ducks and numerous other aquatic birds.

1. *Echinostoma ilocanum* (Garrison, 1908)

HISTORICAL AND GEOGRAPHIC DISTRIBUTION

Echinostoma ilocanum was first described by Garrison in 1908 under the name *Fascioletta ilocana* from twenty-one specimens obtained after a vermifuge treatment to a native prisoner in Manila, Philippine Islands. Later Garrison reported five other cases which were diagnosed from fecal examinations. All of the cases came from the Northwestern provinces of the Island of Luzon. Odhner, in 1911, studied the morphology of this parasite in detail from specimens sent him by Garrison, and placed it in the genus *Echinostoma* Rud. This infection was again reported in 1918 by Hilaria and Wharton from five natives from the province of Zambales, Luzon. It is found frequently in dogs of Canton, China, and in rats of Manila.

MORPHOLOGY

Echinostoma ilocanum is a small, oblong trematode ranging from 4 mm. to 6 mm. in length and from 0.75 mm. to 1.35 mm. in breadth. The anterior part of the body may be well covered with scale-like spines, but as these are very unstable and the least handling causes them to be lost, they may occur only in irregular patches along the margin of the body. The collar is provided with fifty-one spines arranged in two alternating rows uninterrupted dorsally. The oral sucker is small, having a diameter of about 0.18 mm. The acetabulum is between two to three times as large and is situated about 0.7 mm. from the anterior end of the body. The eggs are operculate, oval, and vary from 92 μ to 114 μ in length and from 53 μ to 82 μ in breadth. They are undeveloped when they leave the host, a characteristic typical for the echinostomes.

LIFE-CYCLE

Very little was known of the life-cycle of *Echinostoma ilocanum* before 1933. According to Tubangui and Pasco (1933) the cercaria develops in *Gyraulus prashadi,* a small fresh-water planorbid. When mature, it escapes from this host during the day. If it comes in contact with any exposed portion of another snail, it makes its way into the pulmonary chamber and there encysts. Apparently any of the common Philippine fresh-water snails, including the primary intermediate host, is acceptable as a secondary intermediate host, but the most important snail in transmitting the infection to man is *Pila luzonica.* This snail is customarily eaten raw in the endemic areas of Luzon. It may be eaten straight from the shell by laborers in the field, or uncooked with salt, or as "bagong" with or without vinegar or lemon, in the home.

11. *Echinostoma revolutum* (Fröhlich, 1802)

Echinostoma revolutum (Figure 102) is the common echinostome in the rectum and cæcum of wild and domestic ducks and other aquatic birds and fowl, and has been obtained occasionally from man in Formosa. The life-cycle of this species was followed in detail by Johnson (1920), who found that the miracidium of this fluke escapes from the egg in about three weeks under favorable conditions, and, after penetrating the snail host, *Physa occidentalis,* it develops directly into a mother redia which produces a generation of rediæ in which cercariæ develop. These cercariæ may encyst without escaping from the snail, or may leave this host only to reënter the same speci-

men or another species to form the cyst. The infection is carried to
the primary host when the infected snail is eaten by ducks and geese.
Infection in man is usually attributed to eating raw, salted or insufficiently boiled *Corbicula producta,* in which snail the cercariæ encyst
but do not develop.

III. *Incidental Echinostome Infections in Man*

In addition to the above mentioned species, a number of other
echinostomes have been reported from man in various countries. They
are incidental human parasites. Among these
species are *Euparyphium malayanum* (Leiper,
1911) from the Malay States and India; *E. jassyense* Leon and Cuirea, 1922, from Roumania;
Artyfechinostomum sufrartyfex Lane, 1915, from
Assam; *Echinochasmus perfoliatus* (v.Ratz, 1908)
Dietz, 1910, (Figure 103)
from Japan; and *Himasthla
mühlensi* Vogel, 1933, from
Germany. In known in-
stances, the above species
are common parasites of
dogs, cats and aquatic birds.
Infection in the final host
is acquired by eating molluscs or fresh-water fish
harboring the metacercaria.

VII. Family HETEROPHYIDÆ

This family consists of
very small trematodes,
usually not over 2 mm.
long, with oval or pyriform
bodies, thickly covered with
small scale-like spines, de-
creasing in numbers in the
posterior region. In addition to the oral and
ventral sucker, a sucker-like structure, the
gonotyle, surrounding the genital pore, may be
present. The testes are oval or slightly lobed, horizontal or oblique,
and are located near the posterior end of the body. There is no cirrus
sac. The ovary is oval, anterior to the testes and median in position.

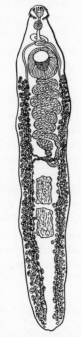

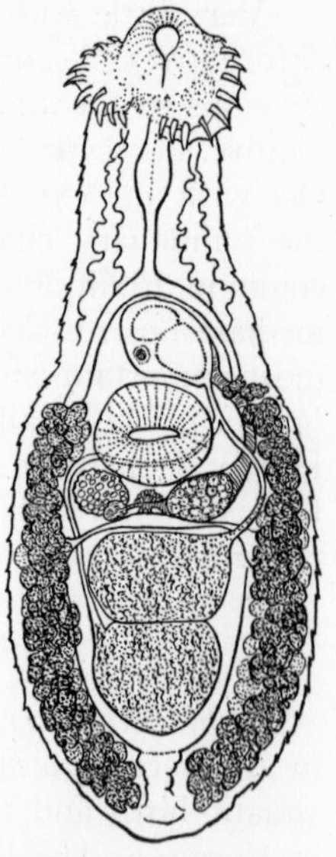

FIG. 102.—*Echinos-
toma revolutum.* (Re-
drawn from Johnson)

FIG. 103.—*Echinochas-
mus perfoliatus.* (Re-
drawn from Ujiie)

The vitellaria are lateral and limited to the lower third of the body. A seminal receptacle and Laurer's canal are present. The uterus is loosely coiled and contains relatively few eggs. The adults are intestinal parasites of mammals and fish-eating birds. Examples, *Heterophyes heterophyes* (von Siebold, 1852) in man, dogs and cats; *Monorchotrema taichui* Nishigori, 1924, in birds and occasionally in man.

1. *Heterophyes heterophyes* (von Siebold, 1852)

HISTORICAL

Heterophyes heterophyes was first discovered in 1851 by Bilharz in the intestine of a boy who died in Cairo, Egypt. A year later it was named *Distoma heterophyes* by von Siebold. Cobbold, in 1866, created the genus *Heterophyes* and made this worm a type for his new genus. The name *Heterophyes heterophyes* was applied in 1900 by Stiles and Hassall, according to the rules of zoölogical nomenclature. A second case of this infection was not encountered until almost forty years later by Blanchard (1891) and it appeared as though the incidence might be very light. Looss (1896), however, reported three cases in Egypt, two at autopsies and the third from a fecal examination and later concluded that this parasite occurred commonly in man in Egypt and that many cases escaped notice in fecal examinations due to the small size of the ovum.

Leiper (1913) found two cases which were diagnosed as infections with *Heterophyes heterophyes* in the Seamen's Hospital in London, one in a Chinaman and the other in a Japanese. In one case, 200 worms were obtained. O'Connor (1919) reported this parasite in two white soldiers who had been in Egypt for only a short time. Onji in 1910 found a peculiar trematode egg in human feces in the Yamaguchi Province, Japan, which he thought might be the ova of *Clonorchis*. Together with Nishio, he described (1915) the adult form under the name *Heterophyes nocens,* and gave an account of its life history. The characters given for this parasite are almost identical with those of *Heterophyes heterophyes*. It is probable that they are one and the same species.

DISTRIBUTION AND FREQUENCY

Heterophyes heterophyes is frequent in man, cats and dogs in Egypt, Palestine, Japan, China, Korea, Formosa and the Philippine Islands. It may also occur in other fish-eating mammals.

DESCRIPTION OF THE ADULT

Heterophyes heterophyes (Figure 104) is a very small trematode measuring from 1 mm. to 1.7 mm. in length by 0.3 mm. to 0.7 mm. in breadth. It has an oval, elongate shape and is gray in color when passed in fresh feces; a brown spot marking the position of the uterus is visible on the mid-ventral surface. The ventral sucker is located immediately in front of the middle of the body and the protrusible gonotyle (Figure 105) lies close behind and a little to one side of the ventral sucker. It has an average diameter of 150 μ, and bears a circlet of about eighty cone-shaped plates which are about 20 μ in length. This circlet of plates is broken for a short distance on the side of the genital sucker toward the ventral sucker. The gonotyle possesses no adhesive functions. The eggs are light brown, operculate, thick-shelled and contain a fully developed, ciliated, embryo when oviposited. The egg may have a knob resembling that of *Clonorchis,* but is less prominent. The average size is from 20 μ to 30 μ by 15 μ to 17 μ.

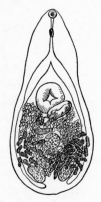

FIG. 104.—*Heterophyes heterophyes.* Adult. (Redrawn from Witenberg)

POSITION IN THE FINAL HOST

Heterophyes heterophyes inhabits the middle third of the small intestine and often occurs in very large numbers. It is usually free within the lumen of the intestine but has been found between the villi and sometimes attached to the mucous membrane near the bases of the villi. *Heterophyes heterophyes,* in most cases, appears to be harmless to the host, although diarrhea, abdominal discomfort, nausea and tenderness below the right costal margin are said to have disappeared after the expulsion of a number of these flukes. Oleoresin of ospidium is the preferred drug against this parasite.

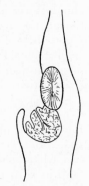

FIG. 105.—*Heterophyes heterophyes.* Longitudinal section through the ventral sucker and gonotyle. The gonotyle is shown retracted. (Redrawn from Witenberg)

Onji and Nishio (1915) found encysted cercariæ in the muscles and on the peritoneum of fresh-water fish, *Mugil japonicus,* and noted that these fishes were eaten raw in endemic centers. By feeding infected fish to experimental animals, these authors were able to follow the details of development from the metacercariæ to the adult. The first intermediate host was discovered but recently. According to Khalil (1933) the cercaria develops in *Pirenella conica,* a common snail of Lake Manzala, the endemic area in Egypt. Although the inhabitants, fisher folk, continually pollute the water of this lake, the cercariæ mature only in summer. The secondary intermediate host, *Mugil cephalus,* is generally salted for food, "fessikh," and eaten after the third day in salt. The metacercariæ may live up to seven days in the salted fish.

11. *Metagonimus yokogawai* (Katsurada, 1912)

HISTORICAL

Yokogawa discovered in 1911 larval trematodes encysted in the gills, under the scales and in the muscles of certain fresh-water fish. He carried out feeding experiments and succeeded in getting these cysts to develop in puppies. After learning the character of the eggs of the adult produced experimentally, he recognized that the eggs of the same species were found in human feces in Formosa and had been taken for those of the liver fluke, *Clonorchis sinensis.* Katsurada described the fluke in 1912 and suggested that this parasite was probably widely distributed in Japan, since he had found its eggs in seven out of nine fecal examinations made of his assistants. It was soon discovered that this species occurs frequently in Japan and is more prevalent and widely distributed in that country than the liver fluke, *Clonorchis sinensis. M. yokogawai* is now known to occur in Japan, Korea, China, Formosa, Dutch East Indies, the Balkans and Palestine in man, dog, cat, swine and fish-eating birds.

DESCRIPTION

Metagonimus yokogawai (Figure 106) is a small fluke of about the same size as *Heterophyes heterophyes.* The uterus occupies the middle of the body and the two testes are arranged posteriorly. The common genital pore lies to the side of the acetabulum and is not surrounded by a collar of spines. The body is covered with minute

spines which are particularly prominent about the oral sucker. The
eggs are operculate and although resembling those of *Clonorchis
sinensis,* the operculum is not set into a groove of the shell as in the
latter species. The eggs measure 28 μ
in length by 16 μ in breadth and are
said to have a knob at the pole opposite
the operculum (Figure 80).

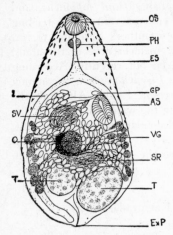

FIG. 106.—*Metagonimus yokoga-
wai.* OS, oral sucker; PH, pharynx;
ES, esophagus; GP, genital pore;
AS, ventral sucker; VG, vitellaria;
SR, seminal receptacle; T, testis;
O, ovary; SV, seminal vesicle; O,
ovary. (Partly after Yokogawa)

POSITION IN THE FINAL HOST

Metagonimus yokogawai is usually
found in the small intestine of man
and dog, especially in the upper and
middle part of the jejunum and rarely
in the duodenum, cæcum and ileum.
The adult worms are found in the
mucus on the surface of the mucous
membrane, while the younger stages
are found deeply imbedded in the
mucosa or submucosa. The length of
life of this parasite is not definitely
known, but probably is about two
years.

The cercariæ develop in the snail,
Melania libertina, and upon their es-
cape from that host penetrate and become encysted in the trout,
Plecoglossus altivelis and other related species. This fish is often
eaten raw or after immersing in soy sauce or vinegar. The cysts
are found most frequently in the subcutaneous tissues about the
scales, gills, fins and tail and rarely in the musculature. Those found
under the scales are usually round, measuring about 0.13 mm. in
diameter, while those in the gills are ellipsoidal in shape having a
length of about 0.15 mm. and a breadth of 0.1 mm.

III. *Heterophyidæ of Lower Mammals*

Tanabe in 1922 described *Stamnosoma armatum* from the small
intestine of birds (the night heron) and mammals in Japan. Nishigori (1924) published an extended account of the life-cycle of a
second species of that genus, *S. formosanum,* also from birds and
mammals in Formosa, but morphologically distinct from *S. armatum.*
The probable natural hosts of these two flukes is the night heron,
Nycticorax nycticorax. Both species were found to be experimentally infective to mammals, including man.

The second intermediate host of *S. armatum* is a cyprinoid fish. The host of the asexual stages is not known. The asexual generations of *S. formosanum* develop in a number of species of snails of the genus Melania and the cercariæ have been found to encyst in several species of fresh-water fish, including *Carassius auratus, Channa formosana, Cyprinus carpis, Gambusia affinis, Pseudorasbora parva,* and *Rhodeus ocellatus.*

Two species in the genus *Monorchotrema* have been described by Nishigori (1924) which are designated as *M. taichui* and *M. taihokui,* the specific names referring to the localities in which the parasites were first found. These flukes are closely related to *Stamnosoma, Heterophyes* and *Metagonimus,* but differ from these genera mainly in that they have but a single, large testis instead of the pair of testes described for the group. *M. taichui* and *M. taihokui* bear a close resemblance to each other, and as their life-cycle, free-swimming miracidial and cercarial stages, and the manner of development in the primary host are also similar, they probably are one and the same species, *M. taichui.*

Monorchotrema taichui occupies the middle and lower parts of the jejunum of its host where it deeply invades the mucous membrane and becomes attached. It has been reported as a natural parasite of the night heron, *Nycticorax nycticorax,* and of the dog, cat and man, of Northern and Central Formosa and the Philippine Islands.

The egg of *Monorchotrema* has a comparatively thick shell with distinct thickened shoulders where the operculum joins the shell, and contains the completely formed miracidium. The ova of *M. taichui* range from 20.7 μ to 23 μ in length by 9.2 μ to 10.7 μ in breadth, and are light brown in color. These ova may be easily mistaken for those of *Clonorchis sinensis* or *Metagonimus yokogawai.*

Species of *Melania, M. reiniana* var. *hidachiens* and *M. obliquegranosa,* serve as the first intermediate host for *Monorchotrema.* Rediæ are produced within the sporocysts, and, after a period of fixe to six weeks, mature cercariæ develop within the rediæ. The cercariæ escape from the snail and encyst on the cartilaginous tissues of the fins and head and on the gills of various fresh-water fishes. Infection in the primary host is incurred by eating raw infected fish.

Recently, Africa and others (1936) have observed several cases of acute vascular changes in the myocardium and a fatal cerebral hemorrhage in man from heterophyid eggs. According to Africa, a certain proportion of the parasites migrate into the deeper tissues of the intestinal wall where their eggs are forced into the general circulation.

VIII. Family TROGLOTREMATIDÆ

These trematodes are characterized by a more or less thick, compact body with the ventral surface flattened and the dorsal surface arched. Suckers may be weakly developed, and the ventral sucker is sometimes absent. The ovary and testes are lobed or coarsely branched and the uterine loops lie chiefly lateral of the acetabulum. The cirrus sac is usually absent. The vitellaria are strongly developed and almost fill the lateral fields on the dorsal surface. They are parasitic in carnivores and birds and generally occur in pairs in cyst-like cavities. The human representative of this family is *Paragonimus westermani*.

1. *Paragonimus westermani* (Kerbert, 1878)

HISTORICAL

Paragonimus westermani commonly known as the human lung fluke, was first found in 1877 in the lungs of a tiger in the Zoölogical Gardens of Amsterdam, Holland, by the director, Westerman. These specimens were sent to Kerbert who described it under the name *Distoma westermani* (Kerbert, 1878). The lung fluke was first discovered in man in 1879 in the lungs of a Portuguese in Formosa. This specimen was described by Cobbold (1880) as *Distoma ringeri*. Manson, in 1880, described eggs found in the sputum of a Chinese suffering from hemoptysis. In 1883 Kiyono, Suga, Yamagata and Nakahama discovered the parasite in the lungs of a Japanese and, recognizing the disease caused by it, described the species as *Distoma pulmonale*. Leuckart (1889) reviewed the morphology of the specimens obtained from both man and the tiger and concluded they belonged to the same species; and Braun in 1899 established the genus *Paragonimus* with *Paragonimus westermani* as the type of the genus. *P. kellicotti* Ward, 1908, was found in 1894 in a cat in Michigan by Ward and later in a dog in Ohio by Kellicott. Stiles and Hassall (1900) found the lung fluke a frequent parasite in hogs slaughtered in Cincinnati, Ohio, and, although these authors recognized the possibility that these worms might represent a distinct variety, they were looked upon as being identical with the Asiatic form. Ward and Hirsch (1915), after a morphological study of the American form with material from man in the Orient, and with three specimens of Kerbert's material from the tiger, con-

cluded that there are three species of the mammalian lung flukes:
(1) the tiger form, *Paragonimus westermani;* (2) the human form,
P. ringeri; and (3) the American form from the dog, cat and pig,
P. kellicotti. Ward and Hirsch based the specific differences mainly
on the size, shape and arrangement of the cuticular spines. Kobayashi (1919) carefully reviewed the structure of the lung flukes
from man and lower animals of Japan and Korea and found that
individual variations are apparently greater than the specific differences recorded by Ward and Hirsch (1915) and concluded that
there is only one species of lung fluke to which the name *Paragonimus westermani* must be given. Later, Vevers (1923) found
differences in the cuticular spines and recognized four distinct
species: (1) *P. westermani;* (2) *P. ringeri;* (3) *P. kellicotti;*
and (4) *P. compactus.* The last named species was described from
Viverra mungos, India, by Cobbold in 1859. Ameel (1934) made a
careful study of the cuticular spines of specimens obtained from
Japan, Formosa, Malay States, Sumatra and North America, and
from original material used by Ward and Hirsch. It appears from
this review that the spines of the adult are not good criteria for
species differentiation and that there is but one species, *P. westermani.*

Life history studies on *Paragonimus westermani* were first made
by Nakagawa (1915). He obtained the adult flukes by feeding
experimental animals fresh-water crabs, *Potamon obtusipes,* in which
he found encysted trematode larvæ. Further studies on the first
intermediate host and the development of cercariæ were made by
Nakagawa (1915-1919), Yokogawa (1917), Kobayashi (1918-
1921), Miyairi (1919) and Ando (1917). These authors have found
that various species of snails of the genus *Melania* serve as the intermediate host of this parasite, and have also determined its course
and development within the body of the final host. Ameel (1934) has
contributed the most recent knowledge on the life history of Paragonimus in North America.

DISTRIBUTION AND FREQUENCY

Paragonimus westermani has a wide geographic distribution and
occurs more or less frequently in local districts of Japan, Korea,
Formosa, China, New Guinea, India, Malay States, Java, Sumatra,
Indo-China, Africa, Brazil, Peru, Venezuela and the Philippine
Islands. A number of cases have been noted in North America among
Oriental immigrants but no definite, native infections in man have
been found in the United States. In Japan the infection is largely
limited to certain mountainous districts along streams. It is widely

distributed in Korea and Formosa. It is rare in China, although there is one endemic area in Chekiang Province (Maxwell, 1931). In the United States the usual host of the adult worm is the mink. Here it has been found most frequently in Michigan, Wisconsin and Minnesota. *P. westermani* has apparently no very definite specificity since it has been recorded from man, cat, dog, tiger, mountain lion, fox, marten, badger, mink, rat and weasel. Monkeys have been experimentally infected as well as rabbits, guinea-pigs, rats and mice, but the development in the last named animals does not proceed to sexual maturity.

MORPHOLOGY

The living specimens of *P. westermani* have no very definite shape as they constantly stretch outward and contract. They may appear more or less like a ribbon when fully elongated, or spoon-shaped when one pole of the body is contracted and the other elongated; or as a sphere when completely contracted. When killed and preserved they have an oval or elliptical form, resembling closely a coffee grain in both size and shape. They are of a reddish brown to a slate color when first removed from the body, but soon become grayish on exposure. The oral sucker is situated at the anterior extremity of the body and opens anteriorly in well extended specimens. In contracted specimens the mouth is ventral. The suckers are usually of about equal size, ordinarily slightly less than 1 mm. in diameter. The ventral sucker, or acetabulum, is situated somewhat anteriorly to the middle of the body and often lies completely invaginated leaving a relatively narrow external opening visible from the body surface. The genital pore lies on the mid-ventral surface close to the posterior margin of the acetabulum. The arrangement of the internal organs is shown in Figure 107.

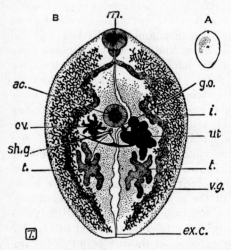

FIG. 107.—*Paragonimus westermani*. A, Natural size. B, detail of internal anatomy: *m.*, mouth surrounded by oral sucker; *ac.*, ventral sucker; *ov.*, ovary; *sh.g.*, Mehlis' gland; *t.*, testis; *g.o.*, genital pore; *ut.*, uterus; *v.g.*, vitellaria; *ex.c.*, excretory pore. (From Manson-Bahr's *Manson's Tropical Diseases*)

LIFE-CYCLE

The eggs of *Paragonimus westermani* usually escape from the host in the sputum. Because of their dark color the sputum often appears rusty, especially when they occur in large numbers. If the host swallows his sputum these ova may also be found in the feces. The eggs of this species are oval, yellowish-brown in color and have a thick shell (Figure 80,₅). They have been found to vary considerably in size, even when obtained from a single host, varying in length from 85 μ to 100 μ by 50 μ to 67 μ in breadth. They show no development when found in fresh sputum, the fertilized cell is in the single-cell stage, and is surrounded by several yolk globules. The development of the miracidium is slow and may require from four to six weeks before it escapes from the shell. Under optimum conditions hatching takes place in about sixteen days.

At least six species of fresh-water snails of the genus *Melania* may serve as the first intermediate host of *Paragonimus westermani*. Of these, *Melania libertina* in Japan and *Melania gottschei* in Korea are perhaps the most important species in the propagation of *Paragonimus* as they are the common fresh-water snails of these countries. *Pomatiopsis lapidaria* is the primary intermediate host in North America. A sporocyst and two redial generations develop within the infected snail.

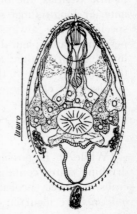

The cercariæ (Figure 108), after their escape from the snail, penetrate into the body of several species of fresh-water crustacea of the genera *Potamon, Sesarma, Eriocheir, Astacus* and *Cambarus*. They encyst in the liver, muscles and especially in the gills.

The fully developed, encysted cercaria within the body of the crab is usually spherical, having a diameter from 0.35 mm. to 0.47 mm. The wall of the cyst is very thick and tough and is surrounded by an outer membranous sac which is produced by a reaction of the host's tissue against the parasite. Within the living cysts the organs of the larvæ are distinctly visible. Man, and other

FIG. 108.—Cercaria of *Paragonimus*. (After Ameel)

susceptible hosts, become infected by eating the raw infected flesh of these crustaceans.

Nakagawa (1918) found that the encysted larvæ of *Paragonimus* were killed when the crabs were roasted until the muscles turned white or were kept in water at 55° C. for five minutes. He also noted that when freed from the tissues of the crab they could survive a 2 per cent hydrochloric acid solution for three hours. One hour in vinegar was sufficient to kill them, and nine hours was sufficient to kill all the larvæ when the crab gills containing the cysts were placed in soy sauce. Yokogawa (1917) found that 10 per cent salt solution killed the encysted larvæ in one hour, 5 per cent in from two to three hours.

POSITION IN THE FINAL HOST

The adult of *Paragonimus westermani* is found most frequently in cysts near the surface of the lungs of the final host. The cyst wall consists of a layer of connective tissue and is produced by the host as a reaction against the parasite. Besides the worm, the cyst usually contains an exudate with eggs of the parasite and Charcot-Leyden crystals. In other instances the worm may have been dead for some time and only its "mummy" remains. In man these cysts usually contain a single worm but in dogs and other mammals they commonly contain two or more.

The adult parasites have been found also in the abdominal and pleural cavities, the brain, orbit and eyelids, omentum, pericardium, anterior longitudinal sinus, spleen and vertebral column. Immature specimens are always encountered outside of the lungs, in the peritoneal and pleural cavities or in soft tissues but never in the lungs. Even if they are directly introduced, when immature, into the lungs by way of the jugular vein, they escape to complete their development elsewhere.

THE MIGRATORY COURSE OF THE LUNG FLUKE IN THE BODY OF THE FINAL HOST

While it is possible that some infections are acquired from drinking water containing living cysts which have been freed from crabs, it is very probable that the majority of infections with *Paragonimus* are incurred by a direct ingestion of the cysts from crustaceans serving as second intermediate hosts, either in connection with the handling of crabs while preparing them for food, or more especially by eating them raw or imperfectly cooked.

After the entrance of the encysted larvæ within the body of the final host, they show a remarkable tendency to migrate, and invade tissues other than the lungs until they are sexually mature. The course of the young flukes in the body of the final host has been studied in detail by Yokogawa (1919) and other Japanese scientists.

The encysted cercariæ, after being swallowed with the flesh of the crab, escape from their cysts in the small intestine of the host. Within several hours, by their own leech-like movements, they penetrate through the intestinal wall and reach the abdominal cavity. The worms pass through the middle and posterior regions of the small intestine. Their movements seem to be influenced by the resistance of the tissues since they penetrate the mucous membrane along the long axis of the intestine, and after passing through the submucosa burrow into the muscular layers moving with the long axes of the fibers. They then make their way along the abdominal cavity and penetrate the diaphragm. They may live for a long time in the abdominal cavity and make their way into other organs before reaching the diaphragm. Therefore, at the time of piercing the diaphragm they may be in an early stage of development or at any stage up to sexual maturity. When young they pass through the muscular parts of the diaphragm pushing aside the muscle fibers. When older they seem to prefer the sinewy parts. They have been found in the chest cavity as early as seventy hours after ingestion. They usually remain much longer in the body cavity, however, and it may be a hundred days or more before they penetrate the diaphragm.

During this time they may burrow into various organs, such as the liver, omentum, mesenteries or spleen. Most frequently they migrate into the liver, probably because it is large and soft and lies directly in their general course. When they enter the liver, they only penetrate a short distance and then turn and escape making characteristic, blind alleys. Most of the young flukes seem to reach the diaphragm by way of the space between the liver and the abdominal wall, since the paths of the worms in the liver are found most frequently on the anterior margin of its upper surface. There is no evidence that the young worms ever migrate to the lungs by way of the blood or lymph vessels of the intestinal wall, omentum or mesenteries. About twenty days or more after infection, the worms enter the chest cavity and penetrate into the lungs. Not all the worms which enter the abdominal cavity will migrate into the diaphragm, however, nor do all those which enter the chest cavity penetrate the lungs. Accordingly, in heavy infections in experimental animals, some worms have been found almost always in the abdominal cavity and surrounding organs and in the pleural cavity and may reach maturity in these locations.

Some of the worms may migrate to the brain but apparently do not remain in this tissue for their development. The course to the cranial cavity is believed to be along the soft tissues of the neck and through the large foramina, especially the jugular foramen, since in human cases, the pathological changes in the brain are almost always in the temporal or occipital lobes near the jugular foramen.

II. *Diseases Caused by Lung Flukes*

PATHOLOGY

The adult flukes ordinarily occur in the lungs of the final host but they may be found in almost every tissue, as pointed out in an earlier paragraph. In the human lungs the cysts are usually flat and contain but one parasite. In the post-mortem examinations of the human lung the cysts are not always easily located since they do not, as a rule, project from the lung's surface. In the lungs of cats, dogs and other animals, however, they stand out clearly as dark-red or brown bodies on the surface of the lung. They are about the size of a filbert and usually contain two worms. The number of flukes in a single human host has usually been under ten and only in a few exceptional cases have more than twenty been found. In dogs and cats, however, the numbers present are usually larger. These cysts represent dilatations of the bronchi, or bronchioles, and contain, besides the worm, a

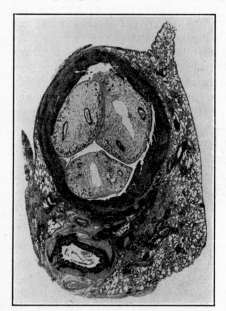

Fig. 109.—Section of lung showing lesions produced by *Paragonimus*. (Copyright by General Biological Supply House, Chicago)

brown exudate in which are found the ova of the parasite and Charcot-Leyden crystals. This material constitutes the characteristic sputum. Sometimes only the "mummy" of the parasite remains and in other instances the cysts may undergo caseation and resemble tubercles. Abscesses and ulcerations occur frequently. The septa between the lesions may break down and thus give rise to cavities which resemble a dilated bronchus. Extensive cirrhotic changes and emphysema may also be associated with these lesions. (Figure 109). Metaplastic changes of the cylindrical epithelium of the bronchi have been noted by several authors.

SYMPTOMS

Patients suffering from paragonimiasis have a chronic cough which is usually most urgent in the morning upon rising. Considerable blood-stained or purulent sputum is ejected in which the ova of the parasite may be found by microscopical examination. The hemoptysis is usually trifling, but in some instances it may be so great as to threaten life. Râles are usually not discoverable. If the infection is abdominal, the abdominal wall feels hard to the touch and there is more or less tenderness. When certain organs are acutely involved, appendicitis, enlargement of the prostate, epididymitis, cirrhosis of the liver and diarrhea from intestinal ulceration may result. Cerebral infections are frequently associated with a peculiar form of Jacksonian epilepsy which may result in paralysis, visual disturbances or aphasia, which are also characteristic of cerebral infections with certain tapeworm larvæ. Paragonimiasis may also be of a more or less generalized type associated with fever, enlargement of the lymph nodes and cutaneous ulcerations.

DIAGNOSIS

The diagnosis of *Paragonimus westermani* is established by the finding of the characteristic ova in the sputum, feces or in fluids obtained by puncture.

TREATMENT

Thus far no specific treatment is known for paragonimiasis, but Ando (1917) has reported that emetine reduces the sexual activity of the parasites.

PREVENTION AND CONTROL

The chief methods which have been suggested are (1) the disinfection of expectorated sputum, (2) the eradication of the various species of snails which serve as intermediate hosts, (3) the eradication of the crabs and crayfish which serve as second intermediate hosts, (4) the prohibition of the use of river water in the infected districts, and (5) the prohibition of eating raw or imperfectly cooked crabs.

Disinfection of sputum of the infected individuals while advisable is not effective as a method of control because the infection is widespread in various domesticated and wild animals. The eradication of the first and second intermediate hosts in exceedingly difficult if not impossible.

The most effective and feasible method of attack against this disease is the attempt by education to prevent the eating of raw or partly cooked crabs. Much publicity has been given to the danger of such food habits in the endemic areas of Japan, Korea and Formosa.

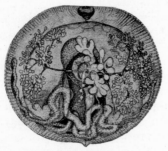

Fig. 110.—*Collyriclum faba.* Adult. (After Tyzzer)

III. *Troglotrema salmincola* (Chapin, 1926)

This species occurs in the small intestine of the dog and other CANIDAE on the Pacific Coast of North America. Its cercaria develops in the snail *Galba plicifera silicula,* and its metacercaria occurs in fishes of the salmon family. The worms reach maturity in the dog's intestine in about five days after eating raw infected fish. This parasite has been associated with a highly fatal disease known as "salmon poisoning" which occurs only in canines. The disease is due apparently to a virus which is transmitted by the flukes. Dogs recovered from an attack have a strong immunity against the parasite and the disease. There is no satisfactory medical treatment known, but the simultaneous injection of virulent blood and serum of hyper-immune dogs produces immunity against the disease.

IV. *Collyriclum faba* (Bremser, 1831)

This parasite (Figures 79, 110, 111) lacks a ventral sucker and was for years classified with the monostomes. The adult worms occur in subcutaneous cysts in passerine birds,

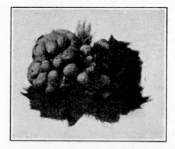

Fig. 111.—Cysts of *Collyriclum faba* showing location of the pore. (After Tyzzer)

chickens and turkeys of Europe and North America. The cysts may be single and are extended in berry-like masses about the vent, legs, abdomen and thorax. Each cyst, or "blister," has a central opening and contains two parasites, a blackish fluid and eggs. The eggs are discharged through the pore. The life-cycle is unknown. Riley and Kernkamp (1924) suggest that the cercaria probably encysts in the larva of some aquatic insect which is used, either as a larva or adult, as food by the final host.

CHAPTER XX

THE DIGENETIC TREMATODES (Continued)

Order *Prosostomata* Odhner, 1905 (Concluded)

III. Suborder AMPHISTOMATA Bojanus, 1817

The members of this suborder may be readily identified by their conspicuous and highly developed acetabulum located at or very near the posterior end of the body. These flukes have thick, muscular, somewhat flattened bodies and are often conical in shape, tapering anteriorly. The cuticula is without spines but is regularly provided with sensory or glandular papillæ. The amphistomes are intestinal parasites of fishes, amphibians, reptiles, birds and mammals. The vast majority of species occur in ruminants and equines. The order consists of three families, (1) GASTRODISCIDÆ Stiles and Goldberger, 1910, (2) PARAMPHISTOMIDÆ *Fischoeder,* 1901, and (3) GASTROTHY-LACIDÆ Stiles and Goldberger, 1910.

I. Family GASTRODISCIDÆ

The members of this family have rather discoidal bodies divided by a transverse constriction into cephalic and caudal portions. The caudal portion bears many large papillæ. There is no ventral pouch. One species occurs in man, *Gastrodiscoides hominis* (Lewis and McConnell, 1876).

1. *Gastrodiscoides hominis* (Lewis and McConnell, 1876)

HISTORICAL

Gastrodiscoides hominis was first described by Lewis and McConnell as *Amphistomum hominis* in 1876 from material sent them by O'Brien and Curren which had been obtained during an autopsy on an Assamese who had died of cholera. It was later placed in the genus *Gastrodiscus*. Giles also reported in 1890 that he frequently encountered this fluke during an investigation of kala azar and beriberi in India. Leuckart reviewed the morphology of this species in 1886-1891 and later Stephens (1906) made futher studies on its structure.

Brau and Bruyant reported the infection from an Annamite in Cochin China which is the first known infection with this parasite outside of India. Leiper (1913) reviewed the morphology of this fluke from material obtained from British Guiana and placed it in a new genus, *Gastrodiscoides*.

DISTRIBUTION AND FREQUENCY

Gastrodiscoides hominis has been reported from the Malay States, Assam, India, Cochin China and British Guiana (Indian immigrants). According to Chandler (1928) this species is common in pigs and occurs sporadically in man in Eastern India. It is probably a normal parasite of the domestic pig and its presence in man but accidental. It has also been reported in deer from the Malay States and in monkeys.

DESCRIPTION

Gastrodiscoides hominis (Figure 112) when alive is reddish. The body is very contractile and when fully extended measures about 1 cm. in length. Preserved, sexually mature adults vary from 5 mm. to 7 mm. in length and from 3 mm. to 5 mm. in greatest breadth, tapering to about 2.5 mm. anteriorly. The body is divided into two distinct regions, (1) the anterior

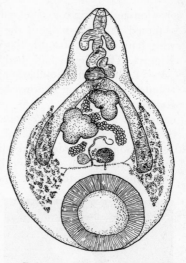

FIG. 112.—*Gastrodiscoides hominis*. (Redrawn from Khalil)

cone and (2) the enlarged, posterior disc which bears the acetabulum on its posterior median margin. The cuticula over the surface of the ventral disc is smooth, no spines are present. The eggs are operculate and have a length of about 150 μ and a width of 72 μ.

POSITION IN THE HOST

The adult of *Gastrodiscoides hominis* is found in the cecum and large intestine of the host. Very little is known of its pathogenicity.

LIFE-CYCLE

The larval stages and intermediate hosts of this species are not known. A general discussion of the life histories of the amphistomes will be given later.

II. Family PARAMPHISTOMIDAE

This family consists of amphistomes in which there is no ventral pouch, and the body is not divided into cephalic and caudal portions. Most of its species occur in domestic animals. One species, *Watsonius watsoni* (Conyngham, 1904) is an incidental parasite of man.

1. *Watsonius watsoni* (Conyngham, 1904)

Conyngham in 1904 described *Watsonius watsoni* from material obtained at autopsy from the jejunum and duodenum of a Negro who had come from the late German West Africa to Northern Nigeria. The Negro had died from inanition and diarrhea. Shipley (1905), Stiles and Goldberger (1910) and Leiper (1913) have contributed much to our knowledge of the morphology of this parasite. Railliet, Henry and Joyeux in 1912 discovered this species in the cecum of a monkey, *Cercopithecus callitrichus,* which suggests that this fluke is only an incidental parasite of man.

Watsonius watsoni is reddish yellow in color when living. It is oval to pyriform in shape and has a length of 8 mm. to 10 mm. and a breadth of 4 mm. to 5 mm. The acetabulum is large, subterminal and with the margin projecting. The eggs are oval, operculated and have a length of 122 μ to 130 μ and a breadth of 75 μ to 80 μ. Nothing is known of its life history.

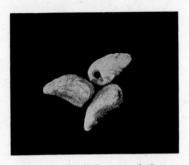

FIG. 113.—*Cotylophoron cotylophorum.* Adult worms. (After Mönnig)

11. *Amphistomes of Lower Vertebrates*

The amphistomes are frequently found in lower vertebrates. Among the commoner North American species are *Diplodiscus temperatus* (Stafford, 1905) from the rectum of frogs; *Allassostoma magnum* (Stunkard, 1916), from the intestine of turtles, *Pseudemys; Zygocotyle ceratosa* (Stunkard, 1916), from the intestine of the duck, *Anas platyrhynchos; Amphistomum cervi* (Schrank, 1790), Fischoeder, 1901, from the rumen of domestic and wild ruminants, and *Cotylophoron cotylophorum* (Fischoeder, 1901), Stiles and Goldberger, 1910 (Figure 113), also of ruminants and which closely resembles *A. cervi.*

The GASTROTHYLACIDAE are for the most part parasites of cattle in India, Ceylon, Siam and East Africa. They are distinguished from the PARAMPHISTOMIDAE by the presence of a ventral pouch.

III. Amphistome Life-Cycles

Although nothing definite is known of the life histories of the amphistomes found in man, it is possible to infer what stages occur from known life-cycles of amphistomes of lower animals. The cercariæ of *Paramphistomum cervi* develop in snails of the genera *Bulinus, Pseudosuccinea* and *Galba.* After they leave the snail they

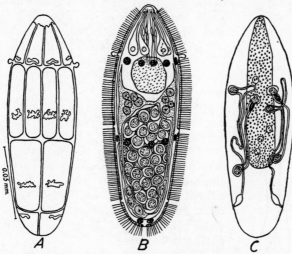

FIG. 114.—*Diplodiscus temperatus.* A. Miracidium, showing arrangement of ciliated epidermal cells. B. Miracidium, showing detail of structure. C. Miracidium, showing gut and excretory system. (After Krull and Price)

encyst upon vegetation. Upon ingestion by a suitable host, the metacercariæ escape from the cyst in the intestine and reach maturity in the abomasum. Snails of the genus *Bulinus* serve as the first intermediate host for *Cotylophoron cotylophorum* in South Africa. Krull (1934) has found that *Fossaria modicella,* a widely distributed species of fresh water snail in western United States, is a suitable host for *C. cotylophorum.* The development of amphistomes is slow.

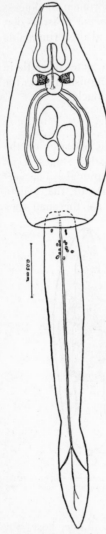

FIG. 115.—*Diplodiscus temperatus*. Cercaria. (After Krull and Price)

Krull (1934) states that six months are necessary for completion of the life-cycle of *C. cotylophorum,* one month for the egg to hatch, one month for the cercarial development in the snail and four months to reach maturity in the final host.

The life-cycle of *Diplodiscus temperatus* has been determined experimentally by Krull and Price (1932), Figures 114, 115. The egg under normal conditions contains a fully developed miracidium when deposited. The body of the miracidium is almost entirely covered with flattened ciliated epidermal cells, twenty in number and arranged in four rows. The posterior half of its body is filled with germ cells which form a single mass which is not attached to the body wall. There is a long sac-like gut and two pairs of unicellular penetration glands, one pair on each side of the anterior portion of the gut. Each gland discharges through a duct which opens at the base of the anterior papillæ. The excretory system consists of two large flame cells and two long excretory ducts, each provided with an excretory bladder. The flame cells are located in the anterior half of the body. Each bladder opens exteriorly through an excretory pore situated between the third and fourth rows of ciliated epidermal plates. Cecariæ develop from rediæ in the snail *Helisoma trivolvis,* a freshwater species found along lake shores, ponds, ditches and rivers.

Living rediæ average about 500 μ long and 168 μ wide. They possess two pairs of appendages. The birth pore is situated dorsally about midway between the oral sucker and the anterior appendages. A single redia may contain as many as twenty cercariæ in varying stages of development.

The body of the cercaria is about 400 μ long and 187 μ wide. The tail is approximately 700 μ long and 70 μ wide at its base. The body is spineless and pigmented on its dorsal surface. A pair of large pigmented eyespots, each with a large lens, are situated on the dorsal side. The oral sucker has a muscular wall with two muscular (pharyngeal) pouches extending from its posterior border. The digestive system is similar to that of the adult (Figure 75F). The large acetabulum is terminal and is directed slightly ventrally. The cystogenous glands are well developed. A small but muscular excretory bladder is situated anterior to the acetabulum which discharges through a dorsal median pore. Three main excretory tubules discharge into the bladder. The posterior median one enters the tail and the other two pass anteriorly into the body proper. The anterior ends of these tubules may be distended by globular concretions.

After the cercariæ escape from the snail host they swim about and may encyst on almost any substratum, but usually they attach themselves firmly to the pigmented areas of a frog where encystment is almost instantaneous. Frogs become infected when they devour their own *stratum corneum* on which cercariæ have encysted. The metacercariæ escape from the cyst in the small intestine of the frog and reach maturity after about three months in the rectum. Infection in tadpoles takes place in a different way. The cysts are loosely attached to the tadpole and, after they are formed, usually drop off into the pond ooze. Tadpoles may be infected while feeding upon ooze. Swimming cercariæ may also be carried into the mouth of the tadpole by respiratory currents. When this happens the cercariæ first suddenly encyst during their passage along the esophagus and later escape from the cyst in the lower small intestine.

Judging from the character of the above life-cycles, it is probable that most of the amphistomes follow the same general lines of development, and that the final host becomes infected with these parasites by ingesting the metacercaria with food or water.

CHAPTER XXI

THE DIGENETIC TREMATODES (Concluded)

Order Strigeatoidea La Rue, 1926

The cercarial forms of these trematodes have forked tails. The flame cell arrangement is reducible to a 1 + 1 pattern. It is probable that some of the species now referred to the PROSOSTOMATA may need transferring to this group when their life histories are known. This order consists of three suborders, (1) STRIGEATA La Rue, 1926, (2) BUCEPHALATA La Rue, 1926, and (3) SCHISTOSOMATA La Rue, 1926. Of these, only the SCHISTOSOMATA contains species of economic or medical importance.

I. Suborder STRIGEATA

The STRIGEATA are monœcious forms. The body is usually divided by a constriction into two parts, the anterior bears special organs of attachment and the posterior portion contains the major parts of the reproductive organs. The genital pore is posterior. The acetabulum is rudimentary or may be lacking. There is a special holdfast organ on the ventral surface posterior to the acetabulum. The cercariæ have a slender tail stem, a pharynx and a true oral sucker. The adults are parasites of snail- or fish-eating vertebrates. There is no human representative. Example, *Diplostomum flexicaudum* Cort and Brooks, 1928.

The adult form of *Diplostomum flexicaudum* (Figure 116) was described by van Haitsma in 1931 from the intestine of herring gulls of Douglas Lake, Michigan. The cercariæ develop from daughter sporocysts in several species of fresh water snails of the genus *Lymnæa*. After leaving the snail, the cercariæ penerate various parts of the body of fishes, particularly the common sucker, *Catostomus commersonii,* and finally lodge within the lens capsule where they grow and metamorphose into metacercariæ. Gulls become infected from eating the parasitized fish.

II. Suborder BUCEPHALATA

The members of BUCEPHALATA are monœcious flukes with nonperforate, degenerate anterior suckers. The mouth is located on the ventral surface, opening through a pharynx into a rhabdocoele intestine. The testes are arranged in a series posterior to the ovary. The genital pore is posterior. A cirrus and cirrus sac are present. The cercariæ (Bucephalus larva) have a thick tail stem and long rami. The adults are intestinal parasites of fish. Example, *Bucephalus papillosus* Woodhead, 1929.

Bucephalus papillosus (Figures 117, 118) inhabits the cecal pouches, stomach and intestine of fresh water bass, sticklebacks and pike. The cercariæ develop from rediæ in *Elliptio dilatatus,* a common river mussel. The escaped cercariæ encyst at the base of the fin rays of small fish. When such parasitized fish are eaten by larger, susceptible fish the cycle of the parasite is completed. Woodhead (1931) regards the mother sporocyst, the redia and the final adult as adult generations. Each are described as possessing well developed nutritive and reproductive systems. According to Woodhead, spermatogenesis takes place in both the mother sporocyst and the redia, as well as in the final adult.

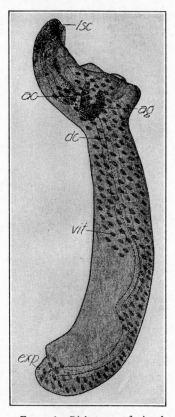

FIG. 116.—*Diplostomum flexicaudum.* Cort and Brooks, 1928. Side view. Major organs of the reproductive system omitted. (After van Haitsma)

ac—acetabulum
ag—adhesive gland of holdfast
dc—digestive cecum
exp—excretory pore
lsc—lateral sucking cup
vit—vitellaria

III. Suborder
SCHISTOSOMATA

The members of this group are monœcious or diœcious blood-inhabiting flukes, without a pharynx and with or without suckers. The cercariæ are forked-tailed with a slender tail stem. The anterior organ of the cercaria is for penetrating and is not a true sucker. They actively penetrate their host through the surface. There is no metacercarial stage. The eggs are not operculate. There is but a single family, the

SCHISTOSOMATIDÆ Looss, 1899. Its members are generally known as schistosomes or "blood flukes."

1. *The Blood Flukes*

These are perhaps the most important trematodes parasitic in man; they cause diseases known as bilharziasis, endemic hematuria or urinary schistosomiasis, and intestinal schistosomiasis, Katayama disease or schistosomiasis of the Far East.

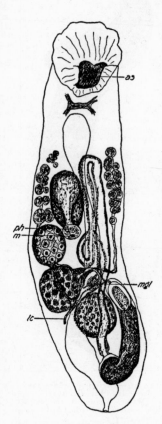

HISTORICAL

Schistosomiasis is a very old disease. In Egypt, hematuria, a common symptom of Egyptian schistosomiasis, has been recognized since the earliest times and the medical papyri contain prescriptions against it. The actual evidence of its presence was brought out by Rüffer (1910) who discovered ova of the parasites in mummies of the twentieth dynasty, 1250-1000 B.C. The discovery of the parasite itself was not made, however, until 1851 by Bilharz.

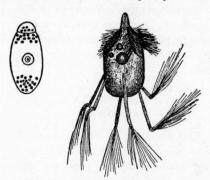

FIG. 117.—*Bucephalus papillosus*. Adult. (After Woodhead)
  as—anterior sucker
  lc—Laurer's canal
  m—mouth
  mgl—Mehlis' gland
  ph—pharynx

FIG. 118.—*Bucephalus papillosus*. Egg and lateral view of the miracidium. (After Woodhead)

Bilharz later established the relation between the blood flukes and the hematuria and dysentery with the accompanying lesions of the bladder and intestine which were so frequent in Egypt. This disease was then known, and is often referred to as "bilharziasis." This work of Bilharz established, for the first time, a connection between a trematode parasite and a human disease. Two types of eggs were found, one with a terminal spine and the other with a lateral spine, but they were considered as from a single species of parasite which produced both bladder and rectal types of the disease. Much confusion followed because of the presence of ova with lateral and terminal spines and it was not until 1907 (Sambon, 1907) that the two species were definitely separated; the separation being based on (1) the position of the spines on the eggs, (2) the different anatomical habitat, (3) differences in pathogenicity and (4) differences in geographical distribution. Sambon retained the name *Schistosoma hæmatobium* for the urinary type of ova with the terminal spine and established a new species, *Schistosoma mansoni,* for the rectal form with lateral spined ova.

In Japan, schistosomiasis is a disease probably as old as Egyptian bilharziasis but exact knowledge regarding it is of quite recent date. In ancient times there was recognized an endemic disease in certain districts of Japan which produced swelling of the liver and spleen. A description of this disease was written in 1847 by Fujii under the name of "Katayama disease." Later Yamagiwa (1890), Fujinami (1904) and others found eggs at autopsies in the liver, mesenteries, lungs and brain of man, and much discussion among the medical men of Japan followed in regard to the relation of the ova of this unknown parasite to the endemic "Katayama disease."

The first actual relation of the causative agent to the infection was obtained by Katsurada (1904). Katsurada found the eggs in the feces of a patient suffering from this disease and a worm in the portal vein of a cat. He also found eggs in the liver of the cat and reported that these were identical with those found in the human disease, and that the worm produced the eggs and was the cause of the disease. He named the worm *Schistosoma japonicum.* Later in the same year the worm was found in the portal vein of a man who had died of the infection.

The discovery of the intermediate stages of the schistosomes and the method of entrance into man is of recent date. All early attempts to infect species of snails or insects with *Schistosoma* were unsuccessful and after repeated attempts to find the intermediate host and larval stages of the Egyptian blood fluke, Looss (1894-1908) advanced the hypothesis that no intermediate host was needed in the life-cycle of this genus, and that man was infected by the penetration of the miracidium through the skin, the intermediate stages developing in the liver of man. Experimental attempts to prove this hypothesis failed and were explained away by stating that since man was the only host for this infection experiments on other animals were without significance. This hypothesis received the support of many parasitologists and undoubtedly delayed the final discovery of the life-cycle of the schistosomes.

In 1909 Fujinami, Katsurada, Nakamura and others proved experimentally that infection with *Schistosoma japonicum* did come about through the skin and adequate protection of the skin was suggested as a prophylactic measure. It was not until 1913, however, that the infective agent was discovered by Miyairi and Suzuki who were not only able to infect mammals from cercariæ from Katayama snails, but also observed the penetration of the hatched miracidia into the same species of snail and followed the development of the larval stages within the snail.

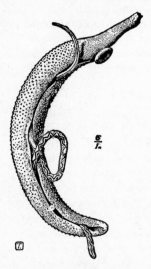

This discovery led to similar investigations on the Egyptian flukes. *Schistosoma hæmatobium* and *S. mansoni* by Leiper (1915-1918) who found the intermediate hosts of these species and studied the larval stages. Further investigations on the life-cycle of *Schistosoma mansoni* have been carried on in the New World by Iturbe and Gonzalez (1917), Lutz (1919) and Faust and Hoffman (1934). The names of various snails which may serve as intermediate hosts for the commoner schistosomes of man are

FIG. 119.—*Schistosoma mansoni*. Male carrying the female in the gynæcophoric canal. (From Manson-Bahr's *Manson's Tropical Diseases*)

listed in Table IV, page 297.

Fisher (1934) described a fourth species of human schistosomes from the Belgian Congo. This species, *S. intercalatum* Fisher (1934), is strikingly similar in all of its known stages to *S. hæmatobium*, but causes a purely intestinal schistosomiasis. It is probable that further investigation will show that many of the cases of intestinal schistosomiasis attributed to *S. hæmatobium* will be found to be infections with *S. intercalatum. Physopsis africana* is the intermediate host.

POSITION IN THE HOST

All of the schistosomes are parasites of the venous system of their final host. *Schistosoma hæmatobium* inhabits especially the mesenteric branches of the portal vein, the vesicoprostatic, the pubic and uterine plexuses and the vesical veins. *S. mansoni* is found most com-

TABLE IV

DISTINGUISHING FEATURES OF THE HUMAN SCHISTOSOMES

	S. hæmatobium	*S. mansoni*	*S. japonicum*
Adult male	Size, 12-14 mm. long Cuticula finely tuberculated Intestinal crura unite late so that united region of intestine is short Testes large, 4 in number	12 mm. long Cuticula grossly tuberculated Intestinal crura unite early so that united region of intestine is long Testes small, 8 in number	9-22 mm. long Cuticula non-tuberculated Intestinal crura unite far back, united region being one-fifth to one-sixth of body length Testes slightly lobate, 7-8 in number
Adult female	Size, 20 mm. long Uterus long and voluminous and contains a number of eggs Ovary in posterior half of body	14-15 mm. long Uterus short, contains usually from 1-3 eggs at a time Ovary in anterior half of body	12-26 mm. long Uterus well-developed, occupies about half of postacetabular region, contains 50-300 eggs Ovary about the middle of the body
Eggs	Terminal spine, 150 x 60, usually deposited in veins of bladder, escape with urine	Lateral spine, 150 x 60, usually deposited in veins of rectum, escape with feces	Abbreviated spine, 80 x 65, deposited in portal system, enter intestine higher than with *S. mansoni*
Intermediate hosts	*Bulinus contortus* (Egypt) *B. dybowskyi* (Egypt) *B. innesi, B. brochii* (Egypt and Sudan) *Physopsis africana* (S. Africa) *P. globosa* (West Africa) *Planorbis dufouri* (Portugal)	*Planorbis boissyi* (Egypt) *P. pfeifferi* (West Africa) *P. adowensis* (Belgian Congo) *P. olivaceous* (Brazil and Dutch Guiana) *P. centimetralis* (Brazil) *P. guadelupensis = Australorbis glabratus* (Venezuela and West Indies) *Physopsis africana* (S. Africa)	*Blanfordia nosophora* (Japan and China) *B. formosana* (Formosa) *Hemibia hupensis* (Yangtse Valley)

monly in the inferior and superior mesenteric veins, the hemorrhoidal plexus and the portal system. The habitat of *Schistosoma japonicum* in the human body is similar to that of *S. mansoni*. The worms are usually mated and headed against the blood current.

Schistosoma japonicum occurs as a natural infection in a relatively large number of mammals, including man, cat, dog, pig and cattle, and can be readily transmitted to laboratory animals, cats, mice, monkeys, guinea-pigs and horses. *Schistosoma hæmatobium* has been observed as a natural infection in the monkey, *Cercocebus fuliginosus*. Characteristically, it is a parasite only of man, but under experimental conditions it can be established in laboratory animals. *Schistosoma mansoni* also may be transmitted experimentally to laboratory animals, but it is known to occur naturally only in man and in the West Indian green monkey, *Cercopithecus sabæus*.

MORPHOLOGY OF THE ADULT WORMS

The male worms are characterized by a body which is widened and infolded behind the ventral sucker into the so-called "gynæco-

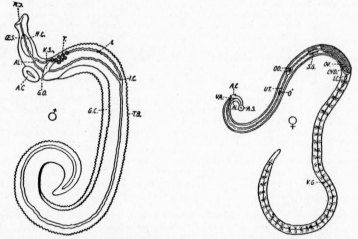

FIG. 120.—*Schistosoma mansoni*, male and female. *A.C.*, ventral sucker; *A.L.*, bifurcation of alimentary canal; *A.S.*, oral sucker; *G.C.*, gynæcophoric canal; *G.O.*, genital pore; *I.*, intestine; *I.C.*, union of intestinal crura; *N.C.*, nerve cord; *O.*, egg; *Œ.S.*, esophagus; *OO.*, oötype; *OV.*, ovary; *OVD.*, oviduct; *S.G.*, Mehlis' gland; *T.*, testes; *T.B.*, tuberculations; *UT.*, uterus; *VA.*, vagina; *V.G.*, vitelline glands; *V.S.*, seminal vesicle. (x 10). (From Manson-Bahr's *Manson's Tropical Diseases*)

phoric canal" in which the female is held at the time of copulation (Figures 119, 120, 121). It is usually light gray or whitish in color and varies from 9 mm. to 22 mm. in length, according to the species, (see Table IV). Extended specimens in the veins may have a length up to 30 mm. The suckers are large and prominent, the oral sucker is funnel-shaped and the acetabulum is distinctly pedunculate and is usually larger than the oral sucker. In the digestive system of both the male and female worms, the mouth is somewhat ventral. The intestine branches immediately in front of the acetabulum and re-unites later in the posterior portion of the body. The length of the united posterior portion forms a characteristic for the species (see Table IV). The excretory system consists of two longitudinal canals which open into the excretory pore which is placed somewhat dorsally at the posterior end. The male repro-

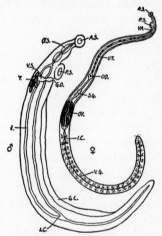

ductive system is made up of from four to eight testes which lie posterior and dorsal to the acetabulum. The vasa efferentia unite to form an elongated seminal vesicle which opens to the exterior through the genital pore, situated immediately below the acetabulum in the median line. There is no cirrus sac. The genital pore is enlarged at the time of copulation, and is applied to the female genital pore for the transfer of spermatozoa.

The female worms are darker in color and vary from 14 mm. to 26 mm. in length, according to the species (see Table IV). They are cylindrical and pointed at each end. The middle portion of the body is generally held within the gynæcophoric canal of the male

Fig. 121.—*Schistosoma japonicum*, male and female; for lettering see legend to Fig. 120 (x 10). (From Manson-Bahr's *Manson's Tropical Diseases*)

and the anterior and posterior portions are free. The posterior free portion is often of a dark brown color. The digestive system is similar to that of the male except as modified by the great difference in body shape. The intestinal cæca are large and prominent and full of dark pigment. The union of the intestinal cæca is back of the ovary. The female reproductive system consists of one ovary situated behind the middle of the body in front of the union of the intestinal cæca. The oviduct arises from the posterior pole of the ovary and as it passes forward is joined by the vitelline duct. The vitellaria occupy the posterior part of the body. The oviduct leads into Mehlis' gland from which the uterus passes forward and opens at the genital pore situated immediately posterior to the acetabulum. Differences in structure of the three species of *Schistosoma* occurring in man are given in Table IV.

GEOGRAPHICAL DISTRIBUTION

As far as our knowledge goes, Japanese schistosomiasis is limited as an endemic disease to the Far East, being quite prevalent in some parts of Japan, Southern Formosa and the Philippine Islands. It is especially prevalent and of economic importance in the rice-growing regions of the Yangtze Valley in China.

The records of the distribution of schistosomiasis in Africa are to some extent confused by the fact that the distinction between *Schistosoma hæmatobium,* and *S. intercalatum* is of recent date.

In South Africa, *Schistosoma hæmatobium* is very prevalent and has a wide distribution, but *S. mansoni* does not occur as frequently. In the Belgian Congo, *S. mansoni* is more prevalent and *S. hæmatobium* is quite rare.

Both species are found in North Africa but *S. hæmatobium* is especially common in Morocco, Algiers and Tunis, as well as in Egypt.

Schistosoma hæmatobium is also met with outside of Africa occurring in Portugal, Mauritius, Mesopotamia, Madagascar and Australia.

It seems probable that *Schistosoma mansoni* was introduced into the western hemisphere with negro slaves from Africa. It is now endemic in Martinique, Guadeloupe, Puerto Rico, Antigua, St. Kitts, Nevis, Montserrat, Vieques, Dutch Guiana, Venezuela and Northern Brazil. Possibly the failure of *S. hæmatobium* to get a foothold in the New World can be explained by the failure of the parasite to find a suitable intermediate host; or it may be that a greater incidence of *S. mansoni* occurred in the regions from which the slaves came.

LIFE HISTORY

In order to get the eggs to the outer world the female schistosome, *in copula,* moves down against the blood stream as far as the size of the smaller venules will permit, deposits one egg at a time and withdraws in the vessel after each deposition so that the vessel has the appearance of a chain of beads, the eggs lying in a single row. In the case of *Schistosoma mansoni* and *S. japonicum* the migration is toward the large intestine and rectum, while with *S. hæmatobium* it is generally to the urinary bladder. When the worm retires the vein contracts to its normal dimensions and the returning blood drives the spine of the egg into the wall of the vein. The eggs then tend to work their way through the mucosa of the bladder, or rectum, as the case may be, so that they are eventually discharged with the urine or feces (Figure 122). The eggs of *S. hæmatobium* (Figure 123) usually are

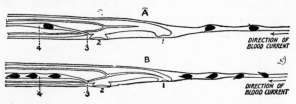

FIG. 122.—Diagram representing deposition of eggs (A) *S. mansoni* and (B) *S. hæmatobium* in blood vessels, and their passage to exterior. 1, oral sucker; 2, ventral sucker; 3, vulva; 4, uterus with contained eggs. (From Manson-Bahr's *Manson's Tropical Diseases*)

passed with the urine and frequently with the feces; the eggs of *S. mansoni* (Figure 124) usually are passed with the feces and only rarely with the urine; while the eggs of *S. japonicum* are passed from the host only in the feces.

In all species of human schistosomes the egg contains a more or less fully developed, heavily ciliated miracidium when it reaches the exterior. The eggs hatch in water within a very few hours and the miracidia immediately set out for the specific intermediate hosts. Under most favorable conditions the miracidium lives but a few hours unless it reaches its snail host.

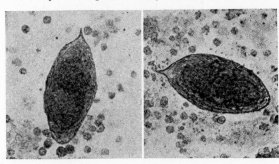

FIG. 123.—Ova of *Schistosoma hæmatobium* with pus corpuscles in urine (x 250). (From Todd's *Clinical Diagnosis,* W. B. Saunders Company)

This miracidium differs from the miracidium of *Fasciolopsis buski* in that it does not lose its cilia when penetrating the snail host but utilizes them in making its way deeper into the tissues. At the base of the gills, or in the tentacle or "horn" of the snail, the cilia are lost within twenty-four to forty-eight hours after penetration, and the miracidium becomes a simple sac, the mother sporocyst. Elongated daughter sporocysts which develop from the germ cells within the mother sporocyst when mature escape through the wall of the mother sporocyst and make their way to the digestive gland or liver of the snail. Here they increase in size, and, when fully developed, they contain a large number of forked-tail cercariæ in different stages of development. The fully developed cercaria (Figure 125) pushes out of the daughter sporocyst, leaves the snail, and swims away in search of the definitive host.

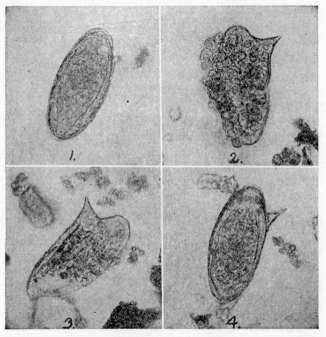

FIG. 124.—Ova of *Schistosoma mansoni:* 1, with spine out of focus; 2, in a clump of red blood cells; 3, apparently unfertilized; 4, usual appearance (x 250). (From Todd's *Clinical Diagnosis,* W. B. Saunders Company)

The cercaria of the schistosomes may develop in a number of fresh-water snails as shown in Table IV.

The cercariæ are very small (about 500 μ in length) and are covered with backward pointing spines. The ventral sucker is well developed. A "head organ" occupies the anterior third of the body. It is roughly pyramidal in outline with the base anterior and concave. It serves as an oral sucker and develops later into the muscular oral sucker of the adult. Two groups of prominent penetration glands, four anterior and six posterior, occupy the posterior third of the body. These glands are unicellular and each has a large nucleus. Their ducts pass forward in two lateral groups and end in the concavity of the head organ between a number of sharply pointed penetration glands.

The digestive system is in a very rudimentary stage of development. The mouth is situated on the ventral surface a little back of the anterior tip. The esophagus extends posteriorly to about the level of the penetration glands where it widens into a heart-shaped structure which represents the beginning of the bifurcation of the intestine. It is non-functional during the free-swimming period of the cercaria.

The only trace of the complicated reproductive system of the adult is a small mass of nuclei on the ventral side posterior to the acetabulum. Since sexual dimorphism is manifest very early in the development of the final host it is evident that there must be a sexual differentiation in the cercariæ, yet no one has actually observed this condition. The cercariæ of the human schistosomes are strikingly similar and cannot be distinguished from each other morphologically.

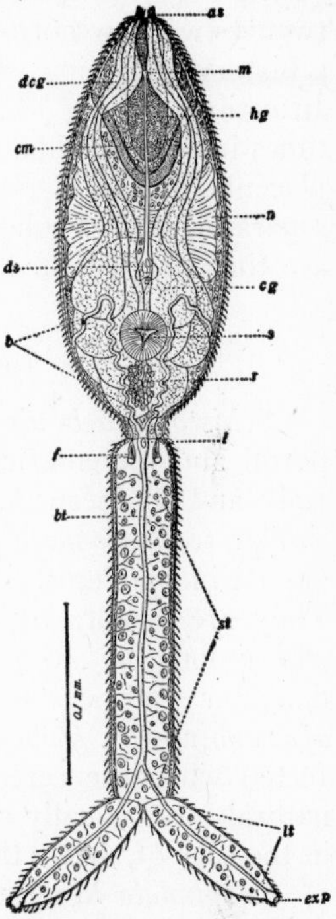

FIG. 125.—Cercaria of *Schistosoma japonicum*, ventral view; *as,* anterior spines; *b,* excretory bladder; *bt,* excretory bladder of tail; *cg,* cephalic glands; *cm,* circular muscles; *dcg,* ducts of cephalic glands; *ds,* digestive system; *exp,* excretory pore; *f,* flame cell; *hg,* head gland; *i,* island in excretory bladder; *lt,* lobe of tail; *m,* mouth; *n,* nervous system; *st,* stem of tail; *s,* ventral sucker. (After Cort)

METHODS OF HUMAN INFECTION

Man acquires schistosomiasis either by drinking water containing cercariæ, or by bathing in infected streams or canals, working in rice cultivation or in following other similar occupations in which the cercariæ are given an opportunity to penetrate the exposed skin. Most cases of infection are by the direct penetration of the host's skin by the cercariæ. Entering the lymphatics or blood vessels the young schistosomes finally accumulate in the hepatic portal vessels, where they attain sexual maturity in from six to eight weeks. After egg production has started the adult flukes make their way down into the mesenteric branches of the portal vein.

A number of prenatal infections with *Schistosoma japonicum* have been observed in both man and lower animals. Narabayashi (1914-1916) found ova of this parasite in the feces of three out of twenty-two new-born babies. The mothers of these children all gave a history of having worked in the rice fields during their pregnancy. Infections arising in this manner have been observed a number of times in experimental animals. The young parasites are carried to the placenta in the blood stream, migrate through the thin membrane separating the circulation of the mother from that of the fetus, and are then carried to the fetus by its own blood vessels.

11. *Blood Flukes of Lower Animals*

Schistosoma bovis (Sonsino, 1876) is a frequent parasite in the portal and mesenteric vessels of cattle, sheep and goats of Africa, Italy and southern Asia. Morphologically, the parasite is strikingly similar to *S. hæmatobium*. It does not occur in man. The eggs are passed in the feces. The eggs vary considerably in size and outline. They are usually oval to spindle-shaped and vary from 130 μ to 280 μ long by 40 μ to 95 μ wide. The cercaria develops from daughter sporocysts in the snails *Bulinus contortus, Physopsis africana* and *P. globosa*. Most laboratory animals may be readily infected when the cercariæ are applied to the skin. Infection in the natural hosts usually occurs by the cercariæ penetrating the skin, but in the case of sheep, they are probably swallowed with water.

S. spindale Montgomery, 1906, occurs in the mesenteric veins of cattle, sheep and goats of India and Sumatra. The eggs measure from 160 μ to 490 μ long by 20 μ to 70 μ wide. The cercaria develops in *Planorbis exustus. S. indicum* occurs in portal, pancreatic, pelvic, hepatic and mesenteric veins of cattle, sheep, goats, camels and wild ruminants of India and Rhodesia. The eggs are oval, bear a terminal spine and measure 120 μ to 140 μ long by 68 μ to 72 μ wide. *S. margrebowiei* Le Roux, 1933, has been reported from the portal system of the zebra and antelope from Africa. Morphologically it is similar to *S. japonicum,* except that the males have four or five testes, and the cuticula is covered with bosses.

Schistosomatium douthitti (Cort, 1914) (Figure 75, D and E) occurs in the hepatic portal veins of the meadow mouse, *Microtus pennsylvanicus,* in North America. It is of particular interest to medical zoölogy because its cercaria is one of several species of non-human schistosomes that often cause a severe papular and frequently pustular dermatitis in persons wading or bathing in fresh-water lakes

(Figure 126), the habitat of the snail hosts, *Lymnæa palustris, L. reflexa, L. stagnalis appressa, L. stagnalis perampla* and *Physa ancillaria parkeri.* The eggs of *S. douthitti* are entirely undeveloped when deposited, but contain mature embryos by the time they have passed through the intestinal wall of the host and appear in the feces. The developed egg measures from 94 μ to 122 μ long and from 74 μ to 98 μ wide. It has a thin, transparent shell and is devoid of markings or a spine. Upon hatching, the miracidium swims actively about in search of a snail host. After penetration of this host, it develops into a mother sporocyst which in turn gives rise to daughter

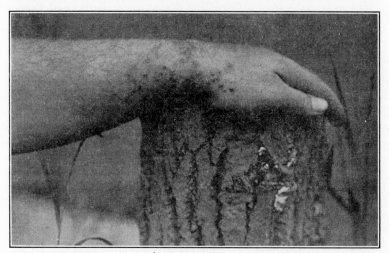

FIG. 126.—Schistosome dermatitis produced by non-human schistosome cercariae.
(Photograph supplied by Dr. W. W. Cort)

sporocysts. The daughter sporocysts give rise to cercariæ which leave the snail and swim about in the water (Figure 84, C_1). The final host is infected by cercariæ penetrating the skin. They follow along the blood stream, finally to the hepatic portal vessels where they develop to maturity in about three weeks (Price, 1931).

The life history of this parasite may be readily followed in the laboratory. Cercariæ may be obtained from naturally infected snails, and laboratory mice can serve as a host for the adult worms.

Schistosomatium pathlocopticum Tanabe (1923) is closely related to *S. douthitti.* This species was reared in laboratory mice from cercariæ found in *Lymnæa palustris* of the fens of Boston. The natural host of the adult is not known.

Bilharziella polonica (Kowalewski, 1896) occurs in the mesenteric and abdominal veins of wild and domestic ducks throughout Europe and has been observed at the National Zoölogical Park in Washington. The intermediate hosts are *Planorbis corneus, Lymnæa stagnalis* and *L. limosa.* It is apparently not very pathogenic. *Trichobilharzia ocellata* (La Vallette-Saint Georges, 1855) is a parasite of wild and domestic ducks of Europe. Its cercaria develops in *Lymnæa stagnalis* and *L. limosa.* This cercaria, morphologically similar to *Cercaria elvæ* Miller, 1923, which has been shown experimentally to produce a dermatitis in man in North America, has been shown by Brumpt (1931) to be a cause of schistosome dermatitis of bathers in France.

PATHOLOGY

The variations in the diseases caused by the different species of schistosomes of man are due chiefly to differences in the place of deposition of the eggs. It will be recalled that *S. hæmatobium* prefers the veins of the urinary bladder whereas *S. mansoni* and *S. japonicum* are more restricted to the veins of the large intestine. The pathological changes brought about by these parasites depend very much on the number of worms harbored and the duration of the infection. The pathological lesions are due almost entirely to the eggs, which act as foreign bodies in the tissue, and to a less extent to the presence of adult worms. Early in the disease caused by *Schistosoma hæmatobium,* the bladder may show either diffuse reddening or hyperemia. Small vesicular or papular elevations are found on the surface of the mucosa, which give it a sandy appearance. Upon section, these elevations are found to contain ova. The eggs are principally deposited in the submucosa and tend to appear in patches. Worms in copula also occur in the veins of this layer. Ulceration may occur and the inflammatory change produced by the egg may give rise to hypertrophy and hyperplasia of the mucosa resulting in papillomata which bleed readily. Occasionally the inflammation extends to the ureter and results in obstruction due to the thickening of its walls. In other instances the seminal vesicle and the prostate of the male, and the urethra and vagina of the female may also be involved. In the case of infections with *S. mansoni* and *S. japonicum* a similar type of reaction takes place in the rectum.

In cases of schistosomiasis japonicum the liver and spleen become greatly enlarged. The liver is cirrhotic and contains many eggs which may be present in the scar tissue or surrounded by foreign-body giant cells. Hematin is prominent in both the liver and spleen. Ova are found in large numbers in the mucosa and submucosa of the intestine, particularly the lower part, where they give rise to ulcers and polypoid masses. The bladder is not affected.

SYMPTOMS

When the cercariæ of the schistosomes penetrate the skin of man, a more or less definite skin eruption follows. Itching precedes the appearance of the lesions, which resemble flea bites. These lesions

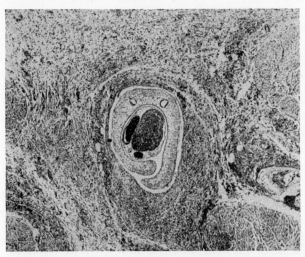

FIG. 127.—Cross-section of male and female *Schistosoma hæmatobium* situated in a distended vein at the juncture of the submucosa and muscular wall of the bladder. This vessel is evidently occluded by the inflammation which the worms' presence has excited. The intestinal ceca of the female are distended with deeply stained material to the right of which is the ovary. (Photograph by Tyzzer)

appear two or three days after exposure to the cercariæ, become smaller after four or five days and disappear entirely in about a week's time. The clinical course of schistosomiasis japonica has been divided into three stages by Faust and Meleney (1924): (1) the stage of invasion and maturation of the parasite, in which the disease is characterized by toxic symptoms, malaise, cough, giant urticaria with edema, intense eosinophilia and abdominal symptoms; (2) the stage of deposition and extrusion of eggs, which is characterized by blood and mucus in the feces, with or without diarrhea and by the continuation of fever and malaise, associated with epigastric pain; ova of the parasite are almost constantly found at this time in the feces; the liver and spleen become enlarged and a progressive anemia develops; the eosinophilia is varied in degree; (3) the stage of tissue reaction and repair in which symptoms of cirrhosis of the liver and portal obstruction appear. Extreme weakness and emaciation follow, and finally death. Frequent superimposed infections often combine this picture with that of the second stage.

Hematuria is the most characteristic symptom in infections with *Schistosoma hæmatobium*. Symptoms of catarrh of the bladder appear in severe forms with occurrence of calculus and urethral obstruction; and in cases of secondary septic infection, a septic cystitis often supervenes. Ova found in the brain and spinal cord have been suspected of causing epileptic and paralytic symptoms. Ova are commonly present in the lungs at autopsy in urinary schistosomiasis (*S. hæmatobium*). Pulmonary schistosomiasis showing clinical symptoms, however, has always been associated with *S. mansoni*. Day (1937) observed a fatal case of pulmonary schistosomiasis (*S. mansoni*) in which the pulmonary circulation was gravely impeded. Numerous granulomata and fibrous nodules embedding ova occurred in the alveolar septa and in the walls of the vessels. The arteries of the lungs were packed with coupled adult worms. Pulmonary carcinoma has been associated with *S. mansoni* infection.

In early infections with *Schistosoma mansoni* the symptoms resemble those of Japanese schistosomiasis. Polypoid growths, similar to those in the bladder, are met with in the mucosa of the rectum.

The condition known as Egyptian splenomegaly, which is a common disease in the Nile Delta, is caused by the repeated invasion of the splenic pulp, over a long period of time, by ova of *S. mansoni* or *S. hæmatobium,* or both, which ultimately produces a condition of permanent hyperplasia and fibrosis (Onsy, 1937).

PROPHYLAXIS

The spread of schistosomiasis is due to neglect of sanitation. In Japan and China, however, human feces are absolutely necessary for the successful fertilization of arable lands. In Egypt all of the arable land lies in the immediate vicinity of the Nile River, or in tracts of land well irrigated from the Nile. Human excreta are not used extensively as crop fertilizer, but are directly deposited in the canals through the religious customs of the people. The majority of the inhabitants are Mohammedans whose religion orders rigid cleansing with water of the urethral and anal openings after defecation or urination. In order that the required ablutions may be performed with ease, the villagers urinate and defecate into or near the stream. The ova from infected individuals are thus either deposited directly into the natural environment of the molluscan hosts or are washed into the canal with water used in cleansing the body.

In Japan prophylactic measures against schistosomiasis have been concentrated on the eradication of the snail host, *Blanfordia nosophora*. Lime in a concentration of 0.1 per cent has been found effective not only in killing the snail host, but in destroying the cercariæ as well. It is spread thickly on the banks and in slowly running water. Chlorinated lime and copper sulphate are also efficacious against the snails but have been found detrimental to crops. Drying is not an effective measure as the snails of this genus are operculate and can withstand great intervals of aridity. Reservoir hosts are eliminated as far as possible from the endemic areas and the possession of dogs and cats is discouraged. Oxen were replaced by horses, as the horse appears to acquire immunity against the parasites.

Adequate protection of the skin is also advised for the farmer who is forced to work in the flooded rice fields or follow other occupations which may expose him to the infection. This measure, however, has not been found practical, for it involves the purchase of clothing to be worn which is contrary to both custom and comfort.

Extensive specific treatment against schistosomiasis is maintained throughout Egypt in out-patient clinics by the Egyptian Government. These clinics are usually crowded each day with patients to receive free treatment and much suffering is thereby temporarily relieved.

Warnings should be made against drinking or bathing in canals or rivers of endemic areas. Only boiled water or water treated with sulphate-of-soda tablets should be used for drinking and water boiled or treated with lysol, creolin or cresol in solutions of 1:10,000 for bathing. Leiper (1916-1918) has shown that the cercariæ of *S. mansoni* and *S. hæmatobium* live in water only about forty-eight hours after the escape from the snail unless the mammalian host is successfully entered but that the snail once infected may remain so for several months. Stored water, free from snails, would then be safe for bathing, as far as any danger from schistosome infections is concerned, but it may still be dangerous from other pollutions unless chemically disinfected or boiled. Chlorine in the strength of 1:1,000,000 appears to have no effect on the cercariæ. Barlow (1935) observed that when water containing schistosome cercariæ. (*S. mansoni* and *S. hæmatobium*) is agitated sharply and then allowed to stand, most of the cercariæ will congregate at the surface. If the water is sprayed immediately with a concentrated solution of copper sulphate, the cercariæ are killed. The copper sulphate then becomes diluted and harmless.

Periodic drying of the canals and irrigation ditches is impracticable as the significant snails can survive a dry period of several months. Canal clearance is effective and is usually financially possible.

So far as we know, there is no serious reservoir of infection with *S. mansoni* and *S. hæmatobium.*

TREATMENT

Preparations of antimony, usually in the form of sodium or potassium antimony tartrate, are successfully used in treating schistosomiasis. Sodium antimony tartrate is generally used in Egypt.

Fuadin (fouadin), a proprietary preparation, has been used successfully in Egypt in the treatment of schistosomiasis. This drug is given intramuscularly without producing unfavorable local reactions.

Medical treatment kills the parasites in the tissues but does not remove the effects of their presence. Therefore it is necessary in advanced cases to excise the papillomatous growths which obstruct the intestinal lumen, and similar growths may be removed from the bladder or from other structures similarly affected.

CHAPTER XXII

CLASS CESTOIDEA

1. General Characteristics of the Class

The CESTOIDEA are all endoparasitic flatworms and are commonly known as "tapeworms." Almost without exception the adult stage is found only in the alimentary tract of vertebrates while the larval forms may inhabit various tissues of both vertebrates and invertebrates (ARTHROPODA). A few primitive forms (CESTODARIA) closely resemble the trematodes in that they have a small, simple body but differ from the trematodes in the absence of a digestive system. The majority of species (CESTODA), especially those occurring in mammals, are well differentiated from the trematodes. They are all more or less like a band or ribbon which is divided by cross-markings into a series of segments or proglottides. The adult worms frequently attain a length of several meters, and may consist of several thousand proglottides. In no stage of development of the cestodes is there any trace of a digestive system. Nutriment is absorbed through the entire surface of the body.

EXTERNAL ANATOMY

An adult tapeworm (Figures 128a, 128b) is typically composed of three fairly distinct regions: (1) the scolex, (2) the neck and (3) the strobila, or the chain of proglottides. The scolex is more or less enlarged, globular or oval in outline and is structurally adapted for adhesion or fixation to the intestinal wall. It is commonly supplied with four cup-shaped suckers (acetabula) placed crosswise at its circumference (Figure 128a). In certain species of tapeworms the scolex carries long, double or quadruple groove-like suckers which are known as bothria (Figure 133). This organ of attachment may also be supplied with hooklets which, when present, are usually numerous and arranged in one or more circular rows around a single protractile organ, the rostellum, located at the tip of the scolex. The scolex is said to be armed or unarmed according to either the presence or absence of these hooklets. The extremity bearing the scolex is generally considered anterior. The posterior extremity is that furthest removed from the scolex.

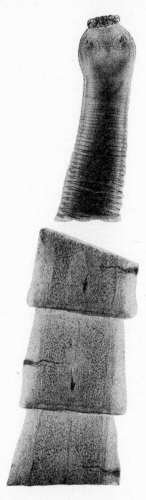

FIG. 128a.—*Taenia pisiformis*. Upper: Anterior extremity showing scolex, neck and early segmentation. Lower: Proglottides from region anterior to middle portion of the strobila. (Copyright by General Biological Supply House, Chicago)

Immediately following the scolex there is usually a slight constriction, which is termed the neck. This portion connects the scolex with the segments and is itself non-segmented. It is the budding zone, composed largely of actively growing germinative tissue, from which new segments or proglottides are formed. The proglottides nearest the neck are the youngest and are quite indistinct and undifferentiated, but as one proceeds posteriorly the proglottides gradually become larger and broader. There also takes place a gradual and progressive development of the organs within each proglottis (organogenesis).

The cestodes, like the trematodes, are hermaphroditic, each proglottis containing all the organs of both sexes, and in some instances two sets occur in each. The reproductive organs are about the only structures remaining in the proglottis and, since there is no connection of these organs in one proglottis with those of the preceding or succeeding proglottis, each proglottis or segment may be considered an individual, and the strobila as a group of individuals which have remained united to form a colony as a result of incomplete separation following asexual reproduction.

The segments near the neck contain only the rudiments of reproductive organs. As one proceeds backwards gradual development can be observed. The male organs are the first formed. Toward the center of the strobila the reproductive organs of both sexes are well differentiated and fully developed. These segments are termed "mature." The various parts of the reproductive systems are similar in character and interrelation to those of the trematodes. In many species, especially those of CYCLOPHYLLIDEA, the uterus becomes crowded with ova toward the terminal portion of the strobila and it largely replaces the other reproductive organs which gradually shrink and may remain only as vestiges. These are known as "gravid" proglottides. These segments, either singly or in groups, finally become separated from the chain, and are carried to the exterior in the host's feces. The PSEUDOPHYLLIDEA, however, do not have ripe segments in the same sense as other cestodes. They possess a uterine pore and continually give off eggs. The uterus does not become branched due to overcrowding with eggs. In this respect the pseudophyllidean tapeworms closely resemble the trematodes.

The proglottides usually show at least one prominent, external opening, the pore of the common genital atrium into which the cirrus and the vagina open. This opening is commonly located on one lateral border or on a surface of the proglottis. In PSEUDOPHYLLIDEA the position of the uterine pore determines the ventral surface of the worm. When the uterine pore is absent, it is customary to call the surface which is nearest the ovary ventral.

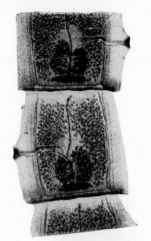
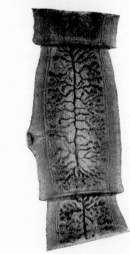

Fig 128b.—*Taenia pisiformis.*
Upper: M a t u r e proglottides.
Lower: Gravid proglottides, the uterus branched and filled with ova. (Copyright by General Biological Supply House, Chicago)

Morphologically, the cestodes closely resemble the trematodes. The body is covered with a homogeneous, elastic and resistant layer, the cuticula, which for the most part is devoid of spines or other appendages, and is produced by special cells situated in the parenchyma. The parenchyma, as in TREMATODA, fills out all the spaces between the different organs and muscles.

Embedded in the parenchyma are located refractile, concentrically striated structures, spherical or broadly elliptical in outline, which are calcareous corpuscles, so named because they contain carbonate of lime. They may vary from 3 μ to 30 μ in diameter according to the species and are chiefly located in the cortical layer.

MUSCULAR SYSTEM

The muscular system of the proglottides is highly developed and is composed of circular, longitudinal, transverse and dorsoventral fibers. A single layer of circular muscles (subcuticular muscles) is followed by a thin sheet of two sets of longitudinal muscles, between which are the subcuticular matrix cells. The inner layer of longitudinal muscles extends to the transverse fibers. The transverse fibers run from one side of the proglottis to the other and reach the cuticula. These occur in two layers and thus divide the parenchyma into two parts. That portion of the proglottis lying enclosed by these fibers is termed the medullary layer and contains all the organs except the principal nerve cords and the excretory tubules. The portion outside the transversal muscle fibers is termed the cortical layer. Dorsoventral fibers extend singly from one surface to the other; these serve to flatten the body.

NERVOUS SYSTEM

The nervous system commences in the scolex where several ganglia are connected by commissures, and form a rostellar ring which is generally referred to as the central part of the entire nervous system. Longitudinal nerve fibres run through the length of the strobila; those at the lateral border are usually the largest.

EXCRETORY SYSTEM

The excretory system of the cestodes is fundamentally the same as that described for the trematodes. Typically it consists of two pairs of longitudinal canals which extend along the lateral borders of the strobila, parallel to the longitudinal nerve trunks. Of these the inner pair is less well developed than the outer pair and may be missing in the older proglottides. The longitudinal canals are commonly connected by a transverse canal which crosses the proglottis close to its posterior border. These main canals receive smaller canals, the branches or collecting tubules of which ramify through the parenchyma and terminate in a flame cell. When the first-formed proglottis has been cast off the longitudinal canals discharge separately; however, if the last segment represents the original proglottis, the canals unite to discharge from a single pore.

REPRODUCTIVE SYSTEMS

The arrangement of the reproductive organs varies greatly in the different genera. As an example, the genus *Tænia* is illustrated (Figure 129).

The male organs consist of from one to several h u n d r e d testes, according to the species, embedded within the parenchyma n e a r the dorsal surface. From each t e s t i s minute ducts, the vasa efferentia, a r e given off which finally unite at about the middle of the proglottis and form the

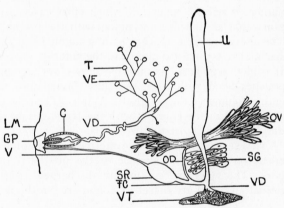

Fig. 129.—Diagram of the genitalia of a tænioid cestode. C, cirrus sac; FC, fertilization canal; GP, common genital pore; LM, lateral margin of the proglottid; OD, oviduct; OV, ovary; SG, Mehlis' gland surrounding the oötype; SR, seminal receptacle; T, testes; U, uterus; V, vagina; VD, vas deferens; VE, vasa efferentia; VT, vitellaria.

vas deferens. The vas deferens, after a more or less convoluted course, leads into the cirrus which is usually enclosed in an elongated cirrus sac. The cirrus opens into a cup-shaped cavity, the common genital atrium, the raised border of which stands out more or less prominently above the edge of the segment and forms the genital papilla. The vagina also opens into the common genital atrium. The genital pore is located either on the lateral margin of the proglottis or on the ventral surface, according to the species. Tapeworms which have two sets of reproductive organs in each proglottis have two genital pores.

The female genital opening, situated posterior to the male genital opening in the common genital atrium, leads into the vagina, a thin straight tube which passes parallel with the vas deferens to the middle of the proglottis where it bends downward into a dilated portion which serves as a seminal receptacle. Immediately beyond this dilatation the vagina connects with the common oviduct and then continues as the fertilization canal to the oötype, where it is joined with the vitelline duct. The ovary is composed of a number of tubular follicles and is usually bilobed. It is situated posteriorly in the proglottis. The vitelline gland is a single, compact body follicular in character and lies posterior to the ovary. Its duct is short. Mehlis' gland which surrounds the oötype has an almost circular outline and is made up of numerous unicellular glands which open separately into the fertilization canal at the place of union with the uterus and vitelline duct. The uterus at first appears as a straight, blind tube of considerable size and runs forward almost to the anterior margin of the proglottis. In older segments the uterus shows very complex branching or pouches filled with eggs and these branches occupy practically the entire volume of the proglottis. While still in the proglottis, the eggs are carried to the exterior with the feces and are set free later upon the disintegration of the proglottis.

In PSEUDOPHYLLIDEA the uterus consists of a single tube which opens on the ventral surface of the proglottis through the uterine pore. The eggs are continually discharged from the worm, as in trematodes, and are therefore found free in the host's feces.

REPRODUCTION

As each proglottis possesses its own genital apparatus, it is probable that autofecundation most frequently occurs, although copulation between the segments of different worms and between different segments of the same worm has been observed. In either mode the spermatozoa pass down the vagina and are temporarily stored in the seminal receptacle. When the eggs and spermatozoa meet, fertilization occurs. The fertilized eggs and yolk material from the vitelline glands pass into the oötype which is surrounded by Mehlis' gland, and here the shells are formed about the eggs which are then passed on into the uterus.

Two distinctly different types of cestode eggs are produced. With forms possessing a uterine pore (PSEUDOPHYLLIDEA) the mature eggs are strikingly similar to trematode eggs. They are oval in outline, yellow or brownish in color, and the shell, which is operculate, contains the fertilized ovum and yolk cells (Figure 130, a). In forms with no uterine pore (CYCLOPHYLLIDEA) the egg-shell is a very thin, delicate structure, has no operculum and there is but a scanty amount of yoke material. As the embryo within these eggs develops, various membranes are formed immediately around it, and constitute what is known as the embryonal shell or embryophore. In TÆNIIDÆ the egg shell proper is soft and colorless and often disappears soon after the formation of the embryophore. As the embryophore is rather thick, brown in color, and composed of numerous rods (Figure 130, c and d) and is the only structure usually seen surrounding the embryo, it is often erroneously called the egg-shell. In HYMENO-LEPIDIDÆ the embryophore is thin and colorless like the egg-shell, which is retained (Figure 130, e). In DIPHYLLOBOTHRIIDÆ the embryophore bears cilia (Figures 137, 138, b and c) by the aid of which the embryo swims about after its escape from the egg-shell. This stage is termed a coracidium.

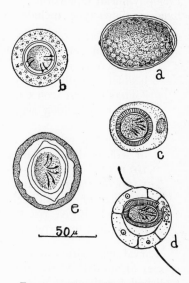

The embryonal development of most tapeworms takes place while the eggs are in the uterus although in PSEUDOPHYLLIDEA cleavage starts only after the eggs have left the host. The embryo when completely formed bears six minute hooks and is termed the onchosphere. Further development of the onchosphere usually takes place only when it is ingested by a suitable intermediate host. Upon entering the alimentary tract of this host, the onchosphere escapes from the embryophore and,

FIG. 130.—Types of cestode eggs. a., *Diphyllobothrium latum;* b, *Dipylidium caninum;* c., *Tænia solium;* d., *Tænia saginata;* (The thin, delicate outer membranes of the eggs of *Tænia* are usually absent, but may be seen on some of the eggs taken directly from the uterus.) e., *Hymenolepsis diminuta.*

with the aid of its hooks, actively bores its way out of the alimentary canal into the body cavity or vascular spaces. It may remain there and undergo further development or, by active or passive migration, reach a preferred tissue where it encysts and passes into a larval stage common to all tapeworms but which varies greatly in structure

according to the species. Among the lower cestodes (PSEUDOPHYL-
LIDEA) this larva is called a PROCERCOID. It develops from the coracidium in the first intermediate host. It is a small, spindle-like, solid
body with a cephalic invagination and a spherical appendage at the
opposite end which carries the embryonal hooks. This appendage is
termed the cercomer. The procercoid gives rise in a second intermediate host to a larva known as a PLEROCERCOID, which is also a
solid body but more elongated and worm-like than the procercoid and
has no hooked appendage (Figures 138-139). The name SPARGANUM
is used generically as a collective term for plerocercoids. It is used
most frequently when the adult stage in the final host is not known.

Larval forms with bladders or vesicles are characteristic of the
cyclophyllidean tapeworms. They are often called "bladder worms."
The commoner types include the following:

CYSTICERCUS: a relatively small bladder enclosing a single scolex,
usually in vertebrates (Figures 131-145).

CYSTICERCOID: a very small cysticercus, practically without a
bladder, usually in invertebrates (Figure 171).

STROBILOCERCUS: scolex not invaginated, but connected to a small
bladder by a long segmented portion, in vertebrates (Figure
153).

MULTICEPS: a relatively large bladder in which a great number
of scolices develop singly from the wall, in vertebrates (Figure
163).

ECHINOCOCCUS or HYDATID: a large bladder which produces
daughter or granddaughter cysts in which brood capsules develop which give rise to numerous scolices from a germinating
membrane, in vertebrates (Figure 155).

Larval tapeworms were considered for many years a distinct
species of animal. A special group, CYSTICA Rudolphi, 1808, was established for them. It was not until 1851, however, when Küchenmeister, by direct feeding experiments, demonstrated that they were
definite stages in the development of tapeworms, that their exact position was known. This experiment by Küchenmeister marks the first
instance of a "feeding" experiment. It introduced a new method of
investigation which was immediately followed by other parasitologists
of the day.

As an illustration of the development of a cestode, the life-cycle
of *Tænia pisiformis,* a common tapeworm of dogs, will be outlined
(Figures 128a, 128b). The adult worm normally occurs in the intestine of the dog but may also occasionally be found in cats. The gravid

segments become detached from the end of the strobila and are carried to the exterior in the dog's feces. These detached proglottides have independent powers of movement and usually show considerable activity when first passed. The proglottis may soon disintegrate but the onchospheres which are surrounded by the protective membrane, the embryophore, may remain viable for a considerable period in the grass or among other vegetation where they may be taken into the alimentary tract of a suitable intermediate host, an herbivore, along with its food. The common cotton-tail, *Sylvilagus flori-danus,* usually serves as the intermediate host of *T. pisi-formis.* In the stomach of the rabbit the onchosphere is freed by the action of the digestive juices upon t h e embryophore and, with the aid of its hooks, the oncho-s p h e r e penetrates the intestinal wall and enters the blood stream.

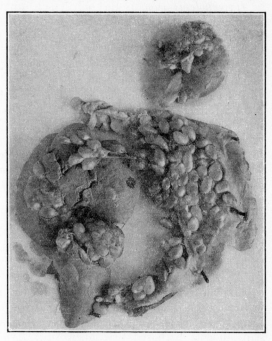

It is carried in the blood stream to the liver where it soon loses its hooks and begins develop-ment as a bladder

FIG. 131.—*Tænia pisiformis.* Cysticerci in the abdominal viscera of a rabbit showing their subserous distribution. To the left is the liver; to the right, the omentum; and above, the kidney. (Photograph supplied by Dr. James Brailsford, The Queen's Hospital, Birmingham)

worm, commonly known as *Cysticercus pisiformis* (Figure 131). Development of the cysticercus is not completed in the liver but in about thirty days after the ingestion of the onchospheres the larva becomes very active and migrates from the surface of the liver. It falls into the abdominal cavity where it remains free for a time, but ultimately becomes attached by an adventitious cyst to the mesen-teries and becomes a fully formed cysticercus. Here it lies without going further in its development unless the infected rabbit is eaten by another animal (dog or cat) which is suitable as a host, in which event the living cysticercus is liberated from its confining cyst by the digestive action of the intestinal juices and the inturned scolex becomes everted and secures attachment to the lining of the intestinal wall. The scolex is not affected by the digestive processes but the cyst proper soon disintegrates leaving only the scolex and neck which, through growth, produce the entire strobila.

Hymenolepis nana is the only tapeworm known not to require an intermediate host. When the egg of this parasite is swallowed by a suitable host, the larva enters a villus of the intestinal wall for a short period of development. Upon maturity, this larva (cysticercoid) drops into the lumen of the intestine, attaches itself to the wall and becomes an adult.

All of the tapeworms, as well as other helminths inhabiting the intestinal tract, show a remarkable ability to resist the proteolytic and dissolving action of the digestive juices. Diastre and Stassano (1903) have demonstrated that *Tænia pisiformis* secretes during life an antikinase which neutralizes the pancreatic juices. After death, however, the worms become quickly disintegrated by the digestive processes of the host.

Abnormalities, malformations and marked variation in a species are extremely common among tapeworms. Fenestration and fusion of the proglottides, double and trihederal scolices and strobilæ, and bifurcation of the strobila have been observed.

LONGEVITY

Many species of tapeworms are known to be but short-lived within the host, while others, under favorable conditions, may live for a very long period. Leuckart (1886) states that one of his Russian students harbored two tapeworms, *Tænia saginata,* for more than five years and mentions other instances where this parasite lasted from twenty to thirty-five years. Riley (1919) has recorded two infections with *Diphyllobothrium latum* of unusually long standing. The first infection was in a Russian Jew who had left Russia some five years previously and had not been exposed to infection since arriving in the United States. The second, a Swedish woman, was definitely known to carry the infection for thirteen years and evidence indicated that the infection had lasted for twenty-nine years.

INJURY TO HOSTS

The degree of injury caused by adult cestodes to their hosts varies considerably with the species involved and the number present. To what extent the host suffers from loss of food which is absorbed by the worm depends largely on the size and the number of worms present and the physical condition of the host. Surely the amount of nutriment required by a large tapeworm for growth and sexual development would be a considerable loss, especially if the host were young, undernourished, or otherwise weakened. Tapeworms may also bring about a reduction or complete occlusion of the intestinal lumen. They produce changes in the intestinal mucous membrane at the place of attachment by the suckers and hooks of the scolex. The scolices of some species of tapeworms (*Stilesia* and *Davainea*) penetrate deeply into the mucosa, giving rise to very definite pathological changes. The wounds thus caused by the penetration of the scolex into the intestinal wall allow the entrance of bacteria which may result in destructive ulceration. Tapeworms often give rise to nervous and mental symptoms, particularly in persons with a predisposition for such disorders. Certain tapeworms have been associated with extreme anemia. Patients may never complain of symptoms if they are ignorant of the infection, but if they know they harbor these parasites almost any kind of symptoms may be educed. The most common complaints are loss of appetite or excessive hunger, nausea, abdominal pains, vertigo, pruritus, cardiac palpitation, anemia, emaciation, and general weakness, all of which usually rapidly disappear after the removal of the worms.

The cystic stages of tapeworms usually give rise to definite and serious conditions, especially in the case of *Echinococcus* which produces large cysts in the liver and other organs, causing symptoms characteristic of a slowly growing tumor. Bladder worms of certain tapeworms have an important bearing upon the sanitary control of meat food products and their presence in the muscles or other parts of the body of cattle, hogs and sheep constitutes the disease known as "measles." The bladder worms of *T. solium* and *T. saginata* have been reported from man. Those of *T. saginata* occur less frequently than *T. solium*. When they are situated in the skin or muscles they are of but slight importance. However, when they occur in the eye or brain they give rise to serious disorders.

ANTHELMINTIC MEDICATION

Treatment for tapeworms, as well as for all helminths, is contraindicated in any debilitation. The condition first should be treated palliatively and the patient's general health brought up as far as possible before the anthelmintic is administered. As most effective drugs used to expel tapeworms are toxic to the host as well as to the parasite one should consider whether the presence of the parasite or the treatment constitutes the greater harm to the patient. Under no circumstances should anthelmintics be administered without the supervision of a physician.

Oleoresin of aspidium has long been known to have a selective action for tapeworms. It is the drug most commonly employed in expelling these parasites from the host. Hall (1923) reports successful removal of tapeworms from dogs with arecoline hydrobromide, and from sheep with one per cent copper sulphate in water.

II. *Collection and Preservation of Tapeworms*

To collect adult tapeworms, the intestine of the host, from the pylorus to the anus, should be removed, laid out straight and opened its entire length. It is then placed in a basin and washed for at least an hour in slowly running water, or in frequent changes of water, at a temperature of about 35° C. If the intestine is of a large host, it is best to open it in convenient lengths, cut off the part opened and examine each part separately. If present, many of the tapeworms will loose their hold on the tissue and will be found free in the sediment. The intestine should be examined with a good hand lens for scolices, immature and small species of tapeworms. Attached scolices should be carefully dissected out with needles under a binocular microscope. If the entire scolex is obtained the determination of the species is less difficult. Under most systems of classification it is impossible to identify cestodes without the scolex. The scolex may be mounted directly in lacto-phenol for immediate examination.

After removal from the intestine, the tapeworms should be placed in a basin of tepid water for about an hour, then kept in 3 per cent formalin. With large specimens the preservative should be changed after three or four days. The addition of a small amount of glycerine will prevent drying should the formalin evaporate. The most satisfactory stains are Delafield's hæmatoxylin, acetic acid alum-carmine and Ehrlich's acid hæmatoxylin. These should be used in diluted proportions, as in the case of trematodes, large specimens being left in the stain overnight. Best results are obtained by over-staining followed by fairly rapid differentiation in 70 per cent acid alcohol. After dehydration they may be cleared in clove oil or carbol-xylol and mounted in Canada balsam or damar. The usual paraffin method is suitable for sectioning. For detailed histological study it is desirable to stain after sectioning.

III. *Classification*

The classification of the tapeworms has been undertaken by a number of investigators. Among the earlier studies are those of Zeder (1800), Rudolphi (1819), Diesing (1863), Carus (1863), Monticelli (1892), Braun (1894-1900) and Lühe (1910). Recently a number of marked revisions and entirely new schemes of classification have been proposed by Poche (1926), Pintner (1927), Southwell (1930), and Fuhrmann (1931). The major groups in the following classification are those of Pearse (1936).

Class CESTOIDEA Rudolphi, 1808, PLATYHELMINTHES, with flat, ribbon-like, unsegmented or segmented bodies, and without cilia (except the onchosphere in PSEUDOPHYLLIDEA).

The alimentary canal is entirely absent and most species are hermaphroditic. The adult stage is usually parasitic in the intestine of vertebrates. The onchosphere contains six or more hooks. Life history, with the exception of *Archigetes* and *Hymenolepis nana,* requires two or mort hosts in one of which the larval form is present, in the other the adult form.

Subclass I. CESTODARIA Monticelli, 1892; CESTOIDEA, with simple, unsegmented bodies containing a single set of reproductive organs; uterine pore present and male genital pore marginal or terminal. The scolex is indefinite or absent, the onchosphere has ten hooks. Intermediate in position between the TREMATODA and CESTOIDEA, resembling TREMATODA in appearance but lacking in alimentary canal and differing from true tapeworms (CESTODA) in never containing more than a single set of reproductive organs. Occur chiefly in the intestine or body cavity of fishes. Of no ecomic importance.

Subclass II. CESTODA van Beneden, 1849; CESTOIDEA with strobila clearly segmented (except in CARYOPHYLLÆIDÆ), each segment containing one or more complete sets of reproductive organs (family DIOICOCESTIDÆ a rare exception). Always a definite scolex or pseudoscolex present. The onchosphere has six hooks.

Order I. PSEUDOPHYLLIDEA Carus, 1863. Emended.* CESTODA, scolex with two, rarely one, never four grooves or bothria, and sometimes four proboscides provided with hooks. Pseudoscolex formation common. Uterine pore on surface of proglottid and uterus in form of rosette-shaped coils or a large sac. Vitellaria composed of many acini scattered widely in cortical parenchyma. Eggs are operculated. The onchosphere is usually ciliated. Contains species of economic and medical importance.

Order 2. TETRAPHYLLIDEA Braun, 1900. Emended.* CESTODA, scolex with four bothridia (lappet-like outgrowths from the scolex) or four suckers, or four proboscides. Bothridia or suckers and sometimes headstalk may be armed with hooks. Primary uterine pore rarely present, secondary uterine pore or pores pierce ventral wall in late stages of egg production and lead to rupture of body wall. Vitellaria in numerous small acini located in lateral margins of proglottides. Eggs non-operculated, onchospheres not ciliated. Parasites in fishes, amphibians and reptiles. Not of economic importance.

Order 3. CYCLOPHYLLIDEA Braun, 1900. Emended.* CESTODA, scolex with four cup-shaped suckers, rostellum present or absent, no uterine pore, proglottides set free after full maturity. Vitellaria concentrated and located usually posterior, rarely anterior to ovary. Eggs with one or more shells, non-operculated; onchospheres not ciliated. Adults parasitic chiefly in higher vertebrates. Of particular economic and medical importance.

* Emendations currently used by La Rue (personal communication).

CHAPTER XXIII

THE PSEUDOPHYLLIDEAN TAPEWORMS

Order *Pseudophyllidea* Carus, 1863

The order PSEUDOPHYLLIDEA consists of a number of families, of which only one, the DIPHYLLOBOTHRIIDÆ Lühe, 1910, contains species of economic and medical importance. This family is divided into two main groups or subfamilies, (1) LIGULINÆ Monticelli and Crety, 1891, and (2) DIPHYLLOBOTHRIINÆ Lühe, 1910. The LIGULINÆ have a very short, and poorly developed scolex, no neck and the segmentation of the adults is often indistinct or lacking. When present, the divisions do not agree with the internal segmentation of the reproductive organs. Their larval stages are found in copepods and fishes, and the adults are largely parasites of birds. They are of but little, if any medical significance. One species, *Digramma brauni* Leon, 1907, has been found twice in man in Rumania (Joyeux and Baer, 1929). The DIPHYLLOBOTHRIINÆ are of considerable medical importance. They have a wide geographical distribution and the adults occur in the intestine of mammals, birds and reptiles.

1. *Diphyllobothrium latum* (Linnæus, 1758)

FREQUENCY AND DISTRIBUTION

Diphyllobothrium latum in the adult stage is a parasite of man, dog, cat, fox and swine. It has also been reported from bears of the Yellowstone Park region and from Minnesota. According to the morphological studies of Scott (1932) and the experimental evidence of Woodbury (1935) this parasite is not *Diphyllobothrium latum*, but a highly variable species, physiologically distinct. *D. latum* is world-wide in distribution and is frequently found among inhabitants of districts surrounding fresh-water lakes where fresh-water fish forms a substantial part of the diet. In Europe there are three foci of infection: (1) the Baltic and North Sea littorals, spreading to the former Baltic Province of Russia, now Esthonia, Latvia, and Lithuania, Northern Sweden, Denmark, Finland, Poland, Eastern Germany and Russia. The incidence is usually high in these countries, (2) the region of the Alpine lakes, spreading to France, Piedmont, Bavaria and Italy; (3) the Danube basin, spreading to Austria, Rumania and Southern Russia. It is one of the most frequent cestodes of man in Turkestan and also occurs often in Japan. In Africa it is reported around Lake Ngami, British Bechuanaland, and in Madagascar.

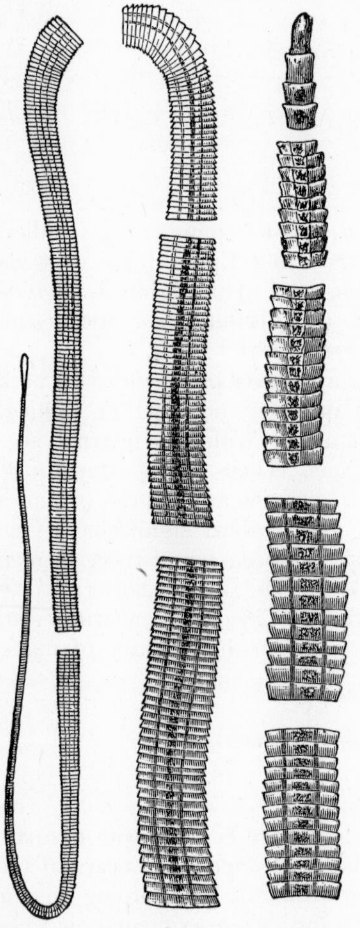

It is generally held that the parasite was introduced into North America by emigrants from Baltic countries to the iron mining districts of Minnesota and Michigan and by the early Jewish emigrants from Lithuania to Winnipeg. The first native case was reported in 1901. Since that time about fifty native cases have been cited from Canada, Minnesota, Michigan, Wisconsin, Illinois, Indiana, Iowa, New York, Massachusetts and Oklahoma. Most of the reported native cases have been Jewish women who have acquired the infection by tasting gefüllte fish (pike or pickerel) as it is being prepared. The main source of infection in North America is fish from the smaller lakes of the north central portion of the United States and of the south central portion of Canada.

FIG. 132.—*Diphyllobothrium latum.* a, showing characteristics of the adult worm, natural size. (After Leuckart)

DESCRIPTION

Diphyllobothrium latum (Figure 132) is commonly referred to as the "broad tapeworm" or "fish tapeworm" of man. This parasite is one of the largest of the tapeworms and commonly attains a length of ten meters. The strobila may be composed of 3000 to 4000 proglottides. It is usually grayish yellow to brown in color. The scolex is more or less elongate, almond-shaped (Figures 133, 134).

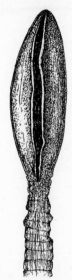

It measures from 2 mm. to 3 mm. in length by 0.7 mm. to 1 mm. in breadth, and is provided with dorsal and ventral brothriæ which may appear laterally due to torsion of the neck. The gravid segments usually measure from 2 mm. to 4 mm. in length by 10 mm. to 12 mm., even 20 mm. in breadth. The uterus is a long, coiled canal and appears as a dark, rosette-like object in the middle field of each of the older proglottides (Figure 135). It is a prominent structure, even in freshly passed specimens, and its characteristic form is of diagnostic value. Gravid segments gradually lose their eggs so that those at the posterior extremity of the strobila may be entirely devoid of them. The gravid segments frequently break off from the parent worm in chains from a few to several feet in length and are passed to the exterior in the host's feces. Figure 136 shows

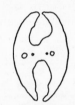

FIG. 134.—*Diphyllobothrium latum.* Outline drawing of scolex in cross section.

FIG. 133.—*Diphyllobothrium latum.* Scolex. Dorsal view.

graphically the arrangement of the parts of the reproductive system. The eggs, when present, occur in large numbers in the host's feces and are easily found in a simple smear preparation. They are large, 55 μ to 76 μ in length by 41 μ to 56 μ in breadth, brownish in color with a small, inconspicuous operculum at one end and a small knob or thickening of the shell at the other (Figures 80, 138). The egg contains a slightly developed embryo when oviposited.

LIFE-CYCLE

Diphyllobothrium latum requires two intermediate hosts for its development, the first, a fresh-water crustacean, a copepod, and the second, a fresh-water fish. The eggs are discharged in large numbers with the host's feces. When the egg reaches fresh water, a ciliated onchosphere develops within a period of a week or ten days if the temperature is favorable. This embryo, surrounded by its ciliated embryophore, escapes from its shell through the oper-

cular opening and swims about freely for several days in the water
(Figure 137). It is a coracidium. The coracidium dies unless it is
ingested by one of a number of fresh-water copepods, *Cyclops
strenuus* and *Diaptomus gracilis* in Europe (Janicki and Rosen,
1917), and *Cyclops brevispinosus, C. prasinus* and *Diaptomus ore-
gonensis* in the United States (Essex, 1927) within which it
undergoes further devel-
opment. Arriving in the
intestine of the copepod
the coracidium loses its
cilia and penetrates the
intestinal wall of its host
with the aid of its hooks
and comes to rest within
the body cavity. Here it
transforms itself into an
elongated organism with

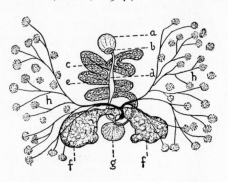

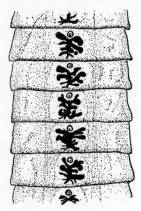

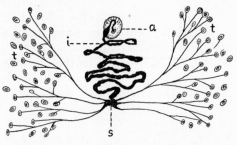

FIG. 135. — *Diphyllobothrium latum.* Gravid proglottides.

FIG. 136.—*Diphyllobothrium latum.* Upper figure,
female reproductive organs. Lower figure, male reproductive organs. a, cirrus sac; b, genital atrium and
pore; c, uterine pore; d, vagina; e, uterus; f, ovary;
g, Mehlis' gland; h, vitellaria; i, vas deferens; s,
seminal vesicle; t, testicular follicles.

cephalic invagination at one end and a circular caudal appendage
carrying the embryonal hooks at the other. Its body is solid and it
is known as the procercoid. When fully grown, it measures about
0.5 mm. in length. No further development takes place unless the
infected copepod is taken in as food by one of several species of
fresh-water fish. When this happens the procercoid becomes free in
the intestine of the fish. It soon penetrates the intestinal wall of

this host and finally encysts in the viscera and muscles after one week to thirty days. This larva is known as the plerocercoid. It is an oval or elongated, spindle-shaped, solid-bodied organism. In Europe the fish commonly found infected with plerocercoids are *Esox lucius, Lota vulgaris, Perca fluviatilis, Salmo umbla, Trutta vulgaris, T. lacustris, Coregonus lavaretus, C. albula, Thymallus vulgaris* and *Acerina cernua.* Vergeer (1928) has found the plerocercoids of *D. latum* in wall-eyed pike, *Stizostedeon vitreum,* sand pike, *S. canadense-griseum,* pike, *Esox lucius* and burbot, *Lota maculosa* from Portage, Lake Michigan.

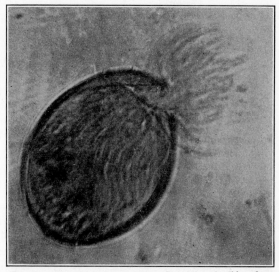

FIG. 137.—*Diphyllobothrium latum.* Coracidium hatching from egg.

The plerocercoids (Figure 139) have a chalky white appearance and are readily seen with the unaided eye. They vary from 1 mm. to 2 cms. in length and from 2 mm. to 3 mm. in diameter. They occur most frequently in the viscera of the fish but are also found encysted in the muscles. When these fish are eaten raw or in an insufficiently cooked condition by a susceptible host, the plerocercoids are set free, the scolex becomes attached to the intestinal wall and quickly grows into the adult tapeworm at the rate of about thirty proglottides a day. Eggs may appear in the host's feces in as short a period as three weeks. Man and other hosts of the adult can be infected only by eating uncooked or improperly prepared infected fish.

PATHOGENICITY

In addition to the symptoms usually associated with adult tapeworms, *Diphyllobothrium latum* has been accused for many years of being a cause of a severe and even fatal anemia with a blood picture indistinguishable from that of true pernicious anemia. Birkeland

(1932), after a careful review of the literature, has found that definite anemia develops in only a small percentage of persons harboring the parasite, and that rapid clinical and hematologic improvement and permanent cure usually follow the expulsion of the tapeworm, although some recovered cases later succumb to pernicious anemia in the absence of the parasite. It is probable that in many instances there is predisposition to anemia and the rôle of the tapeworm is that of a precipitating factor.

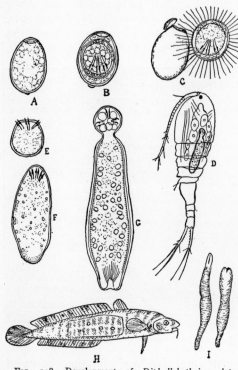

FIG. 138.—Development of *Diphyllobothrium latum* outside of the human body. A, the unripe egg showing the operculum and at the opposite end a rudimentary knob which assists in the diagnosis; B, an egg ready to hatch showing the enclosed hexacanth, ciliated embryo; C, the escape of the embryo (coracidium); D, when ingested by *Cyclops strenuus*, it develops further as shown here in its final stage of development; E, an early stage of the larva after it has lost its ciliated envelope and penetrated into the body cavity of cyclops; F, a growing form; G, the procercoid larva which attains its maximum size after twenty days in body cavity of cyclops; H, a burbot which has become parasitized by ingesting the infected cyclops, the plerocercoids being present in the muscles as well as in the internal organs; I, plerocercoids removed from the fish showing one with scolex extended, the other with scolex invaginated. (Redrawn from Janicki and Rosen)

PREVENTION AND
CONTROL

As *Diphyllobothrium latum* can be transmitted to man only by the eating of fresh-water fish containing living plerocercoids, personal prophylaxis against this infection consists in avoiding improperly cooked, salted, smoked or dried fish or their eggs. Thorough cooking, however, is an adequate protection against *D. latum* for the individual.

Proper disposal of infected feces is a public safeguard. A water carriage system, with the sewage discharged into a lake or river within a relatively few hours without any preliminary chemical or mechanical treatment is dangerous as the eggs

are thus immediately introduced into the habitat of their two necessary intermediate hosts, (1) the copepod, and (2) the fish.

The epidemiological studies of Vergeer (1928)
and Magath and Essex (1931) have shown that the
heavily infected North American lakes are those into
which sewage is emptied from towns. According to
Magath (1933), dogs of the region may be heavily
parasitized but they do not appear to be an important factor in the problem since their feces are usually deposited in situations which permit freezing
and drying, actions which are destructive to the
eggs. Although countless viable eggs doubtless reach
the waters of the Great Lakes, there appears to be
little or no infection in the fish. This may be due to
the absence of a seasonal turnover in these lakes.
The relatively heavy eggs settle to the bottom where
the temperature remains so low that hatching does
not take place. The occasional infected fish taken
from the Great Lakes undoubtedly migrated there
from the small infected lakes.

Only a few observations have been made on the
resistance of the eggs under unfavorable environmental conditions. Helminth eggs with an operculum
are however very susceptible to chemical changes in
the environment. Barlow (1925) has shown that the
eggs of *Fasciolopsis buski* are readily killed in unslaked lime in dilutions up to 1 to 10,000. Essex
(1927) found that the eggs of *D. latum* would not
develop in water after previously exposing them for
a short time to a 2 per cent solution of formol. The
treatment of sewage with formaldehyde or chlorine
is recommended. Freezing infected fish at —10° C.
for twenty-four hours kills the plerocercoid.

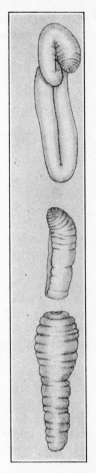

Fig. 139. — *Di-
phyllobothrium
latum.* Plerocer-
coids. x 5. (After
Vergeer)

According to Vergeer (1929) nearly 80 per cent
of the pike consumed in the United States are
caught in Canadian lakes which are known to
harbor heavily infected fish. This export constitutes
85 per cent of the total catch. Inspection of fish placed on the
market for sale has been suggested as a means of public protection
against infection. Such a measure would not be satisfactory since
fish is a very unstable article of diet and any detailed inspection would

cause more economic loss than the importance of the disease in the United States would warrant. Any superficial inspection of fish is not advisable since plerocercoids when occurring in small numbers are easily overlooked.

Each known case of human infection should be thoroughly investigated to determine the species of fish carrying the infection and the source of the infected fish. Resorters and hunters spending their vacations in endemic areas should be warned against the danger of eating insufficiently cooked fish. The only safe measure against *D. latum* is for the individual to cook fish thoroughly before eating it.

11. *Diphyllobothrium erinacei* (Rudolphi, 1819)

1. HISTORICAL

Diphyllobothrium erinacei was known for many years only in its larval stage, the plerocercoid. This plerocercoid was first discovered by Manson in 1882 during an autopsy on a Chinese in Amoy and has since been reported from other parts of the world including Africa, Malay Archipelago, British Guinea, French Indo-China, Annam, Australia and the United States. It is difficult to be certain whether all of these forms reported belong to the same species.

Prior to 1933 this parasite was generally known under the name *Diphyllobothrium mansoni* (Cobbold, 1882). Recently, Iwata (1933) and later Joyeux, Houdemer and Baer (1934), by morphological and experimental studies, showed that *D. mansoni* (Cobbold, 1882) and several other species reported from man and domestic and wild carnivores, *D. reptans* Meggitt, 1925; *D. okumurai* Faust, Campbell and Kellogg, 1929; *D. ranarum* Meggitt, 1925; *D. houghtoni* Faust, Campbell and Kellogg, 1929; *D. decipiens* (Diesing, 1850) and *D. erinacei* (Rudolphi, 1819) are all one and the same species and that, according to the International Code of Zoölogical Nomenclature, the name *D. erinacei* (Rudolphi, 1819) must stand, since it was the first of these names to be given.

DESCRIPTION

The adult worm in the intestine of the dog and other carnivores closely resembles *D. latum* but may readily be differentiated by the egg, which is definitely spindle-shaped and measures from 63 μ to 75 μ in length by 31 μ to 43 μ in breadth. The plerocercoids found in man and various animals are long, white, somewhat ribbon-shaped parasites and may attain a length of 30 cm., a breadth of 0.1 mm. to 12 mm. and a thickness of 0.5 mm. to 1.75 mm. The body is transversely wrinkled but shows no segmentation. On the ventral surface there usually appears a longitudinal median groove. The anterior end is the wider. The plerocercoids are very elastic in the living condition and show but slight movement. The plerocercoids may be found in practically any part of the body, especially in the subcutaneous tissues of the abdomen, inguinal parts, outer genitalia, and in and about the kidneys and the pleural cavity of man. They are also frequently seen about the eye. They occur in a large number of lower vertebrates including monkeys, cats, pigs, weasels, hedgehogs, rats, domestic fowls, snakes and frogs.

LIFE HISTORY

The onchosphere develops within the egg of *D. erinacei* in about eighteen days and emerges in water as a ciliated coracidium. The coracidium, when ingested by one of several species of *Cyclops,* develops into a procercoid within the body cavity of this host. Under normal conditions the plerocercoid stage is passed in the muscles of a frog, toad, or snake, or one of the many susceptible hosts of the plerocercoid which in turn may be food for the final host, the cat or dog, in which the adult stage of the tapeworm is attained. Infection in man is accidentally acquired by swallowing the infected cyclops while drinking.

PATHOLOGY

The plerocercoid may cause small inflammatory swellings and abscesses. When present in the eye, it produces considerable pain, redness and edema with lacrymation and marked depression of the eyelids. Ocular infection apparently is most frequently the result of applying frog poultices to injured surfaces, a custom common throughout different parts of the Far East.

III. *Other Species of the Genus Diphyllobothrium*

Two other species of *Diphyllobothrium, D. cordatum* Leuckart, 1863, and *D. parvum* Stephens, 1908, are known to occur in the adult stage in man. *D. cordatum* Leuckart, 1863, is a natural parasite of the dog, seal and walrus of Greenland and Iceland and probably of bears of the Yellowstone Park area. Its occasional presence in man is only accidental. The scolex of *D. cordatum* is characteristically heart-shaped. *D. parvum* Stephens, 1908, has been found only in man. It was first described from a Syrian in Tasmania and has since been found in Japan, Rumania, Persia and Minnesota. It is a small tapeworm, the largest segments measuring only 5 mm. by 3 mm. When better known, *D. parvum* will probably be found identical with *D.*

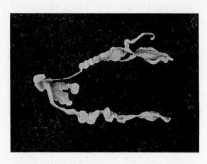

latum. The life histories of these two species are unknown, but it is probable that the plerocercoids are parasites of fish.

Several species of *Diphyllobothrium* have been reported only from lower animals. *D. americanum* Hall and Wigdor, 1918, has been found in dogs in Michigan and *D. mansonoides* Mueller, 1935, has been described from wild and domestic cats and from dogs of the United States. *D. fuscum* was described from dogs in Iceland by Krabbe in 1865. Its life history is unknown.

FIG. 140.—*Sparganum proliferum.* Showing buds and supernumerary heads (x 10). (After Stiles)

IV. *Sparganum proliferum* (Ijima, 1905)

Sparganum proliferum has been reported several times from man in different parts of the world. It was first observed by Ijima in 1905 in Japan and has later been reported several times from Japanese. It has also been found once in man in the United States (Stiles, 1908). Mueller (1937) considers it likely that infections in the United States are traceable to *Diphyllobothrium mansonoides* whose plerocercoids normally develop in mice and the water snake, *Natrix,* but thrive in monkeys.

DESCRIPTION

Sparganum proliferum (Figures 140, 141) may attain a length of from 3 mm. to 12 mm. by 2.5

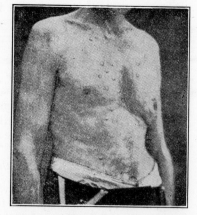

FIG. 141.—Showing acne-like condition and enlarged breasts, due to infection with *Sparganum proliferum.* (After Stiles)

mm. in breadth. The anterior end is narrow and motile and is capable of evagination and invagination. It shows an apical depression. This parasite is characterized by its irregular and bizarre shapes and the supernumerary beads which arise from the parent organism. These beads apparently become detached and wander through the subcutaneous tissue giving rise to acne-like lesions of the skin. They are also known to migrate into the walls of the alimentary tract, mesenteries, kidneys, lungs, heart and brain.

Exceedingly large numbers of these parasites are usually present in the infected individual. Over 10,000 were found in the left thigh alone in Ijima's case. The infections are usually of several years' standing and may result in death.

v. *The Genus Diplogonoporus* Loennberg, 1892

The genus *Diplogonoporus* differs from other DIPHYLLOBOTH-RIINÆ in that its members possess a double set of genital organs with six pores to each proglottis. The scolex is short and broad and is provided with two strong groove-like suckers. The neck is absent. The proglottides are short and broad and clearly show a median field, two uterine fields and two lateral fields. The genital pores, cirrus, vaginal and uterine, occur in longitudinal rows in the uterine field. They are normally parasites of whales and seals.

One species, *Diplogonoporus grandis* (R. Blanchard, 1894), has been reported a few times from Japanese patients. The infection was probably acquired from eating fish containing the plerocercoids. The life history of this parasite is unknown.

CHAPTER XXIV

THE CYCLOPHYLLIDEAN TAPEWORMS

Order *Cyclophyllidea* Braun, 1900

The CYCLOPHYLLIDEA, or tænioid cestodes, are tapeworms characterized primarily by the presence of four cup-shaped suckers upon the scolex. They are further differentiated from the PSEUDOPHYLLIDEA by having the genital pore opening laterally in each segment, the absence of a uterine pore, and their non-operculate eggs in the ripe segments containing a fully developed onchosphere. The onchosphere is never a ciliated larva. The one superfamily, TÆNIOIDEA Zwicke, 1841, contains several families, five of which are of particular economic and medical importance: TÆNIIDÆ Ludwig, 1886; DAVAINEIDÆ Fuhrmann, 1907; ANOPLOCEPHALIDÆ Cholodkowsky, 1902; HYMENOLEPIDIDÆ Railliet and Henry, 1909; and DILEPIDIDÆ Fuhrmann, 1907.

I. Family TÆNIIDÆ

The majority of the more important tapeworms of man and other mammals belong to this family. The uterus in TÆNIIDÆ has a median stem with lateral branches when fully developed and forms an outstanding characteristic. The eggs have a thick, radially striated, inner shell, the embryophore, and a thin, deciduous outer membrane, or true egg shell. The female glands occupy the distal portion of the proglottis with the vitellarium median. The rostellum is usually well developed and is generally armed with a double crown of hooks composed of a circlet of large hooks and one of smaller hooks, the two sets being arranged alternately. The suckers are unarmed. There is one set of genitalia in each proglottis and the genital pores are arranged irregularly alternate along the strobila. There are numerous testes. The ovary is bilobed and is sometimes regarded as two (rarely three) ovaries. The adult worms are parasites of mammals and birds.

1. *Tænia solium* Linnæus, 1758

HISTORICAL

Tænia solium is commonly referred to as the "pork tapeworm of man." It, together with other large tapeworms, has been known since very early times. The larval stage of *Tænia solium*

(*Cysticercus cellulosæ*) in swine has also been known for many years, but its relation to the adult worm remained unknown until the middle of the nineteenth century. About 1860, Küchenmeister pointed out that the scolex of this cysticercus was morphologically identical with that of the adult tapeworm, *T. solium,* in man. This and his earlier "feeding" experiments with *T. pisiformis,* suggested similar experiments with *T. solium.* Van Beneden, Haubner and Leuckart were the first to produce cysticercosis in swine by feeding them gravid proglottides of *T. solium,* but Küchenmeister was the first to definitely establish the relation of the bladder worms to the adult *T. solium* by feeding a condemned criminal twenty bladder worms from a pig. Upon execution of the criminal four months later, nineteen typical, mature specimens of *T. solium* were recovered from his intestine.

Bladder worms were soon reported in man. Although cases of cerebral cysticercosis were noted and described in the medical literature of the day, the seriousness of the condition was almost forgotten until MacArthur (1933-34) and Dixon and Smithers (1935) showed how frequently these bladder worms may be the cause of epilepsy.

DISTRIBUTION AND FREQUENCY

Tæmnia solium has a world-wide distribution which generally corresponds to the distribution of its necessary intermediate host, the pig. Its incidence is in proportion to the amount of raw or insufficiently cooked pork eaten, and the degree of sanitation of the country. Definite data are lacking in most countries on the distribution and incidence of *T. solium.* In many instances cysticercosis is noted far more frequently in swine than is the adult worm in man. The adult parasite appears to be almost nonexistent in man in the United States, but cysticercosis in swine is occasionally encountered at abbatoirs. Colonel MacArthur (1934) and others report cysticercosis astonishingly prevalent among men of the British Army during or after foreign service or residence in India and Egypt. It is probable that cysticercosis in man is far more general and prevalent than present data indicate.

DESCRIPTION

The adult worm averages from two to three meters in length and occasionally specimens up to eight meters or more have been obtained. The scolex (Figure 142) is globular and is about 1 mm. in diameter. A rather short, but distinct rostellum is present which may be pigmented and which is armed with a double row of

from twenty-five to fifty hooks; the larger ones measure about 180 μ
and the smaller ones about 130 μ in length. The suckers measure
about 0.5 mm. in diameter. The neck is fairly thin and measures from
5 mm. to 10 mm. in length. The first segments are small and broader
than long, while those about one meter from the scolex are approxi-

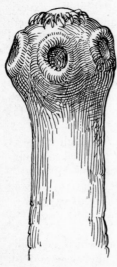

mately square. Ripe proglottides are greater
in length than width, measuring about 12
mm. in length and 6 mm. in breadth. There
is but a single set of reproductive organs in
each proglottis (Figure 143). The genital
pore is marginal and a little below the middle
of the proglottis. The genital pores alternate
more or less regularly from the right to left
margins. The ripe proglottis (Figure 150) is
characterized by the uterus which bears from
five to ten rather thick and somewhat ramified
lateral branches. The onchospheres are round
and from 31 μ to 56 μ in diameter, with a
thick, brown, striated embryophore (Figure
144). The thin delicate egg-shell is rarely
retained after the eggs leave the proglottis.
The ripe proglottides are characteristically expelled passively with the host's feces in chains

FIG. 142.—*Tænia solium.*
Scolex. (Redrawn from several authors)

of from five to six proglottides to a chain.
Natural infections with the adult worm have
been found only in man. Schwartz (1928) has
observed, however, that considerable growth of *T. solium* may occur
in dogs.

POSITION IN THE HOST

The scolex is usually attached to the mucosa of the upper third
of the small intestine with the strobila lying backward. This position can, however, be reversed and the proglottides are then discharge by vomiting.

LIFE-CYCLE

Upon disintegration of the cast-off proglottides, the onchospheres are set free, become scattered about and may be taken
in passively by a susceptible intermediate host with food or water.
It is not necessary, however, that the proglottis become disintegrated
for infection of the intermediate host as the onchospheres are equally
infective within the proglottis. Should the whole proglottis, or sev-

eral proglottides be ingested by the intermediate host the resulting infection would be enormous. Pigs and wild boar are the natural intermediate hosts.

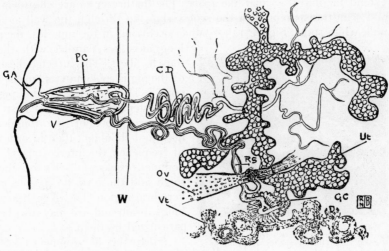

FIG. 143.—*Tænia solium.* Showing the union of the reproductive organs in a mature proglottis. (After du Noyer and Baer). CD, vas deferens; GC, Mehlis' gland; GA, genital atrium; OV, ovary; PC, cirrus sac; RS, seminal receptacle; UT, uterus; V, vagina; W, excretory canal; VT, vitelline gland.

The onchosphere is freed from its embryophore in the small intestine of the intermediate host and, with the aid of its hooks it penetrates the wall of the intestine and gains entrance into the portal vessels or lymphatics and eventually reaches the peripheral circulation. It leaves the circulatory system in the muscular tissue where it develops into a cysticercus. Upon arrival in the musculature, the cells in the center of the larva at first liquefy. It then consists of a mass of peripheral cells with a central portion filled with a clear fluid. A small invagination is formed in the wall at the bottom of which a scolex equipped with hooks and sucker is formed. This is the infective stage for man. Its growth in swine is fairly rapid. At eight days after infection it is but an oval vesicle measuring about 0.033 mm. by 0.24 mm. At twenty days it measures from 1 mm. to 6 mm. by 0.7 mm. to 2.5 mm. and the beginning of the scolex is visible. At

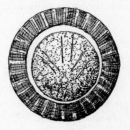

FIG. 144.—*Tænia solium.* Onchosphere. (After du Noyer and Baer)

sixty days it is as large as a pea, complete with hooks and suckers on the scolex. The basal portion of the scolex now increases in length and acquires numerous cross wrinkles and folds which usually extend far into the canal-like space. The mature cysts are ellipsoidal and semi-transparent with the scolex showing through the wall as a milk-white spot (Figure 145). When occurring in the muscles, their long axis lies parallel with the muscle fibers. The infected flesh of the pig is spoken of as "measly pork." The muscles of the pig most often invaded by these cysticerci are those of the tongue, neck and shoulder; then in order of frequency, the intercostals, abdominal, psoas, muscles of the thigh and those of the posterior vertebral region. The liver, heart, lungs, brain and eye may also be parasitized by them.

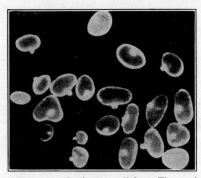

FIG. 145.—*Cysticercus cellulosæ*. The cysticerci have been extracted from their cysts. Natural size. (Photograph by Ransom)

No further development takes place unless the cysticercus is ingested by man, apparently the only definite host. When taken into the alimentary tract of man the bladder is dissolved by the action of the gastric juices. The scolex passes into the small intestine where it fixes itself to the wall of the intestine by its suckers and hooks and the development of proglottides begins. The adult stage, with expulsion of proglottides in the feces, is reached in about two or three months after the ingestion of the cysticercus.

CYSTICERCOSIS IN MAN

Larval infection in man may result from accidental ingestion of onchospheres with food or water or through autoinfection. Development of the cysticerci may take place in any tissue or organ of man, but occurs most frequently in the brain, muscles and subcutaneous tissues.

SYMPTOMS AND PATHOLOGY

In view of the fact that the cysticerci may develop in almost any tissue or organ of the body, the symptoms they produce are both varied and variable. As a rule, cysticerci in the muscles produce no symptoms. In the subcutaneous tissue they may appear as palpable nodules when undergoing degeneration which may be painful at intervals. The important symptoms are those produced by cysticerci in the brain (Figure 146). In most cases of cerebral cysticercosis, mental and nervous symptoms, usually some form of epilepsy, occur. According to MacArthur (1934) and Dixon and Smithers (1935) there is little disturbance in the early stages or as long as the larva remains alive. After its death, however, it degenerates and then acts as a foreign irritant. The tissues about it also undergo active degenerative change with marked cellular infiltration. If the patient survives, the damaged tissues undergo necrosis and the affected area becomes walled off from the normal brain substance by sclerosed neuroglia. Fits are caused, apparently, by cysticerci undergoing active degeneration.

DIAGNOSIS

The diagnosis of infection with adult *Tænia solium* is made on finding characteristic segments in feces of the patient or upon the strobila obtained after treatment. The scolex is of particular value in the diagnosis.

The diagnosis of cysticercosis is established by demonstrating the parasite in a cyst which usually can be excised from the subcutaneous tissues. Specific diagnosis is based upon the scolex, which is identical with that of the adult worm. Palpable cysts are not always present. They are often deep in the muscles and may thus escape detection. A history of nodules that have subsided is suggestive of the infection. An eosinophilia may be present in the early stage but is seldom found when clinical symptoms appear. X-ray examination will detect only calcified cysts. Serologic tests, thus far, have been of only little value in making the diagnosis. Patients previously healthy and of healthy parents who develop fits or mental symptoms during or after residence in countries with poor sanitation should be suspected of suffering from cysticercosis. Other helminths known to cause epilepsy must also be considered. A knowledge of the endemic centers of such parasites is therefore essential.

There is no successful treatment known for cysticercosis. The cysts, when present in the brain, are both numerous (three hundred have been observed in one case) and widely distributed. Removal by surgery is not usually advised.

PREVENTION

In this country, federal inspection of meats includes an examinanation for cysticercosis, and all animals found infected are properly disposed of. However, in view of the fact that this service cannot guarantee pork free from trichina worms, *Trichinella spiralis,* the individual should always safeguard himself by eating pork only when it is thoroughly cooked.

Infection with the adult *Tænia solium* should be regarded as a highly dangerous condition. Infected persons should be treated until all traces of the parasite have disappeared. The danger of auto-infection should be explained to the patient as well as the necessity of proper disposal of feces. It is likely that agencies known to be

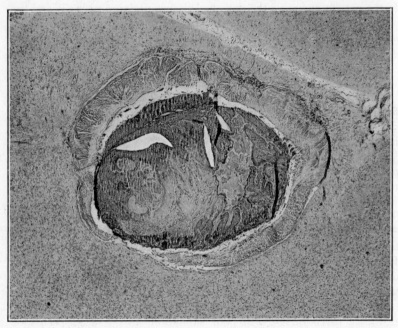

Fig. 146.—*Tænia solium.* Cysticercosis of the brain. Human case. (Photograph by Dr. P. C. Bucy, Chicago)

concerned in the transmission of the cysts of *Endamœba histolytica* are equally effective in transmitting the onchospheres.

All public health campaigns directly or indirectly affect the spread of all tapeworms. In connection with the hookworm campaigns, as carried out by the Rockefeller Foundation and various governments in different parts of the world, there is free anthelmintic treatment, which not only expels hookworms, but is also successful in removing other intestinal parasites including the tapeworms. The campaigns also include a constant drive for sanitation and the construction of privies which tend to keep infected feces out of the reach of the intermediate host. It is of interest to note in this connection that following the hookworm campaign of treatment and sanitation by the Rockefeller Foundation and the Panama Government the incidence of measly swine at the Panama City abattoir dropped from 15 per cent to five per cent. This saving of 10 per cent in condemnations for swine effected an annual saving of $40,000 and illustrates but one of the valuable by-products of a hookworm campaign (Hall, 1928).

11. *Tænia saginata* (Goeze, 1782)

HISTORICAL

Tænia saginata is commonly known as the "beef tapeworm of man." It has been observed from man for as long a time as has *Tænia solium,* but was not identified as a distinct species until 1782. After the discovery that *T. saginata* was a species distinct from *T. solium* studies were soon started on its origin and development. Leuckart (1886) observed that this parasite was especially prevalent in Jews who, like the Mohammedans, are forbidden to eat pork because of religious reasons, and when *T. solium* was found to occur in a Jew, he confessed to having eaten pork. Leuckart also observed that this parasite was frequent in children who had been fed raw beef for dietetic reasons and that the Abyssinians, who eat no swine's flesh, were infected from their earliest years. Guided by these observations, he fed about a meter of ripe proglottides of *T. saginata* to a calf four weeks old. Seventeen days later the calf died and an autopsy showed all muscles, especially the breast and neck, full of cysticerci. Later experiments with other animals showed that cattle only were successful hosts for these cysticerci. Oliver, an Indian army surgeon, was the first to successfully infect human beings with *T. saginata* by feeding cysticerci obtained from beef. In 1869 Oliver (Leuckart, 1886) gave cattle cysticerci to a Mohammedan and a Hindu boy and twelve weeks later obtained from both the proglottides of *T. saginata.* This experiment was later successfully repeated by Perroncito.

DESCRIPTION

The strobilate worm of *T. saginata* (Figure 147) is whitish in color, more or less transparent, and measures from 4 to 10 meters in length. The scolex (Figure 148) is pear-shaped or cubical, from 1 mm. to 2 mm. in diameter and bears four prominent suckers which are frequently pigmented. The scolex is without a rostellum or hooks which differentiate it from the pork tapeworm of man, *Tænia solium*. The mature proglottis is similar in structure to that of *T. solium*. The vagina is provided with a sphincter muscle (Figure 149), which structure is absent in *T. solium*.

The gravid proglottides (Figure 150) are usually from three to four times longer than they are broad, having a length of from 16 mm. to 20 mm. The genital pore is single and alternates irregularly between the right and left margins. The uterus in the gravid proglottides characteristically has from fifteen to thirty lateral ramifying branches. The onchosphere is more or less globular, with the egg-shell frequently remaining intact, and carries one or two filaments. The embryophore is thick, radially striated and somewhat oval, from 30 μ to 40 μ in length and from 20 μ to 30 μ in breadth (Figure 151). The gravid proglottides become detached singly from the strobila and frequently force their way

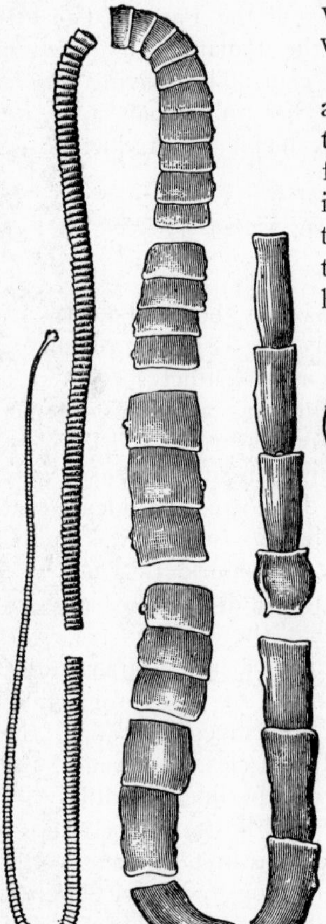

FIG. 147.—*Tænia saginata*. Natural size. (After Leuckart)

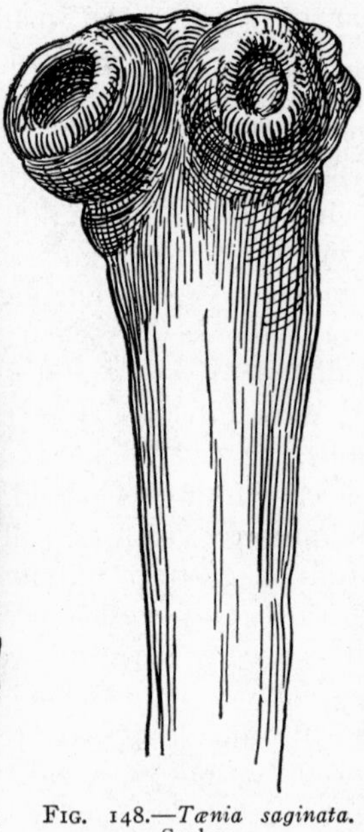

FIG. 148.—*Tænia saginata*. Scolex.

through the anal sphincter. When first passed from the host they show considerable activity and may assume almost any shape. Later on, when quiet, they resemble pumpkin seeds. Because of their ability to force the anal sphincter they are often found in the night clothes and bedding. The chief points of difference between *T. saginata* and *T. solium* are given in the accompanying table.

Tænia solium	*Tænia saginata*
Scolex globular about 1 mm. in length	Scolex quadrangular 1.5 mm. to 2 mm.
Rostellum with two crowns of hooks	Rostellum and hooks absent
Length 3 meters to 5 meters	Length 4 meters to 8 meters
Number of proglottides 700-1000	Number of proglottides about 2000
Branches of uterus in gravid proglottides 5 to 10 in number and dentritic	Branches of uterus in gravid proglottides 15-30, dichotomous
Proglottides expelled in groups passively with feces	Proglottides expelled singly and may force anal sphincter
Larval form, *Cysticercus cellulosæ* of the pig, sometimes in man	Larval form, *Cysticercus bovis,* in cattle
Vaginal sphincter absent	Vaginal sphincter present

Variations, abnormal forms, or malformations of *T. saginata* are very common and have been described as new species. These are now known, however, to be aberrant or immature specimens of *T. saginata. Tænia fusa* Collin, 1876, was characterized by the absence of any external segmentation; and the name *T. fenestrata* Chiaje,

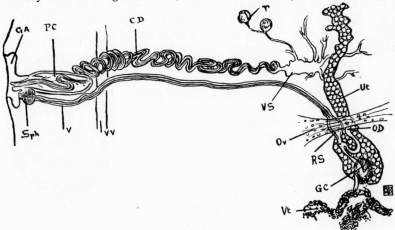

Fig. 149.—*Tænia saginata.* Showing the union of the reproductive organs in a mature proglottis. (After du Noyer and Baer). CD, vas deferens; GA, genital atrium; GC, Mehlis' gland; OD, oviduct; OV, ovary; PC, cirrus sac; RS, seminal receptacle; SPH, sphincter; T, testes; UT, uterus; V, vagina; VS, seminal vesicle; VT, vitelline gland; VV, excretory canal.

1825, was proposed for a specimen with perforated or fenestrated proglottides. Bifurcation of the strobila of *T. saginata* has also been

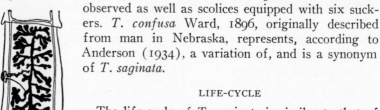

observed as well as scolices equipped with six suckers. *T. confusa* Ward, 1896, originally described from man in Nebraska, represents, according to Anderson (1934), a variation of, and is a synonym of *T. saginata*.

LIFE-CYCLE

The life-cycle of *T. saginata* is similar to that of *T. solium* except that the development of its cysticercus, *Cysticercus bovis,* takes place in cattle instead of swine. The cysticerci may also develop in other ruminants including sheep, goats, antelope, giraffe and llama. They have been reported in man but most of the recorded occurrences are perhaps due to confusion in specific determination. *C. bovis* is smaller than *C. cellulosæ* and its scolex has no hooks. It occurs in various muscles but more especially in the pterygoids, the fatty tissues surrounding the heart, the diaphragm and the tongue. Pre-

FIG. 150.—Upper figure, ripe or gravid proglottis of *Tænia solium;* lower figure, ripe proglottis of *Tænia saginata.*

natal infection may occur in calves.

Man is the only definitive host and acquires the infection from eating raw or insufficiently cooked beef. When the cysticercus is ingested by man the bladder is dissolved away by the action of the digestive juices and the liberated scolex attaches itself to the wall of the small intestine and proceeds to form proglottides. The adult worm is produced in about three months. The diagnosis of *T. saginata* in man is made upon segments passed with the feces and upon the scolex or complete strobila after anthelmintic treatment.

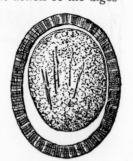

FIG. 151.—*Tænia saginata.* Onchosphere. (After du Noyer and Baer)

GEOGRAPHICAL DISTRIBUTION

T. saginata has a world-wide distribution and its incidence is usually quite high wherever beef is eaten. Its frequency is apparently increasing in the United States, due to the increasing preference for rare beef. *Cysticercus bovis* is commonly met with in slaughtered beef.

Thorough cooking of beef will protect the individual from infection with *T. saginata*. The cysticerci in beef are also killed after twenty-one days in cold storage, or after six days if the meat is held at a temperature not exceeding 15° F.

III. *Other Important Tænia*

Tænia pisiformis (Bloch, 1780) (Figures 127, 128) is one of the commonest tapeworms of dogs and cats and is one that is readily available both for morphological and life history studies. The bladder-worm is known as *Cysticercus pisiformis* and develops in the liver and mesenteries of rabbits. The development of this parasite has already been discussed on page 318.

Tænia ovis (Cobbold, 1869) is a common parasite of dogs. Its bladder-worm, *Cysticercus ovis,* develops in sheep and is essentially a parasite of the intermuscular connective tissue. It is of considerable economic importance because of the losses resulting from the condemnation of carcasses found infected by the Federal Meat Inspection Service. Over 17,000 of the sheep slaughtered during 1917 under Federal supervision were found infected with *C. ovis* (Ransom, 1913). Direct losses which may occur among sheep as a result of the invasion of the parasite may be considerable. As *C. ovis* is not transmissible to man, the precautions taken in the preparation of lamb as food need not be as stringent as those for pork.

Tænia hydatigena (Pallas, 1766) is also a cosmopolitan parasite of dogs and wild carnivora with the larval stage common in sheep. This larva, *Cysticercus tenuicollis,* develops in the liver and, after a certain stage is reached, slips into the abdominal cavity where it is found surrounded by an adventitious cyst attached to the mesenteries or omentum. It does not affect the musculature of the sheep and it is therefore not of the same economic importance as *T. ovis. Cysticercus tenuicollis* may also develop in cattle, goats, deer and pig. Reports of its occurrence in the dog, cat, rodents and man are generally questioned.

PREVENTIVE MEASURES AGAINST DOG-SHEEP TAPEWORMS

All carcasses of dead sheep on the farm or range should be destroyed by fire so that they may not be eaten by dogs or wolves. Dogs should be kept free from tapeworms by systematic medicinal treatment. These measures would also aid in the protection of sheep and other susceptible hosts from various tapeworm cysts which they acquire from dogs.

Tænia tæniæformis Batsch, 1786, commonly known as *T. crassicollis,* is a very common cestode of the domestic cat and has been

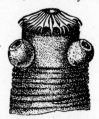

FIG. 152.—Scolex of *Tænia tæniæformis* (x 15). (From Hall. After Neuman)

reported also from a number of different wildcats (Figure 152). Its larval stage, or bladderworm, generally known as *Cysticercus fasciolaris* of rats and mice, is a STROBILOCERCUS (Figure 153). Neither the adult worm nor the larva is of economic importance, but the larva is of particular interest because of its association with sarcomatous growths in the liver of rats. Under natural conditions it is frequently found enclosed in such tumors. Bullock and Curtis (1920) produced a large number of cases of sarcoma of the rat's liver by feeding rats the onchospheres of *T. tæniæformis.* The tumors arose from the encapsulating tissue surrounding the bladder-worms. Miller (1931) has shown that rats with few cysts are protected against infection when fed onchospheres. An active acquired immunity may also be produced in rats by periodic injections with worm material. The naturally acquired immunity is, however, of greater protection than that produced artificially. Kittens and cats with mature parasites, however, are not immune against superinfection when fed cysticerci.

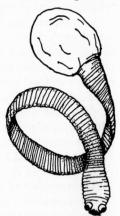

FIG. 153.—Strobilocercus of *Tænia tæniæformis.*

A number of other species of *Tænia* are known from dogs and cats, the more important being *T. balaniceps* Hall, 1910, from dogs and bobcats of Nevada and Southern New Mexico; *T. krabbei* Moniez, 1879, from dogs of Iceland and Alaska; *T. brachysoma* Setti, 1899, from dogs of Italy; *T. brauni* Setti, 1897, from dogs of Eritrea; *T. antarctica* Fuhrmann, 1920, from dogs of the Antarctic regions, and *T. cervi* Christiansen, 1931, from dogs of Denmark. The cysticercus of *T. cervi* develops in the muscles of the deer.

iv. *Echinococcus granulosus* (Batsch, 1786)

DISTRIBUTION AND FREQUENCY

The adult tapeworm is a parasite of the dog, wolf, coyote and other CANIDÆ. It may also occur in cats but it does not develop to maturity and lives but a short time only in this host (Lörincz, 1933). Its larval stage, generally known as the hydatid, can develop in most mammals. The usual intermediate hosts are food mammals, sheep, cattle, rabbits and pigs. These hosts become infected by eating the onchospheres passed with the dog's feces. Dogs become infected with the adult worms by eating the bodies of such intermediate hosts infected with hydatid cysts. Man is also frequently infected with hydatid cysts. This infection in humans is accidental since man cannot transmit the parasite back to dogs except under most unusual circumstances.

Echinococcus granulosus is world-wide in distribution. It occurs most frequently in the cattle- and sheep-raising districts of Australia, Iceland, Argentina, Uruguay, Chile, Algeria, Egypt and Cape Colony. Dogs of North America are seldom infected. It appears to be rather common in our wild animal life, at least in certain sections of the country. Riley (1933) found two of three timber wolves harboring adult worms, and six out of thirteen moose infected with hydatids in northern Minnesota. Hydatid infections in man are fairly frequent in North America. Magath (1937) has found 482 cases of hydatid disease recorded in Canada and the United States since the first case seen in 1808. Of these cases only twenty-two were indigenous infections, the remaining cases occurred among immigrants who probably acquired the infection in foreign countries.

DESCRIPTION

This parasite in the adult stage is the smallest tapeworm of medical importance. Mature worms are from 5 mm. to 8.5 mm. in total length and

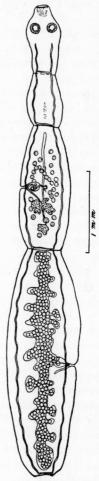

FIG. 154.—*Echinococcus granulosus.* Entire strobila. (After Ortlepp)

have a maximum width across the last and largest segment of about
1 mm. (Figure 154). Usually the entire strobila consists of but
three segments plus a scolex and neck. The scolex is somewhat
globular and carries a prominent rostellum, at the apex of which
is a crown of from 30 to 36 hooks arranged in two rows of fifteen to eighteen each. The hooks of the anterior row are the larger,
varying from 42 μ to 49 μ in length. Those of the second row
measure from 32 μ to 42 μ. Variations in measurements of these
hooks recorded by different observers are due, apparently, to variations in development of worms studied. The suckers are round and
prominent. They are set well back from the rostellum and measure
about 180 μ in diameter. The scolex narrows immediately behind the
suckers to form the neck. The first segment is nearly square and
often but faintly marked off. It contains no definite organization, but
the beginnings of the genital organs may be indicated by a median
patch of darker cells in the posterior portion. The second segment is
mature and contains fully developed genital organs. The last segment
is relatively large, usually longer than the rest of the worm, and only
contains the uterus filled with eggs. The uterus occupies most of the
central area and is provided with 12 to 15 more or less distinct lateral
pouches. The longitudinal vessels of the excretory system are plainly
visible along each side of the worm with cross connecting ducts at
the posterior border of each segment. Calcareous corpuscles are fairly
large and are generally conspicuous in the more transparent parts of
the worm. The shell is brown, relatively thin, radially striated and
contains the hexacanth embryo. The embryophores vary in size from
31 μ by 37 μ to 30 μ by 38 μ. The eggs are smaller, but otherwise
strikingly similar to those of *Tænia saginata*.

Life-cycle. The eggs produced by the adult worm in the intestine
of the dog or other suitable primary host are passed out with the
feces and are ingested, as a rule, by the intermediate host with contaminated food or water. A large number of different mammals may
serve as the intermediate host for *E. granulosus* including man,
monkeys, cattle, sheep, goats, camels, antelopes, pigs, cats, dogs,
panthers, bears, rabbits, squirrels, tapirs, zebras, horses, donkeys and
the giant kangaroo. The peacock and turkey cock also have been
reported as possible intermediate hosts for this parasite but these
need confirmation.

The onchospheres hatch in the stomach and small intestine of the
intermediate host and actively penetrate the wall into the lymphatics
and small radicles of the portal vein, whence they are carried to various tissues where they develop into a hydatid cyst. This larva most

frequently develops in the liver, lungs, kidney, peritoneum, brain or genitalia but occasionally has been encountered in the heart, the long bones and in the orbital cavity. In young pig's liver the onchosphere tends to come to rest in the substance of the hepatic lobule and, according to Dew (1925), shows a striking predilection for those lobules situated close under the peritoneal coat.

The onchospheres may reach the liver as early as twelve hours after ingestion and their presence there causes an early local reaction of the liver tissue by which the hydatid follicle is produced. Vesiculation may commence about two weeks after infection and thus soon form a laminated external membrane and an internal germinative or parenchymatous layer. The growth of the hydatid is exceedingly slow. At the end of five months it may reach a diameter of about 1 cm., but there is at this time no trace of the formation of scolices or other internal structures. As the bladder increases in size, the liver cells in contact with the outer laminated membrane are gradually pressed upon. They undergo atrophy and pressure necrosis and are finally converted into a

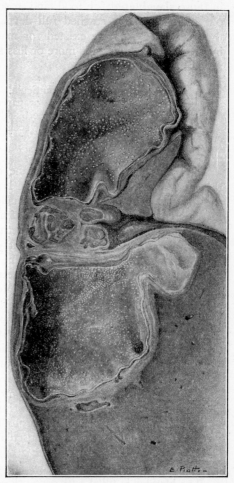

FIG. 155.—Cut surface of a pig liver showing intense infection with fertile hydatids.

fibrous tissue or adventitious layer. A few months later the cyst has increased in size by the accumulation of fluid and begins to produce brood capsules (Figures 155-156).

Completely developed hydatids vary considerably in size. In the hog they are usually from 4 cm. to 5 cm. in diameter while in man they may attain the size of a child's head. This size difference is probably due to age differences. When found in lower animals, it is in those slaughtered for food, and in such cases the hydatids are not old enough to have reached full development. When found in man the infection may have existed for many years. When uninfluenced by pressure the hydatid is more or less spherical in shape and is made up of the following parts:

1. An external laminated cuticula.
2. An internal germinative or parenchymatous membrane.
3. A fluid which distends the bladder.
4. Brood capsules containing scolices.
5. Daughter cysts.

The external cuticular membrane of the hydatid is formed by the original cells of the germinative layer and acts as a support for the delicate germinative or inner nuclear layer. It is more or less hyaline and may attain a thickness of about 1 mm. It is a permeable membrane and apparently has a selective action which insures retention of the specific fluid and the entry, by osmotic processes, of a supply of necessary substances for the growth of the parasite. This cuticular membrane also has a protective action in preventing the entry of noxious substances. The contents of the cysts may remain sterile even after several days immersion in various bacterial cultures. Since this layer is the first formed it becomes greatly stretched as the hydatid increases in size. When it is incised or ruptures, it contracts and rolls up, because of its elasticity, and the cysts turn inside out, thus setting the brood capsules and small daughter cysts free. This is a characteristic of hydatids.

The internal germinative layer is an exceedingly delicate structure measuring from 22 μ to 25 μ in thickness. It is made up of a large number of nuclei embedded in a protoplasmic matrix which is rich in glycogen. It also contains some muscular fibers and calcareous bodies. On its inner surface there appear groups of small papillæ, the brood capsules, in various stages of development (Figures 155, 156).

The bladder is filled with a colorless or somewhat yellowish fluid, which has a specific gravity of 1007 to 1015. This fluid may contain sodium chloride to the extent of 0.5 per cent and phosphates and sulphates of soda, succinates of sodium and calcium, sugar, inosite and albumin which are not coagulated. It therefore functions as a buffer and protects the developing scolices. The hydatid fluid is sterile due to the perfect filtering action of the outer cuticular membrane but should the cyst wall become ruptured the liquid makes an excellent medium for the growth of pathogenic bacteria.

Brood capsules usually appear on the inner surface of the germinative membrane about eight months after the beginning of the cyst formation. They are at first papillary vesicles and are attached to the germinative membrane by a short pedicle. As the vesicle

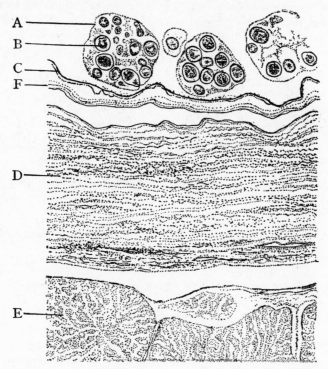

FIG. 156.—Section of a fertile hydatic cyst in the liver of a pig. A, brood capsule; B, scolex; C, germinal layer; D, adventitia; E, liver tissue; F, laminated cuticle.

enlarges there develop on the inner surface a number of small oval bodies or scolices, from five to twenty or more, which, when completely formed, measure about 0.1 mm. in diameter and distinctly show the suckers and a double crown of hooks. Often the scolices break out of their brood capsules and are found free in the hydatid liquid. When these are obtained upon sedimentation of the hydatid liquid they are spoken of as "hydatid sand." Hydatids in which no brood capsules or scolices have developed are frequently found in man. Such specimens are commonly referred to as sterile cysts or acephalocysts.

Very often in human subjects, and occasionally in animals, there is a formation of daughter cysts within the original mother cyst, and these daughter cysts, although smaller, have the same histological structure as the mother cyst. Again, in some cases, these small daughter cysts may contain several smaller cysts or grand-daughter cysts. Several theories have been formulated to explain this phenomenon and it now appears that this daughter cyst formation is the result of some accident or interference with the normal development of the

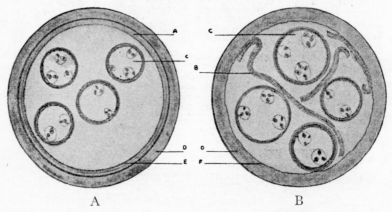

A   B

Fig. 157.—The arrangement of the original mother cyst and daughter cysts. A, the generally accepted view; B, the view according to Dew. A, laminated membrane; B, laminated membrane lying free amongst the daughter cysts; c, daughter cysts containing scolices; D, adventitious capsule; E, germinal or inner nucleated layer; F, rough inner coating of adventitia in typical cases of daughter cyst formation. (After Dew)

parasite. It may be regarded as a defensive reaction to insure the carrying on of the species when the activity of the germinal cells of the parasite is vitally menaced and the continued production of scolices becomes impossible.

Endogenous daughter cysts may arise from the germinative membrane, from brood capsules or from the scolices (Figure 158). Apparently their origin is most frequently the germinative membrane and brood capsules. The delicate germinative membrane is but lightly adherent to the laminated cuticular layer and may separate very readily after slight trauma or other disturbance. It then floats freely in the hydatid fluid and islets of germinal cells may lay down fresh protective laminated layers and produce fluid, forming small daughter cysts. Brood capsules may separate from the germinal layer and float freely in the cyst fluid. An outer, protective layer is then laid down and the cyst increases in size and becomes more rigid. According to Dew (1926) it is probable that such activity is largely limited to young brood capsules which are still growing and give rise to new scolex buds. Nauyn (1862) first described vesicular changes in the scolex leading to the formation of daughter cysts which were also observed by Dévé in 1901. Dévé regards the transformation as a progressive evolution from one state to another. Dew (1926) obtained daughter cysts in rabbits by using active scolices from cysts of sheep, but regards the fully developed scolex as an end product and questions any development of cysts from it.

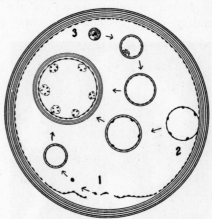

The formation of daughter cysts by the inclusion of islands of original germinative tissue in the laminated cuticular layer leading to the formation of so-called "exogenous

Fig. 158.—*Echinococcus granulosus.* Schematic representation of the development of endogenous daughter cysts. 1, from broken bits of germinative tissue; 2, from a brood capsule; 3, from a scolex.

daughter-cysts" has been described by Leuckart and other authorities. They are said to arise as follows: Bits of the original germinal cells, which in some way have become included in the laminated layer, begin to multiply and form a separate cuticula, and, as the size increases by the formation of additional layers, it becomes vesicular and gradually approaches the external surface of the mother cyst and later comes to lie free between the adventitia and parent cyst. This newly formed cyst may succumb to pressure or increase in size and later acquire its own adventitia. Exogenous daughter cysts occur frequently in secondary echinococcosis of the omentum and of bone. Dew (1926) explains the formation of exogenous cysts by an external herniation of both the laminated and nucleated layers through relatively weak portions of the adventitia as a result of rising intracystic pressure (Figure 159). The pouch thus formed increases in size and finally becomes constricted until it closes off forming a small cyst which remains attached by its cuticula to the original mother cyst. According to Dew the eversions may be multiple and may give rise to tertiary and quaternary cysts.

SECONDARY ECHINOCOCCOSIS

Through traumatic rupture, puncture or imperfect operative technic the scolices, bits of germinal cells, daughter cysts and brood capsules may be set free from the mother cyst and when implanted in other tissues of the body may give rise to secondary cysts. Secondary omental and abdominal hydatids often

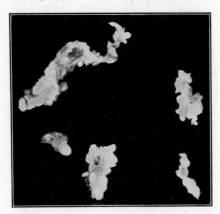

arise following a leakage of a primary cyst into the abdominal cavity and, because of the influence of gravity, they occur frequently in the pelvic cavity. They vary considerably in size, generally have but little support from their adventitia and hang almost freely in the peritoneal cavity. Hydatid emboli may occur when the blood capsules and scolices are carried by the blood stream and form metastases in new situations. When a peripheral cyst of the spleen or liver breaks into one of the systemic veins, the secondary cysts usually occur in

Fig. 159.—Hydatid cyst dissected from decalcified bone. The specimen shows multiple pouchings along bony canals. These latter may become cut off with the formation of small cysts. (After Dew)

the lung. Should the primary cyst occur in the right heart, the metastatic cysts may also occur in the lung, but if it is located in the left heart, the resulting cysts develop mostly in the brain, or the spleen, kidney or liver. The metastatic cysts are as a rule multiple. According to Dew, most hydatids of the brain in young people are single and primary but those occurring in adults are often multiple and secondary to a cyst of the left side of the heart.

ALVEOLAR HYDATID CYSTS

The hydatids thus far described are among the commoner forms encountered in man and other susceptible hosts. They are generally known as "unilocular cysts." A second type, the "alveolar cyst," is rather frequently encountered in certain parts of Europe. It is especially interesting and important because it grows like a neoplasm, thus giving rise to metastases in other organs. These tumors occur almost exclusively in man but somewhat similar cysts are seen occasionally in cattle. The cyst appears like a solid tumor with uncertain boundaries but in section it is porous, consisting of small irregular cavities separated from each other by a more or less thickened connective tissue, and filled with a transparent, jelly-like substance instead of fluid so characteristic of the unilocular cyst. The cavities are small hydatid vesicles and may be identified by the outer laminated cuticula and an inner germinative membrane. They are invariably sterile but occasionally contain brood capsules and scolices. The stroma is usually more or less necrotic and may show some calcification. The cyst grows superficially and invades the healthy surrounding tissue. By direct metastasis, it may give rise to identical cysts in other organs, particularly in the lungs and brain. As the cyst grows and progresses, its center becomes necrosed and may be reduced to a cavity filled with a purulent fluid. Surgical intervention is almost impossible and the infection almost always leads to premature death.

The origin of the alveolar hydatid is not known. It is believed by some parasitologists that it is caused by a different species of tapeworm, *Echinococcus multilocularis,* having a distinct and separate geographic distribution, strictly limited to South Germany, Switzerland and the Tyrol, and to Russia and Siberia. However, isolated cases have been recorded from Italy, France, North Germany and the Argentine which indicates that it may have a world-wide distribution. Others hold that it is the larva of *E. granulosus* and that its peculiar nature is due to excessive growth and function of the germinative layer before the normal, unilocular cyst has been definitely formed. The fact that most alveolar cysts are sterile and therefore cannot carry on the life cycle of the parasite indicates that its development is not normal.

The end product of the hydatid is the scolex and each scolex has the power to develop into the strobilate worm when ingested by dogs or wolves, the primary hosts. As a single hydatid may contain thousands of brood capsules, and each capsule may give rise to a comparatively large number of scolices, the number of strobilate worms resulting from the ingestion of one hydatid may be enormous. In heavy infections the adult worms are so numerous and close together that they appear like a pile on plush. The strobilate stage is reached in the intestine of the dog in from three to ten weeks after the ingestion of the hydatid. Apparently dogs become infected most frequently by eating hydatids from sheep. The adult tapeworm appears to be quite harmless to the dog, but heavily infected animals show an intense intestinal catarrh.

PATHOLOGY

The presence of the hydatid soon provokes an inflammatory reaction and as the cyst increases in size the normal tissue cells are pressed upon and undergo atrophy and pressure necrosis and make up the adventitious layer. Its intimate fusion with the normal tissue prevents enucleation of the adventitious capsule with the contained hydatid cyst at operation.

SYMPTOMS

The growth of an echinococcus cyst is usually so slow that pressure on adjoining structures is rarely noticed until it has attained considerable size. As a rule, it produces symptoms comparable to those of a slowly growing tumor, the severity of which largely depends upon the site of its development. Rupture is, by far, one of the most important possible complications. This may be spontaneous, due to the great pressure within the cyst, or it may be caused by coughing, in case of lung cysts, or muscle strain or any sort of trauma, such as a blow or kick near the site of the cyst. The rupture of a cyst may be accompanied by rupture of blood vessels in the vicinity and, in cases of rupture of lung hydatids, hemoptysis occurs fairly frequently. There is also immediate danger of embolism resulting from fairly large pieces of germinative membrane and brood capsules which escape from the cyst. Following rupture, the cyst and its contents may become septic and symptoms of septic poisoning or localized inflammation may develop. In the majority of hydatid infections, sufficient absorption of antigen from the cyst takes place to render the patient allergic to the fluid within. Consequently, when a cyst ruptures, anaphylactic symptoms may occur which may be serious enough to cause death. Urticaria may develop almost immediately or within one or two days after rupture. This phenomenon was observed so regularly after rupture of a cyst that it led to the discovery of a highly specific diagnostic test, the intradermal or Casoni test.

DIAGNOSIS

If the cyst is near the surface, a fluctuation may be determined which is a characteristic of the hydatid. Until recently suspicion was regularly tested by puncture of the cyst with an exploratory syringe to determine whether the fluid contained characteristic scolices or hooks which would permit a positive diagnosis. Such a procedure is, however, exceedingly dangerous in view of the possible introduction of pathogenic bacteria into the sterile fluid of the cyst and spilling of scolices and brood capsules, thereby producing secondary echinococcosis and toxic symptoms, caused by absorption of the hydatid fluid. If a cyst has ruptured search should be made for evidence of the parasite in the sputum, vomitus, urine, feces, or the discharge from a sinus.

The percentage of eosinophiles in the blood of infected individuals usually is not high and in view of the fact that eosinophilia is a characteristic of most helminth infections, the mere finding of increased numbers of these cells should only suggest the possibility of hydatid disease.

Precipitin, complement fixation and intradermal tests have been developed which have proven to be valuable aids in establishing diagnosis. A positive precipitation test is indicated by a fine flocculent precipitate which forms within a course of 36 hours. The test appears to be specific in about 65 per cent of hydatid cases. The complement fixation test for hydatids is similar in principle to the Wassermann test for syphilis. Alcoholic extracts of hydatid scolices make a stable and sensitive antigen. The test is highly specific in cases where the cyst has ruptured, but may be negative in cases of simple, uncomplicated cysts as frequently occur in children. The intradermal, or Casoni test is generally held to be more sensitive than either the precipitin or the complement fixation tests. It is performed by injecting intradermally a small amount of sterile hydatid fluid on the inner surface of the forearm. An immediate reaction with a delayed phase is obtained in about 95 per cent of cases with uncomplicated cysts.

Dennis (1937) described the preparation of purified and stable hydatid antigen from hydatid fluid obtained from liver and lung cysts of both cattle and sheep. To the chilled fluid, in one-liter amounts, is added crystalline trichloracetic acid to a concentration of five per cent. After several hours at 4° C., most of the antigenic material is precipitated. It is collected by centrifugalization and washed in distilled water. This is then suspended in about 50 c.c. distilled water, and 10 per cent NaOH is added drop by drop, with constant agitation, until solution is completed. The clear supernatant is then chilled and re-precipitated by adding 1/N glacial acetic acid. After about 15 hours' refrigeration the precipitate is collected, washed in distilled water and evaporated over calcium chloride in an oven at 37° C. The dried precipitate is pulverized and stored in a $CaCl_2$ desiccator in the dark. For use, a stock solution (1:1000) is made of the pulverized portion in sterile slightly alkaline physiological saline. This antigen has been found, by its author, to be highly sensitive and can be used in preparing precipitin, complement fixation and skin tests. For the skin test, 0.2 c.c. of a 1 : 10,000 dilution of the antigen is used.

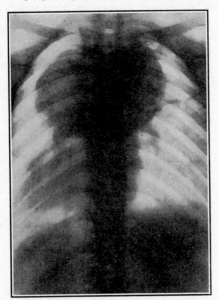

FIG. 160.—*Echinococcus granulosus.* X-ray photograph showing a large hydatid cyst of the superior mediastinum. (Photograph supplied by Dr. James Brailsford, The Queen's Hospital, Birmingham)

X-ray examination is valuable in determining the exact position of a cyst. It may also be of diagnostic help when cysts occur in the lung. Simple, uncomplicated cysts of the lung appear as ovoid shadows with uniform density, regular in outline and without changes in the surrounding tissue (Figure 160). Elsewhere they may be easily confused with a number of pathological conditions. X-ray findings should always be used in conjunction with the results of laboratory tests, clinical findings and the patient's previous history. An accurate knowledge of the geographical distribution of the disease and occupational predispositions of the individual are of fundamental importance in diagnosis.

TREATMENT

Hydatids can be treated only by operative measures. Aspiration may cure simple cysts but is dangerous in that secondary echinococcosis, anaphylactic symptoms and suppuration may result from it. Because of the risks of spilling small daughter cysts, brood capsules or scolices during evacuation of hydatids, a preliminary formalin injection may be made into the cyst contents. This method consists of evacuation under sight by means of a trocar of a quantity of fluid followed by the injection of an equal amount of 2 to 5 per cent formalin. The formalin causes death and fixation of the brood capsules and scolices within a very short time. For lung hydatids other fixative agents such as mercury perchloride or alcohol may be used. This method is most applicable to simple cysts but is of little value in cysts containing daughter cysts.

PREVENTION

Prophylactic measures against *Tænia hydatigena* are equally applicable against *Echinococcus* in dogs. In endemic centers dogs should not be fed on raw meat and all pariah dogs should be killed. In many localities dogs are permitted to enter slaughterhouse premises and to help themselves to refuse. In other instances this refuse is used as a fertilizer and is spread over the fields. The infection can thereby be carried directly to foxes and other wild CARNIVORA which doubtless become important factors in dissemination. Prohibition of dogs from slaughterhouses should be strictly enforced and all cyst-like structures obtained from slaughtered animals should be burned.

Fecal contamination of foodstuffs, particularly uncooked vegetables, is probably the commonest source of infection with hydatids for man. Infection through contact with dogs by acquiring eggs from their fur contaminated with their feces is undoubtedly frequent, either by caressing the dog or by contamination of dishes by the dog. The once high percentage of infection noted among women of Iceland was attributed to the habit of keeping ewes in the houses. Their fleece becomes soiled with dog feces and the eggs may then be transferred to the hands of the women who tend these sheep. Drinking water has been considered a common source of infection, but as helminth eggs sink in water, it is probable that this rarely occurs. Safety is insured, however, from this danger by boiling water for drinking purposes. Cleanliness, especially habitually washing the hands before preparing food and eating, would reduce this infection in man.

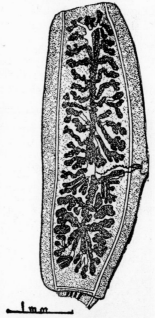

FIG. 161.—*Multiceps multiceps.* Gravid segment. (After Hall)

The recent work of Turner, Berberian and Dennis (1936-37) has shown that dogs may be immunized against infection with *Echinococcus granulosa* by injecting antigens prepared from sheep and cattle hydatids. Similar immunization of sheep does not prevent their infection with hydatid disease, although greater thickness of the adventia and early calcification of the wall of the hydatid cyst develop in immunized animals. It is possible that immunization of dogs will prove of distinct practical value in the control of this parasite.

v. *Multiceps multiceps* (Leske, 1780)

DESCRIPTION

Multiceps multiceps in the adult stage is a common parasite of dogs. The scolex is about 1 mm. in diameter and bears a double crown of twenty-two to thirty-two hooks. The large hooks are from 150 μ to 170 μ long. The small ones measure from 90 μ to 130 μ in length. A gravid segment is illustrated in Figure 161.

The larval stage is commonly known as *Multiceps cerebralis* (Figure 162) which normally develops in the central nervous system of sheep, goats and other ruminants. It has also been found in man.

LIFE-CYCLE

The onchospheres developed by the adult worm in the intestine of the dog pass out and are ingested in contaminated food or water by the intermediate host. The onchosphere is re-leased from its shell in the digestive tract and bodes its way through the tissue into the blood stream. Larvæ which attain the central nervous system develop into the multiceps stage. Others which do not reach there may begin development, but very soon die and undergo degeneration. The larva consists of a membranous vesicle which may vary in size from a filbert to that of a hen's egg and usually takes on a spherical form. The wall is thin, translucent and distended by a colorless fluid. On its surface there are small irregularly grouped spots and each individual spot represents an invaginated scolex. On the death of the sheep, as a result of the pressure from the larva or from other causes, the cyst may be ingested by dogs. When this happens each scolex attached to the vesicle may develop into an adult worm.

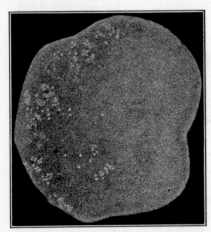

FIG. 162.—*Multiceps multiceps.* Cœnurus from brain of sheep. Enlarged. (After Hall)

PATHOGENESIS

The adult worm in the intestine of dogs is apparently of no pathological importance, but the larval stage in sheep produces a fatal disease commonly known as gid or staggers. Early in the infection the sheep shows dullness and somnolence and there is usually a rapid loss of flesh. Visual disturbances are soon noticed. The head is held in a peculiar position and the animal turns in circles or may stagger and stumble about, repeatedly falling. These symptoms are not continuous. They may appear several times a day with intervals of comparative rest. Treatment by surgery is not satisfactory.

VI. *Multiceps serialis* (Gervais, 1874)

Multiceps serialis, like *M. multiceps,* is a common parasite of dogs. Its larval stage is a parasite of rabbits, hares, squirrels and other rodents. It has been reported several times from man (Bonnal *et al.,* 1933). This larva develops in the connective tissue under the skin and between the muscles, and is further characterized by the production of internal and external daughter bladders which in turn develop numerous scolices (Figure 163). The dog becomes infected by ingesting these scolices from which the strobilate worms develop.

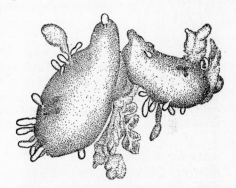

FIG. 163.—*Multiceps serialis* var. *theropitheci.* Two large and several smaller bladder worms. Most of the scolices are evaginated. (After Schwartz)

II. Family DAVAINEIDÆ

The family DAVAINEIDÆ is characterized by the presence of numerous small, hammer-shaped hooks arranged in a double row on the rostellum. The suckers are also usually armed. There may be either a single or double set of reproductive organs in each segment with the genital pores marginal and bilateral or unilateral and irregularly alternating. The uterus is sac-like, persistent; or sac-like or branched, not persistent, replaced either by numerous egg capsules or by a single egg capsule whose formation is preceded by the appearance of a paruterine organ. The onchosphere is surrounded by two thin, transparent membranes. The adults are parasites of birds and mammals, chiefly of scratching birds.

Two genera, *Davainea* Blanchard, 1891, and *Raillietina* Fuhrmann, 1920, contain several species of distinct economic importance which cause severe enteritis and anemia in chickens. *Davainea proglottina* (Davaine, 1860) (Figure 164) is a cosmopolitan tapeworm of chickens, measuring in total length about 0.5 mm. and consisting of from four to nine proglottides. The egg, when ingested by slugs, air-breathing gastropods, of the genera *Limax, Arion, Agriolimax, Cepœa* or *Arianta,* develops into a cysticercoid after about three weeks. Chickens become infected by eating slugs containing mature cysticercoids.

Raillietina (Raillietina) tetragona (Molin, (1858) *Raillietina (R.) echinobothrida* (Mengnin, 1880), and *Raillietina (Skrjabinia) cesticillus* (Molin, 1858) are cosmopolitan parasites of chickens, pheasants, turkeys and guinea-fowl. The house fly, *Musca domestica,* may serve as the intermediate host for *Raillietina (R.) tetragona.* Several species of beetles of the following genera are known to serve as intermediate

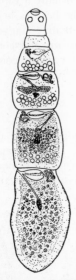

FIG. 164.—*Davainea proglottina.* Young, mature specimen. (After Kotlán)

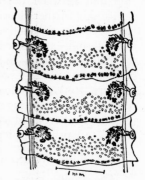

FIG. 165.—*Moniezia expansa.* Mature proglottids, showing interproglottid glands. (After Theiler)

hosts for *Raillietina (S.) cesticillus: Anisotarsus, Chœridium, Selenophorus, Aphodius, Cratacanthus, Calathrus, Stenolophus,* and *Harpalus.* An ant, *Tetramorium cœspitum* has been demonstrated by Jones and Horsfall (1936) to be an intermediate host of *Raillietina (R.) echinobothrida. Davainea proglottina* is the most pathogenic of the poultry tapeworms. The scolex is deeply embedded in the mucosa. Hemorrhagic enteritis frequently occurs in heavy infections.

Three species of the family DAVAINEIDÆ have been reported from man, (1) *Raillietina asiatica* (von Linstow, 1901), from Russian Turkestan; (2) *R. celebensis* (Janicki, 1902), from Formosa and Japan, and (3) *R. madagascariensis* Davaine, 1870, from British

Guiana, Mauritius, Siam, the Philippine Islands, Noissi-Bé and Madagascar. The life histories of these parasites are unknown. The cockroach has been suspected of being a vector.

III. Family ANOPLOCEPHALIDÆ

The ANOPLOCEPHALIDÆ are very muscular cestodes. The scolex is usually rather large, globular and is never armed with hooks. There is no rostellum. The strobila is also relatively large and plump with the genital pores marginal, bilateral, unilateral or irregularly alternate. The genitalia may be single or double in each segment. The uterus lies transversely in the segment and is an elongated sac with pocket-like appendages, anteriorly and posteriorly. The eggs usually have a well-developed pyriform apparatus. The ANOPLOCEPHALIDÆ are common parasites of sheep, cattle, goats and birds.

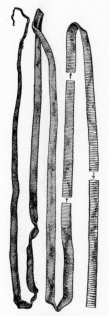

One species, *Bertiella studeri* R. Blanchard, 1891, has been reported several times from man (mostly children) in Mauritius, India, Cuba, St. Kitts, Sumatra, and the Philippine Islands. It is likely that it is a natural parasite of monkeys, orang-utans and chimpanzees which has been transmitted accidentally to man.

Moniezia expansa (Rudolphi, 1810) Blanchard, 1891 and *M. benedeni* (Moniez, 1879) Blanchard, 1891, are very common parasites of young sheep and may also occur in other ruminants (Figures 165 and 166).

FIG. 166.—*Moniezia benedeni*. About one-half natural size. (After Stiles)

The Moniezias are whitish to yellowish in color and may attain a length of several yards. The individual proglottides of the worm are broader than long and each contains two sets of reproductive organs. The genital pores are bilateral. Interproglottis glands are usually well developed and stain readily.

Thysanosoma actinioides Diesing, 1834, or the fringed tapeworm (Figure 167) is a very frequent parasite of range sheep of Western United States, including Minnesota, North and South Dakota, Nebraska, Kansas, Oklahoma, Texas and the states west of these. This parasite may attain a length of 30 cm. but is commonly shorter. It is readily distinguished from other tapeworms by the fact that each of the proglottides has a fringe on its posterior border. There is a

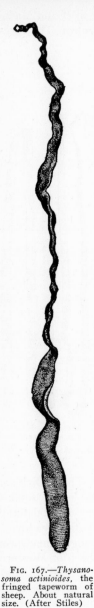

double set of reproductive organs but only a single uterus in each segment, with opposite or with irregularly alternating pores, the pore of one side, with the corresponding cirrus pouch, ovary and vagina having been suppressed. It is frequently found in the gall ducts, gall bladder, biliary canals of the liver and in the duct of the pancreas as well as in the small intestine. It may cause obstruction of the bile ducts and pancreatic ducts and derangement of the liver resulting in impaired digestion, loss of flesh and poor quality of flesh and wall. According to Christenson (1931) *T. actinioides* has been given undue pathogenic importance.

Anoplocephala perfoliata Goeze, 1782, and *A. magna* (Abildgaard 1789) are cosmopolitan tapeworms of horses. Their life-cycles are not known. Tapeworms are rare in horses and are of no economic importance.

For years the life histories of the anoplocephaline tapeworms have remained entirely unsolved. All attempts to discover an intermediate host failed. It was generally believed that development was direct, as is the development of *Hymenolepis nana*. But it was not possible to infect proper definitive host by feeding the eggs of the parasite. Only recently Stunkard (1937) has reported successful rearing of infective cysticercoids of *Moniezia expansa* in the body cavity of free living mites, *Galumna* sp. It is very likely that other tapeworms of this group will be found to have similar modes of development.

IV. Family HYMENOLEPIDIÆ

The HYMENOLEPIDIÆ are small to medium sized tapeworms with proglottides broader than long. The scolex may be either armed or unarmed. When hooks are present they are not hammer-shaped as in DAVAINEIDAE. The suckers are usually unarmed. The neck is short. There is usually only a single set of reproductive organs to each proglottis, with the genital pores marginal and unilateral. One to four testes are normally present in each proglottis.

FIG. 167.—*Thysanosoma actinioides*, the fringed tapeworm of sheep. About natural size. (After Stiles)

The eggs have thin transparent shells. The adult worms are parasites in mammals and birds.

1. *Hymenolepis nana* (von Siebold, 1852)

HISTORICAL

Hymenolepis nana, commonly known as the "dwarf tapeworm," was described by Dujardin in 1845 from rats. It was first discovered in man by Bilharz in 1851 during autopsy of a boy who had died from meningitis in Cairo, Egypt. Von Siebold described the parasite from material sent him by Bilharz, and gave it the name *Tænia nana.* This Egyptian case was the only one reported from man for many years but now it is known that this parasite is cosmopolitan and a very common one of man, rats and mice. It occurs more frequently in children than in adults.

Considerable doubt has existed for years concerning the identity of the species of worms found in man and those found in rodents. Morphologically the rodent form, frequently called *H. fraterna,* is identical with the form from man. Their life-cycles are also identical. They are also interchangeable, but do not develop as readily in the alternate host as they do in the host in which the parents developed (Woodland, 1924). Joyeux (1925) and other workers believe that the parasite from man is derived phylogenetically from the rodent form but now, adapted to man, is a biological species. More recently, however, Shorb (1932) found similar differences in specimens obtained from wild rats and mice. The strain obtained from the former was equally infective for rats and mice, while the mouse strain was distinctly more infective for mice: it developed faster and to a larger size and produced a greater incidence and greater worm burden in mice than in rats. It is evident, therefore, that the forms from mice, rats and humans are the same species, *H. nana,* which has developed different physiological strains. It is probable that this tapeworm originated as a parasite of mice and later became adapted to rats and man.

DESCRIPTION

The strobilate worm (Figure 168) measures from 10 mm. to 45 mm. in length and from 0.5 mm. to 0.7 mm. in breadth. The scolex is globular, about 0.25 mm. in diameter and the rostellum is equipped with a single row of twenty-four to thirty hooks which are from 14 μ to 18 μ in length. The strobila consists of about 200 proglottides. There are three testes in each proglottis and the vas deferens widens to form a seminal vesicle. The uterus is sac-form. The gravid segments are readily digested or rupture within the intestine and the eggs thus set free usually occur in large numbers in the feces of infected individuals. The eggs are globular, more frequently oval and present two membranes, the outer measures from 40 μ to 60 μ in length and the inner from 20 μ to 34 μ. The inner membrane shows filiform projections at each pole (Figure 169).

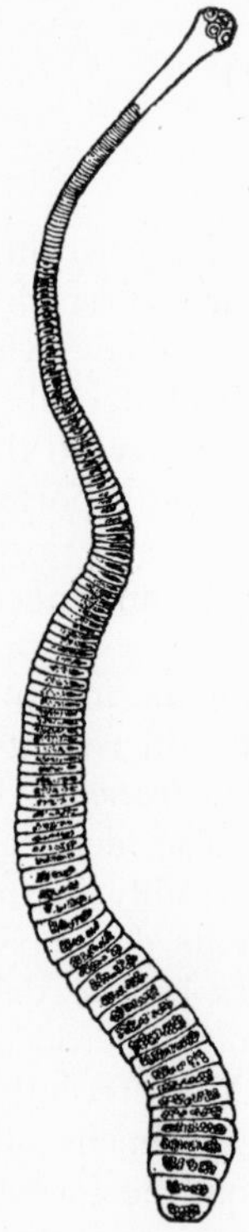

LIFE-CYCLE

No intermediate host is required for the development of *H. nana,* and the eggs are immediately infective as they pass out with the feces. Upon ingestion, the onchosphere becomes free in the small intestine and penetrates into a villus where it becomes a cysticercoid

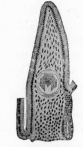

FIG. 170.—Longitudinal section through the intestinal villus of a rat, with the cysticercoid of *Hymenolepis nana.* Magnified. (After Grassi and Rovelli)

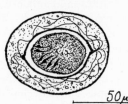

50μ

FIG. 169.—Egg of *Hymenolepis nana.*

FIG. 168.—*Hymenolepis nana,* e n t i r e worm. About 12/1. (After Leuckart)

(Figure 170). In about ninety hours after ingestion the cysticercoid breaks out of the villus, passes into the lumen, soon fixes itself to the intestinal epithelium and develops into the strobilate worm in about ten or twelve days. About thirty days after ingestion its eggs may appear in the feces. This mode of development of *H. nana* may be followed without difficulty in laboratory rats after feeding them the strobilate worms obtained from infected rats.

Hymenolepis nana is further remarkable in its development because it may also be transmitted by an intermediate host (Bacigalupo, 1925). The eggs when ingested by certain insects, including larvae of *Xenopsylla cheopis, Ctenocephalides canis* and *Pulex irritans* and adult *Tenebrio molitor* and *T. obscurus,* develop into cysticercoids which in turn grow into adult worms when the infected insect is eaten by susceptible hosts.

The adoption of the direct mode of transmission by *Hymenolepis nana* undoubtedly accounts for its prevalence in man. Other tapeworms of lower animals which are dependent upon insect transmission rarely occur in man.

PREVENTION

Since auto-infection may occur, personal hygiene is essential in combating infections with *Hymenolepis nana.* In view of the fact that rats and mice may serve as reservoirs for human infection these animals should be destroyed and all food safeguarded from them.

11. *Hymenolepis diminuta* (Rudolphi, 1819)

HISTORICAL

Hymenolepis diminuta is one of the commonest of the rat and mouse tapeworms and is occasionally found in man. It was first discovered by Olfers in 1766 in rats of Rio de Janeiro and was later described by Rudolphi in 1819 under the name *Tænia diminuta.* It was described from man by Rudolphi in 1805. About one hundred cases of infection with *H. diminuta* have been reported from man. The majority of these infections occurred in children under three years of age.

DESCRIPTION

The strobilate worm measures from 20 cm. to 60 cm. in length and up to 3.5 mm. in breadth. The strobila consists of from 800 to 1000 proglottides. The scolex is very small, club-shaped and has a small infundibulum at the apex in which there is a rudimentary rostellum. The scolex is unarmed and the four suckers are small. The arrangement of the reproductive organs is similar to that of *H. nana.* The eggs, when present, are found free in the feces of the host. They are round or slightly oval with an outer shell, yellowish, thickened and maybe striated, and an inner shell, colorless, and somewhat pointed at the poles but without filiform projections. The outer shell measures from 54 μ to 86 μ in length and the inner membrane or embryophore from 24 μ to 40 μ by 36 μ.

LIFE-CYCLE

Unlike *H. nana,* this species of *Hymenolepis* always requires an intermediate host for the completion of its life-cycle. Direct infection is not possible. Grassi and Rovelli (1892) showed that the larval stage of *H. diminuta,* the cysticercoid (Figure 171), develops in the body cavity of a large number of meal-infecting insects. They have been noted in the larva and adult of the moth, *Asopia farinalis,* and in both nymphs and adults of the earwig, *Anisolabis annulipes,* and in adults of tenebrionid beetles, *Tenebrio*

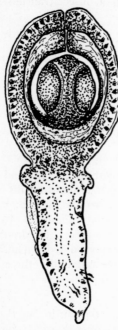

molitor, Akis spinosa and *Scaurus striatus.* Joyeux (1920) found that the larvæ of *Tenebrio molitor* could not be infected with the eggs of *H. diminuta* but that the adult beetle was most susceptible. The dung beetles, *Geotrupes sylvaticus,* were observed also to be readily infected with these cysticercoids as well as larvæ of the fleas, *Leptopsylla musculi, Pulex irritans* and *Ctenocephalides canis.* Nicoll and Minchin (1911) found the cysticercoid of *H. diminuta* in 4 per cent of rat fleas, *Nosopsyllus fasciatus,* and Johnson (1913) found that the flea *Xenopsylla cheopis* might also harbor this larva. Nickerson (1911) fed segments of *H. diminuta* from rats to young myriapods, *Fontaria virginica* and *Julus* sp. In both species cysticercoids were found upon later examination.

Joyeux (1920), however, regards the adult *Tenebrio molitor* and the rat fleas, *Nosopsyllus fasciatus* and *Xenopsylla cheopis* as the natural intermediate hosts.

FIG. 171.—Cysticercoid of
Hymenolepis diminuta.

When the infected intermediate host is ingested by a susceptible host the cysticercoid becomes free in the intestine of the new host and the scolex fixes itself to the intestinal epithelium. It becomes an adult in about eighteen days. It is believed that man becomes infected most frequently from eating breads not well cooked that contain the infected intermediate host. Prevention against infection with *Hymenolepis diminuta* consists in avoiding the ingestion of any of the various arthropods which may serve as intermediate hosts.

Many species of *Hymenolepis* are reported from birds. The reader is referred to Ransom (1909) and Neveu-Lemaire (1936) for a list and descriptions of these species. *Fimbriaria fasciolaris* infects wild and domestic fowl. Its scolex is small and unstable. The worm is anchored by a folded expansion at the anterior end. *Cyclops* is an intermediate host.

V. Family DILEPIDIDÆ

This family is made up of moderate sized tapeworms. The suckers are unarmed but the rostellum is usually armed. The genitalia are single or double and the uterus breaks up into egg-sacs, each containing one or several eggs. There are no paruterine organs. The testes may be numerous. The adults are parasites of mammals and birds.

1. *Dipylidium caninum* (Linnæus, 1758)

DESCRIPTION

Dipylidium caninum (Figure 172) is one of the commonest intestinal parasites of dogs and cats and is occasionally found as a human parasite. The adult measures from 15 cm. to 40 cm. in length and has a maximal breadth of from 2 mm. to 3 mm. The scolex is small and rhomboidal, measuring about 0.55 mm. in diameter. The rostellum is claviform and is capable of retraction into a deep cephalic infundibulum. It is armed with three or four circlets of about sixty hooks. The hooks of the most anterior row are the larger, from 12 μ to 15 μ long. The hooks are easily lost and specimens are often found without hooks or with only a few in place. There are four fairly large, elliptical, unarmed suckers. The neck is very short and

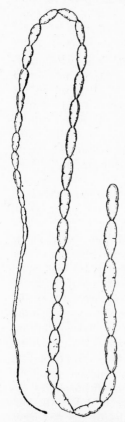

FIG. 172.—*Dipylidium caninum.* Strobilate stage. Natural size. (From Brumpt's *Précis de parasitologie*)

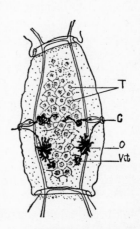

FIG. 173.—Mature segment of *Dipylidium caninum.*

thin. There are usually less than 200 proglottides in the entire chain. The mature or gravid segments are characteristically vase or urn-shaped (Figure 173). Each proglottis has two sets of genital organs and the genital pores lie symmetrically at the lateral margins. The vitellarium is some distance posterior to the ovary. It is irregularly and loosely lobulate. The eggs of *D. caninum* are round and measure from 35 μ to 50 μ in diameter. They are contained in nest-like cavities of the uterus, each including from five to twenty eggs. Eggs are seldom seen in host's feces unless the proglottis becomes disintegrated or broken. Therefore the diagnosis is usually made upon evacuated proglottides.

LIFE-CYCLE

Leuckart believed that an insect intermediate host was necessary for the completion of the life-cycle of *D. caninum* but Melnikoff in 1869 was the first to demonstrate the larvel form in the body of such a host, the dog louse, *Trichodectes canis*. In view of the fact that *T. canis* is not a frequent parasite of dogs and cats, it soon became apparent that this louse could not be the only intermediate host. In 1880, Grassi found that it could also develop in the dog flea, *Ctenocephalides canis,* and in the human flea, *Pulex irritans.*

As in the case of many tapeworms, the gravid segments of *D. caninum* are carried along with the host's feces to the outer world where they disintegrate and the enclosed onchospheres become scattered about. Some of the onchospheres which eventually get into the fur of the dog or cat are ingested by the louse, *Trichodectes,* as it feeds on the skin of the dog, and in its body cavity they develop into the infective stage. In the case of the fleas, however, the eggs are ingested while the fleas are larvæ, feeding on débris. The adult fleas are adapted to feed on blood and are unable to ingest a tapeworm egg. The onchospheres remain more or less unchanged in the adipose tissue and muscles of the flea larva until the adult emerges, at which time they develop into pear-shaped cysticercoids.

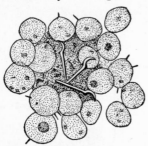

Fig. 174.—*Dipylidium caninum.* Destruction of a cysticercoid by amœbocytes of the flea larva. (After Chen)

When the dog or cat takes up an infected flea by biting itself, or by licking its fur, the cysticercoid becomes free in the intestine and, after attaching itself to the wall of the intestine, quickly grows into the adult worm. Sexual maturity is reached in about twenty days.

A high mortality occurs among cysticercoids during their period of development and growth, in both the flea larva and in the adult flea. Chen (1934) observed that the young cysticercoids are attacked and completely surrounded by leucocytes of the flea shortly after their arrival in the body cavity of the flea larva (Figure 174). They are finally reduced to a mass of yellowish pigment which is disposed of through the epithelium of the ventriculus into the lumen of the intestine.

Infection in man is entirely accidental. Infection in man, as well as in other definitive hosts, can only be acquired by swallowing the infected adult flea or louse. There are now about eighty records of its occurrence in man. Most of the cases are European. It is exceedingly rare in man in the United States. The majority of the infections have occurred in young children, many of whom were of nursing age.

Other cosmopolitan or widely distributed species of the family DILEPIDIDÆ include *Choanotænia infundibulum* (Bloch, 1779), *Amœbotænia sphenoides* (Railliet, 1892), parasites of chickens; *Diplopylidium acanthotetra* (Parona, 1886) in cats and small carnivores. House flies and dung beetles are intermediate hosts for *C. infundibulum,* earthworms for *A. sphenoides,* and numerous lizards, snakes and toads for *D. acanthotetra.*

CHAPTER XXV

CLASS NEMATODA

The NEMATODA are easily distinguished from other helminthes by their round, elongated, non-segmented bodies. They are further characterized by having a relatively large body cavity in which the internal organs are suspended. The body cavity, however, is not a true cœlom as in ANNELIDA and higher animals, since a peritoneal epithelium is lacking. It is formed by the simple breaking down of the connective tissue cells, many of which remain as remnants, especially at the anterior end. The NEMATODA therefore show, in this respect, a closer relation to parenchymatous PLATYHELMINTHES than to the ANNELIDA and higher invertebrates having a true cœlom. The sexes are usually separate and show marked sexual dimorphism.

I. *General Characteristics of the Class*

The NEMATODA, or nemas (Figures 175, 176), have characteristically elongated, cylindrical bodies tapering slightly towards one or both ends and, as a rule, present a smooth, glistening external surface. The anterior end of the worm is usually more or less rounded while the posterior end is pointed. There are both free-living and parasitic nematodes. They have become adapted to almost every conceivable habitat. The free-living forms are abundant in soil and water and occur in arid deserts, lake and river bottoms, and thermal springs, as well as in polar seas and at great depths. Cobb (1914) has estimated that the number of nematodes in the top six inches of an acre of ordinary arable soil, may reach thousands of millions. Many species are parasites of plants and are of considerable economic importance, especially in the sugar beet, citrus and cocoanut industries. It is estimated that over 80,000 nematode species infect the forty-odd thousand species of vertebrates. Insects are also often infected by nematodes as well as molluscs, annelids and crustaceans. Morphologically the parasitic species are strikingly similar to the free-living forms and show but minor modifications resulting from their parasitic habit. This is especially true among the smaller transparent species.

The main points of difference between the free-living and para-

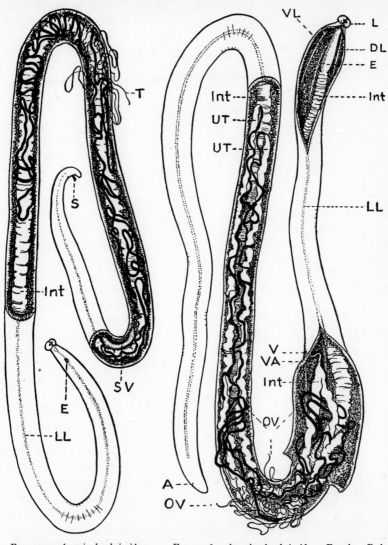

FIG. 175.—*Ascaris lumbricoides.* Male. Middle portion of body wall opened along the side showing a schematic arrangement of the internal organs.

E, excretory pore; Int, intestine; LL, lateral line; S. spicules; SV, seminal vesicle; T, testis.

FIG. 176.—*Ascaris lumbricoides.* Female. Body wall opened at two different levels along the side showing a schematic arrangement of the internal organs.

A, anus; E, esophagus; L, lips; DL, dorsal line; VL, ventral line; Int, intestine; LL, lateral line; OV, ovary; V, vulva; VA, vagina; UT, uterus.

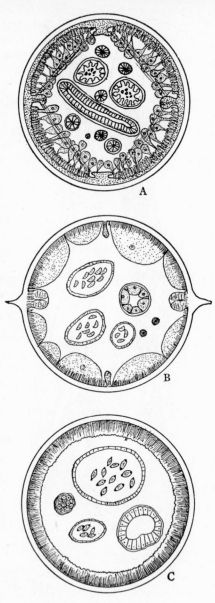

FIG. 177.—Musculature of Nematodes. A, poly-myarian type; B, meromyarian type; C, holo-myarian type.

sitic species lie in the presence of eye-spots, setose tactile organs, amphids and other specialized sensory organs in the free-living forms, and their usual absence in the parasitic ones. When present among the parasitic forms, these sensory organs occur in the free-living developmental stages of the worm but often not in the parasitic adult.

Nematodes range from a fraction of a millimeter to more than a meter in length and are usually white or nearly colorless. The male is usually smaller than the female and is readily distinguished by a recurved posterior extremity, or, in certain species, by special copulatory apparatus such as spicules and a bursa at the posterior extremity.

BODY WALL

The body of the nematode is covered with a hyaline, noncellular layer, the cuticula. It is usually marked by regularly arranged transverse striations or grooves which are often exceedingly fine. The striations are usually superficial. Deep striations c o m m o n l y occur which are called annulations, and the distances between them are known as annules. A few forms have longitudinal striæ, while others bear oblique or cross-hatched markings.

Directly beneath the cuticula lies the hypodermis. The hypodermis is a thin protoplasmic layer internally thickened in four longitudinal lines known as dorsal, lateral and ventral lines or chords. These chords carry the longitudinal nerves of the body and, in many forms, the lateral excretory canals. The hypodermis may be syncytial but the nuclei are confined to the chords. Beneath the hypodermis lies a single layer of partially differentiated longitudinal muscles which line the body cavity. Each muscle cell has only a portion of the protoplasm differentiated into contractile fibers and these fibers lie next and are attached to the hypodermis. The rounded, undifferentiated portion containing the nucleus usually extends into the body cavity. The somatic muscles are separated by the chords of the hypodermis into four primary muscle fields, the dorso- and ventro-sub-median.

The character and arrangement of the somatic muscles as seen in cross section, form a characteristic by which one can identify certain groups of nematodes. Those species in which the muscle cells are numerous and extend well into the body cavity are spoken of as polymyarian (Figure 177a). The ASCARIDÆ, HETERAKIDÆ and the like are polymyarian. In other species the muscle cells are flattened and only from two to three occur in each lateral field; these are known as meromyarian. This grouping of muscle cells is seen in the OXYRUDÆ (Figure 177b). In the third type, holomyarian, the muscle cells are small and closely packed together and usually form a complete wall within the cuticular layer. This type is characteristic of the TRICHINELLINÆ to which belongs *Trichuris trichiura,* the common whip-worm of man (Figure 177c). The arrangement of the somatic muscles is of systematic value, and (according to Chitwood and Chitwood, 1937) appears to have some evolutionary significance, those species with a small number of cells being the more primitive.

Specialized muscles occur in various parts of the body. These include the labial muscles, muscles which extend from the body wall to the esophagus and intestine, muscles of the mouth and of the anus and copulatory muscles, and muscles of the spicules, gubernaculum, etc.

BODY CAVITY

Chitwood and Chitwood (1937) propose to call the body cavity of nematodes a "pseudocœlome." There is no epithelial lining, but there is a delicate connective tissue layer of mesenchymatous origin which more or less completely lines the body wall and covers and supports the internal organs.

Two, four or six large cells, cœlomocytes, probably also of

mesenchymatous origin, are situated in the anterior third of the body cavity. These cells vary considerably in character. They may be round, oval, strand-like, or highly branched and may be ventral, lateral, or dorsal in position. Their function is not clearly understood. Various workers have considered them as excretory cells which store waste products in insoluble form, gland cells, and absorptive or phagocytic cells comparable to the fixed histiocytes of vertebrates.

The body fluid of large ascarids is pink in color. When examined spectroscopically it shows the bands of oxyhemoglobin. Oxyhemoglobin can likewise be demonstrated in the musculature. In certain species where the wave lengths of the bands have been measured it has been found that the measurements are different from those of the oxyhemoglobin of the host (Davey, 1938).

DIGESTIVE SYSTEM

The digestive system of the nematodes is very simple and consists practically of a straight tube running from the mouth at the anterior tip to the anus on the ventral surface at a short distance above the posterior extremity (Figures 175, 176). The mouth is usually surrounded by lips or papillæ and in some species it bears teeth for grasping and tearing loose the host's tissues. The mouth cavity may be simply tubular or funnel-shaped while in some species it is expanded into a cup-shaped capsule which serves as a sucking organ. Behind the mouth cavity there usually occurs a more or less muscular esophagus which shows in cross section a triradial lumen lined with cuticula, and with the muscle fibers perpendicular to the lumen. By contraction, these fibers widen the lumen and the esophagus thereby functions as a pump to draw in food. The cuticular lining is their antagonist. The esophagus usually terminates in a more or less conspicuous bulb or valvular apparatus. Glandular elements are frequently embedded in the muscular wall of the esophagus. The intestine continues posteriorly as a more or less flattened tube with a relatively large lumen. Its wall is composed of columnar epithelium with the cells rich in protoplasm. In the female worm, the intestine narrows into a rectum which is lined by cuticula. In the male worm, however, the genital duct opens into the posterior region of the intestine thus forming a common passageway, the cloaca.

EXCRETORY SYSTEM

The excretory system consists of two lateral canals situated in the lateral chords. These canals pass forward to unite near the anterior extremity of the body and communicate with the exterior through a single excretory pore which is located in the mid-ventral line in the esophageal region. In some forms the canals extend anterior to the sinus, while in others the canals occupy only one lateral chord. In some species the system consists of a single, elongated gland cell without canalicular connections. There are no flame cells as in the PLATYHELMINTHES. There are no circulatory or respiratory systems known for nematodes. The movement of the fluids in the body cavity apparently serves these purposes.

NERVOUS SYSTEM

The nervous system consists of a number of ganglia connected by fibers surrounding the esophagus, the "nerve ring," from which six main nerve trunks pass anteriorly, and a dorsal, a ventral, four submedian and one, two or three pairs of lateral nerves pass posteriorly in the hypodermis. The main trunks pass along in the dorsal and ventral chords. The sensory organs, tactoreceptors, are the papillæ on the lips of the mouth, two cervical papillæ situated laterally in the anterior region and paired caudal or genital papillæ of the male of certain species and of the bursa of others. Frequently a second pair of lateral papillæ situated near the middle of the body are present, and the female may also bear paired caudal papillæ in the region of the vulva. Other sensory structures, chemoreceptors, include two amphids at the anterior extremity, lateral or dorsolateral in position, and, in many species, paired postanal lateral organs, structurally similar to the amphids, called phasmids (Chitwood and Chitwood, 1933).

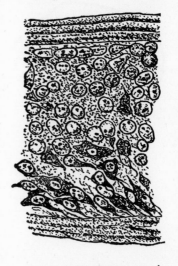

0·05mm

FIG. 178.—*Ascaris lumbricoides.* Germinal zone of ovary. (After Cram)

REPRODUCTIVE SYSTEM

The reproductive system of both sexes in NEMATODA is an exceedingly simple, long, tubular structure in which the various organs are continuous and only slightly differentiated from each other in external appearance (Figures 175, 176). The male reproductive organs are single and occupy the posterior third of the body. The testis is terminal, coiled and thread-like and leads through a vas deferens into a dilated portion, the seminal vesicle. The seminal vesicle is followed by a muscular ejaculatory duct of varying lengths which opens into the cloaca. Spicules are usually present in connection with the terminal portion of the male system and are withheld in pouches in the immediate vicinity of the ejaculatory duct. In many species, the males are equipped with wing-like appendages, a copulatory bursa at the posterior extremity, and cement glands, the secretions of which serve for copulation. The spermatozoa are rounded bodies capable of ameboid motion and in some species are not completely formed in the male, but develop in the female from the sperm mother cells which are transferred to her during copulation. In some species the spermatozoa develop in the same gonad as the egg, while in others parthenogenesis occurs.

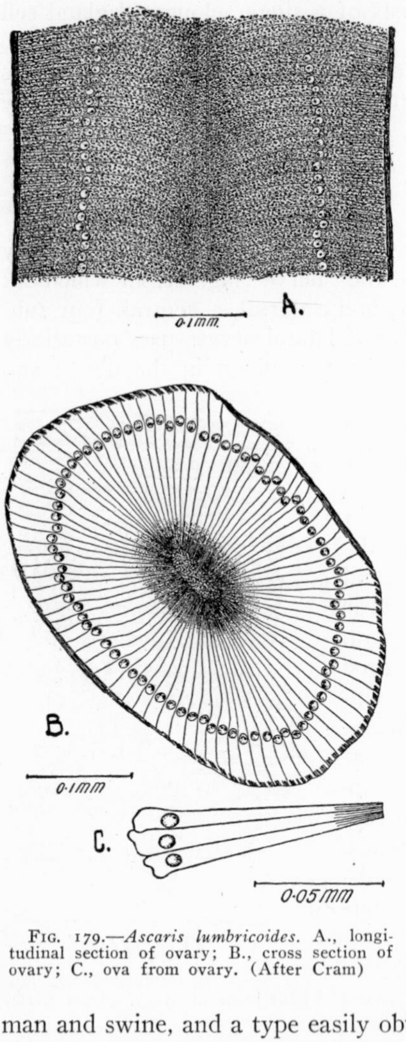

The female reproductive system may be either a single or a bifurcated tube, although most frequently it is bifurcated. The vulva is a small opening on the ventral surface and usually appears as a simple transverse slit. In *Ascaris lumbricoides,* a common intestinal parasite of man and swine, and a type easily obtained at abbatoirs for study, the vulva is situated about one-third the distance from the anterior end of the body and leads into a short muscular vagina from which two uteri branch off and follow a fairly straight parallel course backward to the posterior portion of the worm where each uterus turns

Fig. 179.—*Ascaris lumbricoides.* A., longitudinal section of ovary; B., cross section of ovary; C., ova from ovary. (After Cram)

forward. At this end of each uterus is situated the seminal receptacle, beyond which is the oviduct and then the terminal thread-like ovary which coils back and forth to such an extent that a cross section of the worm shows from twenty to thirty sections of the ovaries. Each ovary is from five to eight times the total length of the worm itself. The free or distal portion of the ovary is the germinal zone and contains a mass of protoplasm with an abundance of nuclei, or germinal vesicles, scattered through it (Figure 178). A short distance from the germinal zone the protoplasm is formed around the vesicle and distinct cells or ova begin to appear. This portion of the ovary is followed by a developmental zone in which the ova have become elongated and are arranged in wreaths around a central stalk or rachis which supplies them with nutriment (Figure 179). Further down, the rachis disappears as the ovary changes to form the oviduct and the ova separate from each other and assume a more or less oval

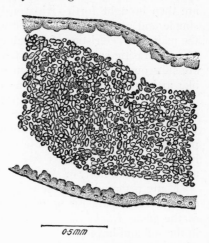

0·5mm

FIG. 180.—*Ascaris lumbricoides*. Longitudinal section of uterus. (After Cram)

form and produce yolk material within their cytoplasm. They are fertilized in the seminal receptacle after which they produce the shell while in the posterior end of the uterus. In *Ascaris* an albuminous substance is secreted from the walls of the uterus which is superimposed upon the shell as the egg passes along its length (Figure 180).

DEVELOPMENT

The development of the parasitic nematodes is exceedingly variable, and although certain species require intermediate hosts, their life-cycles are never as complicated as those of the digenetic trematodes. Most nematodes, like all other helminthes, do not multiply within the body of their hosts. Each adult present is the result of a successful entrance and development of a single infective organism. Multiplication within the host has been attributed to *Strongyloides stercoralis* (Thira, 1919) and *Enterobius vermicularis*. A few parasitic nematodes, however, possess multiplicative periods outside of the definitive host, and these, when present, occur in the free-living generations, as in the genera *Rhabdias* and *Strongyloides* of the family RHABDIASIDÆ.

The eggs of parasitic nematodes may be discharged either before or during segmentation, or with the embryo fully developed. In a few species the embryos hatch within the uterus of the female worm and are then brought forth viviparously. The embryonic development is simple and much alike in all species. The larvæ upon hatching have the main characteristics of nematodes but are not sexually developed. Many parasitic species have certain adaptive larval characters which are subsequently lost. In the course of their development, nematodes, like arthropods, pass through a series of stages marked by molts. A second cuticula is formed beneath the old, which is shed at each molt. There are usually four molts in the development of a nematode with the adult (fifth) stage following the fourth molt. Among the parasitic species some of these molts may take place within the egg before hatching, during its free existence, while within the tissue of an intermediate host, or within the tissues of the definitive host.

Many nematodes appear to be facultative parasites and may live either free or parasitic as opportunities are offered. Several species of the genus *Rhabditis* live abundantly in decaying organic material in the soil and have been reported frequently as parasites of man. To what extent they may become successful parasites is questionable as many of the reported infections appear to have been diagnosed on contaminated waste products of the host.

A number of species parasitic in man and other vertebrates pass through a free-living generation, sexually differentiated into males and females, which alternates with a parasitic parthenogenetic or hermaphroditic generation. In the life-cycle of *Strongyloides stercoralis,* the larvæ produced by the parasitic generation may develop into free-living adult males and females. The free-living female, after copulation, produces eggs. The larvæ which hatch from these eggs feed upon inorganic débris and later metamorphose into non-feeding larvæ, the infective stage. These larvæ when introduced into man or susceptible animals, grow into the adult parasitic generation. *Rhabdias fuscovenosa* from the lung of the garter snake and *Rhabdias bufonis* a common parasite in the lungs of frogs pass through similar stages in their development. These forms are of considerable interest in that they show a close relationship in their free-living generations to *Rhabditis* and certain other non-parasitic nematodes, which suggests possible ancestors from which parasitic species may have evolved.

Most parasitic nematodes have but a single host. Their life-cycles are more or less direct with some stage of development free. They differ, in the various species, mainly in the degree of development attained either before or during the free existence. The hookworms and their close relatives have the embryonic development and the first and second larval stages in the open with the larvæ as feeding stages. The second larva is the end product of the free life and is the infective stage for new hosts. Entrance into the new host is gained by the infective larva boring through the tissues of the host or by food contamination. The life-cycle of *Dictyocaulus filaria,* a parasite of sheep and goats, is somewhat similar to that of the hookworms except that the first and second larvæ, although free, are not feeding stages. These larvæ live on food stored up in the intestinal cells during embryonal development. The post embryonic development up to the first molt is passed inside the eggs of *Ostertagia marshalli.* Its second larva is free but, like that of *Dictyocaulus,* is not a feeding stage. The first and second larval stages of *Nematodirus filicollis* of sheep and cattle and *Oswaldocruzia auricularis* from the frog are passed within the egg and when the larva emerges from its shell it is already in the infective stage.

Many nematodes have no development, outside of the host, beyond the formation of the embryo. The egg alone is free. The eggs of *Ascaris lumbricoides* and *Trichuris trichiura* leave the host in an unsegmented condition. A relatively long period in the open is required before the embryo is formed. The embryonated egg is the end product of the free life for these parasites and is the infective stage for other hosts. When it is ingested by a susceptible host it hatches in the alimentary tract of the host and after a series of molts the adult stage is reached. In other species, such as *Enterobius vermicularis* from man and *Trichosomoides crassicauda* from rats, the embryonic development is completed in the body of the host and when the eggs are passed into the outer world they are immediately infective.

Some nematode species are parasitic in both adult and larval stages and require an intermediate host or a change of hosts to complete their life-cycle. Among these nematodes, certain species have some stage which is free. The guinea worm, *Dracunculus medinensis,* has its first larval stage in the open. The female is viviparous and lives in the connective tissue underneath the epidermis of the host. Her young are expelled into water, whenever an opportunity is offered, and are ingested by certain fresh-water crustaceans (*Cyclops*). Within the body cavity of the *Cyclops* further molts occur after which they become infective larvæ. Further development can take place only after the infected Cyclops is ingested by a susceptible host. *Gongylonema scutatum,* a parasite of horses, sheep and cattle, is free only in its egg stage. The egg of this nematode contains a fully developed embryo when it leaves the body of the definitive host. When it is ingested by certain coprophagous beetles it hatches in the digestive tract and later becomes an infective larva encysted in the body cavity. To complete its development, it must reach its vertebrate host. This is accomplished when the vertebrate host accidentally ingests the infected beetle with other food.

Certain other species requiring a change of host have no stage which is free. The FILARIIDÆ are parasites in the connective or lymphatic tissues. The females are viviparous, and as her young circulate in the peripheral blood they are taken up by certain blood-sucking insects within the bodies of which the larvæ undergo a metamorphosis after which the infective stage is reached. The infection is returned to the vertebrate host when the insect feeds upon that host. In the case of the trichina worm, *Trichinella spiralis,* both adult and larval stages develop within the same host. The sexually mature worms inhabit the small intestine. The gravid female is viviparous and deposits her young directly into the circulating blood and lymph. They are carried by the blood to the musculature where they encyst. Within the cyst the larvæ grow and later show sexual differentiation into males and females. The multiplicative period of these forms, however, is only reached after the muscle containing them is eaten by another susceptible host, at which time they are freed from their cysts in the alimentary tract and the cycle is recommenced.

II. *Collection and Preservation of Nematodes*

Adult parasitic nematodes may occur in almost every organ or tissue, but they are found most frequently in the contents of or adhering to the alimentary tract, particularly the small intestine. It is advisable to open the various organs in a dish of water and to search for specimens in the sediment. The intestines of large hosts should be examined in convenient lengths. The intestinal contents and the evacuated feces should be passed through a mesh or series of sieves having mesh apertures 6, 12, 24 and 40 to the inch. The sieve is washed with a stream of water until only the undigested material remains on the sieves. This material from each sieve is then concentrated and examined for helminths.

Small nematodes should be killed and preserved in hot 70 per cent alcohol to which has been added a small amount of glycerine.

Large nematodes and nematode eggs are satisfactorily killed and preserved in 10 per cent formalin plus a small amount of glycerine. Nematodes killed in formalin or in alcohol can be cleared for immediate study in a solution of carbolic acid and absolute alcohol in proportions of four parts of carbolic acid to one of absolute alcohol. Small nematodes are exceedingly sensitive to changes in osmotic pressure and therefore are difficult to stain and mount. All changes must be very gradual. String siphons, or the more complicated differentiators of Cobb (1890), Magath (1916) and Svensson and Kessel (1926) are valuable aids in this particular step.

Free-living larvæ of parasitic nematodes and free-living nematodes can be isolated from soil with Baermann's apparatus (Cort, Ackert, et al., 1922). This apparatus consists of a glass funnel, the stem of which is closed by a clamp on a piece of rubber tubing, and a sieve lined with a muslin cloth placed in the funnel. The soil to be examined is put in the sieve and warm water is poured into the funnel between the glass and the sieve until the water covers the soil. The nematodes drop into the water and are collected several hours later by drawing off a small amount of water from the stem. The use of this apparatus has made it possible to determine foci and degree of soil infection with hookworms. It can also be used in isolating small parasitic nematodes, particularly larval stages, from tissue which previously has been teased apart or has been passed through a food grinder. Encysted trichinæ are best isolated from tissue by digesting the ground infected muscle in a solution of 0.4 per cent pepsin and 0.3 per cent hydrochloric acid at a temperature of about 38° C. The sediment which contains the freed trichinæ is then concentrated by sedimentation. By washing the sediment several times, the trichinæ can be completely freed from host tissue.

Nematode eggs may be isolated from soil by first treating it for an hour in 30 per cent antiformin solution. To this is then added sodium dichromate. After centrifugation at 1,000 revolutions per minute for two minutes, the eggs can be looped off the surface and transferred to a glass slide for microscopic study (Spindler, 1929). This method has been used extensively to determine foci of *Ascaris* and *Trichuris* infections (Cort, 1931).

III. *Classification*

The student is referred to Yorke and Maplestone (1926), Stiles and Hassall (1926), Baylis and Daubney (1926), and Chitwood and Chitwood (1937), for detailed classifications of NEMATODA. The main divisions followed here are after Baylis and Daubney (1926).

CHAPTER XXVI

NEMATODE PARASITES

Order Ascaroidea Railliet and Henry, 1915

The order ASCAROIDEA consists of both free-living and parasitic nematodes having normally three lips, of which one is dorsal and two are subventral. In certain genera the lips may be much reduced or absent.

Baylis and Daubney (1926) have divided the order ASCAROIDEA into fourteen different families of which four are of particular interest in medical zoölogy. These are the ASCARIDÆ Cobbold, 1864, HETERAKIDÆ Railliet and Henry, 1914, OXYURIDÆ Cobbold, 1864, and the RHABDITIDÆ Micoletzky, 1922.

I. Family ASCARIDÆ

The ASCARIDÆ are parasitic forms, polymyarian, with lips well developed, bearing papillæ and sometimes alternating with three interlabia. There is no buccal cavity. The reproductive organs are highly developed. The male has two spicules and in some species an accessory piece, a gubernaculum, is present. The uterine branches of the female are parallel. Eggs are very numerous and contain an unsegmented ovum when deposited.

1. *Ascaris lumbricoides* Linnæus, 1758

DESCRIPTION

Ascaris lumbricoides (Figures 175, 176, 181) is the common roundworm of man and swine. In the living condition it may be milk-white or somewhat reddish-yellow in color and has a characteristic sheen. It is the largest of the human intestinal nematodes. The females usually vary from 20 cm. to 25 cm. but may attain even greater lengths with a diameter of about 5 mm. The males are smaller and measure from 15 cm. to 17 cm. by 3 mm. in diameter. The cuticula is smooth and rather plainly marked by numerous fine striations. The lips are finely toothed (Figure 182). The dorsal lip carries two sensory papillæ and each of the two ventral lips has one

386

sensory papilla. The anus is subterminal. The posterior end of the male is usually somewhat recurved and bears numerous ventral preanal and postanal papillæ and two short, but prominent, spicules. The vulva is anterior to the middle of the body near the junction of the anterior and middle thirds. The eggs are oval with a thick, trans-parent shell surrounded by an external albuminous coating which is coarsely mammillated. They measure from 50 μ to 75 μ in length by 40 μ to 50 μ in breadth, and are unsegmented at the time of deposition (Figure 183). They are colorless when they leave the uterus of the female but during their short stay in the intestinal tract of the host the albuminous layer acquires a yellowish or deep brown color from the bile. Occasionally eggs are passed without the albuminous coating and frequently unfertilized and atypical fertilized eggs are found Ascaris lumbricoides is known to produce an enormous number of eggs. Cram (1925) estimated that the number of eggs in a single female at one time may be as high as 27,-000,000; and Brown and Cort (1927) and Augustine and others (1928) calculated that the number of Ascaris eggs per gram of feces passed by an infected person may average over 2,000 per female worm.

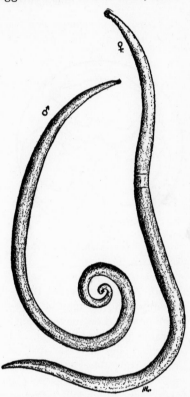

Fig. 181.—*Ascaris lumbricoides,* adult male and female worms, about 2/3 natural size. (From Neveu-Lemaire's *Parasitologie des Animaux Domestiques,* J. Lamarre, Paris)

The ascarids of man and swine are morphologically, toxicologically and serologically identical. Investigations by Koino (1922), Payne, Ackert and Hartman (1925) and the Caldwells (1926) have shown, however, that the infective eggs of the human *Ascaris* probably do not produce mature ascarids in healthy pigs, and that infective eggs of the pig *Ascaris* probably do not produce mature ascarids in man. It has also been noted that in certain localities the incidence of the parasite may be high in pigs but low or absent in humans of the same locality. It is therefore apparent that these two forms are "physiological" or "host" varieties.

GEOGRAPHICAL DISTRIBUTION

Ascaris lumbricoides is a cosmopolitan parasite of man and swine being distributed throughout all countries of the world. It is, how-ever, most frequent in tropical and subtropical countries where all fac-tors concerned are particularly favorable for its dissemination and development.

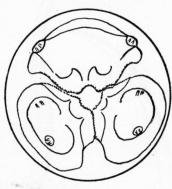

FIG. 182.—*Ascaris lumbricoides.* Head, end-on view (x 56). (Redrawn from Yorke and Maplestone)

LIFE-CYCLE

The eggs of *A. lumbricoides* are unsegmented when they leave the body of the host and under favor-able conditions the embryo is formed in about two weeks (Brown, 1927). Under natural con-ditions the development of the em-bryo may take place in water or soil, or wherever the pollution is spread. As the eggs are thick-shelled they are extremely resistant, and although they may be deposited in environments unfavorable for development they may remain viable for con-siderable periods. Davaine (1863) kept em-bryonated eggs alive for five years and Epstein (1892) was able to produce infections with eggs that had been kept in a culture of feces for a year. Stiles and Gardner (1910) found *Ascaris* eggs viable after 156 days in fecal ma-terial which had become quite dry during that time. They have also been found viable after being in the soil of our Southern States over winter (Martin, 1922). Because of their great longevity the soil exposed to continual pollu-tion may become exceedingly heavily laden with living eggs within the course of time.

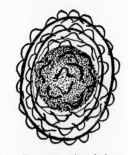

FIG. 183.—*Ascaris lum-bricoides.* Egg (x 500). (Redrawn from Yorke and Maplestone)

Infection with Ascaris results from ingesting eggs containing fully developed embryos. Such embryos have molted once within the egg and are enclosed within a sheath, the old cuticula. The eggs are usually carried to the mouth either with food or water or by accidental transfer of soil containing such ova. They do not regularly hatch in the stomach but pass to the small intestine where they begin this process within a few hours after ingestion. The hatching of *Ascaris* eggs may be observed in most laboratory animals as well as the development which immediately follows. These animals are, however, abnormal hosts and the worms are eliminated from the intestine before they reach sexual maturity.

Formerly it was believed that upon hatching the larvæ settled down in the small intestine and there developed directly into the adult stage. Investigations by Stewart (1916), Yoshida (1919), Ransom, Foster and Cram (1920), Fülleborn (1920-1925) and others have shown, however, that the larvæ of this parasite, as well as those of certain other ascarids, leave the intestine immediately after hatching and then follow a definite path of migration through the tissues of the host, after which they return to the intestine and grow into mature worms.

The newly hatched larvæ burrow into the wall of the intestine and enter the lymphatic vessels or the venules. If the larvæ enter the lymphatics they are carried to the mesenteric lymph nodes and from there may reach the circulation either by entering the blood capillaries and passing into the portal circulation, or pass into the thoracic duct and from there to the right side of the heart. If the portal circulation is entered the larvæ are carried to the liver where they pass from the interlobular veins to the intralobular veins. From the liver they are carried to the right side of the heart and then to the lungs. Within the lungs they break into the alveoli where some further development and growth takes place, after which they pass on to the intestine by way of the trachea, esophagus and stomach. This journey through the host's tissues requires about ten days. The worms become mature in the intestine in about two and one-half months.

Spontaneous hatching of *Ascaris* eggs outside the body has been observed by several workers. The escape of the larva from the shell, as noted by McRae (1935), probably is, in most cases, the result of mechanical injury to the egg-shell and is not comparable to a biological hatching. Infections have been produced experimentally with such larvæ, but it is probable that they seldom cause infection under natural conditions. They are not adapted to free-living life and perish readily.

PATHOGENESIS

The pathological effects from infection with *Ascaris lumbricoides* may be quite variable, due in part to the fact that the larval stages have an extensive course of migration in the body, and in part to the fact that the adult worms also frequently migrate from the intestine into other organs and tissues. In breaking through from the capillaries into the alveoli of the lungs the larvæ produce small hemorrhages which may result in so severe an inflammation that an extensive or generalized pneumonia is likely to occur, especially if the number of worms is large. Such effects have been frequently produced in laboratory animals. The condition known as "thumps," which occurs naturally in young pigs, is frequently a pulmonary infection with *Ascaris* larvæ. Pulmonary symptoms following the experimental administration of *Ascaris* eggs to man have been described by Koino of Japan and others. Koino (1922) swallowed about 2000 embryonated ova of *Ascaris* from man and his brother 400 to 500 embryonated ova of *Ascaris* from swine. In both the symptoms were similar but were much more severe in the first case. Pronounced pulmonary symptoms with blood in the sputum, headache, fever and muscular pains marked the course of the infection. After medication 667 worms were expelled from the former case but none were obtained from the latter subject.

In light infections with the adult worm there is apparently but little if any damage to the host and in many cases their presence is unsuspected until worms are noticed in the stool after defecation. However, many surgical cases, appendicitis, peritonitis, etc., are frequently the result of infection with a single worm. When occurring in large numbers the worms may cause intestinal obstruction by an actual mechanical occlusion. Cases of intussusception due to irritation from ascarids have been observed, some of which have required surgical interference. Adult ascarids frequently leave the intestine, especially during febrile disturbances, and wander up the digestive tract and enter the esophagus, nose, ear or the frontal sinus. They are frequently found in the appendix and in the bile ducts where their presence may be followed by abscesses. They may penetrate through the intestinal wall causing peritonitis and have occasionally invaded the genito-urinary tract causing retention of urine and abscesses in the infected tissue.

Nervous and other constitutional symptoms are often the result of intoxication from substances given off by ascarids. Shimamura and Fujii (1917) separated a highly toxic fraction from the body fluid of several different species of *Ascaris* which produced symptoms similar to anaphylactic shock. Many individuals are very sensitive to contact with *Ascaris,* particularly with the body fluid. Among the symptoms in susceptible persons are irritation of the eyes, nose, throat, edema of the eyes, sneezing, urticaria, lassitude and even prostration. Susceptibility to *Ascaris* fluids is a very common condition among biologists who have been much exposed to contact with the parasite and occasionally may be observed among students during laboratory studies on these parasites.

Ascaris lumbricoides is of great economic importance in hog raising countries. Young pigs are especially susceptible to infection and these often die of pneumonia or "thumps" caused by the larval ascarids in the lungs. It has been estimated that from 10 per cent to 20 per cent of the pig crop in certain sections of the United States was destroyed each year by "thumps" or pulmonary ascariasis before control measures were inaugurated. Other losses occur in the stunting of growth due to early infections with these worms resulting in a loss in quantity and quality of pork production.

TREATMENT

Oil of chenopodium, or its most active anthelmintic constituent, ascaridol, is apparently the most effective drug in removing ascarids. Generally 1 c.c. is effective for adult persons. This drug is decidely irritating, constipating and toxic, and special contraindications include gastroenteritis, pronounced weakness, gastric stasis and constipation. Purgation is essential. Castor oil in adequate amounts, about one ounce, administered with the drug is protective. If the purgative is not given until two or three hours after administration of the chenopodium, a fast-acting purgative, such as salts, should be given rather than the castor oil (Hall, 1923). Santonin, calomel and thymol have been used to remove ascarids but are less effective than chenopodium.

EPIDEMIOLOGY

Because of the enormous egg production of *Ascaris* and the remarkable resistance of the egg to adverse conditions, this nematode is undoubtedly the most prevalent and the most widely distributed of all human helminths. It has been reported from practically every section of the United States, but occurs in epidemic proportions only in the southeastern states among the indigenous population of the Appalachian Mountains and foothills running east, south and west from the main ridges, and in parts of Louisiana and Florida (Otto and Cort, 1934). The southern coastal area, sometimes referred to as the "hookworm belt," has a very low *Ascaris* incidence among the general population, but considerable infection with this parasite exists in several hospitals for the insane of the area (Caldwell, Caldwell and Davis, 1930). Ascariasis is not characteristic of rural sections. It occurs equally frequently in poorly sanitated towns and cities.

In the rural endemic areas of the United States the children of preschool age are most frequently infected and carry the heaviest worm burdens. Cort (1931) and others have noted that the chief factor in the dissemination of *Ascaris* is the careless deposition of stools by the children in the yards close to the house where they are accustomed to play. The eggs passed on to the ground develop to infectivity, even in exposed places, and infection occurs by hand-to-mouth transfer as the children play. Older children of the family and the adult members customarily use whatever toilet facility is available, or remove themselves a considerable distance from their houses to defecate. It has been observed frequently that the introduction of privies into unsanitated areas does not bring *Ascaris* under control, simply because of the failure of young children to use the facilities provided. Medical treatment only temporarily reduces the worm burden. Control lies in the prevention of soil pollution by young children.

PREVENTION

Green vegetables and fruits from gardens fertilized with human excreta have been considered to be a chief source of infection with *Ascaris*. According to Winfield and Yeo (1937), eggs of *Ascaris* seldom adhere to vegetables and infection from such is negligible. Drinking water seldom carries the infection. Sanitation, sewer systems in cities and towns, and sanitary privies on farms, together with personal habits of cleanliness, are effective preventive measures against *Ascaris* infection in man.

The control of ascariasis in pigs is a relatively simple matter in view of the fact that an age immunity is established within a few months, and only the very young pigs are most susceptible to infection. It has been recommended (Ransom, 1921) that the sow and the farrowing pen be thoroughly cleaned shortly before farrowing and that the sow and the young pigs be removed within ten days after birth to clean legume pastures or fields previously sown to other suitable forage crops. The pigs are to be kept there, away from permanent hog lots, for at least four months, during which time they have become relatively immune against this infection. The putting into practice of this simple system has prevented serious losses from ascariasis in the swine industry of the United States.

2. ASCARIDS OF DOMESTIC ANIMALS

Ascaris vitulorum Goeze, 1782, is a fairly common parasite of young calves in parts of southern Europe, Japan and Ceylon. It has also been found in calves of Antigua and Cuba. *A. equorum* Goeze, 1782, is cosmopolitan in horses. The males are 15 to 28 cm. long and the females about 50 cm. long and 8 mm. in diameter. Foals especially suffer from this parasite. The eggs are almost globular and measure about 95 μ in diameter. The preferred drug for *A. equorum* is carbon bisulphid (Hall, 1923). The migrations of these parasites within the body of the host are similar to the course followed by *A. lumbricoides.*

Ascarids are rarely found in sheep. *Ascaris ovis* has been described from sheep in Europe and has been found in sheep in different parts of the United States. It is considered questionable by some authorities whether this parasite represents a distinct species, or whether it is only *A. lumbricoides* in an unusual host.

3. *Lagochilascaris minor* Leiper, 1909

This parasite is one of the smaller ascarids which has been found occasionally in subcutaneous abscesses in man in Trinidad, B. W. I. The males are about 9 mm. and the females about 15 mm. in length. The vulva is slightly anterior to the middle of the body. The lips have a strongly developed cuticular covering and are separated from the body by a groove. The free edge of each lip is deeply indented in the middle, giving the appearance of hare-lips. Well developed interlabia are present. Narrow flanges or alæ extend throughout the whole length of the body. The esophagus is simple. *L. minor* is probably a normal intestinal parasite of cats.

4. *Toxocara canis* (Werner, 1782)

Toxocara canis is the common ascarid of the dog and fox. It is especially frequent in puppies. These parasites are white or somewhat reddish in color and have an arrow-shaped head due to two short lateral cephalic alæ or membranous wings. The head is usually curved ventrally. The posterior portion of the male worm is curved and bears two caudal alæ. The vulva of the female is situated toward the anterior fourth of the body. The males measure from 5 cm. to 10 cm. and the females measure from 9 cm. to 18 cm. in length. The eggs are globular, 75 μ to 80 μ in diameter and have a finely corrugated or pitted shell, light brown in color (Figure 184).

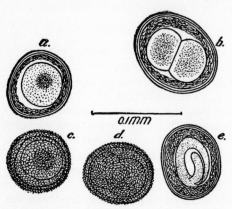

FIG. 184.—Eggs of cat and dog ascarids. *a., b., e., Toxocara mystax; c., d., Toxocara canis.* (From Hall. After Wigdor)

The life-cycle of *T. canis* is similar to that of *A. lumbricoides.* Young dogs are particularly susceptible to infection but, when they reach the age of three or four months, the worms are automatically eliminated and the dogs then remain almost immune to reinfection. Prenatal infection with *T. canis* frequently occurs under natural conditions. The newly hatched larvæ in the intestine of a pregnant bitch show a decided preference for the fetal tissues. The young worms remain in the liver of the fetus until parturition, after which migration takes place from the liver to the lungs and finally to the intestine where the adult stage is reached (Augustine, 1927).

The infection in puppies usually is very heavy and the puppy may show marked emaciation, enlarged abdomen, irregular appetite and often epileptiform seizures. The worms often enter the stomach and cause vomiting, with the vomitus containing many worms.

Toxocara mystax (Zeder, 1800) is a closely related species which is parasitic in cats. It is smaller than *T. canis.* This species has been reported several times from man. Its life-cycle is similar to that of *T. canis.*

The diagnosis of ascariasis in animals can be made by finding the eggs or adult worms in the feces, or adult worms in the vomitus of cats or dogs. Oil of chenopodium appears to be the drug of choice for ascarids in dogs and cats (Hall, 1923; Mönnig, 1934).

II. Family HETERAKIDÆ

The HETERAKIDÆ are medium to small parasites, polymyarian, with lips well defined or so reduced as to appear absent. A buccal capsule may be present or absent and when absent, the anterior portion of the esophagus is usually differentiated as a pharynx. A posterior esophageal bulb is present, except in the genus Ascaridia and a more or less well developed circular preanal sucker is present in the male. The vulva is typically near the middle of the body. Two genera of this family are of particular economic importance, namely *Heterakis* Dujardin, 1845, and *Ascaridia* Dujardin, 1845.

1. *Heterakis gallinæ* (Gmelin, 1790) Freeborn, 1923

DESCRIPTION

This species (Figure 185) is frequently a parasite in the ceca and rarely occurs in the small intestine, colon and rectum of barnyard and wild fowls. It is a small, rigid, white worm, with the anterior end bent dorsally from the region of the esophageal bulb. The mouth is surrounded by three small, equal lips without teeth. Each lip bears two papillæ. Two narrow lateral membranes or alæ extend almost the entire length of the body. The male is from 7 mm. to 13 mm. long and is characterized by a straight tail terminating in a subulate point with two large lateral caudal alæ. There are twelve pairs of papillæ, of which four pairs are between the cloacal opening and the end of the tail, four pairs of ray-like papillæ and two pairs of sessile papillæ are in the vicinity of the cloacal opening and two pairs of ray-like papillæ are in the vicinity of the pre-anal sucker (Figure 186). The spicules are unequal in length, the right being 2 mm. to 2.17 mm. long and the left 700 μ to 1.1 mm.

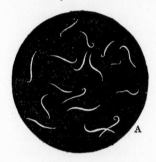

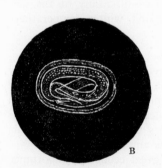

FIG. 185.—*Heterakis gallinæ*. A, adult and several immature worms, about ¾ natural size; B, infective egg showing coiled embryo within shell (about x 200). (After Tyzzer and Fabyan)

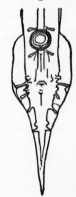

FIG. 186.—*Heterakis gallinæ*. Ventral view of posterior extremity of male showing circular suckers and arrangement of papillæ (x 100). (After Uribe)

long. The female measures from 10 mm. to 15 mm. in length. The tail is long, narrow and pointed and the anus is about 1 mm. from the tip. The vulva is situated slightly posterior to the middle of the body. The eggs have a thick shell, thickening at one end which thickening may enclose a lenticular clear space. They are ellipsoidal measuring from 63 μ to 75 μ in length by 36 μ to 38 μ in breadth and are unsegmented when deposited.

LIFE-CYCLE

Under favorable conditions of temperature and moisture the infective embryo is formed within seven to twelve days. When the embryonated eggs are swallowed by susceptible birds the embryos hatch in the gizzard and pass with its contents to the ceca where the adult stage is reached. Larvæ may enter the ceca as early as twenty-four hours after ingestion of the eggs. These larvæ migrate into the cecal glands. At first, the larva comes to lie within the epithelial layer and later, as size increases, occupies the lumen of the gland. According to Uribe (1922), the larvæ break out of the glands in about five days and complete their development in about thirty days in the lumen of the ceca. Earthworms have been observed to ingest *Heterakis* eggs, and birds may become infected by eating them.

The eggs of *H. gallinæ* are very resistant. Graybill (1921) found eggs viable after sixteen to eighteen days' desiccation and eggs with live embryos after twelve months in moist soil. Many of the embryonated eggs can withstand New England winter temperatures (Uribe, 1922).

PATHOGENESIS

There is but little evidence that *H. gallinæ* itself produces any serious injury to the infected bird. The adult stage lives in the lumen of the ceca and is occasionally found with the head buried in the mucosa or in the cavity of lymph nodules which occur at intervals in the wall of the ceca. It generally feeds upon the cecal contents but occasionally blood may be found in its alimentary tract.

Indirectly *H. gallinæ* is a parasite of great economic importance in that often it is the vector of *Histomonas meleagridis* which causes blackhead in turkeys. Apparently, from the experimental evidence obtained by Tyzzer (1922-1926) the germ of blackhead is carried within the egg of Heterakis and is protected by the shell of the latter. The actual presence of *Histomonas meleagridis* within the egg of Heterakis, however, has not been observed thus far.

Diagnosis is made by finding the eggs in the cecal feces. Rectal injection of oil of chenopodium, 0.1 cc., in 5 cc. bland oil (cottonseed oil) is effective in removing the parasites (Hall, 1923).

2. *Ascaridia lineata* (Schneider, 1866) Railliet and Henry, 1912

Ascaridia lineata inhabits the small intestine of domestic and wild fowls and is the common roundworm of chickens in the United States. Formerly it was assumed that the large intestinal roundworm of domestic fowl in America was *A. galli,* better known as *A. perspicillum,* but Schwartz (1925) after a study of specimens from various parts of this country, pointed out that the North American species is *A. lineata* (Figure 187). Therefore, the various facts published in the United States concerning the life history and pathology of *A. galli,* or *A. perspicillum,* in all probability, refer to *A. lineata.*

A. lineata is white or yellowish in color. The male is from 55 mm. to 68 mm. in length and is characterized by ten pairs of papillæ of which three pairs constitute the first group which are arranged in a linear series on each side of the preanal sucker. A second group of four pairs, three lateral and one ventral, are in the immediate region of the cloaca and three pairs, two lateral and one ventral, are found in a secondary expansion of the caudal alæ toward the tip of the tail. The spicules are unequal, 1.6 mm. to 2.4 mm. in length, with slightly enlarged, rounded points. The female may vary from 60 mm. to 95 mm. in length with the vulva at the union of the anterior and middle thirds of the body length. The eggs are elliptical, 80 μ in length by 50 μ in breadth and have thick, smooth shells.

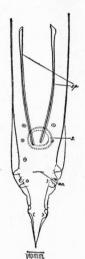

1/10mm.

Fig. 187.—*Ascaridia lineata,* ventral view of posterior extremity of male showing circular sucker and arrangement of papillæ. *an.,* anus; *s.,* sucker; *sp.,* spicules. (After Schwartz)

The eggs of *A. lineata* are passed in the feces. Under favorable conditions an infective embryo is formed within nine or ten days. Such eggs, when ingested by susceptible birds, hatch in the small intestine where the larvæ develop to maturity without a migratory phase in the tissue of the host. Prevention includes the early removal of droppings from penned birds. Ackert has shown that the larvæ may penetrate to some extent the wall of the small intestine and occasionally extend through Lieberkün's glands into the mucosa. Graham, Ackert and Jones (1934) have obtained evidence of an acquired immunity in chickens against this parasite.

III. Family OXYURIDÆ

The OXYURIDÆ are parasitic, meromyarian ASCAROIDEA. The mouth is surrounded by simple, usually inconspicuous lips and there

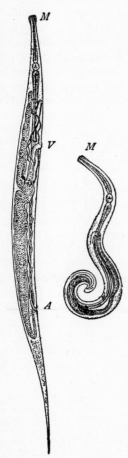

is no buccal capsule. The esophagus is usually provided with a pharynx and always with a distinct posterior bulb, containing three valves. The caudal end of the mature female is always elongated and subulate. The male is without a preanal sucker, except in one genus *Hoplodontophorus* parasitic in *Hyrax,* connies or rock rabbits of Europe, Africa and Southwestern Asia.

1. *Enterobius vermicularis* (Linnæus, 1758)

DESCRIPTION

This species (Figure 188) is commonly known as the pinworm of man. It is a small, white worm with the anterior extremity surrounded by a cuticular expansion. The mouth is surrounded by three fairly distinct lips and the esophagus is provided with an extra or prebulbar swelling and a distinct bulb. Narrow lateral alæ are present which are prominent in cross sections of the worm. The male is much smaller than the female and may easily be overlooked unless special search is made for it. It measures from 2 mm. to 5 mm. in length and the posterior third of the body is curved into a spiral. The tail is blunt and possesses six pairs of papillæ and a single curved spicule, 70 μ long. The female worm measures from 9 mm. to 12 mm. in length and has a long pointed tail. The body is characteristically rigid. The vulva is very prominent and is situated in front of the posterior limit of the anterior fourth of the body. The uteri in gravid specimens are greatly distended which give a plump appearance to the body. The eggs (Figure 80 (19)) are characteristically asymmetrical, and contain a more or less fully developed embryo when deposited by the female. The eggs vary from 50 μ to

FIG. 188.—*Enterobius vermicularis.* On the left, female; on the right, male. *A*, anus; *M*, mouth; *V*, vulva. Greatly enlarged. (After Claus)

60 μ in length and 30 μ to 32 μ in breadth. The shell is hyaline, relatively thick and encloses the embryonic membrane.

HABITAT

Enterobius vermicularis is a parasite in the adult stage of the upper part of the large intestine. It occasionally is found in the female genital organs and bladder. It frequently occurs in the appendix and may be a cause of appendicitis. Early stages of development take place in the small intestine.

DISTRIBUTION

This parasite is world-wide in distribution. It is especially frequent in children, although some of the heaviest infections have been observed in adults. As many as 5,544 have been counted from a single adult after anthelmintic treatment (Hall and Augustine, 1928).

LIFE-CYCLE

The gravid females pass down the rectum and are ejected with the feces, or they may migrate from the rectum into the anal cleft, the genitocrural folds and the neighboring parts. When they are exposed to air, a definite physiological reaction follows in the form of rhythmical contractions of the wall of the vagina which expels the eggs, and, as the worm advances, they are left behind in its trail. The tadpole-like embryo quickly develops into a coiled, nematode-like form which, when swallowed by man, develops directly into the adult stage. The females creep out of the rectum usually at night and in so doing cause intense itching. Scratching, to alleviate the itching, results in the eggs adhering to the hands, especially under the finger-nails. These eggs may sooner or later be conveyed to the mouth directly from the hands, or to food or drink. Eggs may also adhere to the night-clothes and bed linens and thus may be conveyed to persons handling them.

Upon ingestion of the infective eggs, the embryos hatch in the small intestine where the young worms develop to sexual maturity. After the females are fertilized the uteri begin to fill with eggs and the females soon pass down the rectum to discharge them. The duration of the cycle is about two weeks.

Certain writers have reported the simultaneous finding of eggs, larvæ and adults in the intestine, or the existence of *Enterobius* larvæ in fresh feces, or a six to seven week periodicity in the passage of female worms. These observations suggest that the eggs may hatch after deposition in the intestine without passing out of the patient, or in other words, a multiplication of individuals may occur within the intestine of the host.

The observations of Penso (1932) on related species of lower animals support this view. He (1932-33) has observed the eggs of *Passalurus ambiguus,* in the lumen of the intestinal glands of rabbits, and larvæ of *Dermatoxys veligera* in the intestinal mucosa of the hare. His theory is that these and other oxyurids copulate in the intestine of the host, and the females then penetrate the intestinal wall to deposit their eggs. The larvæ upon hatching reënter the lumen of the intestine (as do cysticercoids of the dwarf tapeworm) and grow to maturity. The eggs leave the host only when the female migrates out of the anus, thus passing infection on to another host.

PATHOGENESIS

In migrating out from the rectum the female worms produce an intense itching, and when occurring in large number, a severe anal pruritus may result. The worms may also travel up the vagina and have been accused of being a cause of chronic salpingitis. The itching is more intense at night and may result in loss of sleep and of nervous energy. The patient is often anemic and emaciated from disturbances of appetite and of nutrition and in some cases there are nervous disturbances. Enterobius is frequently found in the appendix and is believed by many observers to have a definite pathogenic rôle in the causation of appendicitis. Harris and Browne (1925) reported *E. vermicularis* in twenty-two appendices out of an uninterrupted sequence of 121 cases of operative appendicitis and concluded that the failure of recognition of *Enterobius* as a factor in the production of appendicitis is due in general to the lack of detailed gross and microscopic study of the appendix.

DIAGNOSIS

Infections with *Enterobius* are diagnosed on the presence of characteristic symptoms and on the finding of the gravid females. A simple examination of the anus will frequently establish the diagnosis but the use of the NIH cellophane type of anal swab (Hall, 1937) is recommended. Eggs are rarely found in the host's feces because of the egg laying habits of the female worm. In infected individuals, however, eggs may frequently be found in scrapings from the fingernails and anal regions.

TREATMENT

Tetrachlorethylene, santonin, chenopodium and thymol have been used with success against *Enterobius,* especially against those forms living in the small intestine. A number of substances have been used as enemas for removing the gravid females from the large intestine. Among enemas which have been recommended (Hall, 1923) are cold water; sodium chloride, vinegar diluted 3 or 4 times with water; 1 per cent acetic acid; 15 to 25 drops of oil of chenopodium shaken up in a liter of water; phenol and glycerin, 5 to 10 minims of each in one pint of hot water; quassia, one ounce steeped in one pint of hot water, and aqueous solutions of hexylresorcinol crystals in dilutions of one part hexylresorcinol crystals to 1,000 parts water. The use of an anal wash or ointment is generally advised to destroy the worms and eggs, to alleviate itching and make less likely the transfer of infective material to the hands, bed clothing and to the mouth.

PREVENTION

Rigid personal cleanliness is essential. Underwear, night-clothes, and bedding of infected persons should be handled with caution and properly laundered to insure the destruction of infective ova. Infected individuals should guard against auto-infection. The anal region should be thoroughly cleansed after defecation followed by the application of an anal ointment. The use of night-clothes which will prevent contamination of the fingers by scratching during sleep is advised for infected children. Separate beds for infected persons will help prevent the spread of the infection.

2. *Oxyuris equi* (Schrank, 1778)

This species inhabits the cecum and large intestine of the horse, ass and mule. The males are about 1 cm. in length and the females vary from 4 cm. to 15 cm. in length. The body is usually white, somewhat thickened and curved. The posterior portion of the female may be much attenuated. *O. equi* produces an anal pruritus in horses such as *Enterobius vermicularis* does in man. To alleviate the itching, the infected animals rub the parts against objects and thus wear off the hair and skin from the base of the tail.

TREATMENT

Hall (1923) recommends 4 or 5 drams of oil of chenopodium followed immediately by a quart of raw linseed oil. Rectal enemas are sometimes used but, according to Hall, they give results inferior to those obtained by the use of oral medication.

3. *Oxyurids of lower vertebrates*

Syphacia obvelata Rudolphi, 1802 (Figure 189) is a common oxyurid in the cecum and large intestine of mice and rats. The female worm measures from 3.5 mm. to 5.7 mm. in length. The eggs are 110 μ to 142 μ in length by 30 μ to 40 μ in breadth. The embryo is not formed at the time of oviposition. This parasite has been reported from an American-Bohemian child living in Zamboanga.

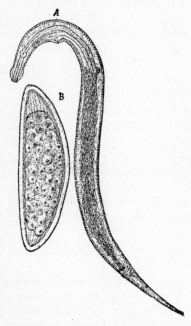

Aspiculuris tetraptera (Mitzsch, 1821) is also a common oxyurid of rats and mice in the United States. This species is somewhat smaller than *S. obvelata*. The eggs are much smaller than those of *S. obvelata* ranging from 84 μ to 90 μ in length by 34 μ to 40 μ in breadth. *Passalurus ambiguus* Rudolphi, 1819, is a common parasite in the cecum and large intestine of rabbits. These oxyurids are usually obtainable for laboratory study.

IV. Family RHABDITIDÆ

The RHABDITIDÆ is composed of small nematodes, free-living or parasitic, or with both free-living and parasitic phases. The buccal cavity may be three-sided, prismatic or tubular, and is usually without teeth. The esophagus generally has a posterior bulb containing valves, and frequently there is a prebulbar swelling. The cuticula is without bristles, or if present, they are very few in number. The female is either oviparous or viviparous, and not infrequently parthenogenetic or hermaphroditic. The reproductive organs are simple.

FIG. 189.—*Syphacia obvelata*. A, Female from the cecum of a mouse; B, egg. Enlarged. (After Riley)

1. *Rhabditis hominis* Kobayashi, 1914

Most species of the genus *Rhabditis* are free-living. They are especially common in decaying matter. The parasitic species occur mostly in insects but a few forms have been reported in man and the dog.

Rhabditis hominis (Figure 190) was first noted in 1914 by Kobayashi (1921) from feces of pupils of a primary school of Japan and has since been observed in human feces in the United States. The female is viviparous and all stages of its development were found in the same specimen of feces. When present in the feces they occur in very great numbers. Sandground (1925) was unable to obtain an infection with *R. hominis* in either the human subject or in laboratory animals and regards it as a free-living coprophagous species which may appear in the feces as a result of soil contamination or by its introduction into the feces by filth flies. The full-grown female measures about 2 mm. in length and the length of the male is about 1 mm.

Among other species of *Rhabditis* reported as parasites of man are *R. pellio* Schneider, 1866, and *R. niellyi* R. Blanchard, 1885. *R. pellio* has been reported from the urine and vagina of a woman from Hungary. It normally lives during the adult stage in decomposing matter in the soil and in its larval stage may be parasitic in

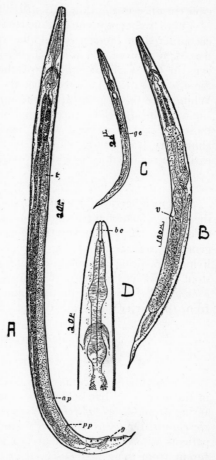

Fig. 190.—*Rhabditis hominis.* A, adult male; B, young female; C, young rhabditiform larva; D, anterior portion of an adult worm showing characteristics of the esophagus (After Sandground)

the nephridia of earth worms. *R. niellyi* was obtained from itching papules on the skin of a boy living in Brest and *R. strongyloides* Leuckart, 1883, has been observed in red, pustular lesions of the skin of a dog. These are normally free-living nematodes and probably gain entrance in the skin only after it has been damaged.

Quite frequently eggs of nematodes parasitic on vegetables are encountered in human feces. One species, *Oxyuris incognita,* was named by Kofoid and White in 1919 upon finding certain nematode eggs in the stools of soldiers of the Southern Department. Later, Sandground (1923) showed that the eggs described by Kofoid and White were the eggs of *Heterodera radicicola,* a common root parasite of radishes, celery, turnips and other vegetables. These eggs, and those of similar species, when ingested by man pass through the alimentary tract uninjured. Unless they are recognized, they might easily be regarded as an indication of a nematode infection.

2. *Rhabdias* Stiles and Hassall, 1905

The members of the genus *Rhabdias* are usually found inhabiting the lungs of amphibians and reptiles. They are heterogenetic nematodes. The parasitic generation consists of females only which are generally regarded as being parthenogenetic in function. The free-living generation are microscopic forms, sexes separate with fairly stout bodies (Chu, 1936). The infective larvæ are sheathed forms. *Rhabdias bufonis* from the frog and toad and *Rhabdias fuscovenosa* from the garter snake are typical examples of this genus.

3. *Strongyloides stercoralis* (Bavay, 1876)

HISTORICAL

Strongyloides stercoralis was discovered by Dr. Normand in 1876 in the feces of French Marines from Cochin China who were suffering from severe diarrhea. Bavay named the parasites *Anguillula stercoralis.* Dr. Normand later found nematodes in the intestines of patients who had died of diarrhea which were morphologically different from those first observed in the feces. These were diagnosed by Bavay as *Anguillula intestinalis.* Both forms were believed to be the cause of the disease, then known as Cochin China diarrhea. Leuckart in 1882 studied the life-cycle of this parasite and demonstrated that the two forms found by Dr. Normand were two succeeding generations of the same species, that *A. intestinalis* lived parasitically in the intestine, and *A. stercoralis* was its progeny which attained maturity in the open and there multiplied.

Fülleborn, in 1914, by experimental methods followed the route of migration of the parasite through the skin, its passage with the blood to the lungs, its active migration through the alveolar tissue and up the trachea to the pharynx and thence to the intestine of the host, where the majority of the females establish themselves and deposit their eggs.

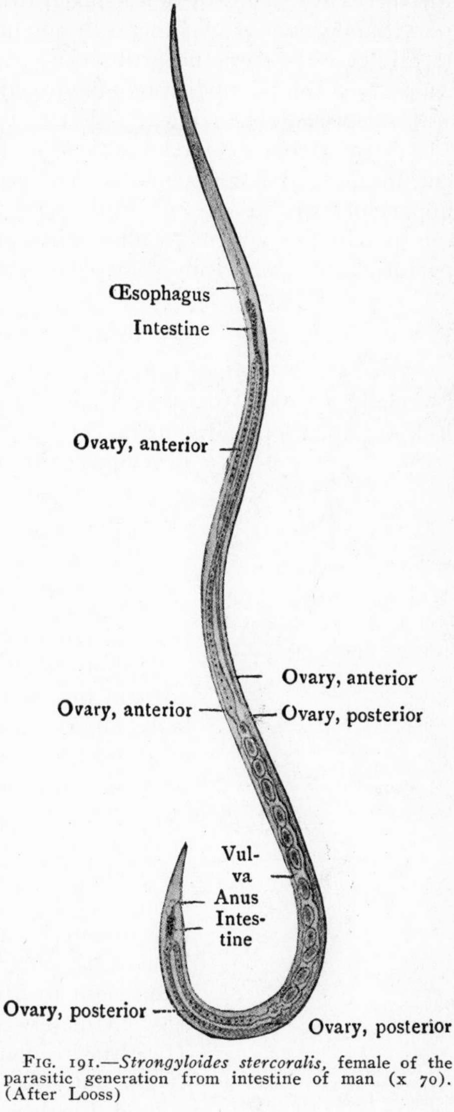

Until recently the parasitic generation was known to include only female worms which were regarded by certain workers to be parthenogenetic in function and by others hermaphroditic (Leuckart, 1882; Rovelli, 1888; Sandground, 1926). In 1932, Kreis reported the finding of parasitic males in material from a human subject and dogs infected with a strain of the parasite in which the free-living generation was constantly absent. Kreis considers that fertilized eggs proceed to direct development while, in the absence of the male worm, the unfertilized eggs proceed to indirect development, i.e., a generation of free-living male and female worms, and that in the indirect type of development the parasitic female is probably parthenogenetic. Faust and co-workers (1933-35), after studying various phases of the life-cycle, including

Fig. 191.—*Strongyloides stercoralis,* female of the parasitic generation from intestine of man (x 70). (After Looss)

the successive stages of development of the parasitic generation, support Sandground's hypothetical contention that the direct development proceeds from unfertilized eggs. Evidence is also presented supporting the possibility of autoinfection, the occurrence of which was suspected by Grassi (1883), Fülleborn (1926), Nishigori (1928) and others. Our knowledge of the parasitic male is, at present, meager; and the points of view regarding the life-cycle of this important parasite are divergent and conflicting. The solution of this perplexing and most interesting problem obviously lies in the performance of carefully controlled experiments.

DISTRIBUTION

Strongyloides stercoralis is world-wide in distribution and is especially frequent in tropical and sub-tropical countries where the lack of sanitation and climatic conditions are most favorable for the development of the free-living generation. It is a natural parasite of man but can develop in dogs, cats and monkeys.

DESCRIPTION

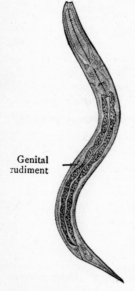

Genital rudiment

Fig. 192.—*Strongyloides stercoralis*, larva from fresh human feces (x 170). (After Looss)

The parasitic generation: The parasitic female is colorless, more or less transparent, and approximately 2.5 mm. in length and 40 μ in maximum width (Figure 191). The body tapers anteriorly and ends posteriorly in a short, conical tail. The cuticula is finely striated. The mouth is surrounded by four indistinct lips. The esophagus is long and slender and occupies the anterior fourth of the body. The vulva is located near the posterior third of the body and leads directly into the uterine branches, which are opposed. The ovaries are reflexed. The uteri contain from eight to fifteen segmenting, thin-shelled eggs characteristically arranged in single file. The parasitic female usually inhabits the wall of the intestine in which the eggs are deposited. Further development and hatching of the eggs take place in the intestinal mucosa and the newly hatched larvæ make their way into the lumen of the intestine. The larvæ are then passed to the exterior with the feces (Figure 192). Because of the early hatching of the eggs within the

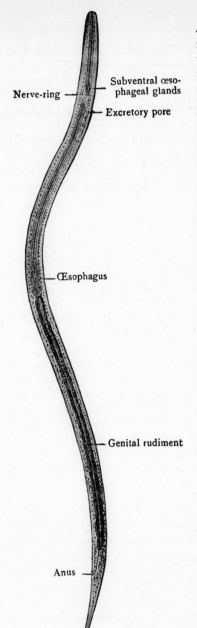

Nerve-ring

Subventral œso-
phageal glands

Excretory pore

Œsophagus

Genital rudiment

Anus

intestine, it is only in cases of severe diarrhea or after purgation
that the ova may be present in the
evacuated feces. The newly
hatched larvæ possess a double-
bulbed esophagus, characteristic of
many free-living nematodes, and
are known as rhabditiform larvæ.
They possess a complete digestive
system but sexual organs remain
undeveloped. The rhabditiform
larvæ feed in the open and later
may metamorphose either into
elongated filariform larvæ or, under certain conditions, into free-
living adult male and female
worms. According to Kreis (1932)
the parasitic male bears no fundamental similarity to the parasitic
female. It has a rhabditiform
esophagus and in all other respects
is practically indistinguishable
from the male of the free-living
generation.

The free-living generation:
The free-living generation of *S.
stercoralis* consists of both sexes
which are typical, free-living nematodes possessing a double-bulbed
(rhabditiform), muscular esophagus. The female worm is smaller
than the parasitic stage, measuring
only about 1 mm. in length. The
male is somewhat smaller. After
copulation the female produces
eggs from which rhabditiform
larvæ emerge which are indistinguishable from the rhabditiform
larvæ produced by the parasitic fe-

FIG. 193.—*Strongyloides stercoralis,* the infective stage of filariform
larva showing long transparent esophagus, slender granular intestine
and characteristic bifurcation of the tail. (After Looss)

male. These larvæ, after a short feeding period, metamorphose into filariform, or infective larvæ (a non-feeding stage) (Figure 193). They are about 550 mm. in length and may be readily distinguished by their long slender esophagus which has a length of almost half the total length of the body and by a distinct cleft at the tip of the tail, seen only with the high power of the microscope. Alicata (1935) has observed that the tip of the tail of filariform larvæ of *Strongyloides papillosus* of sheep and *S. ransomi* of swine is tripartite, two subventral projections and one dorsal. He is of the opinion that the tails of infective larvæ of other members of this group may also show this same character.

LIFE-CYCLE

The rhabditiform larvæ which are expelled from the host feed upon the host's feces and within a short time may metamorphose directly into elongated, infective larvæ, or develop into free-living adult males and females which later copulate and whose end product is an infective filariform larva. Whether the development of the infective larvæ is direct or indirect, they are morphologically identical and possess the same biological characteristics.

Under natural conditions, these larvæ occupy the very upper parts of the soil, and when occurring in great numbers, they form themselves into white, polyp-like masses on the exposed soil aggregates. Infection results when the filariform larvæ penetrate the host's tissues, the opportunity for infection usually being offered when a barefooted individual passes over areas of infected soil. The position of the infective larvæ in the soil makes ideal their transfer to the foot. Infection may also be acquired by drinking water containing the infective filariform larvæ, but it is doubtful if this occurs frequently under natural conditions.

When occasion arises, the filariform larvæ quickly penetrate the skin and enter the peripheral capillaries of the circulation and the lymphatics, and are thus passively carried to the lungs and collect in pulmonary arterioles and capillaries. They break through the alveolar tissue and enter the bronchioles and bronchi, during which time many reach adolescence. They then migrate up the trachea to the glottis, down the esophagus, through the stomach into the upper portions of the small intestine, where the females enter the mucosa, develop to maturity and deposit eggs. The eggs hatch within the tissues. The larvæ, rhabditiform, then migrate into the lumen of the intestine and most of them are carried to the exterior with the feces where they proceed to the free-living stages, the end-product of which is the infective, filariform larva. Some of the rhabditiform larvæ in the intestine may develop to the infective stage, reënter the circulation and establish superimposed infection.

According to Faust (1933), many of the worms remain in the alveolar tissues, a preferred site of the male, and there produce progeny to the filariform stage. A similar condition is reported to occur in the cystic duct. The lungs and the cystic duct are considered important sites for the origin of hyperinfective larvæ.

PATHOGENESIS

S. stercoralis was early believed to be a cause of diarrhea and dysentery. The presence of the worm deep in the intestinal mucosa may produce considerable irritation, especially when occurring in great number, and may intensify a diseased condition brought about by other causes. The intestinal lesions are caused entirely by the female parasite and her progeny. According to Faust (1933) male worms do not invade tissues. The parasites in the lungs may cause considerable hemorrhage and injury to the epithelium of the alveoli and bronchioles. The worms may be attacked and destroyed by a cellular response of the host. Prolonged chronic infections with *Strongyloides* are attributed to the presence of hyperinfective strains. The infective larvæ may produce a more or less severe cutaneous irritation at the site of their entrance to the host, but this irritation usually is unimportant. Diagnosis is based on the finding of characteristic larvæ in the feces.

TREATMENT

Strongyloides is difficult to expel from the host as the female usually lies buried in the mucosa and is thus protected against the vermicidal action of anthelmintics now used in the treatment of roundworm infections. Faust (1932) recommends gentian violet medicinal as a specific. Favorable results were obtained with this drug by Kouri and Sellek (1936) for strongyloidosis in seven patients. Arreza-Guzman (1937) reports unsatisfactory results with gentian violet in the treatment of strongyloidosis in experimentally infected rats. Doses producing toxic symptoms and death of the host failed to injure the worms in the intestine. Other drugs, including oil of chenopodium, thymol, tetrachlorethylene, pyrethrum and glycerine were found equally inefficient against this parasite.

Prevention. Measures used against hookworm infection are equally effective against *Strongyloides*. See page 435.

4. *Strongyloides of lower vertebrates*

Strongyloides canis Brumpt, 1922, was first described from dogs of the Orient by Fülleborn in 1914. This species also occurs in Oriental cats. Morphologically it is indistinguishable from *S. stercoralis,* and it, together with *S. nasua* Darling, 1911, from the coati, *Nasua* sp., are, according to Chandler (1925) varieties of *S. stercoralis.* *S. papillosus* (Wedl, 1856) Ransom, 1911, in sheep, goats, rabbits and antelope, *S. suis* von Linstow, 1905, in the pig, *S. simiæ* Hung See-Lu and Höppli, 1923, *S. fülleborni* von Linstow, 1905, from old world primates and *S. cebus* Darling, 1911, in *Cebus,* sp., are considered by Sandground (1925) and Goodey (1927) as distinct species, while Chandler (1925) regards them as subspecies of *S. papillosus. S. ratti* Sandground, 1925, is said to occur in about 60 per cent of rats caught on refuse dumps in Baltimore and may be a very common parasite of rats in the United States. *S. avium* Cram, 1929, occurs in the ceca of the fowl and turkey and *S. ransomi* Schwartz and Alicata, 1930, occurs in the small intestine of pigs.

CHAPTER XXVII

NEMATODE PARASITES (Continued)

Order *Strongyloidea* Weinland, 1858

The STRONGYLOIDEA consists entirely of parasitic nematodes, the males of which possess a conspicuous terminal or subterminal bursa copulatrix, supported generally by six paired main rays and one median unpaired dorsal ray with accessory branches. All the rays extend outwards from a common center. The esophagus is usually more or less clubshaped posteriorly, but without a definite spherical bulb and without a valvular apparatus.

This order is divided into seven families, according to Baylis and Daubney (1926), of which the STRONGYLIDÆ Baird, 1853, ANCYLOSTOMIDÆ (Looss, 1905) Lane, 1917, METASTRONGYLIDÆ Leiper, 1908, and TRICHOSTRONGYLIDÆ Leiper, 1912, are of particular interest in medical zoölogy.

I. Family STRONGYLIDÆ

This family is characterized by a well developed buccal capsule, the anterior margin of which is without teeth or cutting plates, but usually bears a corona radiata or leaf crown consisting of narrow, flattened leaf-like processes with pointed or rounded tips according to the species (Figure 194). Five subfamilies of STRONGYLIDÆ are recognized by Baylis and Daubney (1926).

1. SUBFAMILY *Strongylidæ* (Railliet, 1893

STRONGYLIDÆ with a relatively large buccal capsule which is more or less subspherical or infundibular. A dorsal gutter forms a ridge in the wall of the buccal capsule and extends nearly to its anterior margin. They are parasites of the alimentary tract of vertebrates. Examples: *Strongylus vulgaris* Looss (1900), *Triodontophorus serratus* Looss (1900) in equines.

2. SUBFAMILY *Trichoneminæ* Railliet, 1916

STRONGYLIDÆ with a cylindrical buccal capsule with relatively thick walls. The dorsal gutter is comparatively short and does not reach the anterior margin of the buccal capsule. There is no ventral cervical groove or cephalic vesicle. The TRICHONEMINÆ are para-sites of the alimentary tract of vertebrates. Examples: *Tichonema tetracanthum* (Looss, 1910), *Gyalocephalus capitatus* (Looss, 1910), in equines.

Strongylus vulgaris (Looss, 1900) and *S. equinus* Mueller, 1780, together with species of other closely related genera, *Triodontophorus* Looss, 1902, *Gyalocephalus* Looss, 1900 and *Trichonema Cobbold, 1874*, are perhaps the most important nematodes parasitic in horses and other EQUIDÆ. These strongyles are practically world-wide in distribution but occur most frequently in the warmer countries where conditions are most favorable for the development of the free-living stages. They often occur in mixed infections and in very great numbers.

The adults of the genera *Strongylus* and *Triodontophorus* are essentially blood suckers and are usually found firmly attached to the wall of the cecum or colon by the buccal armature producing lesions at the point of attachment. When occurring in great numbers they are associated with anemia which in turn is naturally associated with emaciation, edema and ascites. The adults of the genus *Trichonema,* however, are not blood suckers and do not adhere to the mucous membrane. They feed mainly upon the contents of the intestine of the host. According to Kotlán (1919) they may cause a hemorrhagic inflammation of the mucosa when occurring in great numbers.

They, like most other strongyles, have a direct life-cycle. The eggs are passed in the manure and subsequently give rise to an infective

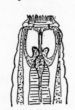

larval stage on the pasture land. About five days are required for the development of the infective larvæ. These larvæ retain the cuticula of the first and second ecdyses (Lucker, 1936). When these infective larvæ are ingested by the horse or other EQUIDÆ, they take different routes in the body and undergo somewhat different lines of development, according to the species involved.

FIG. 194.—Anterior extremity of *Strongylus vulgaris,* showing "leaf crown." (After Riley)

The infective larvæ of *Strongylus vulgaris* make their way to the posterior mesenteric artery where they set up an endarteritis resulting in the formation of an aneurysm. After a certain time in the aneurysm, the larvæ reach the cecum and become encysted in the submucosa where further development takes place. They finally pass to the lumen where they attach themselves to the mucosa and acquire the characters of the adult.

The aneurysms produced by the larval parasites are particularly dangerous as they may rupture causing the death of the host from hemorrhage, or fragments of the clot may break off forming emboli, which may obstruct the blood supply to a portion of the intestine and thereby cause a cessation of peristalsis. The contents of the affected portion undergo fermentation and the intestine then becomes distended with gas. Symptoms of colic may be evident. Occasionally the gas formation may cause a rupture of the intestine, stomach or diaphragm. As these aneurysms persist even after the worms have passed into the intestine, there remains a constant threat to the life and health of the host.

Treatment. According to Ransom and Hall (1920) the strongyles of the large intestine may be readily removed by fasting the animal for thirty-six hours and administering 4 to 5 drams of oil of chenopodium, immediately preceded or followed by a quart of linseed oil.

3. SUBFAMILY *Œsophagostominæ* Railliet, 1915

STRONGYLIDÆ with a cylindrical or large and subglobular buccal capsule and with a transverse, ventral cervical groove and a more or less pronounced cephalic vesicle. Parasites of the alimentary tract of mammals. Examples: *Œsophagostomum columbianum* in sheep and goats, *Œ. brumpti* in man, *Ternidens deminutus* in man and monkeys.

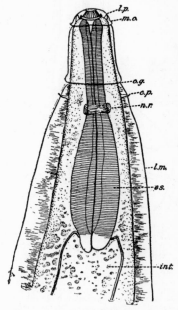

Fig. 195.—*Œsophagostomum columbianum.* Anterior end of the body. Ventral view. *c.g.*, cervical groove; *c.p.*, cervical papilla; *es.*, esophagus; *int.*, intestine; *l.m.*, lateral membrane; *l.p.*, lateral circumoral papilla; *m.c.*, mouth collar; *n.r.*, nerve ring (x 75). (After Ransom)

Œsophagostomum columbianum Curtice, 1890 (Figures 195 and 196), is commonly known as the "nodular worm" of sheep and goats. The female worms attain a length of about 15 mm. and the males about 14 mm. Both sexes have a characteristic solid white color and the head is bent over so as to form more or less of a hook with the body. The eggs measure from 65 μ to 75 μ in length and from 40 μ to 45 μ in width.

This species is very common in sheep in the United States, being especially prevalent in the Southern and Eastern States and less frequent in the Middle West. Its life history is similar to that of other strongyles. When the young worms are first found in the sheep they are encysted in the wall of the intestine. The nodules are most frequent in the Middle West. Its life history is similar to that of other strongyles. When the young worms are first found in the sheep they are encysted in the wall of the intestine. The nodules are most frequent in the wall of the cecum and large intestine but may also occur in the liver and other abdominal viscera. They are at first very small, but gradually increase in size, becoming filled with a mass of greenish caseous material. After the larva has undergone a certain amount of growth and development, it crawls out of the nodule and enters the lumen of the large intestine where it completes its development.

Nodular disease is more or less injurious according to the severity of the infection and the age and vitality of the individual. In severe cases diarrhea and emaciation may be excessive. Affected intestines, so-called "knotty guts," are unfit for sausage casings.

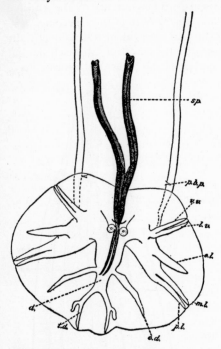

FIG. 196.—*Œsophagostomum columbianum.* Posterior end of body of male with bursa spread out. Ventral view. *d.*, dorsal ray; *e.d.*, externo-dorsal ray; *e.l.*, externo-lateral ray; *l.v.*, lateral-ventral ray; *m.l.*, medio-lateral ray; *p.b.p.*, pre-bursal papilla; *p.l.*, posterior-lateral ray; *sp.*, spicule; *t.d.*, terminal branch of dorsal ray; *v.v.*, ventro-ventral ray (x 75). (After Ransom)

Œsophagostomum radiatum (Rudolphi, 1803) occurs in cattle. The location of the nodules is more often in the small intestine than in the large intestine. *Œ. dentatum* (Rudolphi, 1803), *Œ. longicaudum* Goodey, 1925, and *Œ. brevicaudum* Schwartz and Alicata, 1930, are parasites of pigs. The nodules appear most frequently in the large intestine.

Several species of *Œsophagostomum,* which are natural parasites of monkeys and gorillas, have been reported in man. They are therefore accidental human parasites. Their presence in the cecum and large intestine causes tumors similar to those described under *Œ. columbianum. Œ. brumpti* Railliet and Henry, 1905, was discovered by Brumpt during an autopsy of a native of the River Omo (Lake Rudolph), East Africa, and again later after anthelmintic treatment to a Negress of New Guinea by Joyeux. *Œ. brumpti* also occurs in apes. *Œ. stephanostomum* var. *thomasi* Railliet and Henry, 1909, appears to be a fairly common parasite of man in certain parts of Brazil, and also occurs in the large intestine of the gorilla. *Œ. apiostomum* (Willach, 1891) is a natural parasite of monkeys and has been reported in man in Northern Nigeria.

Ternidens deminutus (Railliet and Henry, 1905) was first found in the large intestine of a Negro of the Comoro Islands. It also occurs in Asiatic monkeys. It is frequently encountered in natives and monkeys in Southern Rhodesia. Its life history is similar to that of other strongyles (Sandground, 1931).

4. SUBFAMILY *Stephanurinæ* Railliet, Henry and Bauche, 1919

STRONGYLIDÆ with a well developed, cup-shaped buccal capsule with a leaf crown at its anterior margin. The bursa of the male is subterminal and poorly developed, with stunted rays. They are parasites in the perirenal fat and kidneys, abdominal viscera and more rarely in the liver and lungs of mammals. Examples: *Stephanurus dentatus* Diesing, 1839, in the perirenal fat of pigs.

(1) STEPHANURUS DENTATUS Diesing, 1839. This species is generally known as the "kidney worm" of pigs and usually occurs in pus pockets in the fatty tissue surrounding the kidneys and along the ureters. The adult worms are lodged in cysts which communicate with the ureters and the eggs are thus discharged with the urine. Immature, or agamic forms, have been found in almost every tissue. They are a cause of heavy loss to swine raisers through the trimming of infected carcasses and the condemnations of "parasitic livers" at abattoirs. Immature forms are equally destructive to cattle livers. The parasite does not develop to sexual maturity in this host, however. The female is about 40 mm. long, the male 30 mm. Their bodies are stout, reddish in color and have a mottled appearance due to the folds of the intestine and reproductive organs which show through the more or less transparent cuticula. The eggs, obtained from urine of infected swine, measure about 95 μ in length and 65 μ in width and show advanced segmentation.

Life history. The development of the free-living stages of *Stephanurus dentatus* is similar to that of other strongyles. The infective stage is reached in about five or six days under favorable conditions of moisture and temperature. Moist, shaded areas of hog lots may teem with these larvæ, particularly about places where the hogs feed. They, like infective hookworm larvæ, are found on the top of the soil, in piles of corn husks, cobs and other debris. The host becomes infected either by ingesting these larvæ with food and water or by the larvæ penetrating the skin (Bernard and Bauche, 1914; Spindler, 1933). After entrance in the body, the young worms are carried about in the circulation and finally come to lodge in the liver where they slowly develop and increase in size. They wander extensively through the hepatic tissue for from one to three months and gradually reach the capsule through which they bore and enter the abdominal cavity, where they wander freely over the surfaces of the viscera. Some of the worms penetrate the peri-renal fat, perforate the ureter and discharge their eggs, which pass out with the urine. Others bore into the spleen, the pancreas, the wall of the stomach and the duodenum, diaphragm and other organs and become enclosed in a cyst. Only those which mature in the perirenal tissues and establish communication with the ureters can pass their eggs to the external world and thus complete the cycle of development.

Control. Spindler (1934) has found that the infective larvæ of *Stephanurus dentatus,* under pasture conditions, live about one month. They are readily killed by freezing, desiccation and exposure to sunlight. There is no appreciable active migration of the larvæ from the place of their development. Plowing infected areas immediately reduces the intensity of soil infection. Feeding pens, water barrels and farrowing houses should be located on well-drained, unshaded soil free from vegetation and debris.

5. SUBFAMILY *Syngaminæ* Baylis and Daubney, 1926

STRONGYLIDÆ with buccal capsule well developed, subglobular, without leaf crowns at its anterior margin but with teeth at its base. The eggs are operculate. The SYNGAMINÆ are parasites of the respiratory tract of birds and mammals. Examples: *Syngamus trachea* (Montagu, 1811) in fowl, *S. laryngeus* Railliet, 1899, in man.

(1) SYNGAMUS TRACHEA (Montagu, 1811). *Syngamus trachea* is a slender, red worm which is frequently found in the trachea and air passages of domestic fowl and wild birds. It is commonly known as the "gape worm" of chickens. The male measures from 2 mm. to 6 mm. and is permanently attached in copula to the female. The female measures from 5 mm. to 20 mm. in length. The eggs measure

about 85 μ in length by 50 μ in breadth and contain a developed embryo at the time they leave the host. They are further characterized by the presence of a roundish opening closed by a delicate membrane at each pole, through which the embryo makes its escape. The eggs may be swallowed by the infected bird and thus appear in the feces or they may also be present in the discharges which are coughed up by the bird. The eggs hatch in the open in about seven days. The newly escaped worm is a 3rd-stage or infective larva (Wehr, 1937). The birds become parasitized by ingesting the infective larvæ with food or drinking water. These larvæ penetrate the wall of the gullet and finally become established in the lungs where they grow to maturity. They occur most frequently near the division of the trachea into the bronchi. The eggs and larvæ may be swallowed accidentally by earthworms, snails and slugs. Taylor (1935) has observed that the larvæ retain their infectivity for the chick in earthworms from upwards of three years. These hosts are not necessary intermediate hosts. They are called "transport hosts."

The presence of the worms may produce a severe catarrh, and occasionally small abscesses are found at the site of attachment of the worm by their buccal capsule to the host. Usually from three to thirty worms are present.

The infected birds cough and shake their heads repeatedly in their efforts to expel masses of mucus and the worms. They frequently open their bills, hence the derivation of the name "gapes," and they have a whistling breath. Young chickens suffer most. Emaciation develops in spite of good appetite and death may be due to asphyxiation. Turkeys are susceptible to infection at any time of life but are little affected by the parasite. They serve as carriers of infection and are looked upon as the normal host of the gapeworm.

Treatment. The worms located in the upper portion of the trachea can often be extracted by the aid of long forceps. Intratracheal injections of about fifteen drops of a 5 per cent solution of salicylate of sodium are said to produce good results.

Prevention. Bodies of all dead birds and feces from poles and roosts should be burned, and sick birds separated from healthy ones. Feeding and drinking places should be kept clean. As *S. trachea* also occurs in a large number of wild birds, including pigeons, blue jays, swallows, starlings, crows, pheasants and partridges, those species frequenting chicken yards, especially crows and swallows, should be fenced out or destroyed. Chickens should be kept separated from turkeys.

Syngamus laryngeus Railliet, 1899, is a widespread parasite in the larynx of ruminants. It was discovered by Dr. King of St. Lucia in the sputum of a Negress suffering from a chronic cough and has since been observed in persons of Puerto Rico, Trinidad, the Philippines and Brazil. Its presence in man is accidental.

II. *Family Ancylostomidæ* (Looss, 1905) Lane, 1917

STRONGYLOIDEA with well developed buccal capsule bearing ventral teeth or cutting plates on its anterior margin. These nematodes are parasites of the alimentary tract in mammals. According to Baylis and Daubney (1926) this family contains two subfamilies, (1) ANCYLOSTOMINÆ (Looss, 1905) Stephens, 1916; and (2) NECATORINÆ Lane, 1917.

I. SUBFAMILY ANCYLOSTOMINÆ (Looss, 1905) Stephens, 1916

ANCYLOSTOMIDÆ with the anterior margin of the buccal capsule armed ventrally with from one to four pairs of teeth and with the mouth directed obliquely dorsally. Example: *Ancylostoma duodenale* Dubini, 1843, in man.

(1) ANCYLOSTOMA DUODENALE Dubini, 1843. *Historical. Ancylostoma duodenale,* or the so-called Old World hookworm of man, was not discovered until 1838, but there is much evidence that the disease caused by it has been of very long standing. Hippocrates, about B.C. 440, described a disease that might well be due to hookworms; those suffering from it ate stones and earth, had great intestinal disturbances and were jaundiced. The striking pallor of miners is also noted in the words of Lucretius and Lucan (B.C. 50 and A.D. 50), and it was believed that gold gave off evil exhalations which turned those digging for it the same color as the metal itself. Khalil (1922) believes the earliest valid record of Ancylostoma and ancylostomiasis was made in the Arabian "Laws of Medicine" dated 525 Hegira or A.D. 1131, by Avicenna. Roundworms were found high in the small intestine by Avicenna and it was noted that these worms were frequent in boyhood and adult life and diminished in old age. From 1611 to 1800 epidemics of a disease in Brazil were described under various names, such as anemia, dropsy, intestinal disturbances and weakness, all of which are symptoms which coincide with those of hookworm disease, and it was noted that it was particularly a cause of death among negro slaves.

Before the hookworm was finally discovered in man, a number of related species had been described from animals. Goeze in 1782 discovered roundworms in the intestine of a badger which he described as *Ascaris criniformis*. He noted a membranous expansion at the posterior end of the male with two rib-like structures which he called hooks. Froelich in 1789 found similar worms in the intestine of foxes, and because of the membranous expansion of the tail of the male and the so-called hooks, he called them "Haakenwürmer" or "hook-worms," and gave the name *Uncinaria* to the genus.

Hookworms in man were first discovered in 1838 by Angelo Dubini, an Italian physician, during an autopsy on a peasant woman who had died of pneumonia in a Milan hospital. But little attention was given to this discovery until four years later when Dubini discovered a second infection with these worms, which he named *Agchylostoma duodenale*. He found this parasite in 20 per cent of the cases examined and in some of these the worms were so numerous that he ascribed death to their presence in the absence of other lesions. Soon after Dubini's discovery, *Ancylostoma* was found in Egypt and it was associated with the extremely prevalent chlorosis in that country. Hookworms were found in 1866 by Wucherer in Brazil in the bodies of patients who had died of tropical anemia and subsequent observations by Brazilian physicians established that these parasites were the cause of a severe and widely prevalent disease.

In 1878 Grassi and Parona discovered that hookworm disease could be recognized from eggs passed in the feces, and from then on it became the custom to search for hookworm eggs in the feces of suspected cases.

As the disease was largely confined to tropical and subtropical regions it attracted but little attention among medical men in countries north of the Alps until 1880, when an epidemic of anemia developed among the laborers at the Saint Gotthard tunnel in Switzerland. Perroncito, an Italian scientist, recognized the parasitic nature of the so-called "tunnel-disease" and proved to those of opposite opinions that the anemia could be cured by vermifuges that expelled the worms. After the completion of this tunnel the laborers sought work in Central European mines and brick fields and carried the infection with them. The disease became most severe in the gold and silver mines of Hungary, in the coal mines of Germany, Holland, Belgium and France, in the lead mines of Spain, in the tin mines of England and in the sulphur mines of Sicily.

The exact method by which man becomes infected with *Ancylostoma* remained unknown until the close of the century. It was early believed that the larvæ could withstand great periods of desiccation and might be transported by air currents or in dust. It was also held that animals, especially the horse, were reservoir hosts and in some mentation, however, it became evident that domesticated animals are not carriers of *Ancylostoma duodenale* or *Necator americanus,* the important hookworms of man.

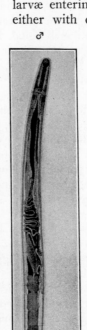

FIG. 197.—*Ancylostoma duodenale.* Male and female adults. (After Looss)

Leichtenstern and others showed experimentally that infection may result from infective larvæ entering the body by way of the mouth either with contaminated food or water. The usual mode of entrance was discovered, however, quite by accident. Looss, in 1898, during his studies on *Ancylostoma* in Egypt, spilled a hookworm culture on his hand and noticed that a dermatitis soon developed at that spot. Later he found hookworm ova in his feces and concluded that he had been infected through the skin. He then proved experimentally this theory of dermal infection and traced the migration of the larva from the time it enters the body until it finally becomes established in the small intestine, the habitat of the adult worm (Looss, 1911).

In 1902, Dr. Stiles described a new species of hookworm, *Necator americanus,* in man from the United States and Puerto Rico. Hookworms in the Americas had been observed much earlier (1888) in Brazil but they were not recognized as a distinct species. It was soon discovered that much of the anemia in certain southern states and Puerto Rico was due, not to malaria, but to this new species of hookworm (Ashford and Gutierrez, 1911) and sooner or later various State Boards of Health took active measures against it. The pioneer work of Stiles and others led to the creation of the Rockefeller Sanitary Commission in 1909 for the purpose of combating hookworm disease, and in 1915 the work of

mines of Hungary horse-haulage was discontinued. Through experi-
that organization was merged with that of the International Health
Board of the Rockefeller Foundation which has coöperated with
governments throughout the world in the fight against hookworm
disease as well as carrying on other public health activities.

Distribution and frequency. *Ancylostoma duodenale* occurs in
practically all countries which lie in the tropical and sub-tropical
zones, extending from parallel 36 degrees
north to parallel 30 degrees south. It is
dominant in Europe whence it is believed
to have been carried to Africa, Asia and
the Americas. It usually is found in mixed
infections with *Necator americanus,* commonly known as the New World hookworm, but occurs alone in Egypt. In the
United States *Ancylostoma duodenale* occurs only in miners and not among the
surface population.

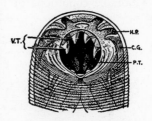

FIG. 198.—*Ancylostoma duodenale.* Showing hook-like central teeth. C.G., cephalic gland;
H.P., head papillæ; P.T., pharyngeal teeth; V.T., ventral
teeth (x 50). (From Manson-
Bahr's *Manson's Tropical Diseases.* After Looss)

Description. *Ancylostoma duodenale*
(Figures 197-199) is characterized by its
well developed buccal capsule with two
pairs of curved teeth on the ventral wall equal in size, and one pair
of dorsal teeth or triangular plates. The body of the living worm is
usually white or gray in color and occasionally the posterior two-
thirds is bright red due to fresh blood in the intestinal tract.

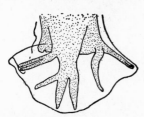

FIG. 199.—*Ancylostoma duodenale.* Side view of bursa. Enlarged. (Redrawn from Looss)

The males measure from 8 mm. to 11
mm. in length by 0.4 mm. to 0.5 mm. in
breadth. The dorsal ray in the bursa is
divided at its distal end into two smaller
rays, which in turn are again divided into
three unequal portions (Figure 199). The
female measures from 10 mm. to 13 mm.
in length by 0.6 mm. in breadth. The vulva
is situated near the posterior third of the
body. The eggs are elliptical in shape with
a transparent shell and when freshly de-
posited contain two or four and rarely eight blastomeres each. They
vary considerably in size, measuring from 56 μ to 60 μ in length by
34 μ to 40 μ in breadth. It is estimated that each female worm produces about 240 eggs per c.c. of formed feces (Augustine *et al.,*
1928).

Position in the host. The adult hookworms inhabit the small intestine where they fix themselves by the mouth to the mucosa. The length of life in the intestine is probably about five or six years. *A. duodenale* develops more or less completely in young dogs and cats, but these animals are unnatural hosts for this species and the worms soon die out.

Life-cycle. The eggs laid by the females pass out in the human feces onto the soil. The embryonic development is rapid and, under favorable conditions of temperature and moisture, the larvæ hatch

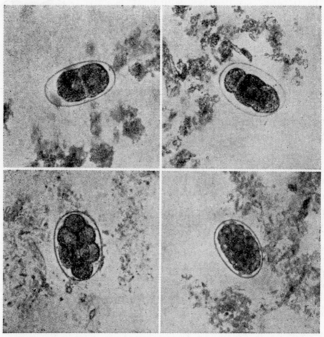

FIG. 200.—Hookworm eggs in different stages of development as found in feces (x 250). (From Todd's *Clinical Diagnosis*, W. B. Saunders Company)

out within about twenty-four hours. The newly hatched larvæ (Figure 201a) measure on the average 0.25 mm. in length and bear a close resemblance to the rhabditiform larvæ of *Strongyloides stercoralis,* but may be differentiated from the larvæ of the latter species by their longer and narrower buccal cavity. The young hookworm larvæ feed on the excrement in which they hatch, and food taken into the body is stored up within the cells of the intestinal tract. By the third day the larva has attained a length of about 0.4 mm. and undergoes its first molt. Growth then continues up to 0.5 mm. to 0.7 mm.

when the character of the esophagus changes and becomes slender and filariform in appearance. The second molt occurs at this time and the larva becomes the infective organism (Figure 201b). The old skin may either be retained or shed depending largely on the physical character of its immediate environment. Further growth and nutrition ceases unless this larva successfully enters its host.

The infective hookworm larvæ may be taken into the body with drinking water or contaminated food, but their usual method of entrance is by boring through the skin and entering the lymphatics or veins and they are then passively carried by the blood to the heart and thence to the lungs. They break out of the alveolar capillaries into the pulmonary alveoli and crawl up the bronchi and trachea and are finally swallowed. They then pass down the esophagus through the stomach to the intestine where they undergo a third molt within four or five days. The fourth or last molt occurs after about the thirteenth day, at which time the worm acquires its adult characteristics. Ova appear in the feces in from three to four weeks after infection.

Experimental studies with the dog hookworm, *Ancylostoma caninum* have shown that when infection occurs by mouth the larvæ usually do not migrate, but develop directly in the intestine (Foster and Cross, 1934).

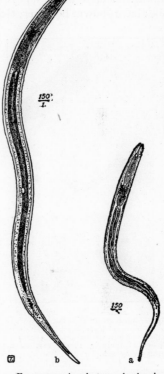

Fig. 201.—*Ancylostoma duodenale.* a, newly hatched or rhabditiform larva; b, mature or filariform larva, the infective stage. (From Manson-Bahr's *Manson's Tropical Diseases.* Partly after Looss)

Biology of the free-living stages. Very little accurate information was available on the life of the free-living stages of hookworms until Baerman (1917) devised a simple method by which nematodes could be isolated from considerable quantities of soil. With this apparatus it has been possible to study the activities of the developmental stages in their natural environments and to determine exact sources of human infection. The methods of counting helminth eggs in feces, as devised by Stoll (1923) and the Caldwells (1926) have placed experimental studies on the biology of the free-living stages on a quantitative basis. The following discussion is based largely on the researches of Cort and his associates carried on from 1921 to 1926 in the West Indies and China and of Chandler (1926-28) in India. In most instances these observations were made on *Necator americanus*. Comparative studies on *A. duodenale* and closely related species have shown, however, that the requirements for development and cies have shown, however, that the requirements for development and the habits of the free stages of this species are practically identical with those of *N. americanus*.

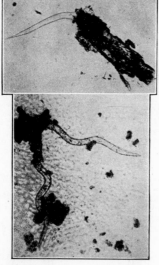

FIG. 202.—*Necator americanus.* Upper photograph showing sheath of a filariform larva cast when the larva penetrated vegetable débris; lower photograph, sheath cast in a sticky clay soil.

In all countries where hookworm is prevalent the people are more or less primitive and unaccustomed to sanitation. They habitually defecate on the surface of the ground, usually in an area which is in some way more or less protected from view, such as in coffee or banana groves, corners of cultivated fields, corners of houses and along the sides of roads or paths. In time certain of these places become well defined defecation areas. Hookworm eggs, as well as the later developmental stages, are not capable in themselves of leaving the area in which they were deposited by the host and, unless they are mechanically carried to other areas by outside forces, they develop at that spot to the infective stage, providing the physical conditions are favorable. Domesticated animals frequently are given a wide range and in one way or another may be factors in hookworm dissemination. Ackert and Payne (1921) demonstrated that when human stools containing hookworm eggs are eaten by pigs, the eggs pass through this animal unharmed and may subsequently develop into normal infective larvæ, but that a high proportion of the eggs devoured by chickens are destroyed, presumably by grinding in the gizzard. Chandler (1924) showed that hookworm eggs devoured by dogs and rats were uninjured by passage through the digestive tract of these animals. As these animals feed to a great extent on human feces in many tropical countries, they may be of considerable importance in the spread of hookworm eggs.

Conditions influencing the development of the larvæ. The temperature, moisture and the nature of the soil are the most important factors in the development of the hookworm larvæ. Temperature and moisture conditions of the tropical and subtropical countries are usually optimum for a greater or less portion of the year for hookworm development. The nature of the soil has an important influence on the degree of development and may be the determining factor, in the incidence and intensity of hookworm infection in areas otherwise favorable. Heavy clay soils are unsuitable for the development and survival of hookworm larvæ, whereas light, sandy or alluvial soils are favorable, and it is on such soil that hookworm in-

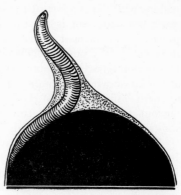

FIG. 203.—Diagramatic representation of an infective hookworm larva extending itself from a soil particle. Showing the aquatic nature of such larvae. (Redrawn from Payne)

fection is most frequent and most severe. Hookworm eggs do not develop under water, presumably on account of the exclusion of oxygen, and it is for this reason that the infection is light or absent in extensive rice producing areas (Cort *et al.,* 1926).

The position of hookworm larvæ in the soil. The first or rhabditiform larva is a feeding stage, and it is usually found near its supply of food, the feces of the host or decaying organic matter.

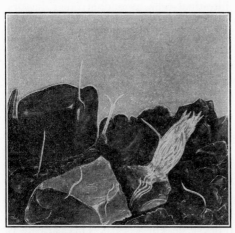

FIG. 204.—Characteristic positions of infective hookworm larvae on moist soil.

When it develops into the filariform or the infective larva it no longer feeds, and acquires tropisms which are characteristic of this stage. Its chief and only purpose is to carry the infection back to the host. The infective larvæ migrate in a vertical plane to the very top soil particles from which they extend themselves, singly or in polyp-like masses with the support of the surface film of soil water (Figures 203, 204). So dominant is the upward movement that the larvæ remain practically at the spot where the infected feces were deposited, unless disseminated by outside agencies, animals, or washing rains; and for this reason a particular spot may contain thousands of infective hookworm larvæ whereas another spot one foot away may be entirely free of them. This position of the infective larvæ in the soil is most advantageous to them in their transfer to the naked foot of man as he walks on the infected ground.

The infective larvæ are markedly thermotropic, and when transferred to the naked foot or other exposed parts of the body, their activity is greatly aroused and almost immediately they begin boring into the skin. Entrance is usually made by way of the hair follicles, but they can bore into any part of the skin as well. Damp soil clinging to the feet is an aid to the larvæ in penetrating the skin, for it not only keeps them moist but also helps keep the larvæ tight against the skin.

Length of life of infective hookworm larvæ. Unless the infective larva successfully enters man its length of life is limited by the supply of food stored in its intestinal cells, providing other factors are favorable. In water, under laboratory conditions, they have been kept alive for as long as eighteen months (Nicoll, 1917; Ackert, 1924). In the soil, however, under natural conditions, frequent droughts, changing temperatures, heavy rains, natural enemies such as bacteria, protozoa and fungi are continually acting upon the larvæ and their numbers become greatly reduced within a short time. A few of a given lot may survive for several months, but it is doubtful if these have sufficient vitality to gain entrance to their host when such an opportunity presents itself (Ackert, 1924). The death-rate of a given lot of larvæ is always greatest within the first ten days. The unsheathed forms are less resistant to adverse conditions and are the first to succumb.

Hookworm disease, treatment and prevention. See pages 431 to 438.

(2) ANCYLOSTOMA BRAZILIENSE de Faria, 1910. This parasite is commonly found in certain wild and domestic animals, particularly dogs and cats in various countries including the southern United States, Brazil, the Federated Malay States, the Philippine Islands and the Fiji Islands. It has been found, in the adult stage, in man of the Orient. Its infective larval stage has been discovered to be the

cause of a "creeping eruption" in man in Florida by White and Dove (1928) see page 437). This species is smaller than *A. duodenale* and the internal pair of ventral teeth are much smaller than the corresponding teeth of *A. duodenale*. The outer cusps are large and end in a very sharp point. The egg is not distinguishable from those of other hookworms in man.

(3) ANCYLOSTOMA CANINUM Ercolani, 1859. This species is common and practically cosmopolitan in the dog and cat. It is particularly frequent in young animals. It is about the same size as *A. duodenale* but has three pairs of teeth on the ventral surface of the buccal capsule, whereas *A. duodenale* has two pairs. Prenatal infections are not unusual. In prenatal ancylostomiasis, as in prenatal arcariasis, the larvæ re-

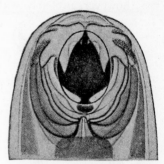

FIG. 205.—*Ancylostoma braziliense.* Showing characteristics of mouth parts. (After Looss)

main in the organs until after parturition (Foster, 1932). Puppies born to resistant mothers are markedly susceptible to infection. *A. caninum* is the cause of a serious disease in these animals and in some parts of this country it is responsible for the death of from 25 per cent to 40 per cent of the puppies born (Stiles, 1903). It has been observed by Wells (1931) that a single worm may remove at least 0.84 cm. of blood daily from its host. The daily loss of blood may be great, particularly in heavy infections. *A. caninum* is also a cause of "creeping eruption" in man.

2. SUBFAMILY *Necatorinæ* Lane, 1917

ANCYLOSTOMIDÆ with the anterior margin of the buccal capsule usually bearing ventral cutting plates but without teeth. The mouth is directed antero-dorsally. Example: *Necator americanus* in man.

(1) NECATOR AMERICANUS (Stiles, 1902). *Historical. Necator americanus* is commonly termed the "New World hookworm" but is perhaps as much an "Old World" species as *Ancylostoma duodenale*. It was probably introduced into America from Africa by slaves. The disease in the United States caused by this species was long recognized before the worm itself was discovered. Pitt in 1808 ascribed dirt-eating and anemia (now recognized symptoms of hookworm disease) then prevalent among the lower class white and Negro population of the southern United States to deficiency in nourish-

ment. Similar symptoms were described in slaves in Jamaica by Thomas in 1820.

The first reported case of hookworm disease in the United States is that of Blickhahn (1893) of St. Louis. The infection in this case was, however, probably with *Ancylostoma duodenale* as the patient was a brickmaker from Westphalia. Soon endemic cases were noted, especially in Texas. From 1896 on an increasing number of cases were reported and it was noted that the infections were with a heretofore undescribed species of hookworm.

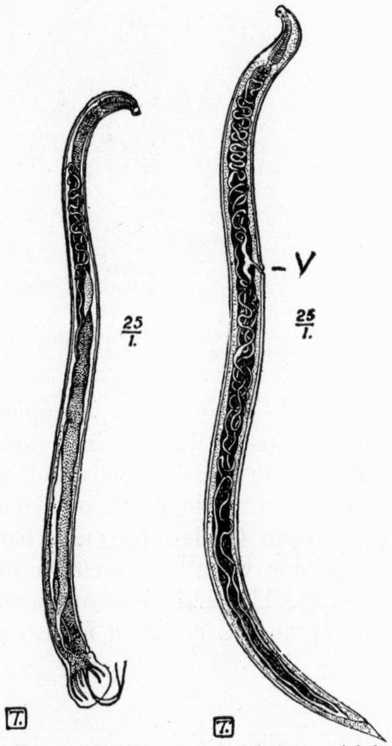

FIG. 206.—*Necator americanus.* Adult male and female. V, vulva. (From Manson-Bahr's *Manson's Tropical Diseases.* After Placencia)

This species was described as *Uncinaria americana* by Stiles in 1902, from material received from A. J. Smith and T. A. Claytor in the United States and from Ashford in Puerto Rico. Stiles showed that this parasite was widely distributed throughout the Southern States and pointed out the great burden of hookworm disease on a large part of the southern population. Ashford in 1899 (Ashford and Gutierrez, 1911) recognized these worms as a cause of anemia in Puerto Rico but thought the species was *Ancylostoma duodenale*. It will be recalled that hookworms and hookworm disease had also been noted much earlier in Brazil, but a species difference was not observed.

Distribution and frequency. Necator americanus, like *A. duodenale,* is largely confined to the tropical and subtropical world. It is frequently found in mixed infections with *Ancylostoma.* It is particularly prevalent in Southern North America, Central and South America and throughout the West Indies. It is the only adult hookworm thus far known to occur in man in the southern United States and, according to Chandler (1928), it is about the only hookworm of man in southern India.

N. americanus, like *A. duodenale,* is typically a parasite of rural populations where little or no sanitation exists, and where temperature, moisture and soil conditions favor the development of the free-living stages of the parasite. In the United States this species is of economic importance only in the South and Eastern sandy coastal plains and in bordering mountain districts where soil conditions are favorable for larval hookworms. Due to the extensive and persistent control campaigns of the Rockefeller Foundation and State Health Departments, the incidence of hookworm infection and the prevalence of hookworm disease have been greatly reduced. In 1903 hookworm disease was considered the commonest of the severe diseases of the South. Today, the extreme case is rare. There are, however, sections of the area where sanitation is still inadequate, and here hookworm remains a major public health problem.

There is a marked difference in the intensity of hookworm infection in white and black races in the southern United States where the two races live side by side on adjoining farms, under very similar economic and sanitary conditions. The infection is generally more frequent and more severe in the white race. While there is as yet no satisfactory explanation for the much lighter infections in the Negro it may be due to physical differences in the two races, namely the much greater thickness of the epidermis of the Negro which makes more difficult the entrance of infective larvæ, or perhaps to a racial

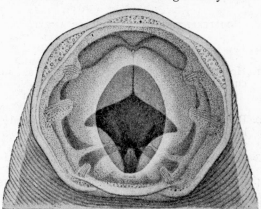

Fig. 207.—*Necator americanus*. Showing cutting plates and the dorsal ridge, and deep in the cavity the edges of the ventral lancets. Enlarged. (After Looss)

immunity possessed by the black but not by the white race. This question should be further investigated.

According to Stoll (1923) a female *Necator* produces about 9,000 eggs per day, or about forty-four eggs per gram of formed feces. It is generally believed that the average length of life of the adult *Necator* in the intestine is from four to five years.

Morphology. The mouth capsule of *Necator americanus* (Figure 207) is smaller than that of *A. duodenale* and the two pairs of curved

ventral teeth characteristic of the latter species are replaced by a pair
of ventral cutting plates. *N. americanus* is also smaller than *A. duo-denale*. It is white to grayish-yellow in color

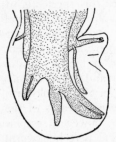

and commonly shows blood in the intestine. The
male measures from 7 mm. to 9 mm. in length
and is about 0.3 mm. in diameter. The dorsal
ray of the bursa copulatrix is divided at its
base and each branch is bipartite at the tip instead of tripartite as in *A. duodenale* (Figure
208). The female measures from 9 mm. to 12
mm. in length and from 0.3 mm. to 0.4 mm. in
diameter. The vulva is located anterior to the
middle of the body. The eggs are practically indistinguishable from those of *A. duodenale*
(Figure 200). The main points of difference in
morphology between *A. duodenale* and *N. americanus* are given in the
accompanying table.

FIG. 208.—*Necator americanus*. Side view of bursa. (Redrawn from Looss)

DIFFERENTIAL CHARACTERS OF ANCYLOSTOMA DUODENALE AND
NECATOR AMERICANUS

A. duodenale	*N. americanus*
1. Head continues in same general curve of body	1. Head turned contrary to general curve of body, giving a perma-nent hooked appearance to an-terior end of the worm
2. Buccal capsule with two pairs of hook-like teeth, about equal in size	2. Buccal capsule without teeth but with one pair of cutting plates
3. Vulva posterior to middle of body	3. Vulva anterior to middle of body
4. Small spine at posterior extrem-ity of female	4. No spine at posterior extremity of female
5. Bursa copulatrix fan-shaped	5. Bursa copulatrix more rounded
6. Dorsal ray of bursa tripartite	6. Dorsal ray of bursa bipartite
7. Larger than *Necator*	7. Smaller than *Ancylostoma*

Life-cycle. Shortly after the discovery that the hookworm in
America was a new species, investigations were undertaken on its
life history and on the disease caused by it. Claude A. Smith repeated
Looss' experiments on *A. duodenale* with *N. americanus* and found
that infection resulted from skin penetration. Detailed clinical studies
were made by Ashford (1911) and his co-workers in Puerto Rico.
The more recent investigations on the biology of the free-living stages
and epidemiological studies include those of Cort, Ackert, Payne,

Smillie, Stoll, Chandler and Augustine which have been discussed
under the life-cycle of *A. duodenale*.

Hookworm disease. The hookworms feed particularly upon the
tissues of the host, and, in tearing bits of the mucosa from the
intestine by their powerful mouth parts, produce small hemorrhages
at the site of injury (Figures 209, 210). The bleeding is maintained
by the deposition in the wounds of a secretion by the hookworms

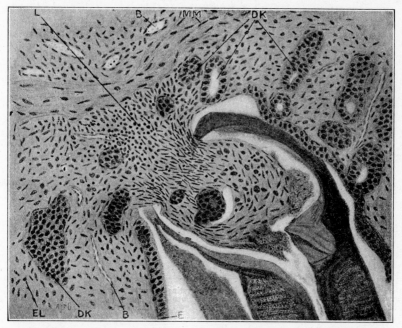

FIG. 209.—A sagittal section of the head end of a hookworm, *Ancylostoma duodenale*,
grasping a piece of mucous membrane, L; EL, eosinophile leucocytes; DK, intestinal
glands; B, blood vessels; E, epithelial cells. Enlarged. (After Oudendal)

which inhibits the coagulation of the blood. And as the worms change
their position again and again and when there are thousands present,
the loss of blood from the intestines may be considerable. It is generally held that the severe anemia in hookworm disease is a complex
result of such chronic blood loss (Rhoads *et al.*, 1934; Foster and
Landsberg, 1934; Pena and Rotter, 1935; Lane, 1937).

A severe hookworm dermatitis frequently results when the infective larvæ pass through the skin which is locally known as ground
itch, mazamorra, water sores or sore feet of coolies. This dermatitis
is most frequent in the rainy season in the tropics and during the

spring and autumn months in the southern United States where moisture and temperature conditions are at the optimum for larval development. It occurs most frequently on the feet, particularly between
the toes, for it is these parts which are constantly exposed to the
larva-laden earth. Vesiculation and pustulation or even ulceration
often result which may persist for several weeks.

Symptoms. Hookworm disease is characterized by a more or less
severe anemia and faulty development. The skin takes on a light

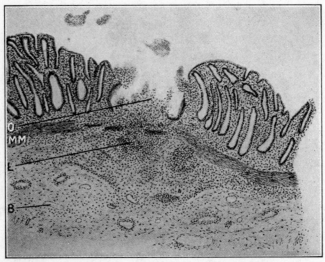

Fig. 210.—Diagonally cut section of the intestine showing an ulcer caused by *Ancylostoma duodenale.* U, ulcer; MM, muscularis mucosæ; L. lymphocytes; B, blood vessels.
Enlarged. (After Oudendal)

orange-yellow coloring which first arises in the temples and later on
extends over the whole body. The patient has a typical apathetic
expression (Figure 211), and is often undersized, with dry skin,
scanty hair, edema of the face and legs, shortness of breath and
weakness and with mental development retarded.

All individuals having hookworm ova in their feces do not, however, show characteristic symptoms. This is in part due to differences
in individual resistance and to the number of worms harbored. As
shown by Smillie and Augustine (1926) children with twenty-five
Necator americanus show no measurable injuries and are apparently
as healthy and alert as individuals free from hookworms and therefore may be regarded as carriers. Children with from twenty-six to
100 hookworms, *N. americanus,* show no variation from the normal

in rate of growth in weight and height but may have slightly lowered hemoglobin and slight mental retardation. Many individuals in this group are borderline cases and may be classed among those with mild hookworm disease. Children with more than 100 hookworms, *N. americanus,* however, usually show marked retardation in normal growth in height and weight, a more or less severe anemia, and may show a marked degree of mental retardation (Smillie and Spencer, 1926). This group is regarded as having true hookworm disease. It

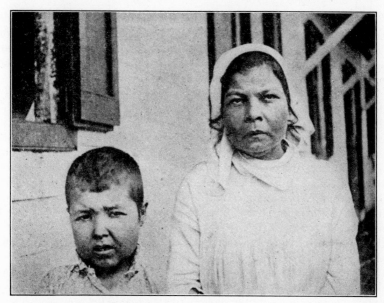

FIG. 211.—Typical facial expression of individuals suffering from hookworm disease. (From Ashford and Guiterrez)

is generally believed that *A. duodenale* is more malignant than *N. americanus* and that relatively few worms of the former species may cause a definitely diseased condition.

Diagnosis. The diagnosis is made by finding the eggs of the parasite in the feces. However, the eggs of the various hookworms are almost indistinguishable from each other, and hence the identification of the species present must be made upon the adult worms, usually obtained after vermicidal treatment.

A number of methods have been devised for a rapid detection of hookworm eggs. Of these, Willis' method (Willis, 1921) is the easiest to follow and is one of the most accurate of the simpler methods.

Willis' method. By this method a small amount of feces, about 1 to 2 grams, is thoroughly mixed with concentrated salt solution. The container is then filled to the brim with the salt solution and a clean, grease-free glass slide of such size that it will more than cover the container used, is placed thereon and allowed to stand for several minutes. The slide is then carefully removed, inverted and examined under the low power of the microscope. Care must be taken in removing and inverting the slide so that none of the adhering brine is lost.

Willis' method is likewise effective in detecting most nematode and cestode eggs discharged with the feces but cannot be used for concentrating operculate eggs of trematodes and cestodes. Operculate eggs burst in the salt solution and do not rise to the surface of the preparation.

The direct centrifugal flotation or D.C.F. method of Lane, fully described by him (1932), is without question the most certain of the direct methods for detecting light infections. One c.cm. of feces is used. After centrifugation in water, the residue is thoroughly agitated in concentrated salt solution. The eggs, if present, are thus brought to the surface, and a cover-glass is placed upon the mouth of the tube between four special metal horns surrounding the centrifuge guard. The tubes are then again centrifuged and the glass cover slide examined as a "hanging drop" preparation under the low power of a microscope for eggs. It is advisable to have the special instruments, centrifuge, tubes, etc. described by Lane when this method is in constant use.

The method of Stoll (1923) and Stoll and Hausheer (1926) was devised for counting hookworm eggs. It has been used extensively in experimental studies on the biology of the free-living stages of hookworms and to evaluate control measures. The steps in Stoll's technic are as follows:

(1) Weigh by difference 3 grams of the feces into a large-sized tube or centrifuge tube graduated at 45 c.c.

(2) Add decinormal sodium hydroxide to the 45 c.c. level.

(3) Add ten small (3 mm.) glass beads, close with a rubber stopper and shake vigorously until a homogeneous suspension is obtained.

(4) Immediately transfer 0.15 c.c. of the suspension to the center of a 2 x 3 inch slide and cover with a 22 x 40 mm. No. 2 cover-slip.

(5) Count all the ova in the slide preparation with aid of a mechanical stage and a low power of the microscope. The number of ova found, multiplied by 100, represents the number of ova per gram of feces used.

Since the original method was devised, Stoll has made certain improvements in the technic which facilitate its operation. Special

Pyrex Erlenmeyer flasks with marks at the 56 c.c. and 60 c.c. levels are used instead of test-tubes graduated at 45 c.c. The quantity of feces is also measured by displacement instead of weighing. The flasks are first filled with decinormal sodium hydroxide to the lower 56 c.c. mark and the feces are added until the diluent level reaches the upper 60 c.c. level. Samples of 0.075 c.c. are withdrawn from the suspension for the count instead of 0.15 c.c. as formerly employed and a 25 mm. square cover-slip is used instead of the 22 x 40 mm. size. The average of two such counts is multiplied by 200 (rather than 100 as originally planned) to secure the number of ova per cubic

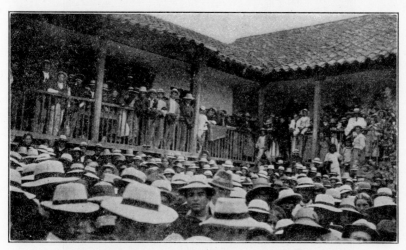

Fig. 212.—Group assembled to hear a public health lecture and receive treatment for hookworm disease, Colombia, S. A. (Photograph by permission of the Rockefeller Foundation)

centimeter, or the sum of two such counts may be multiplied by 100 to arrive at the same number. Other requirements in the original technic are not modified, such as thorough comminution of the specimen and adequate shaking before withdrawing the amount to be examined. This method has been found to yield average counts correct within less than 10 per cent of the absolute number of ova present in the fecal specimens.

Treatment. Thymol was tried by Bozzolo in 1879 as a vermifuge for hookworm anemia among the bricklayers in northern Italy and has since been used extensively for this purpose (Lane, 1936). However, it has been almost replaced by oil of chenopodium or ascaridol, tetrachlorethylene and hexylresorcinol.

Prevention. Since the spread of hookworm disease is due entirely to neglect of sanitation, its prevention and control requires the installation of adequate latrine accommodations and the habitual use of them by the people who are to be directly benefited. Anthelmintic treatment relieves immediate suffering, but without sanitation reinfection occurs and the benefit from the anthelmintic is only transient.

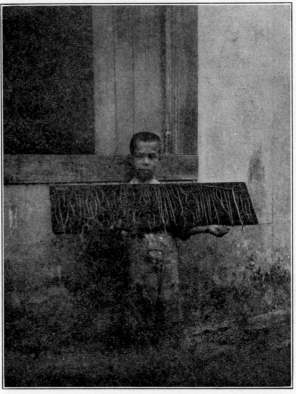

FIG. 213.—Besides getting rid of his hookworms this boy also became free of his ascarids after one treatment with oil of chenopodium. (Photograph by permission of the Rockefeller Foundation)

Proper disposal of human feces and the education of the people as to the mode of transmission are the chief measures of permanent control of hookworm infection.

It was formerly thought that infection might commonly result from water or food contamination with infective larvæ but these are now known to be unimportant sources of infection, and it is highly probable that each parasite in the intestine has entered through the skin. Therefore shoes, even though of crude design, are more or less effective in preventing the entrance of the larvæ. Smillie (1922) found that the hookworm infection in the native, unshod workers of the Brazilian coffee estates was about nine times heavier than that in the Spanish colonists, who, although they worked side by side with the natives, always wore shoes of crude design. In the Southern United States hookworm infection is most frequent and usually heaviest in rural children up to about fourteen years of age. At this time constant wearing of shoes begins. From then on little or no hookworm infection is acquired, and the old parasites gradually die (Smillie and Augustine, 1925). This single factor of wearing shoes is, in all probability, largely responsible for the absence of heavy hookworm infection in rural adults of the Southern United States.

Creeping Eruption. The names creeping eruption, dermatitis linearis migrans and creeping disease have generally been associated with skin lesions caused by various fly larvæ and by a nematode, *Gnasthostoma spinigerum.* Kirby-Smith, Dove and White (1926) and Dove and White (1926) demonstrated that this disease may be caused also by the infective larvæ of *Ancylostoma braziliense* and *A. caninum,* frequent parasites of dogs and cats. The eruption is exceedingly prevalent in the Southern United States, especially in Florida. It is characterized by a linear, tortuous and serpiginous eruption due to the larva migrating within the skin and is accompanied by intense itching. The most recent lesion caused by the worm is indicated by a very narrow reddish line which later becomes slightly raised and palpable. The surface then becomes dry and a thin crust is formed. According to Kirby-Smith and others (1926) the parasite may travel from a fraction of an inch to several inches a day, advancing as a rule more rapidly at night. Scratching to alleviate the itching often results in bacterial infections and raw surfaces. About 50 per cent of the cases seen by Dr. Kirby-Smith are believed to have originated at the beach at points above the high tide water mark. Several cases definitely attributed the origin of their infection to contact with damp sand when they were wet with perspiration and while working in the sand in repairing automobiles or making plumbing connections underneath houses. Creeping eruption most frequently occurs during the summer months following periods of rainy weather, which is to be expected in view of our knowledge of the development of the free-living stages of the hookworms. The infection may persist for a very long time; Fülleborn (1926) has reported one case of twenty years' duration.

Ethyl acetate applied on cotton or gauze or used in a flexible collodion has been found effective in many cases, as well as refrigeration with ethyl chloride, carbon dioxide snow or crushed ice with salt. Dakin's solution (chlorinated soda) may be employed for the secondary infections which are frequently associated with creeping eruption.

Prophylactic measures taken against "ground itch" are equally effective against creeping eruption. As these hookworms are natural parasites of dogs and cats, frequent anthelmintic medication of these animals would greatly reduce soil infection and thereby render less likely the infection in man. All stray dogs and cats should be disposed of.

(2) NECATOR SUILLUS Ackert and Payne, 1922. This species was discovered in pigs of Trinidad, B. W. I., where over 89 per cent of these animals are said to be infected. Morphologically it is quite similar to *N. americanus,* but cross infection experiments carried on by Ackert and Payne (1922) indicate that *N. suillus* is a distinct species.

(3) BUNOSTOMUM TRIGONOCEPHALUM Rudolphi, 1808. This hookworm is a frequent parasite in the small intestine of sheep and goats in Europe and the Southern United States. The male is from 12 mm. to 17 mm. in length and the female is from 19 mm. to 26 mm. in length. A closely related species, *B. phlebotomum* Railliet, 1902, occurs in cattle and has been associated with the so-called "salt sickness" of Florida. This disease is characterized at first by low fever, loss of appetite and progressive emaciation and anemia.

(4) UNCINARIA POLARIS Looss, 1911. *Uncinaria polaris* appears to be a fairly frequent parasite of foxes in North America and may prove to be of considerable economic importance in the fox-raising industry. The male measures about 8 mm. and the female about 11 mm. in length. *U. criniformis* (Rud. 1809) or *U. stenocephala* Railliet, 1884, is a somewhat smaller species which has been repeatedly noted in European foxes and dogs. Apparently, this latter species does not exist in this country. Oil of chenopodium is, according to Riley and Fitch (1921) the preferred drug in the treatment of foxes for hookworms.

III. Family METASTRONGYLIDÆ

STRONGYLOIDEA with the buccal capsule much reduced or absent. The bursa of the male may be relatively well developed or vestigial with more or less typical rays. The METASTRONGYLIDÆ are parasites

of the respiratory and circulatory systems of mammals. Examples:
Dictyocaulus filaria in sheep and goats, and *Metastrongylus apri* in
the pig.

I. DICTYOCAULUS FILARIA (Rudolphi, 1809)

Description. Dictyocaulus filaria (Figure 214) is commonly
known as the "thread lung worm" and is found in the air passages,
bronchi and bronchioles of the lungs of sheep, goats, cattle and other
ruminants. *D. filaria* is widely distributed over the
world and is fairly common in the United States,
especially in our Southern States where climatic
conditions are more favorable for the development of the free stages. Early development takes
place in the mesenteric lymph glands. The immature worms enter the circulation and finally become concentrated in the lungs where they break
out of the capillaries and continue their development in the air passages. Prenatal infection may
occur. It is a rather long worm, the male measuring from 3 cm. to 8 cm. and the female from 5
cm. to 10 cm. in length. The intestine shows as a
dark hair-line throughout the length of the worm.
The eggs are elliptical and vary from 112 μ to
135 μ in length by 52 μ to 67 μ in breadth and
contain a fully developed embryo at the time they
leave the female worm.

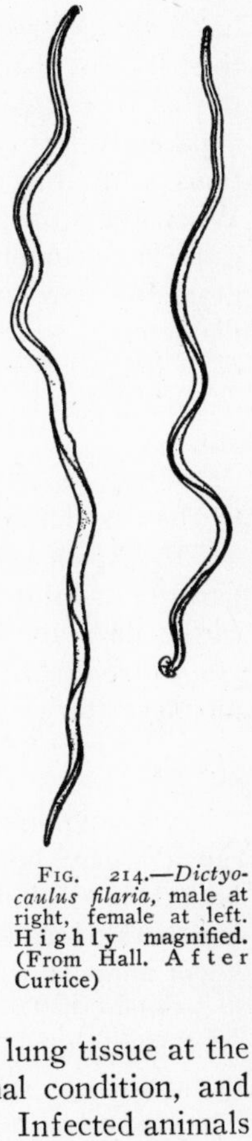

Life-cycle. The eggs hatch in the lung of the
host and the first larvæ leave the lungs by way of
the trachea and get onto the pasture either in the
saliva or in the feces. This larva molts twice within a short time, according to temperature and
moisture conditions, and in about ten days it is in
the infective stage. The infective larva crawls up
grass blades when they are wet and is then taken
in by grazing sheep or cattle.

FIG. 214.—*Dictyo-
caulus filaria,* male at
right, female at left.
H i g h l y magnified.
(From Hall. A f t e r
Curtice)

Pathogenesis. The presence of the worms and
their eggs and larvæ may set up an irritation of the lung tissue at the
point at which they are located causing a catarrhal condition, and
bacterial infection of the weakened lung may follow. Infected animals
usually show larvæ in saliva taken from the back of the tongue or
from the pharynx.

Dictyocaulus viviparous (Bloch, 1782) is a cosmopolitan parasite in the lungs of cattle and deer. *D. arnfieldi* (Cobbold, 1884) is parasitic in bronchi of horses and other EQUIDÆ.

Prevention. Segregation of infected animals and pasture rotation are of value. Moist pastures should be avoided.

2. PROTOSTRONGYLUS RUFESCENS (Leuckart, 1865)

This species occurs in the small bronchioles and in the lung tissue of sheep, goats and rabbits and is commonly termed the "hair lung worm." It is a smaller worm than *Dictyocaulus filaria* and the body has a characteristic brownish-red color, due to the color of the intestine. Its life history is not definitely known, but it is probably similar to that of *D. filaria*. The hair lung worm is widely distributed but is apparently less common in the United States than *D. filaria*. Infections with this species may terminate in a verminous pneumonia. When the worms are aggregated in the pneumonic areas they may cause a pneumonia with areas resembling tubercles. These show as grayish-yellow tumors from a few millimeters to two centimeters in diameter in which are the reddish worms, eggs and embryos. Secondary bacterial infections sometimes occur.

3. METASTRONGYLIDS OF OTHER ANIMALS

Ælurostrongylus abstrusus Railliet, 1898, is parasitic in the lungs of the cat. The mouse is a required intermediate host.

Metastrongylus elongatus (Dujardin, 1845) is a fairly common parasite of bronchi of pigs and wild boars and occurs rarely in sheep, cattle, deer and man. The infective stage develops in earthworms. *Angiostrongylus vasorum* (Railliet, 1866) occurs in the heart, pulmonary arteries and in the eyes of the dog.

IV. Family TRICHOSTRONGYLIDÆ

STRONGYLOIDEA with a rudimentary buccal capsule, or the buccal capsule may be absent. The bursa copulatrix has well developed lateral lobes but the dorsal lobe is small or rudimentary. The members of TRICHOSTRONGYLIDÆ are for the most part parasites of lower animals, ruminants and herbivores, and their occurrence in man is accidental.

This family includes two subfamilies: (1) The TRICHOSTRONGY-LINÆ Leiper, 1908, and (2) the HELIGMOSOMINÆ Travassos, 1914. The members of HELIGMOSOMINÆ are of no economical importance, and are, for the most part, parasites of rodents. They are slender forms with the buccal capsule absent or rudimentary and the female reproductive system consists of a single tube. The vulva is situated close to the anus. As far as we know their development is direct and similar to that of the hookworms. *Nippostrongylus muris* Yokogawa, 1920, in wild rats of the United States is a representative species. This species is readily obtainable for laboratory study.

The TRICHOSTRONGYLINÆ differ from the HELIGMOSOMINÆ in that the female genital tubes are paired. The vulva is situated toward the posterior end of the body. The development is probably direct in all species.

1. HÆMONCHUS CONTORTUS (Rudolphi, 1803)

Description. A number of strongyles are parasites in the abomasum, the fourth or digestive stomach and in the duodenum of ruminants. Certain of these species are of considerable economic importance, particularly *Hæmonchus contortus.* This parasite is whitish or of a reddish color which is attributed by most authors to blood which it has sucked up. Two lateral, spine-like papillæ are situated near the anterior end of the body. The male is from 1 cm. to 2 cm. in length and the bursa copulatrix consists of two long lobes and an asymmetrical dorsal lobe. The female is from 2 cm. to 3 cm. in length and has a spiral striping. The vulva is situated in the posterior fifth of the body and is marked by a more or less prominent linguiform process which projects backward. The eggs are elongated, oval and measure from 75 μ to 95 μ in length by 40 μ to 50 μ in breadth and are segmenting when deposited.

Life-cycle. The development is direct. The infective stage is a sheathed larva. It crawls up wet grass blades and here becomes ingested by grazing sheep and cattle. They are highly resistant forms and can withstand severe cold and long periods of dryness. The eggs and first larvæ are, however, less resistant.

Distribution. H. contortus is world-wide in distribution, occurring wherever there are sheep, cattle or other suitable host animals. It has been reported as a parasite of man in Brazil and Australia.

Pathogenesis. This species is very injurious to young sheep, especially when occurring in large numbers. It evidently feeds uoon the blood of its host, attacking the mucous membrane of the abomasum. The infected animals become dull and anemic showing emaciation and irregularities of digestion. Diarrhea may be present.

The genus *Trichostrongylus* Looss, 1905, contains several species which are common and important parasites in the small intestine of sheep and cattle, and rarely in man. *T. probolurus* (Railliet, 1896) ; *T. colubriformis* (Gilles, 1892) ; and *T. vitrinus* (Looss, 1905) occur in sheep and goats and have been reported in man. *T. orientalis*

Jimbo, 1914, occurs as a parasite of man in Japan, Korea, and Formosa. *T. extenuatus* (Railliet, 1898) is a common and widely distributed parasite of ruminants in the United States and is considered by some authors to be a cause of gastro-enteritis in calves. *T. capricola* Ransom, 1907, occurs in goats and sheep of the United States and is apparently more frequent in these animals than *T. extenuatus*. Also of common occurrence are several species of the genera Ostertagia Ransom, 1907, and Cooperia Ransom, 1907. *Obeliscoides cuniculi* Graybill, 1923, is common in domestic and wild rabbits of the United States. It produces ulceration of the stomach wall.

2. NEMATODIRUS FILICOLLIS (Rudolphi, 1802)

The nematodes of the genus *Nematodirus* are commonly termed the "thread-necked strongyles" on account of the anterior portion of the body being more slender than the posterior. They are found in the small intestine of sheep and cattle. *N. filicollis* occurs in the small intestine of sheep, cattle, goats and other ruminants and is of rather common occurrence in the United States but usually not in large numbers. It therefore probably does not seriously affect its host. Attention is again called to the fact that the infective larva of *N. filicollis* develops within the egg before hatching, thus differing from other forms such as the hookworms and *H. contortus,* in which the first larva hatches and, after a feeding stage, develops in the open into the filariform or infective larva.

Treatment. Copper sulphate and sodium arsenate in the proportion of 4 to 1 have been used effectively against *H. contortus* and other "stomach worms" of sheep. According to Hutyra and Marek (1926) the dose is 0.625 gm. for adult sheep, 0.5 gm. for yearlings, 0.375 gm. for lambs six to ten months old, 0.25 gm. for lambs four to six months old, and 0.2 gm. for lambs two to four months old, given on the empty stomach. Carbon tetrachloride in doses of 10 c.c. followed immediately by 128 gms. of magnesium sulphate, according to Hall and Shillinger (1925) is highly effective in removing stomach worms, *Hæmonchus contortus,* nodular worms, *Œsophagostomum* sp. and small trichostrongyles, *Ostertagia* sp., from sheep and is especially effective against the blood-sucking *Nematodirus* sp.

Prevention. Pasture rotation is essential. Cattle and sheep should be kept out of each pasture for at least one year before it is used again. Young animals are most susceptible to the infection and should therefore be furnished the safest pasture lands. Frequent anthelmintic treatment is advised.

CHAPTER XXVIII

NEMATODE PARASITES (Continued)

Order *Filarioidea* Weinland, 1858

The FILARIOIDEA are parasitic nematodes with paired lateral lips, or with or without prominent lip-like structures. The esophagus is without a bulb but is divided into a muscular anterior portion and a glandular posterior portion. The eggs are embryonated when laid or may hatch within the uterus. They differ from other nematodes previously studied in that they require an intermediate host for development and transmission.

This order, according to Baylis and Daubney (1926), is made up of six families: (1) FILARIIDÆ Claus, 1885; (2) PHILOMETRIDÆ Baylis and Daubney, 1926; (3) SPIRURIDÆ Örley, 1885; (4) CAMALLANIDÆ Railliet and Henry, 1915; (5) CUCULLANIDÆ Barreto, 1916, and (6) GNATHOSTOMIDÆ Railliet, 1895, all of which contain species of medical importance.

I. Family FILARIIDÆ

FILARIOIDEA with usually filiform and much elongated bodies. The females are not more than three or four times as long as the males. The head is characterized by two lateral and four submedian papillæ, and the mouth is usually without lip-like structures. There are usually two spicules, dissimilar and unequal. The vulva is almost always in the esophageal region. The adults inhabit the connective tissue, blood-vessels or serous cavities of vertebrates.

1. SUBFAMILY FILARIINÆ Stiles, 1907

FILARIIDÆ with a simple mouth, not bounded by a chitinous peribuccal ring or epaulette-like structures and without trident-like chitinous structures on each side of the anterior end of the esophagus. The spicules are unequal and dissimilar. The adults are parasites in the connective tissue, blood-vessels or serous cavities of vertebrates. The larvæ produced by the adult parasites are generally found in the circulating blood and are generally known as microfilariæ. As far as is known, the required intermediate host is either a mosquito or a bloodsucking fly. The FILARIIDÆ infecting man belong to this sub-family. Examples, *Wuchereria bancrofti* (Cobbold, 1877) in man, and *Dirofilaria immitis* (Leidy, 1856) in the dog.

(1) WUCHERERIA BANCROFTI (Cobbold, 1877). *Historical.* This species was known for a long time only in its larval stage in the blood of man. It was first discovered in 1863 by Demarquay in Paris in the hydrocele fluid of a patient from Havana. These larvæ were next observed in 1866 by Wucherer in chylous urine from a number of cases in Bahia, Brazil. Lewis, in 1872, dis-covered the larvæ in the blood of man in India and found that they were usually present in persons suffering from chy-luria, lymphatic enlargements and ele-phantiasis, and occasionally in apparently healthy individuals. To these larvæ he gave the name *Filaria san-guinis hominis.* The adult was discovered in 1876 by Bancroft in Brisbane and Cobbold gave it the name *Filaria bancrofti.* Manson in 1878 observed that the microfilariæ were ingested by certain mos-quitoes while feeding upon the blood of infected individuals. He later described the metamorphoses of the parasite while within the mos-quito's body. Manson also noted the phenomenon of filarial periodicity, and, because the larvæ appeared most frequently at night in the cir-culating blood, the name *Filaria nocturna* was given them. This larva is now generally referred to as *Microfilaria bancrofti.*

FIG. 215.—*Wuchereria bancrofti.*
a, male; *b,* female. Natural size.
(From Manson-Bahr's *Manson's Tropical Diseases*)

Distribution and frequency. Wuchereria bancrofti is practically world-wide in distribution but, like the hookworms, is largely con-fined to tropical and subtropical countries. Its dissemination neces-sarily depends on the extent of the migrations of the infected indi-vidual and on the presence or absence of its intermediate hosts. It is especially frequent in India, South China, Samoa and on the Western Pacific Islands. O'Connor (1923) reports that over 61 per cent of the individuals past sixteen years of age in the Ellice Islands show evidence of the infection. The infection is also a very common one throughout the West Indies, in South America and in West and Central Africa, O'Connor (1932). There is one endemic area in the United States, Charleston, S. C. Johnson (1915) found that 19 per cent of the patients admitted to the Roper Hospital in Charleston harbored microfilaria, and Francis (1919) found thirteen, or 35 per cent, of the inmates at "The Old Folks Home" with microfilaria in their blood. It is very probable that the infection was introduced into

Charleston, as well as into other parts of the Americas, by Negro slaves from a heavy focus of infection in Africa.

Description. The adult forms of *Wuchereria bancrofti* are white, more or less transparent, thread-like worms with a smooth cuticula. The male is about 40 mm. in length by 0.1 mm. in breadth and possesses two spicules. The larger spicule measures 500 μ in length and has a short, thick proximal portion and a long whip-like distal portion ending with a hook. The shorter spicule is 200 μ in length and is grooved on its ventral surface. A crescent-shaped gubernaculum, or accessory piece, is present. There are fifteen pairs of post anal papillæ. The female measures from 65 mm. to 100 mm. in length by 0.2 mm. to 0.28 mm. in breadth. The anterior end is tapering with the head distinct and followed by a narrower neck. The posterior portion is narrow and ends abruptly rounded. The vulva is situated about 0.6 mm. to 1.3 mm. from the anterior tip. The eggs measure about 40 μ in length by 25 μ in breadth and contain formed embryos when in the upper part of the uterus. The eggs possess an embryonal covering or vitelline membrane, but not a true shell. Hatching apparently occurs in the uterus or shortly after oviposition.

The adults are parasites of the lymphatic tract of man only. They may occur at any level of the system but are found most frequently in the limbs, scrotum and the inguinal regions. The two sexes usually are found coiled together in the periglandular tissues, the lymphatic vessels of the capsule and the cortical sinuses. In heavy infections they may also occur in the medulla.

The microfilariæ. In fresh preparations the microfilariæ appear as exceedingly active, thread-like bodies and can be detected with a low power of the microscope as they lash their way among the blood corpuscles. Unless the slide is properly prepared and stained very little definite structure can be determined. After staining with hematoxylin a certain amount of structure can be made out (Figure 216). The larva is enclosed in a sheath. This sheath is not apparent on larvæ in the circulation. It is formed on the slide in the clotting and drying blood. The larva is mechanically held in the medium, and in its efforts to push on and back out the outer covering is stretched. It usually does not escape. The covering is retained as a distinct sheath and apparently, like that of infective strongyloid larvæ, is the result of an incomplete ecdysis. The head is rounded. The tail is distinctly pointed. The body of the larva is composed mainly of exceedingly small cells. At about one-fifth of the entire length of the body backward from the head is a hyaline V-shaped space which is termed the "V-spot." A smaller, second spot is visible a short dis-

tance from the end of the tail which is known as the "tail-spot." The
V-spot probably represents the undeveloped excretory system and the
tail-spot the anus or cloaca, as the case may be. The excretory cell is
located directly behind the V-spot. There is also a break in the
column of nuclei somewhat anterior to the V-spot which indicates
the position of the nerve ring.

Observations on related species (*Dirofilaria immitis* and *Vag-
rifilaria columbigallinæ*) show that microfilariæ are exceedingly active

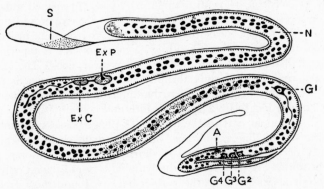

Fig. 216.—*Wuchereria bancrofti.* Microfilaria showing "fixed" structures. (Redrawn
from Feng). A, anal pore; N, nerve ring; Ex C, excretory cell; Ex P, excretory pore;
G, 1, 2, 3, 4, genital cells; S, sheath.

and able travelers. They readily pass through lymph nodes and
traverse the capillaries, moving both with and against the blood
stream. Their every movement has the effect of maintaining them in
the circulation. Unless they are sucked up by a proper mosquito, no
further development occurs. They are finally filtered out of the circulation in the liver and spleen where they are disposed of by the
cells of the reticulo-endothelial system (Augustine, 1937).

Periodicity. The microfilariæ of *M. bancrofti* usually appear in the
peripheral blood at night, and for this reason they are said to have a
nocturnal periodicity. In the Americas, India and China they are
found in greatest numbers between ten o'clock in the evening and
two o'clock in the morning, while during the day they may be entirely
absent from the blood. In the Philippine Islands and neighboring
islands in the Pacific the microfilariæ of *W. bancrofti* do not have a
nocturnal periodicity but appear during both the day time and night
time in the blood stream in equal numbers.

Many theories have been advanced to explain the remarkable
phenomenon of filarial periodicity. Most of these lack supporting

evidence. Lane (1929-1937) holds that periodicity is due to simultaneous development and parturition of microfilariæ by female worms and their daily destruction by the host. The anatomical studies of O'Connor (1931-1932) on female worms removed at different times over twenty-four hours from surgical cases and autopsies support Lane's conception of Bancroftian periodicity.

O'Connor found all female worms from a given case to be in the same stage of uterine development; and that parturition occurs about midday. Evidence of daily destruction of microfilariæ is, at present, limited. Observations indicate that many microfilariæ are disposed of in the liver and spleen by action of the reticulo-endothelial cells. All evidence indicates that such microfilarial destruction causes no protein shock to the host.

Life-cycle. In order to complete the life-cycle the microfilariæ must be taken up by one of various mosquitoes of the genera *Culex, Aëdes,* and *Anopheles.* Of these, *Culex fatigans* and *Aëdes variegatus* are the usual intermediate hosts. The mosquito in sucking blood into its stomach takes in the microfilariæ as well. Shortly after entering the mosquito's stomach the microfilariæ loose their sheaths. A few of the unsheathed larvæ penetrate the wall of the stomach to enter the abdominal cavity and arrive in the thorax in about one hour after being ingested by the mosquito. Most of the larvæ, however, remain in the stomach for about eighteen hours. They then aggregate at the anterior end of this organ and enter the anterior part of the midgut, penetrate its walls and enter the thoracic muscles (Figure 217) (O'Connor and Beatty, 1936). They lie between the wing muscles and

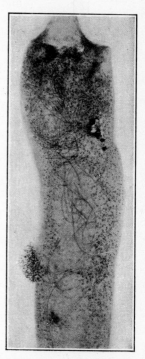

Fig. 217.—*Wuchereria bancrofti.* Larvæ in masses at the anterior end of the anterior and tubular part of the midgut of *Culex fatigans* about 16 hours after a single infective blood meal. (After O'Connor)

there undergo metamorphosis. They first assume sausage-like forms and possess a rudimentary digestive tract (Figure 218). These larvæ measure about 0.5 mm. in length. They soon elongate. The digestive tract is completed and three subterminal caudal papillæ appear. At about the tenth day they reach about 1.4 mm. in length. They then travel forward through the thoracic muscles into the proboscis and there lie more or less coiled up and await an opportunity to get back into man, which opportunity presents itself when the mosquito feeds upon an individual. Matured larvæ (Figures 219, 220) are occasionally found in the mosquito's head, abdomen, legs, antennæ and palpi but it is doubtful whether any are infective for man unless they are actually in the proboscis. When the infected mosquito feeds upon another individual the larvæ are attracted by the warmth of the body and make their way down the proboscis sheath, the labium. They break through its terminal portion, known as Dutton's membrane, and crawl onto the surface of the host's

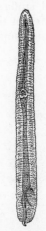

FIG. 218.—*Wuchereria bancrofti.* Young larva dissected from the thoracic muscles of *Culex fatigans.*

skin. The larvæ then penetrate the skin at or near the puncture caused by the stilette bundle of the mosquito and pass by the way of the lymphatics to lymph glands where they grow into the adult stage.

While the mosquito is the sole vector of *Wuchereria bancrofti,* as in malaria, the transmission is accomplished with much less certainty and promptness in the case of filariasis. There is no multiplication of the filaria larvæ in the intermediate host. There develops but one infective larva from each microfilaria sucked in by the mosquito, whereas the malaria parasite

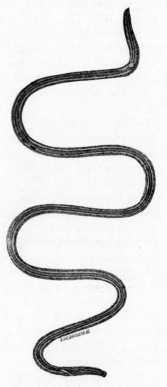

FIG. 219.—Showing structure of mature larva at time of escape from the proboscis of *Culex fatigans.* Magnified. (After Francis)

multiplies enormously and the chance of the infection being returned to man is by thousands of times more likely. The actual number of microfilariæ sucked up by the mosquito is also relatively small in comparison with the number of malarial organisms in the blood which may be taken up in a similar manner. A high mortality may also occur among the microfilariæ which actually reach the stomach of the mosquito. At every step of the transmission of *W. bancrofti* by the mosquito only a small number are involved. Conjugation of the sexes is essential to multiplication and that conjugation takes place only within the lymphatic system by the adult worms. When the infective larva leaves the proboscis of the mosquito it is of one sex or the other and, although it may successfully become established in a lymph gland, multiplication cannot take place until one of the

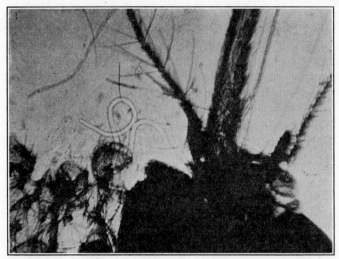

Fig. 220.—*Wuchereria bancrofti.* Infective larva dissected from the labium of *Culex fatigans.* (Photograph supplied by Dr. Henri Galliard, Hanoi)

opposite sex lodges within that same lymph gland. It is therefore possible that an individual might harbor a relatively large number of adult parasites and yet show no microfilariæ in his blood because the adults are so distributed that the two sexes never meet. It is quite evident that successful infections are only the result of mass biting by mosquitoes and the spotted geographic distribution of this and related species is due to these factors.

Pathogenesis. It is generally held that living microfilariæ are not pathogenic but that the serious disorders are brought about by dead microfilariæ and living and dead adult worms. These disorders in every case can be traced to interference with the lymphatic system.

Living worms apparently cause little damage other than varying degrees of blockage of the afferent approach of the vessels in which

they lie. When the parasite dies it becomes a foreign body. Degeneration of the body follows, which may terminate either in its absorption
by giant cells or in calcification. Microfilariæ may be disposed of in
a similar manner in lymph glands. The end result is fibrosis with complete occlusion of the parasitized vessel. The degree of infection
necessary to produce symptoms is probably high. Lymphangitis, abscess, hydrocele, lymph scrotum, chyluria and elephantiasis of the
leg, scrotum, vulva, arm and breast are among the more serious
consequences of the infection (Figure 221). Elephantiasis is the
result of long and widespread lymphatic obstruction.

Pyogenic bacteria, staphylococci and streptococci, have been isolated fairly frequently from blood and from the region of lymphe-
dema (Grace and Grace, 1932). Their responsibility in the disease
syndrome is not clear. Drinker and associates (1937) have shown
that loss of lymph circulation predisposes to streptococcic infection,
that these bacteria cause attacks of severe chill and high fever and
usually can be isolated only in the early stages of the seizures.

The diagnosis of infections with *W. bancrofti* is made by finding
the characteristic microfilariæ in the blood. Many cases, however,
having clinical symptoms show no microfilariæ in blood nor in the
contents of the dilated vessels. In such instances the infection is
usually of long standing and either the adult worms have died or the
lymphatics draining the affected area have become obstructed by
the worms and their products to such an extent that the microfilariæ cannot pass along the vessels to enter the circulating blood.
For the examination of blood for microfilariæ six or eight large
drops of blood are allowed to drop from the tip of the finger onto
an ordinary clean slide and evenly spread before clotting over the
surface of the slide. The blood films are dried in a level position,
protected from insects and dust, but should be freely exposed to the
air. They are then dehemoglobinized in water in order to get a
colorless film and when the laking of the hemoglobin is complete, the
slides are examined while still wet on a mechanical stage and under
a low power of the microscope. The microfilariæ, if present, appear
as glistening objects and are readily distinguishable.

For morphological study and identification of the microfilariæ
the dehemoglobinized preparations may be stained with Delafield's
hematoxylin for five minutes, steamed over a flame as in staining tubercle bacilli, and then washed in tap water. They should
then be differentiated momentarily in acid alcohol, washed again in
tap water until blue, dehydrated in absolute alcohol, cleared and

mounted in Canada balsam. Calcified worms may be located by x-ray examination (O'Connor, 1930).

Treatment. Thus far no satisfactory medical treatment for filariasis has been perfected. Elephantiasis of the scrotum may be successfully treated by operative measures (Auchincloss, 1930). Excision of focal spots may bring about relief (O'Connor, 1935). Roentgen therapy applied locally has given encouraging results in the treatment of lymphangitis, adenitis and chyluria (Golden and O'Connor, 1934). A change to cooler climates has often proven beneficial.

Prevention. Filariasis is characteristically common in the overcrowded dwellings of poor people. Better housing is essential in control. In view of the fact that *W. bancrofti* is transmitted to man solely through bites of mosquitoes, its prevention is primarily one of mosquito

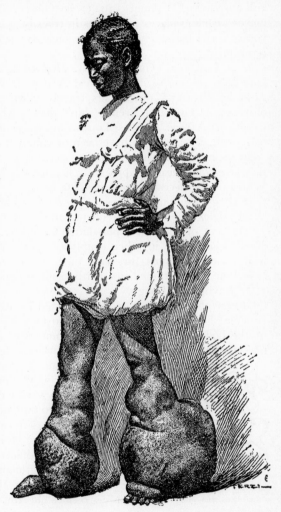

Fig. 221.—Elephantiasis of lower limbs. (From photograph by Sambon)

control and measures taken against these insects in malaria and yellow fever control are equally effective against this parasite. *Culex fatigans* is a domestic mosquito and breeds in cisterns, rain barrels, and tin cans. *Aëdes variegatus* also breeds in fresh water in the husks and shells of cocoanuts, in crevices and holes in trees, in bottles and tin cans. O'Connor (1923) has observed that the Pacific rat makes breeding places for Aëdes in trees by gnawing and gutting the young cocoa-pods. These pods become dry and soon form hanging reservoirs.

(2) LOA LOA (Guyot, 1778). *Historical. Loa loa* is commonly known as the eye worm of West Africa. It was noted as early as 1598 by Pigafetta during his travels in the Congo. It was later observed by Guyot, a French ship's doctor while cruising the West Coast of Africa. It was known by the name "loa" among the natives. *L. loa* is said to have been of common occurrence among the Negroes in South America during slave days but disappeared when the slave traffic ceased, apparently because of the absence in the New World of the necessary intermediate host.

Distribution and frequency. Loa loa is indigenous only in tropical West Africa where it is a frequent parasite in man. In certain sections 75 per cent of the native population have been found infected. It is noted occasionally in other countries among Europeans and Americans who have lived for some time on the West Coast of Africa. Infection has continued in such persons for as long as fifteen years after leaving the Congo.

Description. Loa loa is characterized by its nodular or wart-like cuticula. These bosses rise from 9 μ to 11 μ above the general surface of the body and are usually more numerous in the female. In the male they may be absent at the extremities. The male measures from

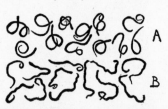

FIG. 222.—Showing characteristic altitudes of microfilariæ of A, *Wuchereria bancrofti* and B, *Loa loa.* (Redrawn from Manson in Brumpt)

30 mm. to 34 mm. in length and about 0.35 mm. in breadth. The female varies considerably in length up to 70 mm. and is about 0.5 mm. in breadth. The average length of the female is probably about 50 mm. The microfilariæ are present in the circulating blood during the day only, appearing in the blood about eight o'clock in the morning and disappearing about nine o'clock in the evening. They, like the microfilariæ of *W. bancrofti,* are sheathed forms. They may be differentiated from the latter in dried and stained preparations by their stiff, ungraceful and angular attitude (Figure 222). The microfilariæ of *W. bancrofti* assume more sweeping and graceful curves. The nuclei forming the central column in

the microfilariæ of *Loa loa* are larger and stain less deeply than those of *W. bancrofti*.

Position in the host. The adult of *Loa loa* is primarily a sub-cutaneous tissue parasite. It is frequently observed just beneath the skin of the fingers, the eyelids and conjunctiva. It commonly makes excursions through the subdermal connective tissues and has been observed to travel at the rate of an inch in two minutes.

Life-cycle. Manson and Sambon early suspected that the flies of the family TABANIDÆ, the horse-flies, were agents in the transmission of *Loa loa,* and Leiper (1913) demonstrated that the microfilariæ may complete their development in *Chrysops dimidiata* and *C. silacea.* The developmental stages of *Loa loa* in these flies closely follow those of *W. bancrofti* within the mosquito. They develop to infectivity in about ten days and are then found at the root of the proboscis. The infective larva breaks through the proboscis sheath and falls upon the skin of the person when the infected fly feeds. The Connals (1921) have found nearly 4 per cent of the wild flies of Calabar infected with *Loa loa.*

Pathogenesis. Aside from the itching and irritation caused by these migrations the parasite apparently produces no serious damage in its host. The worms may be readily extracted through a small incision. It is generally believed that the localized edemas, known as Calabar swellings, are due to the presence of adult worms. These swellings appear suddenly and then gradually disappear. They may attain the size of a hen's egg and may occur on any part of the body, but frequently appear on the hand and forearm. They are said to be painless and never suppurate.

Other species of FILARIINÆ occurring in man are *Acanthocheilonema perstans* Manson, 1891; *Onchocerca volvulus* (Leuckart, 1893); *O. cæcutiens* Brumpt, 1919; *Dirofilaria magalhæsi* (R. Blanchard, 1895); and several poorly known species which are temporarily included under the genus *Filaria.*

(3) ACANTHOCHEILONEMA PÉRSTANS (Manson, 1891). *Acanthocheilonema perstans* is widely distributed throughout Africa, especially along the western coast and the Congo. In certain districts 90 per cent of the population are infected. *A. perstans* is normally a parasite of man but may occur also in the chimpanzee. The adults of this species inhabit the mesentery and the perirenal and retroperitoneal tissues and the pericardium. The body is smooth and without markings. The microfilariæ are not sheathed and show no strict periodicity. The insect vectors of *A. perstans* are *Culicoides austeni*

and *C. grahami,* blood-sucking flies. *A. perstans* is apparently non-pathogenic.

(4) ONCHOCERCA VOLVULUS (Leukart, 1893). *Onchocerca volvulus* lives in subcutaneous tumors, especially in intercostal spaces, the axillæ and popliteal spaces. This species is also African in distribution and is especially frequent in the valley of the Congo and along the West Coast. In Sierra Leone, Blacklock (1926) has found 45 per cent of the persons examined infected with this parasite. It is especially prevalent in hilly countries covered with brush and grass and having abundance of streams and rivers. The microfilariæ are sheathless and are found in the skin, especially in the skin of the waist

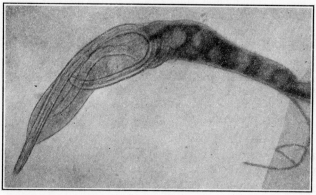

FIG. 223.—*Dirofilaria immitis.* Larva in a Malphigian tubule of *Aëdes ægypti* 9 days after an infective blood meal. (Photograph supplied by Dr. Henri Galliard, Hanoi)

region. They are never found in the peripheral blood like *W. bancrofti* and *L. loa.* The microfilariæ of *O. volvulus* present a great variation in size; the majority of forms in the skin measure from 250μ to 300μ in length by 5μ to 9μ in breadth. Blacklock (1926) has recently shown that the microfilariæ develop in the thorax of the black fly, *Simulium damnosum. O. cæcutiens* Brumpt, 1917, occurs in Central America and is apparently very common in the higher altitudes of these countries. It produces subcutaneous tumors especially frequent in the occipito-frontal and temporal regions of the scalp, and is also associated with punctate keratitis and loss of vision. The larval development of *O. cæcutiens* takes place in *Simulium avidum, S. mooseri* and *S. ochraceum* (Strong, Sandground, Bequaert and Ochoa, 1934).

Sandground (Strong et al, 1934) was unable to find constant morphological differences between *Onchocera volvulus* and *O.*

cæcutiens. He is of the opinion that probably they are synonyms. It likewise appears that *O. flexuosa* (Wedl, 1856), from the red deer of Central Europe, and *O. gibsoni* (Cleland and Johnstone, 1910), in cattle and zebra of India, Australia, Ceylon and the Malay region, are indistinguishable from *O. volvulus. O. cervicalis* (Railliet and Henry, 1910) occurs in the cervical ligament of horses and mules of various countries. It appears to be a common parasite of horses in the United States and is considered by some authorities to be a cause of fistulous withers and poll evil. Species of the genus *Culicoides* are probably the vectors.

(5) DIROFILARIA MAGALHÆSI (R. Blanchard, 1895), *Dirofilaria magalhæsi* was discovered in the heart of a Brazilian child. The life-cycle of *D. magalhæsi* is not known but its transmission is probably by certain blood-sucking insects. A closely related species, *D. immitis,* (Leidy, 1856) commonly occurs in tangled masses in the right ventricle of the heart of dogs. It is world-wide in distribution. The micro-filariæ of *D. immitis* are sheathless and appear in the peripheral blood of the dog at all times but are most numerous at night. When taken up by certain mosquitoes, particularly of the genera *Anopheles, Aëdes,* and *Culex,* they migrate to the malpighian tubules and there under-go larval development (Figures 223, 224). They pass to the labium and are returned to another dog in a manner like that in which *W. bancrofti* is re-

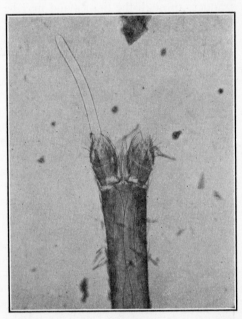

FIG. 224.—*Dirofilaria immitis.* Larva escaping from the labium of *Aëdes ægypti* 16 days after an infective blood meal. (Photograph supplied by Dr. Henri Galliard, Hanoi)

turned to man. Heavily infected dogs show severe emaciation, jaundice and weakness; there is a persistent cough which is aggravated upon the least exercise. Fuadin is the drug of choice (Wright and Underwood, 1934). Repeated intramuscular or intravenous injections with this drug render the female worms sterile and eventually destroy some or all of the adults in the heart and pulmonary artery.

(6) Mansonella ozzardi (Manson, 1897). This species was discovered by Ozzard in the blood of aboriginal Carib Indians of British Guiana. It occurs in Yucatan, Panama, St. Lucia and neighboring islands. The microfilariæ closely resemble those of *Acanthocheilonema perstans,* but have sharp tails, while those of the latter species are more or less rounded. They are non-periodic. The adult forms occur in the mesentery and visceral fat. The life-cycle is not fully known, but apparently a species of *Culicoides* is its vector.

(7) Setaria equina (Abildgaard, 1789). *Setaria equina* appears to be a relatively frequent parasite of the peritoneal cavity of horses and other equidæ, and has also been observed in cattle. It often wanders through the tissues and may be found in other parts of the body and sometimes invades the aqueous humor. It is then commonly termed "snake in the eye." In the eye it may cause inflammation with bulging and opacity of the cornea. It may be removed by operative measures. The males measure from 6 cm. to 8 cm. and the females from 9 cm. to 12 cm. in length. The posterior extremity of the male ends in a characteristic corkscrew spiral. The embryos are present in the blood vessels of infected animals. The life-cycle of this species is not known but it is probably transmitted from one host to another by some biting insect which becomes infected with the embryos in the blood stream. *S. labiato-papillosa* (Alessandrini, 1838) is a closely related species occurring in the peritoneal cavity, ovaries, renal capsule and diaphragm of cattle. The stable fly, *Stomoxys calcitrans,* is the intermediate host. *Stephanofilaria stilesi* Chitwood, 1934, causes a dermatitis in cattle of Central and Western United States. It has also been found in goats and swine. It occurs in the epithelial layers of the skin. The early lesions are small papules which later increase in size and coalesce to form lesions with crusts up to 25 centimeters in diameter. The diagnosis may be established on finding adult worms in the lesions or microfilariæ in deep skin scrapings. A closely related species, *S. dedoesi* Ihle and Ihle-Landenberg, 1933, causes similar lesions in cattle of the Dutch East Indes.

filariæ are very common in birds in the United States, particularly in crows and English sparrows. A single drop of their blood may contain thousands of microfilariæ. The microfilariæ may be kept alive for hours in heparinized blood by rimming the cover glass with vaseline, and permanent preparations may be made by methods given for *Wuchereria bancrofti.*

II. Family PHILOMETRIDÆ

FILARIOIDEA with more or less elongated body, the anterior end of which is rounded and sometimes bears a cuticular shield. The mouth is simple, without lips, but is surrounded by six or eight papillæ. The anus may be absent in the adult. The male is much smaller than the female, with two equal, finely pointed spicules. A gubernaculum, or accessory piece, is present. The vulva is very inconspicuous or absent and the vagina is rudimentary or absent in gravid females. The uterine branches are directly opposed and form a continuous tube, with the ovaries situated at opposite ends of the body. The female is viviparous. These nematodes are parasitic in the body cavity, serous membranes or connective tissue of vertebrates. Example: *Dracunculus medinensis* (Linnæus, 1758) in man.

I. DRACUNCULUS MEDINENSIS (Linnæus, 1758)

Description. The female of this species is commonly known as the "guinea worm." This parasite has been known since the most remote period and very probably is the "fiery serpent" which troubled the Israelites by the Red Sea, mentioned by Moses (*Numbers,* xxi). The adult female is unusually long and may attain a total length of over 1 meter, although the average is perhaps not over 60 cm. with a diameter of about 1.5 mm. A cuticular shield or "helmet" is present at the anterior end. The cuticula is smooth and presents a milky-white appearance. The alimentary tract be-low the esophagus is atrophied and is largely replaced by the long uterus which is filled with motile larvæ. The vulva is situated immediately behind the cephalic shield and during parturition the uterus is prolapsed through this opening.

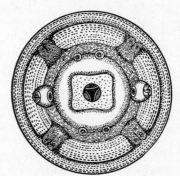

FIG. 225.—*Dracunculus medinensis.* Anterior extremity of male, head-on view. (After Moorthy)

The male worm had remained practically unknown until Moorthy and Sweet (1936) obtained specimens from experimental dogs. The specimens were recovered from the region of the esophagus, beneath the right scapula, the right orbit, the meninges, scalp, the thoracic and abdominal walls and from the extremities. The males are from 12 mm. to 29 mm. long by 0.4 mm. in diameter. The mouth (Figure 225) is small and is surrounded by an internal circle of four to six well-developed papillæ and an external circle of four double papillæ. The anus is 250 μ from the posterior extremity. There are six postanal and four preanal papillæ. The spicules are subequal, 490 μ to 730 μ long. A gubernaculum is present

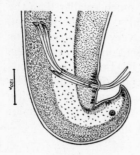

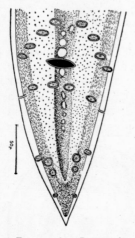

(Figure 226). Moorthy (1936) is of the opinion that copulation takes place early since males were not found later than six months after infection.

Geographical distribution. Dracunculus medinensis is widely distributed and is a common parasite of man in tropical Africa, Arabia, Dutch East Indies and India. It has been reported a few times from man in the United States. Unquestionably, these infections were acquired abroad. It occurs also in a large number of domesticated and wild animals including the dog, cat, pole cat and wolf of the Old World, and has been found in the silver fox from Iowa, the raccoon from New York and Ontario, and the mink from Nebraska. The freedom of man from this infection in this country is probably due to high standards of sanitation.

Position in the host. The adult female worm occurs most frequently in the subcutaneous connective tissues of man, especially of the arm, leg and shoulders (Figure 227). More than twelve worms have been noted in the same person within a week or ten days.

Life-cycle. The female worm when about to produce her young migrates to the parts of the skin which are likely to, or frequently do, come in contact with water,

Fig. 226. — *Dracunculus medinensis.* Tail of male. Upper figure, lateral view; lower figure, ventral view. (After Moorthy)

such as the arms and legs of laundresses, or the backs and shoulders of water carriers. A small vesicle soon appears and ulceration follows. A small hole may be seen at the base of the ulcer from which a portion of the anterior end of the worm may protrude. When the affected parts come in contact with water a milky fluid is discharged directly from the hole in the ulcer, or from the vulva if the worm is exposed to that extent. This fluid contains thousands of motile larvæ which may swim actively about in the water (Figure 228). The larvæ are at first from 650 μ to 750 μ in length by 17 μ in breadth and are characteristically flattened forms with a long slender tail, well adapted for swimming. They are actively hunted and ingested by several species of *Cyclops*. Shortly after ingestion, the young worms penetrate the wall of the stomach and pass into the body cavity. Within the body cavity of *Cyclops* the larvæ undergo two molts, acquire a cylindrical shape, and in from four to six weeks become infective for man. Infection in susceptible hosts results from swallowing infected *Cyclops* in drinking water. The complete development of the worm in man is exceedingly slow and it is not until the worm is about a year old that it seeks the surface of the body to discharge the young.

Pathogenesis. Urticaria, cyanosis, dyspnœa, vomiting and diarrhea are noted at the time the female worm establishes connection with the surface of the body. These symptoms are probably of an anaphylactic nature. Usually the parasite is innocuous if not interfered with. Should the worm break and the larvæ become discharged into the tissues, violent inflammation and fever, followed by abscess formation and sloughing, may develop and result in death from septicemia. Ulcers also may arise should the worm fail to reach the surface of the skin to bring forth her young. Fre-

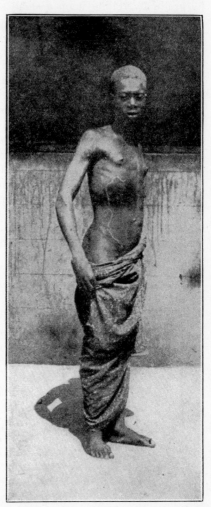

Fig. 227.—*Dracunculus medinensis*. Showing the adult worm beneath the skin of the chest and abdomen. (Photograph by Macfie)

quently her body becomes calcified and may then be felt for years as a hard, twisted cord beneath the skin.

Treatment. For ages it has been the custom to extract the worm by gradually rolling it on a small stick. A few turns are given the stick each day until the worm is entirely drawn out. This method is dangerous, however, because the worm frequently breaks while still within the tissue and this may be followed by severe inflammation, abscess formation and conditions previously mentioned. It has been observed that the worm may be killed by injecting it with a 0.1 per cent solution of either mercury bichloride or acriflavine and after twenty-four hours it may then be extracted without difficulty. If injected with a 10 per cent collargol solution it is made visible by the X-ray and may then be dissected out. Frequent douching of the ulcer and the part occupied by the worm with cold water hastens complete expulsion of the larvæ, after which the worm may emerge spontaneously or may be extracted without resistance.

Prevention. Water supplies should be protected from pollution by guinea-worm patients. According to Moorthy (1932) wells may be kept free from adult *Cyclops* for a month by adding three pounds of perchloron and one-half pound copper sulphate per 100,000 gallons of water. Aqueous extract and juice from young bamboo shoots have a definitely lethal action on guinea-worm larvæ and *Cyclops*. In addition, fish, *Barbus puckelli,* voraciously feed upon *Cyclops* and larvæ and may be of value in control. It has been observed by Moorthy that the infective *Cyclops* are sluggish in their movements and that this fish appears to feed better on infected rather than non-infected *Cyclops*.

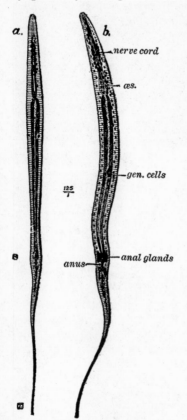

FIG. 228.—*Dracunculus medinensis.* showing characteristics of larvæ. *a.,* side view; *b.,* front view. (From Manson-Bahr's *Manson's Tropical Diseases.* After Looss)

III. Family SPIRURIDÆ

FILARIOIDEA with the mouth bordered by two lateral lips. A buccal capsule is usually present. The esophagus consists of a short anterior muscular portion and a long and thicker posterior glandular portion. The male is equipped with two usually unequal and dissimilar spicules. The position of the vulva is variable but is never very close to the anterior end. The eggs are thick-shelled and contain an embryo when deposited. The adults are parasites of the esophagus, stomach and intestines of vertebrates while the larvæ, as far as is known, are parasites of arthropods. According to Baylis and Daubney (1926) this family contains five subfamilies: (1) SPIRURINÆ Railliet, 1915; (2) ARDUENNINÆ Railliet and Henry, 1911; (3) ACUARIINÆ Railliet, Henry and Sisoff, 1912; (4) PHYSALOPTERINÆ Stossich, 1898; and (5) THELAZIINÆ Baylis and Daubney, 1926. They are, for the most part, parasites of birds, reptiles and lower mammals. The ARDUEN-NINÆ and THELAZIINÆ contain a few species which are rare or accidental parasites of man.

1. SUBFAMILY SPIRURINÆ Railliet, 1915

SPIRURIDÆ with lips followed by a cuticular collar which is prominent dorsally and ventrally and may form dorsal and ventral shields overlapping the lips. The buccal capsule is without spiral or annular thickenings. The male is typically with four pairs of preanal papillæ; and a gubernaculum, or accessory piece, is usually present. Examples: *Habronema megastoma* (Rudolphi, 1819) in horses, and *Protospirura gracilis* Cram, 1924, in cats.

(1) HABRONEMA MEGASTOMA (Rudolphi, 1819). *Description.* *Habronema megastoma* is a small, whitish nematode which occurs in the stomach of the horse. It appears to be of wide distribution and in the United States is especially prevalent in the southern portion where conditions favor its development. The female measures from 10 mm. to 13 mm. in length and the male from 7 mm. to 10 mm. These worms live in nodules or tumors in the stomach and parts of their bodies may be seen projecting from small apertures at the summit of the tumor. Many of the worms may also be found free in the contents of the stomach. The worm-swellings are particularly common in July and may seriously interfere with the functioning of the stomach if situated near the pylorus.

Life-cycle. The embryos of *H. megastoma* pass out in the manure and become ingested by maggots of the house-fly (*Musca domestica*) as they feed in the manure. The infective stage is reached about the

time the fly emerges from the pupal stage and is transferred to the
final host when the infected fly comes in contact with the horse's
lips or when the fly is swallowed by the horse, the latter opportunity
arising when the benumbed flies fall into the feed boxes, mangers
and drinking troughs while the temperatures are low in the early
morning. The larvæ thus ingested escape from the flies in the stomach
of the horse and there continue their normal development. It is generally believed that the summer sores arise as the result of the horse
lying down on floors or soil covered with manure, thereby bringing
abraded areas in contact with young larvæ in the manure. Infective
larval worms from the fly when transferred to a wound cause an
increase in the severity of the sore.

Habronema muscæ (Carter, 1861) and H. microstoma (Schneider, 1866) also occur in horses of this country. The larval development of H. muscæ likewise takes place in the house-fly. This fly can
also serve as the intermediate host for H. microstoma but the development of this latter species usually takes place in the stable-fly,
Stomoxys irritans. According to Roubaud and Descazeaux (1922)
the larvæ of H. megastoma are exclusively parasitic in the malpighian
tubules of the house-fly, whereas the larvæ of H. muscæ and H. microstoma are parasitic in the cells of the adipose tissue of their intermediate hosts.

2. SUBFAMILY ARDUENNINÆ Railliet and Henry, 1911

SPIRURIDÆ with trilobed but not prominent lips, and without
dorsal and ventral cuticular shields. The buccal capsule, or pharynx,
is typically with annular or spiral thickenings in its walls. Asymmetry
is frequently present in the cervical and caudal alæ, and in the papillæ
and other structures of the male. There are four pairs of preanal and
one or two pairs of large postanal papillæ present. Gubernaculum
present. Examples: Gongylonema pulchrum (Molin, 1857) in the
horse, ox, goat and sheep, and Arduenna strongylina (Rudolphi,
1819) in the stomach of pigs.

GONGYLONEMA PULCHRUM (Molin, 1857). Gongylonema pulchrum
(Figure 229) is a common parasite of sheep, cattle, goats and pigs
in the United States, and occurs less frequently in horses. It inhabits
the mucosa of the esophagus. It is usually found in the thoracic
portion where it is lodged immediately beneath the epithelium. It
rarely occurs in man but has been taken from the lips and mouth of
several persons in the United States. The body is long and white,
or yellowish-white in color. The anterior extremity of the body is
studded with irregular longitudinal rows of cuticular bosses. The

tail of the male is rolled up and has two asymmetrical alæ and two very unequal spicules. The vulva of the female is located immediately above the anus. The ova have a thick shell and contain an embryo at the time of deposition.

Life-cycle. The eggs of *G. pulchrum* are passed with the host's feces, and, when ingested by various species of dung beetles, hatch in the intestinal tract. The newly hatched larvæ penetrate the gut wall and pass into the body cavity of the insect where the infective stage for the ruminant host develops within about one month. The final host accidentally ingests these insects along with grass, and thus becomes infected. Gongylonema larvæ have been found by Ransom and Hall (1915) in various species of dung beetles collected from sheep manure, including *Aphodius femoralis, A. granarius, A. fimentarius, A. coloradensis, A.*

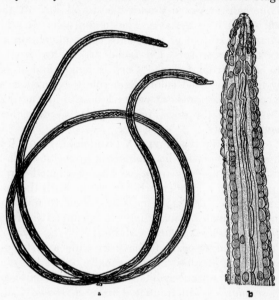

FIG. 229.—*Gongylonema pulchrum* from human host. a, adult worm (x 15); b, anterior end of same specimen (x 140). (After Ward)

vittatus, Onthophagus hecate and *O. pennsylvanicus.* Cockroaches, *Blattella germanica,* can be infected experimentally.

Gongylonema ingluvicola Ransom 1904, has been reported in the mucous lining of the crop and occasionally in the undilated portion of the esophagus from chickens bought in the markets at Washington, D. C. This species appears to be cosmopolitan in distribution.

Gongylonema neoplasticum (Fibiger and Ditlevsen, 1914) occurs in the anterior portion of the digestive tract of rats, including the mouth, tongue, esophagus and fundus of the stomach. This parasite was considered a cause of gastric carcinoma in rats. Delbet (1936), however, could produce no lesions in parasitized rats fed on a good diet. Cancers developed only in the infected rats which were fed on white bread, magnesium and vitamin A deficiencies. The embryonic development takes place in the cockroach, *Blatta orientalis*. Within twenty days after the ingestion of the eggs by this insect the fully developed larvæ may be found coiled up in the muscles of the prothorax and limbs. *Blattella germanica* and *Tenebrio molitor* may also serve as intermediate hosts for *G. neoplasticum*.

SPIROCERCA SANGUINOLENTA (Rudolphi, 1819). *Spirocerca sanguinolenta* occurs in tumor-like formations of the esophagus, aorta and stomach of the dog. The tumors may vary in size from that of a hazelnut to that of a pigeon's egg and contain a purulent fluid and one to seven worms. The female worms are from 6 cm. to 8 cm. and the males from 3 cm. to 5 cm. in length and are easily distinguished by their blood-red color. As a rule they produce no serious disturbances but may cause extensive lesions in the aortic wall. The eggs are passed with the dog's feces. Species of dung beetles are the intermediate hosts.

ARDUENNA STRONGYLINA (Rudolphi, 1819). This species is found in small tumors in the submucosa of the stomach and small intestine of pigs. It appears to be widely distributed throughout the United States. It is a slender, whitish worm, with the body often curved in a semicircle. The male measures from 10 mm. to 13 mm. in length and the female from 12 mm. to 20 mm. It is frequently found with *Physocephalus sexulatus* (Molin, 1860), a very closely related species. *P. sexulatus* appears to have as wide a distribution in the United States as *A. strongylina* but usually occurs less abundantly. It apparently has the same habits of injuring the mucosa as *A. strongylina*. *P. sexulatus* is differentiated from *A. strongylina* by the swelling of the cuticula at the anterior end and has three lateral alæ on each side. The tail of the male has narrow symmetrical alæ while in *A. strongylina* the alæ on the tale of the male are asymmetrical. These parasites are known to be the cause of a serious gastritis in pigs. Dung beetles, species of the genera *Onthophagus, Aphodius* and *Gymnopleurus,* act as intermediate hosts.

3. SUBFAMILY ACUARIINÆ Railliet, Henry and Sisoff, 1912

SPIRURIDÆ with quite distinct, but very small conical lips. The anterior tip is provided with "cordons," "epaulettes" or other homologous structures. The buccal capsule is thin-walled and without thickenings. There are typically four pairs of pedunculated preanal papillæ in the male. The spicules are unequal and usually quite dissimilar.

There is no accessory piece. The eggs are ellipsoidal, with a thick shell and embryonated at time of oviposition. The ACUARIINÆ are parasites of the digestive tract of birds. Their life histories are, for the most part, unknown, but probably involve intermediate stages in arthropods or other small invertebrates which probably eat the eggs passed with the feces of the host. When such infected intermediate hosts are eaten by birds the larval worms grow to maturity.

Acuaria spiralis (Molin, 1858) (Figure 230) is found in papillomatus growths in the proventriculus and in the esophagus of chickens, ducks, pigeons, turkeys and pheasants. Larval development of this species takes place in sow-bugs, *Porcellio scaber* and *Armadillidium vulgare*. *A. hamulosa* Diesing, 1861, occurs in fleshy growths on the surface and in the wall of the gizzards of chickens, turkeys and pheasants. Grasshoppers, *Melanoplus femurrubrum* and *M. differentialis,* serve as intermediate hosts for this parasite. The larvæ become infective, third stage, in about twenty-two days. They occur chiefly in the muscles of the grasshopper. Africa and Garcia (1936) extracted an undetermined species of the genus *Cheilospirura* from a nodule in the conjunctiva of the lower right eye of a Philippino suffering from chronic catarrhal conjunctivitis and keratitis. The presence of spirurids in man is very rare and probably accidental.

Tetrameres americana Cram, 1927, is a fairly common parasite in the proventriculus of chickens and the bobwhite quail of North America. Marked sexual dimorphism is found in this species. The mature female is of a brilliant red color, almost globular in shape with two small projections, one of which, the head, is at one pole and the other, the tail, at the opposite pole. The body measures about 4 mm. in length by 3 mm. in diameter. The male worm retains the elongated, slender body characteristic of nematodes and is practically colorless. The adult female lies buried in the proventricular glands with the tail protruding

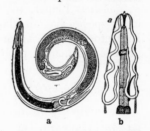

Fig. 230.—*Acuaria spiralis.* a, female. (After Piana in Cram) b, head end. (From Cram. After Seurat)

into the duct, thus facilitating the passage of eggs into the lumen. The head is buried into the fundus of the gland where she sucks blood. The males leave the gland shortly after copulation and die. The worms are particularly pathogenic at the time they enter the wall of the proventriculus. Grasshoppers, *Melanoplus femurrubrum* and *M. differentialis,* serve as intermediate hosts (Cram, 1931). Several species of the genus *Tetrameres* have been reported from wild and domestic fowl from various countries. *T. crami* Swales, 1933, occurs in domestic ducks of Canada.

4. SUBFAMILY PHYSALOPTERINÆ Stossich, 1898

SPIRURIDÆ with two large and entire lips with forwardly-projecting teeth on their inner surface and frequently followed by a cuticular collar which is entire and does not form dorsal and ventral shields. There is no buccal capsule. The males have large, bare caudal alæ, joined anteriorly across the ventral surface and the caudal papillæ are pendunculated. The vulva of the female is anterior to the middle of the body. Their life histories are, for the most part, unknown, but probably involve intermediate stages in insects or other hosts. Parasites of the digestive tract, generally the stomach of reptiles, birds and mammals. Examples: *Physaloptera truncata* Schneider, 1866, inhabits the proventriculus of chickens and pheasants. *P. constricta* (Leidy, 1856) occurs in water-snakes. *P. rara* Hall and Wigdor, 1918, is recorded from the stomach of dogs in the United States. Most recognized species are European, African or South American in distribution. The North American species are not adequately known.

Two species of *Physaloptera* have been found in man, (1) *P. caucasica* von Linstow, 1903, by Menetriés in Caucasia and (2) *P. mordens* Leiper, 1908, by Turner in the Transvaal, Africa. The latter species has also been found by Leiper in man of the Uganda Protectorate. It is, apparently, a normal parasite of monkeys and its presence in man is probably accidental.

5. SUBFAMILY THELAZIINÆ Baylis and Daubney, 1926

SPIRURIDÆ with inconspicuous lips and dorsal and ventral cuticular shields absent. Buccal capsule short and not well developed and without annular or spiral thickenings in its wall. The male with or without caudal alæ but typically with numerous preanal papillæ. Spicules usually very unequal. The tail of the female generally ends bluntly. The life histories are not adequately known but they probably all involve intermediate stages in other hosts. Examples: *Oxyspirura mansoni* (Cobbold, 1879) is found under the nictitating membrane and occasionally in the nasal cavities and sinuses of chickens, turkeys and peacocks; *Cystidicola stigmatura* (Leidy, 1886) Ward and Magath, 1916, in the air bladder of salmoid fishes and, *Thelazia callipæda* Railliet and Henry, 1910, in the eye of the dog.

T. callipæda has also been reported from the eye of a Chinese by Stuckley in 1917. *T. californiensis* Kofoid and Williams, 1935, is the first case of eye infection by *Thelazia* in man in America. An insect intermediate host is required for development. Cockroaches serve as intermediate hosts for *O. mansoni*.

A number of forms whose relationships are uncertain have been appended to THELAZIINÆ by Baylis and Daubney. Among these is *Spinitectus gracilis* Ward and Magath, 1916, a common parasite in the intestine of fishes of the United States including the black crappie, sheepshead and white bass. This parasite may be recognized by the presence of a series of transverse rings on the cuticula bearing backwardly directed spines which diminish in size and number posteriorly.

IV. Family CAMALLANIDÆ

FILARIOIDEA without lips, and with the mouth a dorsoventral slit followed by a large buccal capsule whose wall is either separated into two lateral scallop-shell-like valves or is continuous. The vulva is prominent and is situated in the middle portion of the body with the vagina directed posteriorly. The uterine branches are opposed with the posterior branch ending blindly without an ovary. Parasites of the alimentary tract of reptiles, amphibians and fishes. Examples: *Camallanus ancylodirus* Ward and Magath, 1916, in North American carp; *C. oxycephalus* Ward and Magath, 1916, in North American white bass and black crappie; and *C. trispinosus* (Leidy, 1851), in tortoises.

The life-cycle of this group may be illustrated by that of *Camallanus lacustris* Zoega, 1776, as worked out by Leuckart. *C. lacustris* in the adult stage is parasitic in the intestines of several species of fish. The female is viviparous. The larvæ pass out with the feces and swim about in water where they may sooner or later become ingested by the fresh-water crustacean, *Cyclops*. They bore through the gut wall of the *Cyclops* into the body cavity and there undergo metamorphosis. No further development takes place unless the infected *Cyclops* is in turn eaten by a suitable fish host. When this occurs the larvæ are set free from the body of the *Cyclops* by digestion and within ten to fourteen days the worms are fully matured and pair. In some species of *Camallanus* a second intermediate host is required.

Species of *Camallanus* are usually not difficult to obtain and make excellent material for morphological and life history studies.

V. Family CUCULLANIDÆ

FILARIOIDEA with two large lips each bearing three papillæ, and surrounding the mouth, a dorsoventral slit. The esophagus is in two portions but is without a distinct glandular portion and is usually dilated anteriorly to form a large muscular "false buccal cavity." The spicules are equal and an accessory piece is usually present. A preanal, sucker-like organ is typically present in the male. The vulva is situated in the middle region of the body, or posteriorly. The vagina runs forward from the vulva. The CUCULLANIDÆ are, for the most part, parasites in the alimentary tract of fishes and turtles. *Cucullanus clitellarius* Ward and Magath, 1916, in the lake sturgeon, and *Dacnitoides cotylophora* Ward and Magath, 1916, in the intestine of the yellow perch, *Perca flavescens,* and wall-eyed pike, *Stizostedion vitreum,* are representative species in North America.

VI. Family GNATHOSTOMIDÆ

FILARIOIDEA with large trilobed lips having the cuticula of their inner surfaces thickened and usually raised into longitudinal toothlike

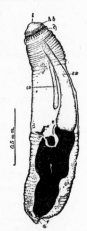

FIG. 231.—*Gnathostoma spinigerum. a,* anus; *c,* cuticular collar; *cs,* cervical sac; *es,* esophagus; *hb,* head bulb; *i,* intestine; *l,* lip; *r,* rectum. (After Faust)

ridges which meet or interlock. Male with caudal alæ supported by broad pedunculated papillæ. The vulva is situated in the posterior half of the body. The vagina of the female runs forward from the vulva and there are from two to four uterine branches. The eggs have thin colorless shells and are ornamented with fine granulations. Parasites of the stomach and intestine of fishes, reptiles and mammals. North American representatives of the family are *Gnathostoma horridum* (Leidy, 1856) from the stomach of alligators and *G. sociale* (Leidy, 1858) from the stomach of a mink. Yorke and Maplestone (1926) regard *G. sociale* a synonym of *G. spinigerum* Owen, 1836 (Figure 231), which occurs in stomach nodules of cats of the Far East and has been occasionally found in man causing subcutaneous abscesses, tumors or a "creeping disease." According to Prommas and Daengsvang (1937) this parasite requires two intermediate hosts, the first, *Cyclops,* and the second, fresh water fishes, *Ophicephalus striatus* and *Clarias batrachus.* The adult stage is reached in the wall of the cat's stomach in about six months after the ingestion of infected fish. *G. hispidium* Fedeschenko, 1872, is a normal parasite in the intestine of cattle and hogs of Europe and Asia. Its larvæ have also been encountered in cutaneous lesions in man. All specimens of *Gnathostoma* obtained from man have been immature and it is evident that these worms cannot settle down to develop to maturity in any organ of an unsuitable host like man, but wander in the body, especially on the surface, and there cause cutaneous lesions.

CHAPTER XXIX

NEMATODE PARASITES (Continued)

Order *Dioctophymoidea* Railliet, 1916

The order DIOCTOPHYMOIDEA consists of medium to large nematodes with the body sometimes spiny. Each of the four muscular fields are divided longitudinally into two by the insertion of well developed suspensory muscles of the alimentary canal. The mouth is hexagonal and is surrounded by one, two or three circles each of six papillæ. The esophagus is relatively long, simple and club-shaped. The tail of the male is furnished with a "bursa," a closed bell-shaped, copulatory organ which is not supported by rays. A single long spicule is present. The anus of the female is terminal. The female genital system consists of but a single tube. The eggs are barrel-shaped with modified poles and with a thick, pitted, albuminous coating. The adults are parasites of the digestive tract, kidneys and body cavity of mammals and birds and larval development occurs in an intermediate host.

I. Family DIOCTOPHYMIDÆ

I. DIOCTOPHYME RENALE (Goeze, 1782)

Dioctophyme renale (Figure 232) is one of the largest of the nematodes. The male measures from 14 cm. to 40 cm. in length by 4 mm. to 6 mm. in diameter. The female may attain a length of 1 m. and a diameter of from 5 mm. to 12 mm. The body is of a blood-red color. This species is most frequently found in the pelvis of the kidney, more rarely in the abdominal cavity, of the dog, and has been also reported from the seal, otter, wolf, horse, cattle, marten and polecat. There are a few authentic cases of infection with this parasite in man (Neveu-Lemaire, 1936).

D. renale grows to an enormous size within the kidney and produces a purulent material within which the worm lies tightly coiled. Only one kidney is infected, and usually with but a single worm. The infected kidney eventually becomes a mere thick-walled cyst while the uninfected kidney is usually found to have undergone a compensatory hypertrophy. The diagnosis is made by finding characteristic ova in the urine.

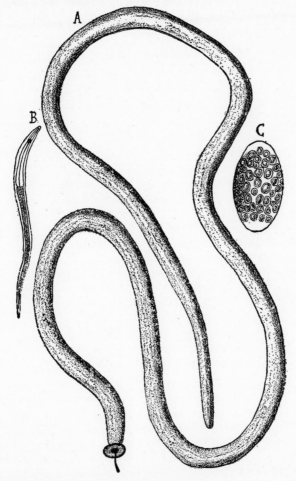

Fig. 232.—*Dioctophyme renale.* A, male, natural size; B, larva; C, egg (x 370). (From Neveu-Lemaire's *Parasitologie des Animaux Domestiques,* J. Lamarre, Paris)

Life-cycle. The embryonal development takes place in water or moist soils. The embryos are highly resistant and may remain alive for a year or more. The source of the infection in dogs or other hosts is not definitely known. Direct infection experiments with embryonated ova have been unsuccessful and it has been thought that fish might serve as an intermediate host. This hypothesis is supported by the finding (Ciurea, 1920) of a female specimen of *D. renale* entangled in the intestine of a dog which had been fed fish, *Idus idus,* from the Danube River. It is difficult, however, to explain infection in horses and cattle from this source.

CHAPTER XXX

NEMATODE PARASITES (Continued)

Order *Trichinelloidea* Hall, 1916

The members of this order are characterized by a body more or less clearly divided into an esophageal portion and a posterior portion which contains the other organs. The muscular tissue of the posterior part of the esophagus is somewhat reduced and the esophageal glands outside the contour of the esophagus form a single or double row of cells (Figure 235). The anus is terminal or subterminal in both sexes. The male is provided with a single spicule, enclosed in a sheath or is without a spicule. The vulva of the female is located near the termination of the esophagus and the female reproductive system consists of only a single tube. This order contains but one family, the TRICHINELLIDÆ Stiles and Crane, 1910. It is made up of three subfamilies, (1) TRICHINELLINÆ Ransom, 1911; (2) TRICHURINÆ Ransom, 1911; and (3) TRICHOSOMOIDINÆ Hall, 1916.

I. Subfamily TRICHINELLINÆ

TRICHINELLIDÆ, males of which are without spicule or spicule-sheath. The eggs are without a true shell but are surrounded by a delicate membrane. The adults in the intestine give rise to larvæ which become encysted in the musculature of the same host. Females viviparous. Example: *Trichinella spiralis* (Owen, 1835).

1. *Trichinella spiralis* (Owen, 1835)

HISTORICAL

Trichinella spiralis, commonly termed the "trichina worm," was first known by its larval stage encysted in the muscular system of man. These cysts were noted by Tiedemann in 1821 in Germany and by Peacock in London in 1828. Hilton in 1832 considered the cysts to be of parasitic nature and Paget, a student at St. Bartholomew's Hospital, made dissections of the cyst and sketched the parasite. He called his discoveries to the attention of Owen, who described the parasite in 1835, giving it the name *Trichina spiralis*. It was soon found in man throughout Europe and North

473

America and was discovered in the pig by Leidy in Philadelphia. Leuckart and others commenced feeding experiments and it was discovered that the larvæ become adults within a few days in the intestine, and that the female is viviparous. The parasite was considered harmless to man until 1860, when Zenker found the adult worms in the intestine of a young girl who had died in a Dresden hospital, supposedly of typhoid fever. At autopsy the intestine did not show characteristic typhoid lesions but numerous adult trichinæ

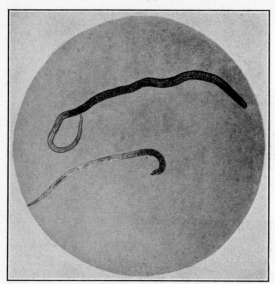

FIG. 233.—*Trichinella spiralis.* Adult specimens from intestinal contents. Upper figure, female; lower figure, male. (After Hemmert-Halsweck)

were found. The history of the case revealed that she had been taken ill shortly after eating pork and, at the same time, several others who had also eaten of the same pork were sick, and pieces of the meat were full of the *Trichinella* larvæ. Numerous other similar cases were observed, many of which occurred in epidemic form. From 1881 to 1898 serious epidemics occurred, particularly in Germany, and during this time American pork was excluded from the German markets because of the alleged frequency with which it was found infected with *Trichinella.* A systematic inspection of pork was then started which led to our present-day system of Federal meat inspection. An examination for trichinous pork, however, is not now included in this inspection for reasons which will be discussed later.

DESCRIPTION

(Figures 233, 234, 235.) The adult males measure about 1.6 mm. in length by 0.04 mm. in breadth and are characterized by the body tapering anteriorly and by the two lateral hemispherical lobes at the posterior extremity which serve during copulation. The adult female measures from 3 mm. to 4 mm. in length by 0.06 mm. in breadth. The vulva is situated in the anterior fifth of the body. Fertilized ova in various stages of development may be seen in the ovary which occupies the posterior extremity, and, as the female is viviparous, larvæ may be seen in the upper third of the uterus. Newly escaped larvæ, about 0.1 mm. in length, may be seen in fresh preparations.

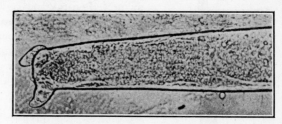

FIG. 234.—*Trichinella spiralis.* Posterior extremity of male showing copulatory appendages. (After Hemmert-Halsweck)

The adult worms inhabit the small intestine of various mammals while the larvæ are found encysted in the voluntary muscles of the same animal which harbors the adult. The life span of the adult worms is a matter of only four or five weeks, whereas the encysted larvæ may remain alive for years in the muscles before they die and become calcified.

GEOGRAPHICAL DISTRIBUTION AND INCIDENCE

Trichinella spiralis is world-wide in distribution and, as it is transmitted from host to host solely as the result of one host eating the flesh of another, its frequency in man depends upon the frequency of the infection in hogs used for food, and upon the extent to which raw or insufficiently cooked pork is eaten. It is, however, a characteristic helminth infection of the Northern Hemisphere and is almost unheard of, as a natural infection, in the tropics. The disease rarely occurs among Americans, English and French who habitually thoroughly cook their pork. Fatal epidemics have occurred particularly among Germans, Austrians and Italians who are fond of raw pork, especially in sausage form and raw spiced hams. From recent studies it appears that trichinosis is astonishingly frequent in the United States. Examinations of diaphragms obtained at autopsy (Queen, 1931; Hinmann, 1936; McNaught and Anderson, 1936) show an incidence varying from 3.5 per cent in New Orleans to 24 per cent in San Francisco, to 27.6 per cent in Boston. Our severest epidemics have been traced directly to home-grown hogs fed garbage from sources which permit a high content of uncooked meat scraps. The pork was usually made at home into highly spiced sausages which were eaten either raw or after imperfect cooking.

Trichinosis occurs most frequently in swine fed on raw garbage. Recent critical surveys by the U. S. Bureau of Animal Industry show that less than 1 per cent of our grain-fed hogs are trichinous, whereas over 4 per cent of those fed on raw garbage are infected. Swine fed on cooked garbage are practically free from trichinæ.

LIFE-CYCLE

The life-cycle of *Trichinella spiralis* may be easily followed by feeding trichinous muscle to a series of white rats or guinea pigs followed by examinations of different individuals at stated intervals. The encysted larvæ are already in an advanced stage of development and when ingested with raw or insufficiently cooked meat they escape from their cysts in the stomach. They reach sexual maturity in the small intestine within as short a period as forty-eight hours. Mating then occurs. After fertilization the female worms burrow more or less deeply into the mucosa of the intestine so that they commonly reach the lymph spaces of the villi. The female is viviparous and deposits the larvæ in successive batches directly into the lymph spaces, or in different parts of the mucous membrane from which they gain entrance into the lymph spaces. They are eventually carried to the blood stream, and then by the blood stream through the lungs to all parts of the body. They are most numerous in the circulating blood between the eighth and twenty-fifth day after infection. Those larvæ which are carried to voluntary muscles leave the capillaries and quickly penetrate into the primary muscle bundles. It is usually those muscles with the richest blood supply which are most

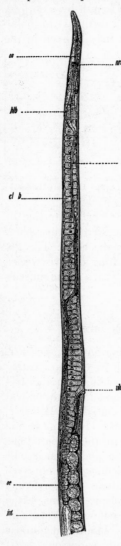

Fig. 235.—Anterior extremity of *Trichinella spiralis* showing the relation of the esophagus and cell body. (After Chitwood) blb, pseudobulb; clb, cell body; int, intestine; oe, esophagus; nrvr, nerve ring; vlv, vulva.

heavily parasitized, such as the diaphragm, intercostal, laryngeal, tongue and eye muscles and the greatest invasion takes place about the tenth day after infection.

Larvæ which fail to enter a muscle fiber are surrounded by a focus of intense acute inflammatory reaction and are destroyed. Such is the fate of larvæ lodging in the brain, heart, liver, pancreas, etc., and also of those in the skeletal muscles which fail to get the protection of the sarcolemma. The cells involved in the destruction of the parasite are polymorphonuclear leukocytes, endothelial leukocytes, lymphocytes and eosinophiles. Giant cell formation is frequent.

The larva when it enters the muscle fiber measures about 0.1 mm. in length and 0.006 mm. in breadth. It is provided with a spear, a movable boring apparatus at the anterior end, by which it is aided in its penetration of a muscle fiber. It comes to lie along the long axis of the fiber and quickly grows in length reaching a total of about 1 mm. within ten to

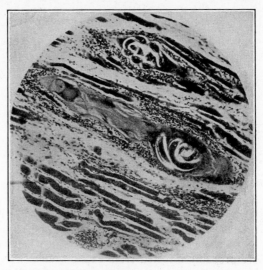

Fig. 236.—Active trichinosis. Early stage of encystment, showing acute inflammatory reaction around parasitized muscle fibers. (After Hemmert-Halsweck)

fourteen days and then assumes the characteristic spiral form of the encysted parasite. The invaded muscle fiber rapidly undergoes more or less degeneration. A lemon-shaped cyst wall of collagen fibrils is formed around the larva. The cysts have an average size of about 0.5 mm. in length by 0.25 mm. in breadth and usually contain one, sometimes two or three larvæ each. Calcification of the capsules may occur as early as six months but usually cyst walls are not completely covered until after one to two years. The newly formed cysts are invisible to the unaided eye, but, after calcification has taken place, they may give a characteristic fine sanded or granular appearance to the cut surface of the infected muscle, especially in massive infections (Figures 236, 237, 238).

A considerable amount of development of the larvæ takes place within the cyst. The reproductive organs are formed, but are not matured, and the larvæ show sexual differentiation. It is for this reason that the larvæ become mature so quickly after ingestion by the host.

Most animals may be experimentally infected with trichinæ but those of omnivorous or carnivorous habits are most frequently parasitized under natural conditions. From the public health standpoint the only animals in this country which are sources of infection and propagators of the disease are hogs, rats and bears. Man becomes infected from eating trichinous pork, and

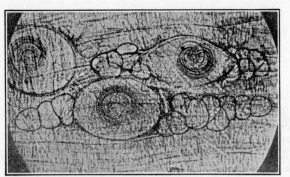

Fig. 237.—Encysted trichinæ showing depositions of fat at the poles of the cysts. (After Hemmert-Halsweck)

hogs become infected from eating the carcasses of other infected hogs, offal from slaughter houses and perhaps occasionally from infected rats. Rats, in turn, acquire the parasite by eating the flesh of trichinous hogs or other rats which happen to be infected. Bears are probably infected from eating young infected pigs.

COURSE OF THE DISEASE

The severity of trichinosis depends upon the number of infective parasites ingested. A few may cause no noticeable symptoms. Most cases, however, are usually characterized by the presence of more or less severe gastro-intestinal disturbances, muscular pain and tenderness, fever and chills, facial edema, urticaria and prostration. Recovery is slow. Vague rheumatic pains, noticed particularly upon rising, may persist for about a year. Death, due to exhaustion, pneumonia or cardiovascular complications, occurs from the fourth to the eighth week after infection.

Trichinosis manifests such a variable symptomatology that the diagnosis is often obscured when the patient is first seen. This is characteristic of mild and sporadic cases. The adult worms and larvæ in the intestine may cause vomiting, abdominal pain, fever, chills, diarrhea, constipation or successive constipation and diarrhea which have been diagnosed typhoid, malaria, colitis, peptic ulcer, appendicitis, gastro-intestinal catarrh and food poisoning. Hiccough, cough, laryngitis, severe muscular pain, difficult breathing, impaired vision, rose spots and cutaneous eruptions, fever with the temperature curve similar to that of typhoid, positive Kernig's sign, facial edema and edema of the eyes are characteristic symptoms during the time the larvæ are in the criculation and the muscles. These symptoms have been diagnosed acute nephritis, conjunctivitis, mumps, periph-

eral neuritis, tetanus, p l e u r i s y, influenza, upper respiratory infection, pneumonia, syphilis, undulant fever, scarlet fever, arthritis, erysipelas, pelvic inflammatory disease, rheumatic fever, angioneurotic edema and lead poisoning. Larvæ which become lodged and disposed of in the heart cause cardiovascular complications which have been diagnosed as myocarditis, rheumatic myocarditis, endocarditis and other pathological heart con-

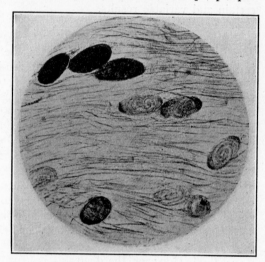

Fig. 238.—Encysted trichinæ in varying degrees of calcification. (After Hemmert-Halsweck)

ditions. Larvæ disposed of in the central nervous system may give rise to neurological symptoms which have been diagnosed meningitis, encephalitis, tuberculous meningitis and poliomyelitis.

There is no typical course in trichinosis. Even in severe cases the order of events may be irregular. Gastro-intestinal symptoms are prominent in the disease picture but may be absent in many cases. Minot (1915) observed several cases of trichinosis with respiratory symptoms so severe, when first seen, as to lead to a serious consideration or actual diagnosis of a purely pulmonary condition. Eye symptoms often predominate to the extent that the patient first consults an ophthalmologist. Heart and nervous conditions may likewise obstruct the entire picture of trichinosis.

The most characteristic and constant symptom is a gradual rise to a high level followed by a gradual decline in the eosinophile count in the circulating blood. Eosinophilia usually appears about the second week of the infection, but may be absent in the blood smears of severe and fatal cases, or in patients who have a complicating secondary infection (Spink, 1934). The total white blood cell count ranges from 7,000 to 17,000 per cubic millimeter.

A single infection appears to confer some immunity against *Trichinella spiralis* for a limited time, but attempts by various workers to immunize laboratory animals artificially have given uncertain and variable results.

DIAGNOSIS

Like many other infectious diseases, the diagnosis of trichinosis is relatively easy when it occurs in epidemic form and when suspected. It is quite generally recommended to examine the patient's blood, spinal fluid, feces or biopsy of muscle for direct evidence of the parasite. These attempts to demonstrate the parasite are so frequently unsuccessful that they are of doubtful value as aids in diagnosis.

Herrick and Janeway (1909) were the first to demonstrate the larvæ in the circulating blood of man. The bloods of three patients of a family of eight ill with trichinosis were examined for larvæ. After more than an hour's search, four larvæ were found in the blood of one. The success of this method has not increased with the years.

Trichinella larvæ were first observed in the spinal fluid by van Cott and Lintz in 1914. Others have since demonstrated them in spinal fluid. However, the diagnosis is usually correctly made before the parasites may be found in the spinal fluid and, since it is such an infrequent finding, one is not warranted in recommending a lumbar puncture as a routine clinical procedure in the diagnosis of trichinosis.

It is generally advised to examine the feces during the stage of diarrhea for adult worms. This method may have had its origin in the ease with which adult worms are usually found in the intestinal contents at autopsy. The adult worms are, however, usually destroyed beyond recognition before they reach the exterior.

A usual procedure employed in diagnosing trichinosis is the microscopic examination of excised skeletal muscle for larvæ. In view of the high incidence of the disease in this country, the finding of larvæ surrounded by thick connective tissue capsules or calcified capsules showing no inflammation is evidence that such are old larvæ and unrelated to an acute condition. Sections of muscle obtained during the acute stage of the illness reveal larvæ with surrounding inflammation and muscle destruction. *Trichinella* larvæ are found in less than half of the biopsies. In most instances, the diagnosis has been made on the presence of myositis rather than on the presence of the parasite itself. Diagnosis by muscle biopsies is therefore exceedingly uncertain.

Serologic tests, skin and precipitin reactions, have been employed only recently in the diagnosis of trichinosis. Guinea pigs are generally used in preparing the antigen. The muscles from an animal which has been infected with *Trichinella* 4 or 5 weeks previously are passed through a food grinder and then digested in a solution of pepsin and hydrochloric acid. The trichinæ settle out in the container and are then washed repeatedly with water until they are free from host tissue. These larvæ are dried, placed in ether for 24 hours, and then dried in a vacuum. They are ground in an agate mortar. To this, 100 parts of Coca's solution ($NaCl$, $NaHCO_3$ and phenol) are added. After 3 or 4 days, the whole mixture is filtered through a Seitz filter and sterilely transferred to small vaccine bottles. For the precipitin tests, the antigen is used in this 1:100 dilution. Higher dilutions are necessary for skin tests.

The precipitin test is performed by overlaying 0.3 cc. of clear serum in a small tube with an equal amount of a 1:100 dilution of the trichinella antigen. A control tube contains 0.3 cc. of serum overlaid with Coca's solution. The tubes are placed in the water bath for 1 hour at 37.5° C. A positive test shows a white ring at the junction of the serum and antigen. The precipitin reaction in trichinosis usually becomes positive about the fourth week of the disease. It is especially useful if the test is at first negative and then later in the disease is found positive. In a few instances, a ring is found in both tubes and, rarely, false positive reactions may be observed after the administration of quinine and probably certain other drugs.

The intradermal skin test is made by injecting 0.1 cc. of a 1:10,000 dilution of the trichinella antigen into one arm, and a similar amount of Coca's solution into the other arm. Immediately following the injections there is an erythematous flare, which quickly subsides. Within 5 minutes after the injection of positive reactors, a blanched wheal appears, sometimes with pseudopodia running out from it, with a pronounced area of erythema surrounding the wheal. The reaction reaches its maximum in one hour, and then gradually subsides. This is the immediate type of reaction which has been accepted as diagnostic for trichinosis. The skin test does not usually become positive until the second week of the disease, and may be elicited months and years after the acute illness has subsided. Like the precipitin test, the skin test is especially useful if the test is at first negative and then later becomes positive. Skin tests performed on the second to the fourth day of the illness result in no immediate response, but twenty-four hours later there may occur a delayed, tuberculin-like type of reaction. This reaction has been elicited only during the first week of the illness; after that the response is of the immediate type (Spink, 1937). So far as is known, the presence of other helminths does not affect these reactions (Kaljus, 1936).

In the use of these tests, one must not lose sight of the fact that no biologic test is infallible. Any test employed should be considered in connection with other evidence.

The presence of an ascending eosinophilia is the most reliable laboratory aid in the diagnosis of trichinosis. Eosinophilia usually appears about the second week of the infection. Frequent examinations of stained blood smears are often necessary. Eosinophilia may be absent in the blood smears of severe and fatal cases, or in patients who have a complicating secondary infection. The recognition and correct diagnosis depend on a careful history of the patient's illness, a complete physical examination, repeated examinations of blood smears for eosinophiles, and the use of skin and precipitin tests.

TREATMENT

The treatment of trichinosis is entirely symptomatic. No drug is known to be effective against either the adults or the larvæ.

PREVENTION

Although trichinosis is relatively common in pigs, the chances of infection in man may be entirely avoided by eating pork only after it has been thoroughly cooked or thoroughly cured. For detailed account of the effects of pork-curing processes on trichinæ, the reader is referred to Ransom (1920). Microscopic inspection of pork is not a safeguard against trichinosis. Trichinous pork has been examined microscopically as many as eighty times before the parasites were found. Stiles has shown that nearly one-third of the cases of trichinosis occurring in Germany between 1881 and 1898 were caused by hogs inspected and passed as free from trichinæ (Ransom, 1915). Because of the unreliability of microscopic inspection for trichinæ it is not included in the system of meat inspection in this country. Therefore the Government mark, "U. S. Inspected and Passed," on pork does not guarantee that the meat is trichinæ free and it should be thoroughly cooked before it is used for food. When properly cooked, trichinous pork is as wholesome as non-trichinous pork. One of the most important of all measures against trichinosis in man is the education of the individual as to the danger of eating raw or insufficiently cooked pork. It would seem that one of the most effective means of bringing this information to the public is through the school.

Inasmuch as trichinosis in swine in this country appears to have its source in garbage and offal, it would be advisable to encourage the feeding of cooked garbage and cooked offal, particularly garbage collected from market districts and known to contain raw meat scraps.

For the present, the control of trichinosis obviously rests with the housekeeper, which means that all pork should be cooked thoroughly before it is eaten.

II. Subfamily TRICHURINÆ

TRICHINELLIDÆ. Males with one spicule, or exceptionally with only a spicule-sheath. The eggs are lemon-shaped, with a thick shell and polar opercula and are unsegmented when deposited. The development, so far as known, is direct. Example: *Trichuris trichiura* (Linnæus, 1771) in man.

1. *Trichuris trichiura* (Linnæus, 1771)

DESCRIPTION

Trichuris trichiura is generally known as the whip-worm of man. It is most frequently found in the cecum and the appendix and more rarely in the large intestine of man. It has also been found in monkeys and LEMURIDÆ. The whip-worm is world-wide in distribution, but like many other helminths, it is most frequent in the tropical and subtropical countries.

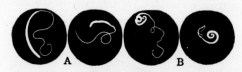

FIG. 239.—*Trichuris trichiura*. A, females; B, males. The posterior portion of the male is usually coiled as is shown at the right. Photographs of mounted specimens. Natural size. (From Todd's *Clinical Diagnosis,* W. B. Saunders Company)

The whip-worm (Figures 239, 240) is of a grayish or pinkish color. The anterior portion of the body is much attenuated, hence the derivation of its common name, "whip-worm." The anterior portion is longer than the posterior portion, or body proper. The males measure from 30 mm. to 45 mm. and the females from 30 mm. to 50 mm. in length. The adult worms are provided with a lancet-shaped spear at the anterior extremity which probably serves the purpose of working an entrance into the host's tissue (Figure 240). The eggs are characteristically barrel shaped, brown in color, measure from 51 μ to 54 μ in length by 22 μ in breadth and are unsegmented at time of deposition (Figure 241).

LIFE-CYCLE

The development of the embryo is very slow and may require from six months to a year before it is completely formed. The

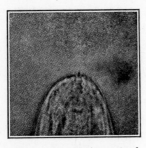

FIG. 240.—Anterior end of *Trichuris trichiura* showing protrusion of spear. (After Li)

eggs are very resistant and, like those of *Ascaris,* may live for a long period in the open. The method of infection is direct and once the ripe egg is ingested by man or another suitable host the embryo escapes from the egg-shell and, according to Hasegawa (1924), penetrates the villi of the intestine, especially the villi of the cecum, and there rests for two or three days near the glands of Lieberkühn. It then passes into the lumen of the cecum where development proceeds to maturity. Eggs may appear in the host's feces thirty-six days after infection. *Trichuris* eggs are less resistant to drying than *Ascaris* eggs.

PATHOGENESIS

The whip-worm is commonly found with its whip-like anterior portion embedded superficially in the mucous membrane. This species

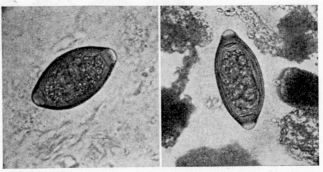

FIG. 241.—Eggs of *Trichuris trichiura* in feces (x 500). (From Todd's *Clinical Diagnosis,* W. B. Saunders Company)

has been associated with appendicitis but it is generally believed to be of no great importance in human pathology.

The whip-worms are difficult to remove by anthelmintics on account of their position in the host. The latex of a wild fig tree, *Ficus glabrata,* of Central America and Colombia is known to be effective against *Trichuris* when used in the fresh state. This drug may be taken in large doses, 30 ml. or more, without any apparent discomfort to the patient.

Prevention. Measures taken against *Ascaris* are equally effective against *Trichuris.*

Other species belonging to this genus are *Trichuris vulpis* in the dog and wolf; *T. suis*

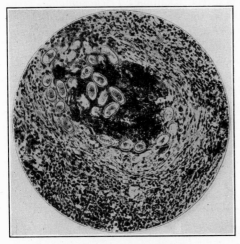

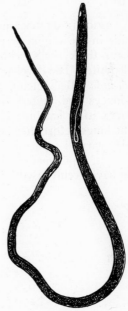

FIG. 242.—Section of rat liver showing intense cellular reaction against the eggs of *Capillaria hepatica.* (After Weidman)

FIG. 243.—*Trichosomoides crassicauda.* Mature female with male in uterus. (After Hall)

in the pig; *T. ovis* in sheep and cattle; *T. leporis* in rabbits.

The genus *Capillaria* Zeder, 1800, is frequent in birds and mammals, not including man. This genus is characterized by the esophageal portion being shorter than, or rarely equal in length to the posterior portion. Representative species are, *Capillaria brevipes* in the small intestine of sheep, *C. annulata* in and beneath the thickened lining of the gizzard of pheasants and *C. hepatica* (Bancroft, 1893) in rats and rodents. The life-cycle is direct.

C. hepatica is a frequent and sometimes fatal parasite of rats and other rodents. It occurs in the liver, where it causes great destruction of tissues from accumulations of its eggs (Figure 242). This species has been reported once from man, a British soldier in India, who had died from septic pneumonia secondary to a liver abscess caused by the accumulation of these worms and their eggs. Eggs of *C. hepatica* have been encountered occasionally in human feces. Whether these represent true infections or are cases of food contamination is not known.

III. Subfamily TRICHOSOMOIDINÆ

TRICHINELLIDÆ; male without spicule or spicule-sheath and parasitic in the vagina or uterus of the female (Figure 243). The eggs have thick shells with polar opercula and contain embryos when deposited. The development is direct. Example: *Trichosomoides crassicauda* (Bellingham, 1840), in the urinary bladder, pelvis of the kidneys and ureters of rats. According to Yokogawa (1920) the larvæ after hatching in the stomach and intestine of the rat pass to the lungs before they become established in the bladder, and are probably carried from the lungs to the bladder in the blood vessels. Calculosis, papillomata and malignant growths of the bladder are believed to have been caused by these worms and their eggs.

CHAPTER XXXI

NEMATODE PARASITES (Concluded)

Appendix to *Nemathelminthes*

I. *Gordiacea*

I. GENERAL DESCRIPTION

The GORDIACEA are long, thin worms generally known as "horse hair snakes." They are larger than most nematodes and are more uniformly cylindrical, with blunt rounded anterior ends, and with the caudal end swollen, lobed or curled in a loose spiral. They usually show some coloration. Their resemblance to the nematoda is, however, only superficial, and in finer details of structure they have little in common with them. There are no lateral lines and the body is opaque. The cloaca, or common outlet of the reproductive and alimentary systems, is present in both sexes and is situated near the posterior extremity of the body. The male never possesses spicules. The body cavity is lined by epithelium. The gonads are not continuous with their ducts. The ova are discharged into the body cavity and then pass into the ducts. In sexually mature worms the alimentary trace is atrophied.

The adults live free in water and are frequently found in the country in drinking troughs, ponds, streams and puddles of water formed by heavy rains. The larval forms are, however, parasitic and frequently occur in land insects which have aquatic stages.

2. LIFE-CYCLE

The female deposits long strings of eggs on aquatic vegetation and these develop into small larvæ, characterized by a proboscis armed with hooks. The newly-hatched larva swims about in the water for a time and enters into an aquatic insect, usually the nymph of the mayfly. After a period the still immature worm passes into new hosts, namely, beetles, crickets and grasshoppers, where it continues development in the body cavity. The mode of transfer of the infection to these hosts is not clearly known, but in the case where the first host is the nymph of a mayfly, and the second a carnivorous beetle, it has been suggested that in a season of drought, when the pools become dry, the mayfly larvæ become the easy prey of beetles, and when feeding upon them the beetles take in the young hair snakes. Development continues within the body cavity of the new host until the worm is almost full grown, when it escapes into the water and becomes sexually mature. As the final host is usually a terrestrial insect it is necessary that this host be drowned in water in order that the adult worms can reach their natural environment. It is for this reason that the hair snakes are found most frequently in bodies of water following a rainstorm or flood.

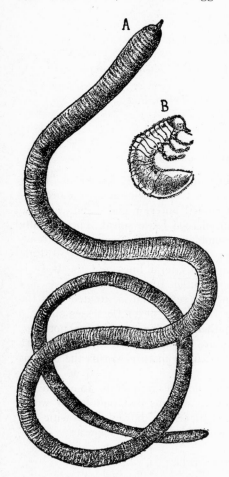

FIG. 244.—*Macracanthorhynchus hirudinaceus.* A, female, natural size; B, larva of *Melolontha melolontha,* an intermediate host. (From Neveu-Lemaire's *Parasitologie des Animaux Domestiques,* J. Lamarre, Paris)

A number of adult GORDIACEA have been reported as human parasites. In most instances the worms were said to have been vomited or passed with the stool. In all probability these were cases of contamination. More recently Sayad, Johnson and Faust (1936) report the removal of a small, sexually immature specimen, probably *Gordius robustus,* from an abscess of the lower eyelid of a man residing in Florida. It is likely that this infection came from drinking water containing newly hatched larvæ. This is, probably, the first authentic case of human parasitism by a gordiid worm.

II. *Acanthocephala*

1. GENERAL DESCRIPTION

The ACANTHOCEPHALA include the "spineheaded worms." The adults occur only in the intestine of vertebrates and are commonly attached to the intestinal wall by means of a protrusible proboscis which is almost invariably covered with hooks. The ACANTHO-CEPHALA, like the GORDIACEA, bear only a superficial resemblance to the nematoda. They characteristically present a roughened surface and have a more or less spindle-shaped form. At no stage in their life history is there any trace of an alimentary system. The reproductive system is very complex. In the female there is no persistent gonad. The egg masses are formed early and, after fertilization, these break up into individual spined embryos, each of which becomes surrounded by three embryonic membranes. They are usually oval in form. The ACANTHOCEPHALA are common parasites of fishes and birds but may also occur in other vertebrates, including man.

2. LIFE-CYCLE

The life-cycle of ACANTHOCEPHALA is poorly known but probably there is always an alternation of hosts during development. For example, the embryos of *Macracanthorhynchus hirudinaceus* Pallas, 1781, a common parasite of pigs, develop in terrestrial beetle larvæ, and those of *Moniliformis moniliformis,* which usually occurs in rats and other rodents, develop in the cockroach. In aquatic species it is inferred that the ripe embryos become ingested by a suitable host, probably a crustacean in the body cavity of which they develop to the stage infective for the final host.

FIG. 245.—Egg of *Macracanthorhynchus hirudinaceus*. Magnified. (Partly after Leuckart)

Macracanthorhynchus hirudinaceus (Figure 245) has been reported from man in Russia and *Moniliformis moniliformis* (Bremser, 1811) of rats, mice and the dog appears to be a facultative parasite in man. Several species of the genera *Echinorhynchus* and *Neoechinorhynchus* occur in American fishes. *Onciola canis* (Kaupp, 1909) occurs in dogs in Texas and Nebraska and *Plagiorhynchus formosus* van Cleve, 1918, in American passerine birds and chickens. The ACANTHOCEPHALA are not of economic importance.

The student is referred to van Cleve (1936) for recent systems of classification.

Section III

ARTHROPODS
OF
PARASITOLOGICAL IMPORTANCE

BY

FRANCIS M. ROOT

AND

CLAY G. HUFF

Grateful acknowledgment is made to Dr. W. A. Hoffman for aid upon the Ceratopogonidæ; to Dr. M. A. Stewart for the revision of the chapter on Siphonaptera; to Dr. P. F. Russell for advice upon the section on the malaria-carrying *Anopheles;* to Dr. S. Adler for advice on *Phlebotomus;* to Dr. W. E. Dove for the use of figure 305; to Dr. D. G. Hall, Jr., for the use of figure 283; and to Dr. G. H. Bradley for the use of his key to the American anophelines.

CHAPTER XXXII

INTRODUCTION

I. *Arthropods of Parasitological Importance*

In Sections I and II of this book attention is directed to animals which are of interest because of their ability to produce directly harmful effects upon the animals in which they live. In the following section we are concerned with invertebrate animals, belonging chiefly to the phylum ARTHROPODA, which are of interest to us not so much because of their abilities to produce harmful effects upon their hosts directly but rather because of their abilities to transmit from one individual host to another diseases caused by other parasitic forms of life. This branch of parasitology is most commonly referred to as Medical Entomology. This term is misleading, however, unless we apply it in a restricted sense; for the subject to which we have referred above does not fall entirely within the field of entomology nor is it of medical interest only. Some of the most important disease-carrying parasites, such as ticks and mites, are not insects. Nor is the importance of arthropods in causing or transmitting disease by any means to be restricted to those concerned with human disease. We, therefore, lack a correct and comprehensive name for the study of arthropods of parasitological importance, although for most purposes it will be convenient to continue to use the term Medical Entomology. The study of the insects and other arthropods which cause or carry diseases of wild or domestic animals is often referred to as Veterinary Entomology in contrast to the forms of strictly medical importance. In the following section it seems desirable to consider all of these forms as belonging to one field of study, since the same basic principles underlie their study, whether the parasites concerned transmit human or animal diseases. In fact, we know that the same arthropods often transmit identical diseases of man and animals, or transmit them back and forth between animals and man.

The phylum ARTHROPODA, consisting of invertebrate animals with paired, jointed appendages on the segments of the head, the thorax and sometimes the abdomen and with a chitinous exoskeleton, is divided into the following five classes:

Class INSECTA (true insects)
Class ARACHNIDA (ticks, mites, spiders, scorpions, etc.)
Class CRUSTACEA (crabs, lobsters, shrimps, water-fleas, etc.)
Class MYRIAPODA (centipedes and millipedes)
Class PROTRACHEATA (Peripatus)

The forms which are of parasitological importance include especially several types of true insects and certain ticks and mites, but one
might also treat under the head of Medical Entomology those spiders,
scorpions and centipedes whose bites or stings can produce symptoms
in human beings and the crabs and water-fleas (Cyclops) which act
as intermediate hosts for helminth parasites of man.

While there is no doubt of the advisability of including this field
as one of the divisions of Parasitology, there may be much discussion
as to whether we can, strictly speaking, call these arthropod vectors
Parasites. In the last analysis, the difficulty lies in defining how long
an organism must remain on its host to be called a parasite. In the
first chapter of this book we have defined a parasite as an organism
that lives on, in or with some other living organism from which it
derives some benefit, and have recognized as periodic parasites those
parasites which make short visits to their hosts to obtain nourishment
or other benefits. The question is, how long must these visits last?
At first glance one would probably declare that a tick was undoubtedly a parasite, but a mosquito was not. And yet most ticks behave
toward their hosts exactly as does a mosquito. Both attach themselves
to the host by piercing its skin with their mouthparts and, if not disturbed, remain attached until they have filled themselves with blood.
The difference is that while the mosquito can engorge in a few minutes, the tick must remain for days or even weeks before engorgement
is complete. In either case, however, when filled with blood the arthropod leaves its host and digests the blood-meal and lays its eggs in a
free-living condition. The transient nature of the parasitic habit of
many such forms as mosquitoes introduces a complicating factor into
the study of the arthropods of parasitological importance which is not
so important, or may be completely lacking, in the study of the parasitic protozoa and worms. These latter parasites are usually *within* the
host and hence are largely isolated from other similar animals. Most
of the parasitic arthropods, on the contrary, are free-living during
much of their lives and hence their importance is not so apparent. The
problems of seeking out from the many closely related forms those
which are of importance in disease transmission, of proving or dis-
proving the part played by these in transmission, and later, the

continual necessity for identifying the incriminated species place additional burdens upon parasitologists who study the parasitic arthropods. For this reason, classification and identification necessarily play greater parts in this study. It is also true that one who studies these arthropods needs an accurate knowledge of the bacteria, filterable viruses, protozoa, and helminths which are transmitted by them.

II. *External Structure of Insects*

Insects are completely enclosed in a non-cellular integument which is more or less chitinized and which is often called the exoskeleton, since it performs both the protective function of a skin and the supporting function of a skeleton. In order to permit freedom of movement this integument is not uniformly chitinized throughout, but consists of a number of hard plates or *sclerites,* connected with each other by flexible, slightly chitinized membranes.

Insects are supposed to have developed from ancestors more or less resembling the segmented worms, and in the beginning the insect body probably consisted of a large number of similar segments, each with a pair of jointed appendages. In the insects of the present time, however, the segmentation is obvious only in the abdomen, and the division of the body into the three regions of head, thorax and abdomen is much more important than the original segmentation.

The head consists of a box-like capsule formed, as we can see if we study insect embryology, by complete fusion of seven original segments. The appendages of these segments are retained, for the most part, and form the antennæ or feelers, the compound eyes, and the mouth parts, which usually include a pair of mandibles, a pair of maxillæ and a labium formed by the fusion of a pair of maxilla-like appendages. The maxillæ and the labium may have sensory *palpi* attached to them. The structure of the mouth parts varies a great deal, depending upon the type of food taken by the insect. From one to three ocelli or simple eyes may be present on the dorsum of the head in addition to the compound eyes.

The thorax consists of three segments (prothorax, mesothorax and metathorax), which may or may not be fused together. The appendages of these three segments are the legs, each made up of a number of joints (called, proceeding from base to tip, coxa, trochanter, femur, tibia and several [usually five] tarsal joints). In addition to the legs, the mesothorax and metathorax each has a pair of wings in most insects. This is not always true, for in the Order DIPTERA, so important from the medical viewpoint, the metathoracic wings are always reduced to tiny rudiments of no value in flight, and in ectoparasitic insects like fleas and lice wings are entirely absent.

The size and degree of development of the thoracic segments depends a great deal upon the development of the wings. In wingless forms like the fleas the three thoracic segments are all small and about the same size. In winged insects the prothorax is often smaller than the other two segments and in the flies or DIPTERA, the meso-thorax, bearing the only functional wings, is very large, while both prothorax and metathorax are much reduced in size.

Each thoracic segment has chitinized plates or sclerites dorsally, laterally and ventrally. If there is only one in each region the dorsal sclerite is called the *notum,* the ventral one the *sternum* and each of the lateral ones a *pleuron.* Often these sclerites are more or less distinctly divided into several portions by scars or *sutures,* at least in one or two of the thoracic segments. The notum may be divided into *prescutum, scutum, scutellum* and *postscutellum.* The pleuron is usually divided into an anterior *episternum* and a posterior *epimeron,* but in most of the DIPTERA the very large meso-thoracic segment has these sclerites still further divided, the episternum being separated into a dorsal *mesopleura* and a ventral *sternopleura,* the epimeron into a dorsal *pteropleura* and a ventral *hypopleura.* The sternum is usually a single plate but may be divided into *sternum* and *sternellum* in some insects.

While the head of an insect is a special region bearing sense organs and mouth parts and the thorax is a region specialized for bearing locomotor appendages, the abdomen is not a specialized region but only the remaining segments of the body. The number of segments in the abdomen varies in different insects, but the usual number appears to be ten. The last one or two segments are usually somewhat modified for sexual purposes, forming the external genitalia or *hypopygium* of the male and the *ovipositor* of the female. Each abdominal segment usually has a single dorsal sclerite (*tergite*) and a single ventral sclerite (*sternite*) connected at the sides by *pleural membranes.* In most insects, the appendages of the abdominal segments are absent except in the terminal segments which are modified for copulation and oviposition.

III. *Internal Structure of Insects*

Internally insects differ most strikingly from vertebrates in the position of the nervous system, the development of the circulatory system and the method of functioning of the respiratory system. (See Figure 246.)

The nervous system consists of a chain of ganglia, connected by commissures, lying ventrally, just inside the ventral body wall. Originally there was one ganglion or pair of ganglia for each body segment, but in present-day insects the seven head ganglia have fused into two and the abdominal ganglia are usually reduced in number because a certain amount of fusion has taken place in that region also. Besides the two main ganglia of the head there is usually a

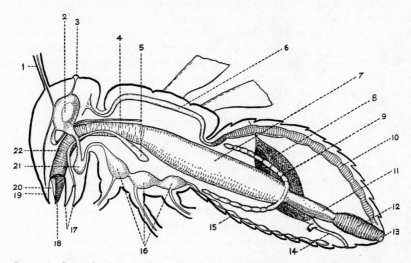

FIG. 246.—Internal structure of a typical insect. (Redrawn from Berlese "Gli Insetti")

1—Antennæ	12—Rectum
2—Supra-esophageal ganglion	13—Anus
3—Ocellus	14—Gonaduct
4—Esophagus	15—Abdominal nerve ganglion
5—Salivary gland	16—Thoracic nerve ganglia
6—Aorta	17—Maxillæ
7—Midgut	18—Mandible
8—Gonad	19—Labrum
9—Malpighian tubule	20—Mouth
10—Dorsal pulsating vessel	21—Sub-esophageal ganglion
11—Intestine	22—Pharynx

large pair of optic ganglia in close connection with the compound eyes. Usually the three thoracic ganglia are larger than the head ganglia. From each ganglion nerve strands are given off to the adjoining tissues and appendages.

There is no well-developed circulatory system in insects. The blood fills the body cavity (*hæmocœle*) and is kept more or less stirred up by the pulsations of a single dorsal vessel which takes in blood posteriorly and ejects it anteriorly.

The respiratory system consists of a branching system of internal air-tubes (*tracheæ*) which open to the exterior through one or more pairs of *spiracles* and carry air directly to all tissues of the body. There is a pair of large tracheæ running the full length of the body and communicating with the spiracles either directly or by short side-branches. From the large tracheal trunks are given off smaller tracheæ which branch again and again until the ultimate branches or tracheal capillaries reach all the cells of the body. In some aquatic insect larvæ the tracheal system is open to the air, as in the adults; in others the tracheal system is closed and oxygen is obtained from the water by means of *tracheal gills,* much like blood-gills in their structure except that the capillaries are represented by fine tracheæ.

The digestive system is well-developed, but a large part of it consists of invaginated ectodermal tissue. Only the stomach or *ventriculus* is endodermal. Salivary glands are usually present, but are not connected with the digestive system except for the fact that their duct ends in connection with the mouth parts. In some insects a *crop* for the storage of food is present.

Excretory organs are represented by a variable number of *Malpighian tubules,* which are attached to the alimentary canal just about at the point of junction of ventriculus and intestine.

The reproductive system is comparatively simple. There is a pair of testes or ovaries, whose ducts soon unite to form a common duct leading to the genital opening. The male may have accessory glands and a seminal vesicle for the storage of spermatozoa and the female may have shell glands, cement glands, and a seminal receptacle.

In the abdomen is found a loosely connected tissue of large cells called the *fat-body,* which may be very prominent in insects entering upon hibernation and presumably represents a reserve food supply.

IV. *Life Histories of Insects*

All insects produce eggs, although in some insects the eggs hatch within the body of the female. In the more primitive insects, grasshoppers or bugs for example, the *larva* which hatches from the egg closely resembles the parent except in size, proportions and the absence of wings and reproductive organs, and takes the same food as the adult. As the larva grows it has to shed its skin or *moult* at intervals, finally becoming an *adult* with functional wings and sex organs after the last moult. Such a life history is said to be a case of *incomplete metamorphosis,* since there is no striking change in appearance when the larva becomes an adult.

In the more highly specialized insects, such as butterflies or flies, on the other hand, the larva which hatches from the egg is a worm-like organism which looks very different from its parent and has entirely different food-habits. As this larva grows and moults several times it retains essentially the same appearance until, at the next to the last moult, it suddenly changes into an enclosed or protected *pupa,* which does not feed, but again sheds its skin to liberate the adult after a variable interval. Such a life history is said to exhibit *complete metamorphosis,* since there is a complete change in appearance in passing from the larva to the adult. Although some pupæ (those of mosquitoes, for example) are quite active, most pupæ are relatively or entirely quiescent, so that the pupa is sometimes spoken of as a resting stage. This is true, superficially, but if we were to look into the inside of the pupa we should find it in a period of intense activity, during which almost all of the larval structures are broken down and the structures of the adult built up. This seems to be, in fact, the reason for the pupal stage. The larvæ of these specialized insects have become so different from the adults, in adaptation to their different habitat and food, that they are no longer able to change directly into the adult, by shedding their skins and have to take this externally quiescent pupal period to concentrate upon the task of remodelling all their structures for an entirely different sort of life.

The fact that insect larvæ are completely enclosed by a more or less chitinized integument, which must be shed or moulted periodically in order to permit of growth, is often very convenient for the entomologist in studying life histories. In the case of mosquitoes, for example, it is easily possible to isolate a larva and preserve for study the larval skin, the pupal skin and the adult mosquito. The larval and pupal skins retain all their characteristic hairs and other appendages and are often even better material than preserved larvæ or pupæ for the study of their structure and distinguishing characteristics. They also have, of course, the additional advantage that one may be sure of studying the larval, pupal and adult structures of the same individual specimen.

V. *Relationship to Disease*

Insects, and some other arthropods, may cause injury to man and animals in two ways. As mentioned previously, they are of very great importance because of their ability to transmit disease-producing organisms. Others of them are able to bring about harmful effects directly by their attacks. In the case of some diseases the transmissions are effected entirely mechanically by the arthropods concerned. Thus we know that house flies may carry the organisms of typhoid directly from the feces of a patient to the food of other persons. In such a transmission there is no multiplication of the organism during the transfer, and the fly is not acting as a true host to the typhoid bacillus. This mechanical type of transmission may occur by contamination of the external surface of the insect and the subsequent contact of this contaminated surface with food or with some part of the host which the disease organisms may attack, or the organisms may be ingested with the food of the insect and later given up through regurgitation or defecation. In a larger number of transmissions of important disease-producing organisms, the insect serves as a host for the organisms, allowing their multiplication or development, or both, and then passing them on to other persons or animals. In most cases these insects also have acquired their infections through their food, that is, by sucking blood or other fluid which contains the organisms, or by ingesting feces containing the organisms. However, they may transfer the organisms back to another host in a number of ways. They may pass the organisms on to another host by fecal contamination, as mentioned above, by injection of saliva, by deposition on the skin, or finally, the insects themselves may be eaten by a second host. An arthropod which transmits a disease from one vertebrate host to another is spoken of as a *vector* of that disease.

Upon the recognition of the above possibilities a classification of disease transmissions by arthropods has been proposed (Huff, 1931) as follows:

A. BIOLOGICAL

      I. CYCLO-PROPAGATIVE—the organisms undergo cyclic change and also multiplication.

     II. CYCLO-DEVELOPMENTAL—the organisms undergo cyclic change but do not multiply.

    III. PROPAGATIVE—the organisms undergo multiplication but no cyclic change.

B. MECHANICAL—the organisms undergo neither cyclic change nor multiplication.

The arthropods which are capable of injuring their hosts directly do so (1) by means of venoms or poisons introduced into them by bites, stings, stinging hairs, vesicating fluids, etc., or (2) by destroying the tissues of the host. Examples of the first group are the bites of spiders, the stings of bees, the stinging hairs of certain caterpillars, and the fluids from blister beetles; while the flesh-eating maggots of flies are examples of the second group. (See Chapters XLV and LII.)

The ability to cause or transmit disease is directly related to the structure, physiology and habits of the arthropods involved. The arthropods with mouthparts adapted to bloodsucking are especially important in the transmission of those pathogenic organisms which are found in the blood or other body fluids. Other arthropods, such as most of the bugs (HEMIPTERA), have piercing or sucking mouthparts, but have not developed the habit of feeding on man or animals. Consequently they are of negligible importance in transmitting disease amongst these groups. Some arthropods may be adapted in structure and habit for feeding on blood, but lack a susceptibility to the organisms living in this medium, and consequently cannot serve as transmitting hosts for the latter. Many flies are attracted to fecal matter but fail to be effective transmitting agents because they do not also have the habit of visiting the food of man. This need for the correlation of several characteristics in order to be an efficient vector explains why only a relatively small number of arthropods transmit disease. Quite naturally, we shall be most interested here in those characteristics of arthropods which make them suitable for disease production and tranmission.

In addition to the rôle known to be played now by arthropods in the transmission of disease there is the possibility that some of the parasites of man and animals may have been parasites of arthropods originally. Thus there seems to be good evidence that the hæmoflagellates, the piroplasmas, the malarial parasites, the relapsing fever spirochætes, and the rickettsiæ evolved first as parasites of arthropods and were transferred to vertebrates when the arthropods become parasitic upon vertebrates. (See Huff, 1938.)

CHAPTER XXXIII

THE DIPTERA (FLIES, MOSQUITOES, ETC.)

I. *Importance*

Of all the groups of arthropods which are concerned with the production or transmission of disease the Order DIPTERA, or true flies, are of paramount importance. This order includes a great variety of blood-sucking forms responsible for the transmission of such important diseases as malaria, yellow fever and African sleeping sickness, and also contains a number of non-blood-sucking forms of sanitary interest, such as the ordinary house-flies and blow-flies.

II. *Characteristics*

The most characteristic thing about the DIPTERA is that only one pair of wings (the fore-wings) is functional, the hind wings being reduced to tiny club-like structures known as the *halteres*. In consequence of this, the mesothorax, bearing the functional wings, is enlarged dorsally at the expense of the other two thoracic segments, so that in dorsal view nearly all the visible parts of the thorax belong to this segment.

The mouth parts of the DIPTERA are always adapted for sucking up liquids, but their structure varies a great deal in different groups and sometimes even in the two sexes of the same species. Some forms feed on vertebrate blood, others on the blood and body juices of other insects, and many more on the nectar of flowers or on any exposed food substance which is in a liquid state or can be liquefied by the regurgitation of fluid from the crop.

In the more primitive DIPTERA, such as horse-flies or mosquitoes, the mouth parts include paired *mandibles* and *maxillæ* and an ensheathing *labium* as well as two other structures, the *epipharynx* and the *hypopharynx,* which together form a tube through which blood or other liquids can be sucked up. The hypopharynx also contains the salivary duct, which opens at its tip. A pair of *palpi* are attached to the bases of the maxillæ, but in the DIPTERA labial palpi are never present. As we run through a series of families in the

DIPTERA we find first the mandibles and then the maxillæ reduced and then entirely absent until in the most highly developed DIPTERA, such as the house-flies and tsetse-flies, the mouth parts include only labium, epipharynx, hypopharynx and the maxillary palpi, which are now attached to the base of the labium.

III. *Classification*

In classifying the DIPTERA, that is, in arranging the various different forms in a natural evolutionary series, we make use of several different tendencies which may be seen in the group. The first division depends on the structure of the larva and pupa. In the suborder ORTHORRHAPHA the larva has a well-chitinized head capsule and the pupa is enclosed in its own heavily chitinized pupal skin. The adult escapes from the pupal skin by a longitudinal dorsal slit in the thoracic region. In the more specialized suborder CYCLORRHAPHA the larval head is not enclosed in a chitinized capsule, and the pupa which

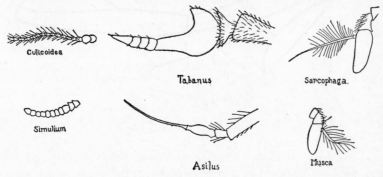

Culicoides

Tabanus

Sarcophaga.

Simulium

Asilus

Musca

Fig. 247.—Antennæ of Diptera; *Culicoides* and *Simulium* representing the Nematocera, *Tabanus* and *Asilus* the Brachycera, and *Sarcophaga* and *Musca* the Cyclorrhapha. (Original. Root)

does not have a well chitinized skin, is enclosed and protected by a *puparium* formed by a further deposit of chitin upon the last larval skin. The adult escapes from the puparium by pushing off a circular cap at the anterior end by repeated protrusions of a fluid-filled vesicle, the *ptilinum,* which projects from the anterior surface of the head of the adult, just above the bases of the antennæ. After the adult has emerged the ptilinum is withdrawn within the head, leaving only a scar to mark the place where it was evaginated. In some flies with a small ptilinum this scar is only a crescent-shaped affair above the bases of the antennæ (the *frontal lunule*). In others where the ptilinum is larger, the scar is continued ventrally on each side of the depression in which the antennæ lie, these continuations being called the *frontal sutures.*

Although this division of the Order DIPTERA into two suborders is a fundamental one for classification, it is not a very convenient one to use in identifying specimens. For identification it is easier to make use of the tendencies toward reduction or simplification which appear in the structure of the antennæ and the venation of the wings.

The most primitive forms of insects have long antennæ composed of a considerable number of elongated joints. As we pass to higher and higher forms we find the joints becoming shorter and thicker and the number of joints reduced, until in the higher flies we reach a standardized condition in which the antennæ consist of

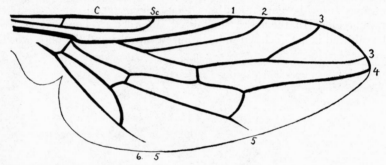

FIG. 248.—Wing venation of *Scenopinus;* C, costa; Sc, subcosta; 1 to 6, first to sixth veins. (Original. Root)

two short basal joints and a larger third joint from whose dorsal side near the base there arises a slender filament, the *arista,* which probably represents several joints fused together (see Figure 247).

The wing venation also offers very convenient characters for identifying flies. Along the front edge of the wing there runs a strong vein, the *costa,* which may extend entirely around the wing margin or may end abruptly at or before the tip of the wing. Just behind the costa lies another vein, the *subcosta,* which usually joins the costa somewhere along the anterior margin of the wing. Behind the subcosta come a series of six more longitudinal veins which are simply called the first, second, third, fourth, fifth and sixth veins. The first, fourth, fifth and sixth veins arise at the base of the wing, but the second and third do not. In many wings it can be seen that the second vein arises as a branch of the first and the third vein as a branch of the second, but in such a wing as that of a mosquito, for example, this is not always obvious. The longitudinal veins are joined to each other by a small number of short *cross-veins*. Beneath the base of the wing are often found rounded, membranous prolongations extending posteriorly and called the *squamæ*.

In passing from lower to higher groups of DIPTERA, we find that the tendency of evolution in the order is toward a reduction in number of veins produced by the fusion of adjoining veins, beginning at their tips. This process may be appreciated best by comparing the positions of the sixth vein and the posterior branch of the fifth in the wings of *Anopheles, Chrysops, Scenopinus,* and *Musca* (Figures 250, 271, 248, 275).

The legs of DIPTERA are of the usual insect structure, with five tarsal joints. The last joint usually bears at its tip two *claws* and often two hairy pads or *pulvilli*. Ventrally, in the mid-line, we often find an *empodium*, which is usually a branched or unbranched bristle-like structure, but sometimes forms a third hairy pad like the pulvilli.

The following tabulation will show the general scheme of classification of the Order DIPTERA and the position in it of those families which contain species of importance to parasitologists.

Order DIPTERA
    Suborder ORTHORRHAPHA
        Section NEMATOCERA—CULICIDÆ—Mosquitoes
                    CERATOPOGONIDÆ—Midges
                    PSYCHODIDÆ—Moth-flies
                    SIMULIIDÆ—Black-flies
        Section BRACHYCERA—TABANIDÆ—Horse-flies
    Suborder CYCLORRHAPHA
        Tribe ACALYPTRATÆ—OSCINIDÆ—Eye-flies
        Tribe CALYPTRATÆ —ŒSTRIDÆ—Bot-flies
                    SARCOPHAGIDÆ—Flesh-flies
                    CALLIPHORIDÆ—Blow-flies
                    MUSCIDÆ—House-flies
                    ANTHOMYIDÆ
                    HIPPOBOSCIDÆ—Tick-flies

In the following key an attempt has been made to give sufficient information to enable the student to distinguish the families which contain species of medical importance, but a number of families of flies which are of no interest from the parasitological viewpoint have been omitted. A complete table of families of DIPTERA is given by Curran (1934).

KEY TO THE FAMILIES OF DIPTERA WHICH ARE OF PARASITOLOGICAL
INTEREST

1. Abdomen distinctly segmented; wings usually present 2
   Abdomen sac-like, without distinct segmentation; wings sometimes reduced or absent .... (CYCLORRHAPHA PUPIPARA) 17
2. Antennæ long and composed of more than six joints; tips of sixth
   vein and posterior branch of fifth widely separated
   .... (ORTHORRHAPHA NEMATOCERA) 3
   Antennæ short and composed of three or four joints; the last
   joint may be simple or divided into annuli and, if simple, may
   have either a terminal bristle or a dorsal arista; tips of sixth
   vein and posterior branch of fifth close together or fused.... 7
3. Wing venation well-developed, so that nine or more veins or
   branches of veins reach the margin of the wing 4
   Wing venation reduced, so that less than nine veins or vein
   branches reach the wing margin 6
4. Wings without cross-veins except near base........ *Psychodidæ.*
   Wings with one or more cross-veins at or beyond middle of wing 5
5. Ocelli absent; mesonotum divided into scutum, scutellum and
   postscutellum; no extra seventh vein present in the wing
   .... *Culicidæ.*
   Ocelli present (*Rhyphidæ*) or mesoscutum divided into prescutum
   and scutum by a V-shaped suture and usually a seventh vein
   present in the wing .... (*Tipulidæ*).
6. Short, stout flies with stout antennæ which do not bear circlets of
   long hairs on most of the segments.............. *Simuliidæ.*
   Usually more slender flies; antennæ slender, with circlets of long
   hairs on most of the segments, this being especially noticeable
   in the males .... *Chironomidæ.*
7. Third vein forked; antennæ projecting anteriorly; frontal lunule
   and frontal sutures always absent
   .... (ORTHORRHAPHA BRACHYCERA) 8
   Third vein not forked; antennæ usually bent downward; frontal
   lunule present and often frontal sutures also (CYCLORRHAPHA) 9
8. Last joint of antenna divided into from four to eight annuli;
   squamæ large; discal cell of wing longer than broad
   .... *Tabanidæ.*
   Last joint of antenna not divided into annuli (many families, including *Asilidæ, Leptidæ, Bombyliidæ*) or else squamæ small
   or discal cell of wing small and as broad as long
   .... (*Stratiomyidæ*).
9. Frontal lunule present; frontal sutures absent
   .... (CYCLORRHAPHA ASCHIZA) 10
   Frontal lunule and frontal sutures both present
   .... (CYCLORRHAPHA SCHIZOPHORA) 11
10. A false vein in wing between third and fourth veins and parallel
    to them .... *Syrphidæ.*
    No false vein in wing .... (*Pipunculidæ*).
11. Squamæ small or rudimentary; subcosta often reduced (ACALYP-

TRATÆ—many families, including *Drosophilidæ, Sepsidæ, Scatophagidæ*).

Squamæ large: subcosta always well developed... (CALYPTRATÆ). 12

12. Mouth-parts reduced; mouth opening small .... *Œstridæ.*

Mouth-parts well developed; mouth opening large 13

13. A row of strong bristles on the hypopleura 14

Hypopleura bare or with fine hairs 16

14. Postscutellum with a double convexity; abdomen very bristly
.... (*Tachinidæ, Dexiidæ*).

Postscutellum with a single convexity; abdomen bristly only
near tip 15

15. Antennal arista plumose for only about half its length; body
usually gray and black .... *Sarcophagidæ.**

Arista plumose nearly to tip; body usually metallic bluish or
greenish .... *Calliphoridæ.**

16. Tip of fourth vein straight .... *Anthomyidæ.*

Tip of fourth vein angled or curved toward the third vein
.... *Muscidæ.*

17. Head not folding back onto dorsum of thorax; palpi not broad
and leaf-like; ectoparasitic on birds and mammals
.... *Hippoboscidæ.*

Head folding back onto dorsum of thorax (*Nycteribiidæ*) or
palpi broad and leaf-like (*Streblidæ*); both ectoparasitic on
bats only.

* Curran (1934) places these two groups in the family *Metopiidæ.*

CHAPTER XXXIV

FAMILY CULICIDÆ—SUBFAMILY CULICINÆ—TRUE MOSQUITOES

I. *Characteristics*

The family CULICIDÆ is made up of the subfamily CULICINÆ (true mosquitoes) and two other subfamilies, the DIXINÆ and CHAOBORINÆ (or CORETHRINÆ), which include species resembling mosquitoes in many respects but not blood-sucking in habit and without parasitological significance.

The true mosquitoes (subfamily CULICINÆ) may be distinguished from all the other small flies which superficially resemble them by the following combination of characters: (a) wing venation as in Figure 250, (b) mouth parts or *proboscis* much longer than the head, (c) longitudinal veins and posterior border of wings fringed with flat, striated scales. Some TIPULIDÆ, for example, have long proboscides, and some of the CHAOBORINÆ resemble mosquitoes in the venation and scalation of the wings, but only the true mosquitoes exhibit the combination of all three of these characteristics.

II. *Structure of Adult*

The head of a mosquito bears five prominent appendages, two antennæ, two palpi and a proboscis (see Figure 252). Each antenna consists of a small ring-like basal joint, a large bulbous second joint or *torus,* and thirteen *flagellar segments,* all slender and elongate. Each of the flagellar segments bears a circlet of hairs, which are comparatively short in females, but very long in most male mosquitoes. The bushy, plumose antennæ of the males make it easy to distinguish the sexes of mosquitoes. The palpi (really, of course, maxillary palpi) consist of from three to five joints in different species and sexes of mosquitoes. They may be very short or longer than the proboscis and these differences in length are very important in differentiating the malaria-carrying mosquitoes from the other species. The proboscis is always much longer than the head and is usually straight. The visible portion of the proboscis of the mosquito is really the ensheathing labium, which has a deep groove on its dorsal surface. In the female mosquito six slender *stylets* lie in this groove, representing a pair of mandibles, a pair of maxillæ, an epipharynx and a hypopharynx. When the mosquito bites it is only the stylets which pierce the skin, the labium remaining outside and being bent into the shape of a U as the stylets penetrate more deeply. In the male mosquitoes the mandibles are usually absent and the maxillæ reduced

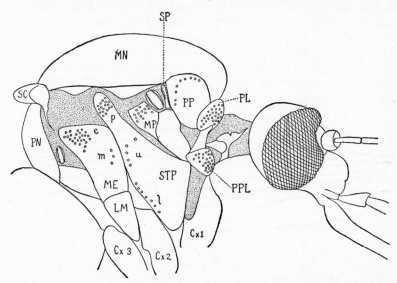

FIG. 249.—Lateral view of the thorax of *Psorophora,* to show the locations of sclerites and groups of bristles. The position of the bristles is indicated by tiny circles, representing the scars which they leave when removed. SC, scutellum; PN, postnotum; PL, prothoracic lobe; MN, mesonotum; PPL, propleura (bearing propleural bristles); PP, posterior pronotum (bearing pronotal bristles); SP, spiracular sclerite (bearing spiracular bristles); MP, mesopleura (bearing post-spiracular bristles); STP, sternopleura (bearing p, pre-alar bristles; u, upper sternopleural bristles; and l, lower sternopleural bristles); ME, mesepimeron (bearing e, upper mesepimeral bristles; and m, mid mesepimeral bristles); LM, lateral metasternal sclerite; Cx1, Cx2, Cx3, coxæ of first, second and third legs. (Original. Root)

in size. For this reason male mosquitoes are actually incapable of biting.

The thorax of a mosquito is composed of a number of sclerites, most of which belong to the middle thoracic segment. The presence or absence of groups of bristles on various sclerites of the thorax is much used at present as characters for differentiating the various genera. Figure 249 shows a lateral view of the thorax of a mosquito with the names usually applied to the sclerites and the groups of bristles which they bear. The thorax bears one pair of functional wings and three pairs of legs.

The venation of a mosquito wing is shown in Figure 250. There is comparatively little variation in different species. The costa extends all around the wing, although in speaking of the costa or the costal region of the wing we usually mean only that part of the costa which forms the anterior border of the wing, from the base of the wing to the tip of the first vein. The subcosta and the first, third and sixth veins are not forked. The second, fourth and fifth veins are forked. Cross-veins seem to be present connecting the costa and subcosta, the subcosta and the first vein, the first and second veins, the second and third veins, the third and fourth veins and the fourth vein and the anterior branch of the fifth. The apparent cross-veins connecting the first vein to the second and the second to the third often look just like the other cross-veins, but are really the bases of

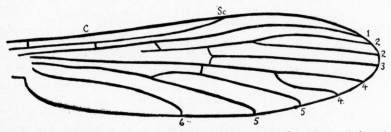

FIG. 250.—Wing venation of *Anopheles*. C, costa (costa); Sc, subcosta (subcosta); 1, first vein (Radius-one); 2,2, second vein (Radius-two and Radius-three); 3, third vein (Radius-four plus five); 4,4, fourth vein (Media-one and Media-two); 5,5, fifth vein (Cubitus-one and Cubitus-two); 6, sixth vein (Anal). (Original. Root)

the second and third veins, which arise as branches of the first and second veins, respectively. The spaces between the forks or branches of the second and fourth veins are often called the *first* and *second fork cells,* and those parts of the second and fourth veins which lie between their bifurcations and the cross-veins connecting them with the third vein are termed the *stems* or *petioles* of the fork cells.

In the key to adult mosquitoes of the tribe CULICINI it will be noticed that the shape of the individual scales of the wing must often be studied. The presence or absence of bristles and hairs on the *base of the first vein* (that part of the first vein which lies between the base of the wing and the *humeral cross-vein* connecting the costa and subcosta) is also of considerable importance.

In the legend for Figure 250 are given both the terminology of the veins used in this book and also another system invented by Comstock and Needham and used by many authors. The latter names are placed in parentheses.

The legs of a mosquito are long and slender and of the type usual in the DIPTERA, with five tarsal joints. Sometimes the first tarsal joint is called the metatarsus, but usually the tarsal joints are simply referred to as first, second, third, fourth and fifth, the first being the one which is attached to the tibia and the fifth the terminal joint which bears the claws. For brevity it is often convenient to omit the word joint or segment; thus if we speak of the first hind tarsal we mean the joint next to the tibia on the hind leg.

The abdomen of a mosquito is long and slender and consists of ten segments, of which eight are well developed and easily seen, while the last two are modified for sexual purposes. The last segment of the female abdomen bears a pair of short *cerci,* while in the male the last two segments and their appendages form the external genitalia or *hypopygium.* The numerous modifications of the male hypopygium are of great value in classifying and even in identifying mosquitoes, but are not convenient for field work and cannot be treated in detail in a book of this size.

III. *Life History*

The female mosquito lays her eggs either on or in water or in situations which will be covered with water at some later time. Mosquito larvæ are usually found only in water, although they may survive for a few days in merely moist surroundings. The larval stage is the growth period of the mosquito. This growth necessitates a periodic moulting or shedding of the skin of the larva. These moults divide the larval life of a mosquito into four periods or stages, leading us to speak of larvæ as being in the first, second, third or fourth larval stage. Since the hairs and other structures which are used in identifying mosquito larvæ usually differ in different larval stages, descriptions of mosquito larvæ and keys for identifying them usually refer only to the full-grown or fourth-stage larvæ.

When the fourth-stage larva moults, there emerges a comma-shaped pupa, which is very active but takes no food. After a few days the pupa comes to the surface of the water and its skin splits open dorsally to liberate the adult, which remains for a short time on the raft formed by the air-filled pupal skin and then flies off. Mating between the sexes probably occurs in nature soon after the emergence of the females. In some species, the yellow-fever mosquito, for example, mating occurs readily in the laboratory. In other species, such as the malarial mosquitoes, it is usually very difficult to obtain mating in captivity, probably because the males of these species

normally form mating swarms which hover in sheltered places await-
ing the coming of the females.

IV. *Structure of Larvæ*

A mosquito larva is a worm-like creature without legs or wings.
Its head is enclosed in a chitinized capsule, but the large unsegmented
thorax and the nine-segmented abdomen are covered for the most
part by a membranous integument. The head bears compound eyes
and antennæ dorsally and the mouthparts ventrally. In addition to
mandibles, maxillæ and *labium* a mosquito larva also has a pair of
large hairy structures, the *mouth brushes,* which project anteriorly
beyond the anterior margin of the head. These are used by most
mosquito larvæ to create currents in the water which bring the small
floating plants or animals on which they feed to the mouth. Some
few mosquito larvæ feed on the larvæ of other mosquitoes, and in
these each hair of the mouth brushes is converted into a stiff comb-
like structure which aids it in securing a firm grip on its victims.

The head, thorax and abdominal segments of mosquito larvæ
all bear numerous paired hairs, whose form and position vary in
different species and are used in identifying the larvæ. The region of
the body which is most important in identifying mosquito larvæ is the
tip of the abdomen. The openings of the respiratory system of the
larva are situated dorsally on the next to the last abdominal segment.
In all mosquito larvæ except those of *Anopheles,* the actual openings
are at the tip of the more or less elongated, chitinized *air-tube,* which
projects dorso-posteriorly. The air-tube has one or more pairs of
ventral hairs or *hair-tufts* and usually bears also a row of spines,
called the *pecten,* on each side, ventrally, near its base. In larvæ of
Anopheles the air-tube is rudimentary and consists only of a ribbon-
like chitinization which is triangularly expanded at each end to bear
the *pecten* (often called the *comb* in descriptions of *Anopheles*
larvæ). The true *comb* is present laterally on the eighth abdominal
segment of nearly all other mosquito larvæ and even in the first-stage
or newly-hatched larvæ of *Anopheles.* It consists of a line or triangular patch of *comb-scales* which are often more or less fringed
with spinules and may or may not be attached to the posterior margin
of a chitinized plate.

The ninth or anal segment of the abdomen of a mosquito larva is
usually more slender and elongate than the other segments. It is
usually more or less completely encircled by a chitinous *plate.* The
anus is at the tip of the ninth segment and around it arise four
transparent, usually sausage-shaped structures, the *anal gills.* The

ninth segment also bears at its tip two pairs of *dorsal* and one pair of *lateral hairs* or *hair-tufts*. In most mosquito larvæ there is also a line of unpaired, mid-ventral hair-tufts, which are referred to as the *ventral brush.*

As has been noted above, the respiratory system of a mosquito larva has external openings and the great majority of mosquito larvæ have to come to the surface of the water periodically for air. In the larvæ of a few species, however, the anal gills are unusually large, and the larvæ rarely if ever come to the surface, so that it seems probable that they are able to extract what oxygen they need from the water by means of these gills. In the genus *Mansonia,* moreover, the larvæ thrust the sharp tips of their air-tubes into the air-containing tissues of certain aquatic plants and thus escape the necessity of coming to the surface for air.

V. *Structure of Pupæ*

In the mosquito pupa, the head and thorax are fused into a single roundedly triangular mass from which projects the elongate, curved, segmented abdomen, ending in a pair of leaf-life *paddles.* On the sides of the main mass may be seen the cases which contain the antennæ, wings and legs of the adult. The respiratory system opens to the exterior through two more or less tubular *breathing trumpets,* which arise near the mid-dorsal region of the thorax. Since pupæ usually yield adults within a few days it is not so important to be able to identify pupæ as it is in the case of larvæ, but the pupæ do offer characters by which they may be distinguished. The shape of the breathing-trumpets and of the paddles at the tip of the abdomen, and the hairs and hair-tufts on the abdominal segments are particularly valuable for this purpose.

VI. *Classification of Mosquitoes*

According to Edwards's classification, the sub-family CULICINÆ is divided into three tribes. Two of these tribes, the ANOPHELINI and the CULICINI, include species which are disease carriers and others which are important pests. The other tribe, the MEGARHININI, are of very little importance from the parasitological point of view. Tribe CULICINI is divided into five groups.

The following keys to tribes by adult and by larval characters are constructed from characters given by Edwards (1932) and Dyar (1928).

KEY TO TRIBES OF CULICINÆ AND GROUPS OF CULICINI (ADULTS)

1. Abdomen without scales, or at least with sternites largely bare
   ....Tribe *Anophelini*
   Abdomen with both tergites and sternites completely clothed with
   scales 2
2. Proboscis rigid, outer half more slender and bent backwards
   ....Tribe *Megarhinini*
   Proboscis more flexible, of uniform thickness (unless swollen at
   tip), outer half not bent backwards.............Tribe *Culicini* 3
3. Pulvilli present, broad and distinct; slight development of scales
   ....*Culex* group
   Pulvilli absent 4
4. Bristles usually present on pronotum; hairs of abdomen absent
   (except bristly fringe on hind margin of 7th segment)
   ....*Sabethes* group
   Bristles absent on pronotum; some hairs usually present on all
   abdominal segments 5
5. Sixth vein short, ending opposite fork of 5th vein or basal to it
   ....*Uranotænia* group
   Sixth vein extending beyond fork of 5th vein 6
6. Claws of female simple, pulvilli absent, thorax very bristly; wing
   scales usually enlarged ....*Theobaldia* group
   Claws of female toothed; abdomen of female pointed with long
   cerci ....*Aëdes* group

KEY TO TRIBES OF CULICINÆ (LARVÆ)

1. Spiracles sessile, air-tube absent ....Tribe *Anophelini*
   Spiracles at tip of air-tube, which is at least as long as broad.... 2
2. Mouth-brushes prehensile, each composed of ten stout rods; eighth
   segment laterally without comb ....Tribe *Megarhinini*
   Mouth-brushes rarely prehensile, composed of 30 or more hairs;
   eighth segment with comb ....Tribe *Culicini*

The groups of Culicini do not separate well on larval characters.
Therefore, a key to the genera of the western hemisphere is given.
(See Chapter XXXVIII.)

CHAPTER XXXV

TRIBE ANOPHELINI—THE MALARIAL MOSQUITOES

I. *Characteristics*

Since the distinction between the malarial mosquitoes (tribe ANOPHELINI) on the one hand and other mosquitoes, particularly those belonging to the tribe CULICINI, on the other is very important, it is worth while to discuss these differences in some detail. There are a number of characters which may be used, but most of them are not infallible in every case, although true enough in general.

I. THE ADULT STAGE

Resting attitude. In most cases, anopheline mosquitoes may be distinguished in life at first glance by their characteristic attitude (see Figure 251). The whole body and proboscis form a straight line at an angle to the surface on which the mosquito rests. The resting attitudes of other mosquitoes are different in different genera, but in general the culicine mosquitoes rest with the proboscis not in line with the abdomen and the body roughly parallel to the substratum.

However, not all anophelines have the characteristic anopheline attitude. In the southern United States it will be noticed that the resting attitude of *A. quadrimaculatus* is intermediate between the typically anopheline pose of *A. crucians* or *A. punctipennis* and that of a culicine. In India one of the worst malaria-carriers has been given the name of *A. culicifacies* because of its *Culex*-like resting attitude. In South America there are two rare anophelines, one of which, *Chagasia fajardoi,* has a "hump-backed" resting attitude like that of the culicine genus *Mansonia,* while the other, *Anopheles nimbus,* is said to rest in the same peculiar attitude as the members of the tribe SABETHINI.

Wing spotting. It is often said that the wings of anopheline mosquitoes are spotted, while those of other mosquitoes are unspotted. This is the rule, but there are numerous exceptions on both sides. The most primitive anophelines have absolutely unspotted wings. Others, like *A. quadrimaculatus,* have all the wing-scales dark colored, but at certain places on the wing the scales are more crowded than at others, giving the impression of four indistinct dark spots when looked at with the naked eye or a hand lens. In the majority of anophelines, however, the wings show very definite dark and light spots, due to the fact that the scales along the wing veins are dark-colored in some areas and white or cream-colored in others.

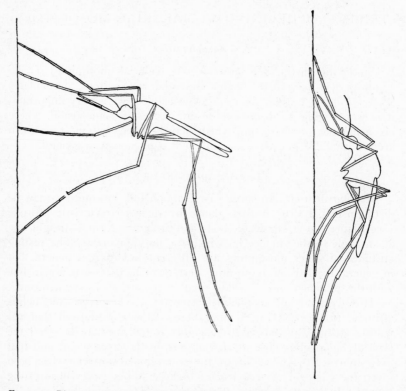

FIG. 251.—Diagrams of the typical resting attitudes of adult females of *Anopheles* (left) and *Culex* (right). (Original. Root)

In most culicine mosquitoes the wing-scales are all dark. But a good many species have the veins clothed with a mixture of dark and light scales and in a few forms, such as the species of the sub-genus *Lutzia* and the species of *Culex* related to *C. mimeticus*, there are alternating areas of dark and light scales just as in the typical anophelines. In many species of *Theobaldia*, also, the wings present indistinct dark spots not unlike those of *A. quadrimaculatus*.

Form of scutellum. In most anophelines the posterior margin of the scutellum is evenly rounded and has a regular row of bristles. In most other mosquitoes the scutellum is definitely tri-lobed posteriorly, with a clump of bristles on each of the three lobes. It must be noted, however, that the rare anophelines of the genus *Chagasia* have the scutellum tri-lobed, and that the species of *Megarhinus* have the scutellum evenly rounded, as in *Anopheles*.

The form of the palpi. The form of the palpi is the best character for differentiating anopheline mosquitoes from the others, but it has the disadvantage that the palpi are different in the two sexes of the same species (compare Figure 252). Male mosquitoes, of course, may be readily distinguished from females in nearly every case by their bushy, long-haired antennæ, and by the presence of the hypo-

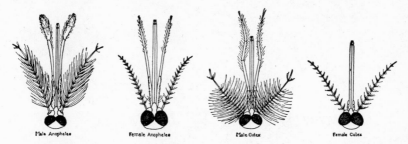

FIG. 252.—Heads of male and female adults of *Anopheles* and *Culex*. (Original. Root)

pygial structures at the tip of the abdomen. Most male mosquitoes have the palpi longer than the proboscis, although a few aberrant species in many different genera have short male palpi. In male *Anopheles* the last two joints of the palpi are broad and flat, giving the palpi a clubbed appearance, while male culicines have the last two joints of the palpi tubular, like the other joints, so that the palpi are slender throughout. It should be noted, however, that in some culicine genera, *Theobaldia* for example, the last two joints of the male palpi may be slightly greater in diameter than the other joints, producing a very slightly clubbed appearance. The male palpi of the peculiar anopheline genus *Chagasia* are like those of *Theobaldia*.

In the females, the distinction is more obvious. All female anophelines have palpi which are more than half as long as the proboscis, and usually they almost equal it in length. In the female culicines, the palpi are almost always decidedly less than half as long as the proboscis. The only exceptions are the species of

Megarhinus, which can be readily differentiated from anophelines by other characters.

2. THE EGG STAGE

Anophelines drop their eggs singly onto the surface of the water and although the eggs of different species vary a good deal in detail, they are almost always boat-shaped, pointed at both ends, with flat dorsal surface and convex ventral surface, and they practically always have lateral air-chambers or "floats," which aid in keeping them at the surface (see Figure 259).

Culicine mosquitoes show a good deal of variation in the way in which they lay their eggs and in their shape. In general, culicine

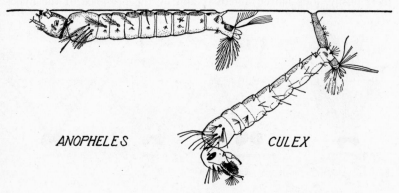

ANOPHELES   CULEX

FIG. 253.—Positions assumed by larvæ of *Anopheles* and *Culex* at the surface of the water.
(Drawn from life. Huff)

mosquitoes which breed in permanent bodies of water deposit "rafts" or clumps of several hundred eggs on the water surface (examples, *Culex, Uranotænia*). Those culicine mosquitoes which breed in temporary pools (*Aëdes, Psorophora*) or in water held by plants (*Megarhinus,* SABETHINI) lay their eggs singly, usually in places which are dry at the time but will later be covered with water. Among the mosquitoes which have become domestic in their habits both of these methods of oviposition may be observed. The domestic species of *Culex* (*C. pipiens* and *C. fatigans*) lay large egg-rafts on the surface of the water. The yellow-fever mosquito (*Aëdes ægypti*) lays its eggs singly, sometimes on the surface of the water, but more often on the side of the container, just above the edge of the water.

The eggs of culicine mosquitoes are of various shapes, but usually are ellipsoidal or elongate-conical, and without any definite "floats."

3. THE LARVAL STAGE

Attitude at surface of water (Figure 253). Anopheline larvæ are usually readily recognizable in life by the fact that when they come to the surface for air they lie horizontally, just below the surface film and touching the surface at several different places. Culicine larvæ usually hang vertically or obliquely when at the surface, touching the surface film only with the tip of the air-tube. The larvæ of some species of the culicine genus *Uranotænia* and of certain

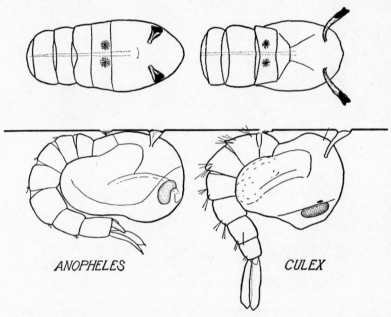

ANOPHELES   CULEX

FIG. 254.—Appearances of pupæ of *Anopheles* and *Culex* from above (top row) and from the side (bottom row). (Drawn from life. Huff)

Chaoborinæ (especially *Eucorethra*) resemble *Anopheles* larvæ superficially to a certain extent.

Development of air-tube. Culicine larvæ always have a well-developed air-tube on the dorsum of the eighth abdominal segment. In anopheline larvæ the air-tube is reduced to such a rudiment that for practical purposes it may be said to be absent. It should be noted that in anopheline larvæ the two spiracular openings on the dorsum of the eighth abdominal segment are surrounded by five flap-like structures, the posterior pair of flaps being larger than the others and more or less fused together. These flaps tend to close together when the larva leaves the surface, retaining a bubble of air above the spiracles, so that no water can enter the tracheal system. They correspond to the five little flaps at the tip of the air-tube of culicine larvæ, which open out, star-like, when the tip of the air-tube reaches the surface.

The shape of the head, decidedly longer than it is wide, will also serve to differentiate *Anopheles* larvæ from those of all culicines

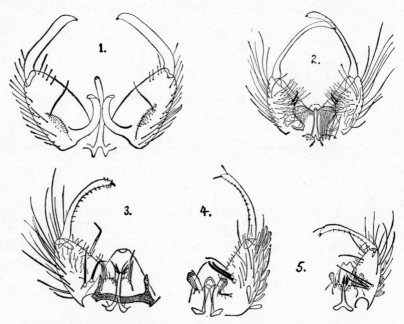

FIG. 255.—Male terminalia of the genera and subgenera of anopheline mosquitoes. 1, *Bironella;* 2, *Chagasia;* 3, *Anopheles* (*Anopheles*); 4, *Anopheles* (*Nyssorhynchus*); 5, *Anopheles* (*Myzomyia*). (Original. Root)

except *Uranotænia*. The presence of palmate hairs on thorax and abdomen (see page 527) is also a characteristic of anopheline larvæ.

4. THE PUPAL STAGE (Figure 254)

The breathing trumpets. Anopheline pupæ can usually be recognized on microscopic examination by the form of the breathing trumpets, which are short and broad with a large terminal opening which is continued by a split down the front. In pupæ of *Culex* the breathing trumpets are long and tubular, with a small terminal opening. In other culicine genera, such as *Aëdes,* the pupal breathing trumpets may be short and conical, but usually do not have a split down the front nor such a large terminal opening as in *Anopheles.*

Paddles at tip of abdomen. A more certain character, but one more difficult to see, is furnished by the fact that in *Anopheles* pupæ the paddles at the tip of the abdomen have a small hair on the surface of the paddle near its tip, in addition to a larger terminal hair. Culicine pupæ usually have a large terminal hair on the paddle, but never show the small accessory hair.

II. *Classification of Anophelini*

The tribe ANOPHELINI includes the two small and unimportant genera *Chagasia* (three species in tropical America) and *Bironella* (one species in Papua) and the large genus *Anopheles,* which is further subdivided into three subgenera, *Anopheles, Nyssorhynchus* and *Myzomyia.* The subgenera may be still further subdivided into groups of species. The division into genera and subgenera is based primarily upon the structure of the male hypopygium, particularly on the structures present at the base of the *side-piece,* or basal joint of the clasping appendages. These differences may be briefly summarized as follows (compare Figure 255).

1.   Inner side of side-piece with a lobe bearing 2 or more spines ....   *Chagasia*
2.   Ventral surface of side-piece with a massive spur arising near its base...   *Bironella*
3.   Ventral surface of side-piece with 1 to 6 strong spines (*parabasal spines*) near its base ....   *Anopheles*
    3a. Two (rarely one or three) parabasal spines present ....   subgenus *Anopheles*
    3b. One parabasal spine present and also two *accessory spines* arising on the ventral surface of the side-piece at about the middle of its length .... subgenus *Nyssorhynchus*
    3c. A clump of from four to six parabasal spines present ....   subgenus *Myzomyia*

III. *Geographical Distribution of Anopheles*

Some species of the genus *Anopheles* will be found in almost every region of the globe. Certain subgenera and groups, however, are more or less restricted to certain regions. The subgenus *Anopheles* includes: (a) a few rare and primitive tropical species; (b) two groups of species (Anopheles group and Patagiamyia group) which are particularly characteristic of the north temperate region, although some species of these groups are found in the tropics; (c) two highly specialized groups of tropical species one of which (Myzorhynchus group) is found only in the Old World, the other (Arribalzagia group) only in the American tropics. The subgenus *Nyssorhynchus* is confined to the tropical and subtropical regions of the New World, the subgenus *Myzomyia* to the corresponding parts of the Old World. *Anopheles gambiæ* was reported from Natal, Brazil by Shannon (1930). It is the first species of the subgenus *Myzomyia* to be reported from the Western Hemisphere and undoubtedly represents a recent importation.

The emphasis in this book will be upon the anophelines of the New World. Students who desire to become acquainted with the Old World forms may consult the papers on them listed in the bibliography (See particularly Christophers, 1924; Covell, 1927; and Edwards, 1932).

IV. *Identification of American Species of Anopheles*

In the identification of adult anophelines, particularly the females, it is necessary to rely on color characters, mainly on the coloration of the wings, palpi and legs. Since all these appendages owe their color to their covering of scales, it is often difficult to identify specimens which are so old or have been so carelessly handled that many of the scales have been rubbed off. In tracing the evolution of the color patterns of *Anopheles* we find that in the more primitive species the scales on wings, legs and palpi are usually all dark in color. As we pass to more and more specialized forms we find light-scaled areas appearing, at first few in number and small, then becoming more numerous and more extensive. Usually the light-scaled areas are found in certain definite places, varying in their degree of extension but not in their location. Slight shifts of location of white areas do sometimes occur, however. Frequently it is found that two adjacent light-scaled areas have extended until they have fused together, obliterating the dark-scaled area between them. In a few groups of species there seems to have been a sort of fragmentation of the white spots, so that two, three or even four small white areas appear where most species show only one large one. This is particularly well shown in the wing-pattern of the species of the Arribalzagia group (see Figure 258).

The areas which are most useful for identification are, on the wing, the costa (which term means only that part of the costa which lies along the anterior margin of the wing between the wing base and the tip of the first vein), the third vein, and the sixth vein; on the legs, the tarsal joints, especially of the hind legs; and on the palpi the two terminal joints. The key which follows is intended primarily for female specimens. Males can usually be identified by it also, except that the different form of the male palpi and the reduced scaling of the male wings make characters based on these structures less reliable than in the case of females.

The key includes all the American groups of anopheline mosquitoes, but some of the rarer and less important species have been omitted or lumped together.

KEY TO IDENTIFY ADULT FEMALES OF AMERICAN ANOPHELINE MOSQUITOES

1. Wings either entirely dark-scaled or with a mixture of light and dark scales, but without definite light-scaled and dark-scaled areas 2
   Wings with definite light and dark spots produced by alternating light-scaled and dark-scaled areas 3
2. Tarsi conspicuously white-banded .... (*Chagasia*) 7
   Tarsi all dark .... (Anopheles group) 9
3. Second, fourth and sixth veins of wing entirely dark-scaled, without any light areas .... (Kerteszia group) 33
   These veins with some light-scaled areas 4
4. Sixth vein with four or more small dark spots
   .... (Arribalzagia group) 17
   Sixth vein with only one, two or three dark spots or areas...... 5
5. Costa of wing with light areas only at tip of first vein or at tips of first vein and subcosta .... (Patagiamyia group) 13
   Costa with more than two light-scaled areas 6
6. Third vein either nearly all dark or with three distinct dark spots .... (Myzorhynchella group) 26
   Third vein mainly white, with a small dark spot near each end
   .... (Nyssorhynchus group) 28

Genus *Chagasia*

7. Wings entirely dark-scaled .... *C. fajardoi.*
   Wings with a mixture of light and dark scales 8
8. Last four hind tarsal joints with only one black band each
   .... *C. bonneæ.*
   Last four hind tarsal joints each with two black bands
   .... *C. bathanus.*

Genus *Anopheles*
Subgenus *Anopheles*, Anopheles group

9. Hind tibia with a broad white band at its tip......... *A. eiseni.*
   Hind tibia all dark 10

10. Mesonotum with narrow median and lateral silvery stripes
....*A. nimbus.*
Mesonotum without such narrow silvery stripes 11
11. Wings with four indistinct darker spots 12
Wings not indistinctly spotted
....................*A. barberi, A. walkeri* and *A. atropos.*
12. Wing fringe all dark ....*A. quadrimaculatus.*
Wing fringe coppery or yellowish at tip of the wing
....*A. maculipennis.*

Patagiamyia group

13. Hind tibia with a broad white band at its tip........*A. eiseni.*
Hind tibia without a white band 14
14. Femora and tibiæ with small yellowish spots; some of the wing
scales almost circular ....*A. grabhami.*
Femora and tibiæ not mottled; wing scales all slender......... 15
15. Costa, white only at tip of first vein; sixth vein with three
dark spots ....*A. crucians.*
Costa white at tips of first vein and subcosta; sixth vein with
only one or two dark areas 16
16. Sixth vein with two dark areas; third vein dark, except sometimes at tip; palpi dark ....*A. punctipennis.*
Sixth vein with one dark area; third vein extensively white in
middle; palpi with narrow white rings..*A. pseudopunctipennis.*

Arribalzagia group

17. Fourth and fifth hind tarsal joints all white.....*A. annulipalpis.*
At least fourth hind tarsal joint with some black 18
18. Fifth hind tarsal partly or entirely white or yellow............ 19
Fifth hind tarsal all dark; third and fourth hind tarsals all dark
or with small apical light rings 20
19. Third and fourth hind tarsals with at least two white rings each.. 22
Third and fourth hind tarsals with one apical yellow ring each;
wing scales predominantly black ....*A. shannoni.*
20. Tip of abdomen conspicuously white-scaled dorsally
....*A. peryassui.**
Tip of abdomen not white-scaled 21
21. All light spots on wings very small; middle of third vein dark
....*A. vestitipennis.*
Light wing-spots larger and more distinct; middle of third vein
with an area of mixed light and dark scales....*A. maculipes.*
22. Fifth hind tarsal all white or yellow 23
Fifth hind tarsal with a black ring 24
23. Hind tarsi yellow, with black spots and rings..*A. mediopunctatus.*
Hind tarsi black with white spots and rings....*A. punctimacula.*
24. Dark area at tip of wing about the same size as the dark area
between it and the large dark area just beyond the tip of
the subcosta ....*A. punctimacula.*

* Placed in Group *Manguinhosia* Lutz by Shannon and Davis (1930).

Dark area at tip of wing decidedly larger than the dark area between it and the large dark area just beyond the tip of the subcosta 25

25. Third vein extensively white in middle; broadest wing-scales about one-third as broad as long ....*A. pseudomaculipes.*
Third vein with numerous small light and dark areas; broadest wing-scales nearly half as broad as long, enlarged, with rounded tips ....*A. intermedius.*
Third vein either extensively white in middle or with many small light and dark areas; broadest wing-scales nearly half as broad as long, not enlarged, truncate at tip....*A. apicimacula.*

Subgenus *Nyssorhynchus*
Myzorhynchella group

26. Third, fourth and fifth hind tarsals all white 27
Third and fourth hind tarsals with small black rings
....*A. nigritarsis.*

27. Third vein of wing nearly all dark; tip of abdomen not white-scaled dorsally ....*A. lutzi.*
Third vein with three dark spots; tip of abdomen conspicuously white-scaled dorsally ....*A. parvus.*

Nyssorhynchus group

28. Third, fourth and fifth hind tarsals all white 29
Fifth hind tarsal with a black ring, third and fourth white..... 31
Black rings on fifth hind tarsal and also on either third or fourth hind tarsals or on both
..............*A. rondoni, A. cuyabensis* and *A. triannulatus.*

29. White spot on costa near humeral cross-vein smaller than the black spot just basal to it......................*A. darlingi.*
White spot on costa near humeral cross-vein larger than the black spot just basal to it 30

30. Mid tarsi with definite white rings; second hind tarsal joint often with more black than white...................*A. albitarsis.*
Mid tarsi without definite white rings; second hind tarsal joint usually with much more white than black.....*A. argyritarsis.*

31. White spot on costa near humeral cross-vein larger than the black spot just basal to it 32
White spot on costa near humeral cross-vein as small as or smaller than the black spot just basal to it.......*A. bachmanni.*

32. Next to last joint of female palpi mainly black; second hind tarsal joint usually more black than white.....*A. albimanus.*
Next to last joint of female palpi mainly white; second hind tarsal joint usually more white than black
.............................*A. tarsimaculatus, A. strodei.*

Kerteszia group

33. Third, fourth and fifth hind tarsals all dark......*A. boliviensis.*
Third, fourth and fifth hind tarsals with broad, white, apical rings
....................................*A. bellator, A. cruzi.*

V. *Identification of Anopheles Larvæ*

It is often convenient in survey and control work to be able to identify larvæ of *Anopheles* without waiting to breed out adults. All *Anopheles* larvæ look very much alike, but there are certain

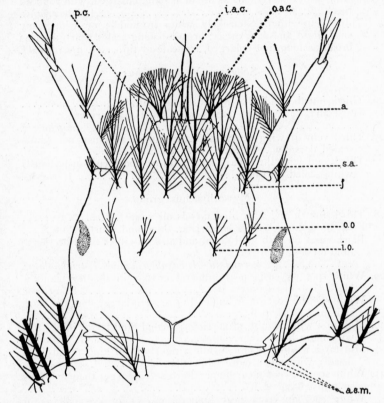

Fig. 256.—Head and anterior edge of thorax of larva of *Anopheles*. i.a.c., inner clypeal hairs; o.a.c., outer clypeal hairs; p.c., pre-antennal hairs; a., antennal hair; s.a., sub-antennal hair; f., frontal hairs; o.o., outer occipital hairs; i.o., inner occipital hairs; a.s.m., anterior submedian thoracic group of hairs. (Original. Root)

differences, mainly in the form and position of various hairs, which enable us to identify many larvæ. The hairs most used for identification are the following.

Head hairs. Inner and *outer* pairs of *clypeal hairs* on the anterior margin of the head. The outer clypeal hairs lie just above the protruded mouth brushes and are sometimes hard to see in preserved larvæ. The other dorsal head hairs, whose positions and names are indicated in Figure 256, are only occasionally of value.

Thoracic Hairs. The most important of the thoracic hairs is the inner hair of the *anterior submedian thoracic group,* which includes the three hairs nearest the mid-dorsal line on each side of the anterior margin of the thorax. The middle and outer hairs of this group are practically the same in all *Anopheles* larvæ, but the inner hairs show characteristic variations in certain species.

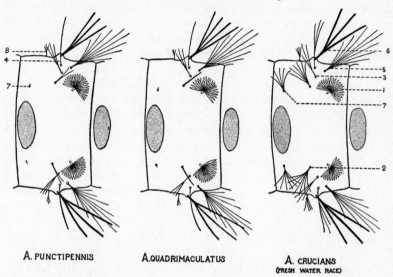

A. PUNCTIPENNIS   A.QUADRIMACULATUS   A. CRUCIANS
(FRESH WATER RACE)

Fig. 257.—Fourth abdominal segments of the larvæ of *Anopheles quadrimaculatus, punctipennis,* and *crucians* (fresh-water race). The numerals follow Martini, 1923. (Original. Root)

1—Palmate hair	5—Hair "5"
2—Ante-palmate hair	6—Long lateral hair
3—Hair "3"	7—Anterior hair
4—Hair "4"	8—Hair "8"

Palmate hairs. The name *palmate hairs* is applied to paired hairs which may be present on the posterior corners of the thorax and on the first to seventh abdominal segments. When fully developed, a palmate hair consists of a short, stout, erect stalk from the top of which a number of slender, flattened *leaflets* radiate out horizontally. The number of pairs of palmate hairs varies characteristically in certain species, but is not a very good character to use, because palmate hairs are readily broken off and leave no scar to mark their former position. In some species of larvæ, also, one finds hairs intermediate between ordinary hairs and the palmate type, so that it becomes difficult to decide just how many pairs of real palmate hairs are present. The shape of the individual leaflets of the palmate hairs is often characteristic of certain species or groups of species.

Other abdominal hairs (compare Figure 257). The long *lateral abdominal hairs* are often of value. All *Anopheles* larvæ have two long, feathered lateral hairs on each side of the first and second segments of the abdomen and a single similar hair on each side of the third segment. The fourth, fifth, and, in certain groups, the sixth segment each have a pair of shorter lateral hairs, and these vary in their branching in different groups and are often useful in field identifications. The *antepalmate hairs,* the hairs nearest the mid-dorsal line just in front of the palmate hairs, on abdominal segments four and five are sometimes useful also.

The pecten. The *pecten* or comb on the eighth abdominal segment shows a characteristic arrangement of the long and short teeth in certain species, but this is a character difficult to study in living larvæ on account of the lateral position of the pecten.

The following keys are not wholly satisfactory, but it is thought that the characters used are constant enough to permit of the correct identification of the majority of larvæ encountered. The following key to the *Anopheles* larvæ of the United States is from Bradley (1936).

KEY TO THE LARVÆ OF THE GENUS ANOPHELES OCCURRING IN THE UNITED STATES

1. Abdomen with plumose lateral hairs on first 6 segments; head hairs simple ....*barberi*
   Abdomen with plumose lateral hairs on first 3 segments only; head with plumose hairs 2
2. Outer clypeal hairs simple, unbranched; elements of dorsal abdominal palmate hairs with long, slender apical portion
   .... *pseudopunctipennis*
   Outer clypeal hairs branched; inner clypeal hairs simple, branched, or feathered; elements of dorsal palmate tuft notched toward tip 3
3. Outer clypeal hairs with few (5 to 8) branches; inner clypeal hairs usually divided into 2 or more branches toward tip; occipital hairs simple ....*atropos*
   Outer clypeal hairs thickly branched, fanlike 4
4. Abdominal segments 4 and 5 with 2 conspicuous hairs anterior to the palmate tuft. (These are of approximately equal size and each has from 4 to 9 branches.) ...*crucians* (fresh-water race)
   Abdominal segments 4 and 5 with but 1 conspicuous hair anterior to the palmate hairs. (This may be single or with 2 to 3 branches.) 5

5. Abdomen with the palmate tufts on segments 3 to 7, inclusive, of similar form but those on segments 3 and 7 noticeably smaller than the others; posterior clypeal hairs long, usually single; antennal branched hair long, being approximately one-half the length of the segment from which it arises; tubercles of inner anterior clypeal hairs wide or close
.............................*crucians* (brackish-water race)
Abdomen with the palmate tufts on segments 3 to 7, inclusive, of approximately equal size 6
6. Tubercles of inner anterior clypeal hairs separated by at least the width of one of these tubercles; antepalmate hairs on segments 4 and 5 usually single, palmate tufts on segment 2 usually well developed ....*quadrimaculatus*
Tubercles of inner anterior clypeal hairs so close together that another tubercle of similar size could not be placed between them 7
7. Inner anterior clypeal hairs not minutely feathered toward tip; antepalmate hairs of abdominal segments 4 and 5 usually double or triple 8
Inner anterior clypeal hairs minutely feathered toward tip; antepalmate hairs of abdominal segments 4 and 5 usually single.... 9
8. Antepalmate hairs of abdominal segments 4 and 5 usually with 2 branches, rarely 1 or 3; posterior clypeal hairs usually with 2 branches from near base; inner anterior clypeal hairs single, unbranched ....*punctipennis*
Antepalmate hairs of abdominal segments 4 and 5 usually with 3 branches, rarely 2 or 4; posterior clypeal hairs usually long with apical branching; inner anterior clypeal hairs unbranched or with 2 to 3 branches beyond middle ....*maculipennis*
9. Hairs 1 and 3 of submedian prothoracic group of approximately equal length; hair O on abdominal segments 2 to 6 poorly developed, usually single or having 1 to 3 branches
....................................*walkeri* (northern race)
Hair 1 of submedian prothoracic group approximately twice as long as hair 3; hair O on abdominal segments 2 to 6 fairly well developed and having 3 to 7 branches...*walkeri* (southern race).

KEY TO THE ANOPHELINE LARVÆ OF TROPICAL AMERICA

1. Very long, feathered lateral hairs present on abdominal segments 1, 2 and 3, followed by long lateral hairs on segments 4 and 5; anterior flap of spiracular apparatus short and stout, more or less semicircular 2
Very long, feathered lateral hairs present only on abdominal segments 1 and 2, no long lateral hairs on segments 3, 4 and 5; anterior flap of spiracular apparatus long and tubular, bearing a long filament at its tip
.........*Chagasia* (*C. fajardoi, C. bonneæ,* and *C. bathanus*).
2. Frontal hairs of head long and feathered 3
Frontal hairs shorter, with few or no lateral branches
....................(Kerteszia group) *A. bellator, A. cruzi.*
3. Long lateral hairs of abdominal segments 4 and 5 single and unbranched 4

Long lateral hairs of abdominal segments 4 and 5 double, triple,
multiple or with lateral branches 11
4. Outer clypeal hairs thinly branched to form a flat, fan-shaped
tuft with less than twenty ultimate branchlets; long lateral
hairs absent on abdominal segment 6 . . . most species of the
Arribalzagia group, including *A. punctimacula, A. apicimacula, A. pseudomaculipes, A. intermedius* and *A. medio-
.... punctatus.*
Inner and outer clypeal hairs both with a single main stem and
a variable number of delicate lateral branchlets, which are
sometimes difficult to see clearly; long lateral hairs present on
abdominal segment 6 as well as on segments 4 and 5
.... (Nyssorhynchus group).   5
5. Distance between bases of the two inner clypeal hairs only about
one-third of the distance between the bases of the inner and
outer clypeal hairs of either side   6
Distance between bases of the two inner clypeal hairs equal to
or only slightly less than the distance between the bases of
the inner and outer clypeal hairs of either side 7
6. Inner hair of anterior submedian thoracic group resembling a
palmate hair, i.e., with about fifteen flat, leaflet-like branches
all arising at about the same level ....*A. strodei.*
Inner hair of anterior submedian thoracic group smaller, with
seven or eight hair-like branches arising along a short main
stem ....*A. argyritarsis.*
7. A long, erect hair present on each of the posterior flaps of the
spiracular apparatus ....*A. darlingi.*
No long hairs on these organs   8
8. Inner hairs of anterior submedian thoracic group long, usually
over half as long as the middle hairs, and of much the same
form, with numerous hair-like branches arising along a short,
thick main stem ....*A. albimanus.*
Inner hairs of anterior submedian thoracic groups short, much
less than half as long as the middle hairs, and with their
branches all arising at about the same level   9
9. Inner hairs of anterior submedian thoracic groups larger, with
broad, usually pigmented, leaflet-like branches; the inner hairs
of the two sides so close together that another similar hair
could not be placed between them without overlapping
....*A. albitarsis.*
Inner hairs of anterior submedian thoracic groups smaller, their
branches narrower or more transparent; those of the two sides
far enough apart so that another similar hair could be placed
between them without overlapping   10
10. Inner hairs of the anterior submedian thoracic groups each with
about eleven, fairly broad, leaflets.........*A. tarsimaculatus.*
Inner hairs of the anterior submedian thoracic groups each with
thirteen to eighteen narrower, almost hair-like leaflets
....*A. bachmanni.*
11. Outer clypeal hairs thickly branched, forming flat, fan-shaped
tufts with very numerous ultimate branchlets............... 12

Outer clypeal hairs thinly branched, forming flat, fan-shaped tufts with less than twenty ultimate branchlets; lateral hairs of abdominal segments 4 and 5 double........*A. vestitipennis.*
Outer clypeal hairs each with a single main stem, with or without delicate lateral branchlets 13

12. Inner clypeal hairs with delicate lateral branchlets near tip; lateral hairs of abdominal segments 4 and 5 double.*A. grabhami.*
Inner clypeal hairs without any lateral branchlets; lateral hairs of abdominal segments 4 and 5 split into from three to five branches ....*A. crucians.*

13. Inner and outer clypeal hairs with a main stem bearing a number of delicate lateral branchlets; lateral hairs of abdominal segments 4 and 5 split into four or five branches...*A. parvus.*
Inner and outer clypeal hairs single, without any lateral branchlets 14

14. Inner clypeal hairs close together; lateral hairs of abdominal segments 4 and 5 double........................*A. eiseni.*
Inner clypeal hairs well separated; lateral hairs of abdominal segments 4 and 5 with a single main stem and a number of well-developed lateral branches........*A. pseudopunctipennis.*

VI. *Notes on Groups and Species of American Anopheles*

1. SUBGENUS ANOPHELES

Anopheles and Patagiamyia groups. These two groups include all of the anopheline mosquitoes of the United States and a few tropical species. In the United States *punctipennis* ranges all over the country, *quadrimaculatus* is found in most of the States east of the Rocky Mountains, but is replaced by *maculipennis* on the Pacific Coast and along the northern border, *crucians* occurs mainly in the Southeastern States and *pseudopunctipennis* is found in the southwest from California to Texas. This last species has the widest range of any in these groups, since it occurs all through Central America, on the west coast of South America, and is widely distributed in the northwestern part of Argentina, where it is said to be the most important vector of malaria. In other parts of its range it is not considered to be an important carrier. In the United States, malaria is carried mainly by *quadrimaculatus* in the Southern States and by *maculipennis* on the Pacific Coast. Individuals of *punctipennis* and *crucians* have been found in nature infected with malaria parasites, but they are not considered to be as dangerous vectors of the disease as *quadrimaculatus* and *maculipennis*. *Anopheles walkeri,* a relatively rare mosquito reported from Virginia, Louisiana, Tennessee, Florida, and certain parts of Canada and eastern United States, has been shown to be susceptible to and capable of trans-

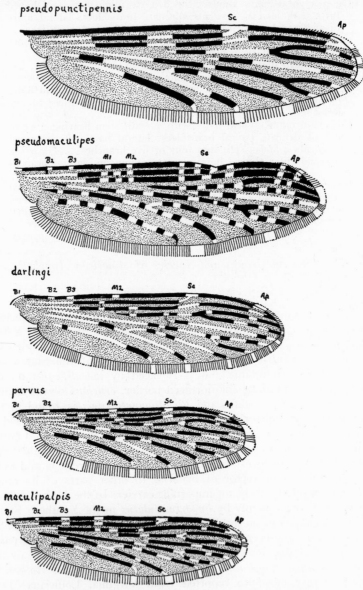

FIG. 258.—Diagrams of the wing patterns of various species of *Anopheles: A. pseudo-punctipennis* (Patagiamyia group). *A, pseudomaculipes* (Arribalzagia group), *A. darlingi* (Nyssorhynchus group), *A. parvus* (Myzorhynchella group), *A. maculipalpis* (subgenus *Myzomyia*). (Original. Root)

mitting benign tertian malaria (Matheson, Boyd, and Stratman-Thomas, 1933).

The larvæ of the species which occur in the United States resemble each other very closely and are difficult to identify. To add to the difficulty, it has been shown that *A. crucians* exists in two races, one breeding in the salt-marshes along the coast from New York to Texas, the other inhabiting fresh-water ponds in Georgia and Alabama. The larvæ of these two races are quite different, but no adult differences have yet been demonstrated. They are about equally susceptible to malaria and neither is a good vector (Boyd, Kitchen, and Mulrennan, 1936).

Arribalzagia group. The species of this group breed mainly in jungle pools. Many of the species are rare, but *punctimacula* is quite abundant in Panama and other Central American countries, *apicimacula* in Venezuela and *intermedius* and *pseudomaculipes* in Brazil. The larvæ of the species of this group are all very similar and difficult to distinguish, although readily identifiable as members of the group by the form of the outer clypeal hairs. In Venezuela Root found it possible to distinguish larvæ of *punctimacula* and *apicimacula* by the pecten teeth, which showed a regular alternation of long and short teeth in *punctimacula,* while the pecten of *apicimacula* always had at least one place where two or three short teeth stood together without intervening long teeth. Although the larvæ are difficult to differentiate, the pupæ of the species studied by Root show characteristic differences in the form of their breathing-trumpets, which is not usually the case in other groups. The species of this group have usually been considered as incapable of transmitting malaria but Simmons (1936) has found *A. punctimacula* naturally infected and believes that it is one of the most common carriers in the Canal Zone. He has also been able to infect *A. neomaculipalpus* experimentally with *Plasmodium vivax* and *P. falciparum.*

2. SUBGENUS NYSSORHYNCHUS

Myzorhynchella group. Includes three species from the interior of Brazil, which are evidently not important vectors of malaria.

Nyssorhynchus group. This group of "white-hind-footed" species includes the most abundant anophelines and the most important malaria-carriers of Tropical America. Many closely-related species or varieties are known in this group and there are very likely others which have not yet been described. We also need further information on the relations of the different forms to the transmission of malaria. The information at present available indicates that *albimanus* is the most important malaria-carrier of the Caribbean littorals and that either *albitarsis* or *darlingi* or both are the most important vectors in the lowlands of Brazil. Davis (1931) found a natural infection rate of 22 per cent in 200 specimens of *A. darlingi* caught in houses in Belém, Brazil. Davis and Kumm (1932) found 26 per cent of *A. darlingi* caught in houses in França, Brazil, to be infected with malaria. Even though *A. albitarsis* was the predominating mosquito from breeding areas, the only *Anopheles* found in houses was *darlingi*. Boyd (1926) has also shown that *tarsimaculatus* is a malaria-carrier, but of less importance than the others mentioned. Rozeboom (1935) has infected *A. bachmanni* with *P. vivax*.

The adult markings of species of this group are unusually variable, and in working out the fauna of a region which has not been carefully studied previously, it is essential to base identifications on larval and hypopygial characters, which are comparatively stable, instead of on the variable characters of the adult coloration.

Kerteszia group. The species of this group are very small anophelines, which breed in the water held by the leaf bases of epiphytic Bromeliads; that is, plants of the pineapple family (BROMELIACEÆ) which grow on the trunks and branches of trees. They are usually rare or local in their occurrence and are probably not important vectors of malaria.

3. SUBGENUS MYZOMYIA

This highly specialized group of mosquitoes contains some of the most dangerous malaria carriers. It is restricted to the Eastern Hemisphere, with the exception of the occurrence in Brazil of *A. gambiæ.* Shannon (1930) discovered this species in Natal, Brazil, and shortly afterwards there was a very severe outbreak of malaria in the vicinity of its breeding grounds. During this epidemic Davis (1931) collected females of *A. gambiæ* from houses, and out of 172 specimens found 108, or 62.8 per cent, infected. The introduction of this species into a new geographical area was undoubtedly brought about either by fast mail steamers which make the trip from Dakar, West Africa, to Natal in four days, or by aircraft. It is an example of the type of hazard introduced into public health by rapid transportation.

VII. *Malaria Carriers in Other Parts of the World*

1. SUBGENUS *Anopheles*

Anopheles maculipennis with its several varieties is generally considered to be one of the most widely distributed anophelines in the world and the most important malaria carrier in Europe. Many of the contradictory claims about this species as a vector of malaria are now reconcilable on the knowledge that it occurs in several varieties separable chiefly on basis of egg pattern (see Figure 259). The type variety is found rather generally distributed over Europe, the larvæ breeding in upland, cold waters and also in the waters of the plains under subtropical conditions. Variety *atroparvus* breeds in cool waters of slight to moderate salinity. Variety *messeæ* prefers cool, fresh waters, more often being found in standing than in running water. It is the predominant form on the European continent. Variety *labranchiæ* breeds in warmer saline waters but can also breed in fresh water. It is found in the Mediterranean region. Variety

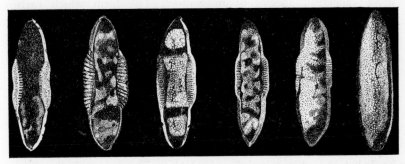

FIG. 259.—Eggs of European varieties of *Anopheles maculipennis* and *A. sacharovi*. Left to right: var. *melanoon;* var. *messeæ;* type variety; var. *atroparvus;* var. *labranchiæ;* and *A. sacharovi* (*elutus*). (Redrawn from Malaria Commission of the League of Nations, 1934)

melanoon is similar in its known habits to *messeæ* and is found in Spain, Italy, and Greece. The type variety and *messeæ* are capable of transmitting malaria but are probably easily deviated from man by stabled cattle. The same is true of *atroparvus,* but this variety undergoes partial hibernation in northern climates and, therefore, is attracted more to warmed houses. *A. maculipennis* var. *labranchiæ* and *A. sacharovi* (*elutus*) seek out bedrooms even in the presence of many domestic animals and are associated with intense malaria. *A. claviger* (*bifurcatus*) occurs throughout Europe, Northern Africa, Asia Minor, and Turkestan. In Palestine it breeds most commonly in wells and cisterns. Malaria was effectively controlled in Jerusalem following the World War by controlling the breeding of this species in wells and cisterns. The varieties of *A. hyrcanus* extend from the Rhone delta to the Levant, across Central Asia to Japan. The variety *sinensis* of this species is probably an important carrier in China.

A. umbrosus occurs in Assam, Andaman Islands, Burma, Malaya, Cochin-China, Borneo, the Dutch East Indies, and the Philippine Islands. It does not carry malaria in India, Cochin-China, or the Philippine Islands.

2. SUBGENUS *Myzomyia*

In Africa, *A. gambiæ* and *A. funestus* are widely distributed and both are very important malaria carriers. There is much to indicate that *A. pharœnsis* is a good vector in Egypt. *A. superpictus,* an undoubted carrier of malaria, is found from the eastern coast of the Mediterranean Sea to the northwestern part of India. *A. stephensi* occurs in Mesopotamia and throughout India where it is one of the most dangerous species of mosquitoes. The form which carries malaria breeds chiefly in wells and cisterns. *A. culicifacies* is distributed throughout India and extends westward to Arabia and eastward to Siam. It is the most important vector of malaria in India although it apparently is not a vector in northeast India. It is the only carrier in Ceylon and was responsible for the epidemic there in 1934-35. *A. fluviatilis* is also found all through India and Siam, occurring chiefly on the plains. *A. annularis* (*fuliginosis*) is an important carrier in Bengal and perhaps in the Dutch Islands. Because of the enormous numbers in which it breeds it may be of greater importance in other parts of its range than it is usually considered to be. It is widely distributed through Malaya, Dutch East Indies, Siam, South China and the Philippine Islands. It is definitely known not to transmit malaria in the Philippines. *A. maculatus* is not a vector in India or Ceylon but is known to be important in Malaya and the Dutch East Indies. It occurs from India to Indo-China and the Philippines. *A. minimus* is the chief vector in Assam and its variety *flavirostris* is the chief carrier in the Philippine Islands. *A. sundraicus,* which in Bengal, Malaya, and the Dutch Indies was formerly called *ludlowi,* is a carrier. The species *A. litoralis* which breeds in salt water in the Philippines and was formerly called *ludlowi* is not a vector, nor is the species now called *A. ludlowi* which breeds in fresh water in Formosa and the Philippine Islands. *A. annulipes* is widespread in Australia where it is suspected on epidemiological grounds of being a good carrier of malaria. No discussion is devoted here to the large number of species of *Anopheles* found in these regions of the world which are thought to play no part or a very slight part in the transmission of malaria.

VIII. *Vectors of Simian Malaria*

The various species of malaria found in monkeys have received considerable study within recent years. Some of these are very similar to species found in man, and since many experiments can be done with these species which cannot be done satisfactorily on human malaria they are sure to assume still greater importance in the future. As with human malaria the vectors have proved to be anopheline mosquitoes. Green (1932) infected *A. kochi, A. maculatus,* and *A. vagus* with *Plasmodium inui cynomolgi.* Sinton and Mulligan (1933) also record finding of sporozoites in mosquitoes of the following species after the latter had been fed upon monkeys infected with the above species of simian malaria: *A. annularis, A. splendidus, A. maculatus* and *A. culicifacies.* A complete transmission was effected by the bite of *A. annularis.*

CHAPTER XXXVI

MALARIA AND MOSQUITO SURVEYS

Surveys of the prevalence of malaria and of anopheline mosquitoes are usually made either to determine whether a control project is feasible or else before and after the application of control measures, to enable one to evaluate their efficacy. If it is intended to abate a mosquito nuisance as well as reduce malaria, the survey must be extended to include other mosquitoes also. But, in the tropics particularly, it is usually advisable to restrict control measures not only to anopheline mosquitoes alone, but even to the few species or varieties of *Anopheles* which can be proved to be the most important malaria vectors of the region. Unless this is done, the project will often prove too costly for adoption.

In order to combat malaria intelligently in any locality it is essential that a certain amount of survey work be done in that locality. It is often unsafe to accept information about the potentialities of a species of *Anopheles* as a vector of malaria, or control measures which have proved successful in other regions, without first making a survey to be sure that these data are really applicable to the locality in question.

The survey should give information on the following points, which will be treated in turn:

I. The prevalence of malaria.

II. The species and varieties of *Anopheles* present, their relative abundance and their breeding-places.

III. Which species and varieties of *Anopheles* are the important vectors of malaria.

I. *The Prevalence of Malaria*

We have as yet no entirely satisfactory methods for determining the proportion of a given population which are actually infected with malaria parasites. There are, however, several methods which will give a measure of the prevalence of malaria satisfactory for comparative use, provided that the two surveys to be compared use the same methods and technic. Since one is usually more interested in comparing the incidence of malaria in two different regions, or in the same area before and after control, than in the actual number of people infected with the disease, these methods are all reasonably satisfactory for practical purposes.

I. CASE INDEX

In a civilized community, the prevalence of malaria may be measured by persuading the physicians to report all their malaria cases during stated periods of time. We must remember, however, that not only may there be errors in diagnosis, but also that in a malarious region the majority of cases of malaria are never seen by a physician, being treated at home by "chill-tonics" and the like.

2. HISTORY INDEX

Among intelligent people, the prevalence of malaria may be approximated by a series of house-to-house visits by an inspector who finds out how many of the occupants of each house have suffered from "chills and fever" during the past year, for example. Here one is sure that no one in the population or the sample of the population selected for study has been overlooked, but errors in diagnosis or interpretation are much greater than in dealing with trained physicians.

3. PARASITE INDEX

This is obtained by making blood smears from the entire population or a sample thereof and examining them for the malaria parasites. It is advisable to record both the percentage of individuals infected with each of the three species of parasites and the percentage of *gamete carriers,* individuals who have more than one gamete to each 500 leucocytes, and are thus presumably capable of infecting mosquitoes. In examining blood smears for survey purposes it is essential to use the same technic throughout, if the surveys are to be comparable. Two surveys of the same individuals and made at the same time would yield widely divergent results if thin smears were used in one and thick smears in the other, or even if the smears were examined for ten minutes before being called negative in one and for five minutes in the other. Microscopists should be given intensive training before the real survey is begun, in order to minimize as far as possible errors due to their progressively increasing skill in detecting the parasites.

4. SPLEEN INDEX

This index is obtained by examining a sample of the population by palpation to determine the percentage of individuals with enlarged spleens. It is usually desirable to examine samples of both adults and of children under ten years in each locality, so as to distinguish between endemic and epidemic malaria. In comparing spleen indices obtained in two different surveys it must be remembered that the number of slightly enlarged (barely palpable) spleens found will vary decidedly according to the position in which the examination is made (standing or lying), whether clothing is loosened or not, and to the skill of the examiner. It must also be kept in mind that diseases other than malaria, notably kala-azar, produce enlargement of the spleen.

It is frequently advisable to combine two of these indices. In the southern United States a combined history and parasite index has sometimes been used, by taking blood-smears only from those individuals who gave a negative history. In the tropics it is usual to palpate the spleen at the same time that the blood-smear is obtained for the parasite index. Such combined indices will almost invariably give higher percentages of infection than either index alone.

II. *Anopheline Surveys*

Although the work of surveying the anopheline fauna of the locality and of determining the dangerous carriers among them should be carried on together, it is convenient to take up these two questions separately.

In order to be sure of obtaining all the species of *Anopheles* found in a given region, both adults and larvæ should be collected, for it sometimes happens that a species is easy to obtain in one of these stages but difficult to find in the other.

Adult mosquitoes are usually caught with a chloroform tube, made by placing rubber bands or a piece of a rubber stopper in the bottom of a large test-tube, pouring over them all the chloroform they will absorb and covering them first with cotton and then with a perforated disc of cardboard or cork. Such a tube should be kept tightly corked when not in use. The adults may be preserved for study by transfixing them with slender pins (the tiny pins called "minuten-nadeln" are often used) and pinning them into a cork-lined insect box or by placing them in pill-boxes with a thin layer of cotton to prevent their shaking about. In either case the specimens need to be fumigated frequently with carbon disulphide to prevent their being eaten up by museum pests. The specimens should be handled as little as possible and only with a pair of fine-pointed forceps.

Adult anophelines should be collected in their daytime resting places, both in houses and stables and in hollow trees or under bridges and culverts near their breeding-places. It is especially important to capture adults in sleeping-rooms, for usually the most dangerous carriers are to be found here. It is also advisable to make catches of adults with animal bait, collecting them at dusk as they come to bite a tame horse or cow. Regularly timed catches of this sort are particularly valuable in following the reduction in numbers of adults during control work.

In searching for anopheline larvæ one needs a dipper (preferably white-enamel-lined and with a hollow handle in which a wooden staff may be inserted), a large-mouthed pipette or medicine dropper for picking out larvæ and pupæ from the dipper, and bottles for carrying them back to the laboratory. In the laboratory there should be a series of small bowls or pans for the larvæ and plenty of gauze-covered lantern chimneys, bottles or test-tubes for breeding out adults from the pupæ.

In dipping for anopheline larvæ, which are usually at the surface of the water, the dipper should skim the surface or be lowered gently into the water so that the surface water will run into it. Experience will soon show that larvæ are usually obtained in the greatest numbers by dipping where the aquatic vegetation is thick enough to shelter them from fish.

Larvæ should be sought in every possible breeding-place, including not only ponds, streams and marshes but also puddles, hoof-prints, barrels, tanks, tree-holes and water-holding plants. Careful records of just what specimens are bred from each breeding-place should, of course, be kept. In a systematic survey it is best to make a detailed map of the territory surveyed, marking the location of every breeding-place discovered, and designating each breeding-place by a number. Collections of larvæ and pupæ can be labeled with the number of the breeding-place where they were secured and with the date of collection or a serial number or letter from which the date may be found by reference to one's notes.

It is usually easy to breed out adults if only large larvæ and pupæ are collected. Small larvæ are more difficult to rear because they must be supplied with food and the water changed regularly before it becomes at all foul. For food one may use very small amounts of dried and powdered insect tissue, yeast or dried blood-serum, by sprinkling them on the surface of the water in the breeding dishes.

If a good culture of unicellular algæ or protozoa can be maintained in the laboratory it makes excellent food for rearing larvæ.

III. *Anopheline Breeding-Places*

If we were to glance over the anopheline fauna of the whole world, we should find that some species of *Anopheles,* somewhere, will breed in almost any conceivable sort of water-collection. Some species have a wide range of habitats, while others are very restricted in their breeding.

The great majority of species probably prefer the comparatively pure, standing, fresh water of pools, ponds, marshes and swamps, but there are many exceptions to this rule. Some few species, like *A. subpictus* of India, are said to prefer polluted water. *Chagasia fajardoi* in Brazil and *A. maculatus* and its allies in the Orient breed in swift-flowing streams, and larvæ of many different species may be found in the vegetation along the edges of flowing streams and ditches. Some species prefer brackish to fresh water. Some require sunlight, others shade. Several anophelines breed only in water-holding plants. Thus *A. barberi* and its relatives breed in the water held by rot holes in trees, the Kerteszia group of tropical America in the leaf bases of Bromeliads and the Oriental *A. asiaticus* in cut bamboo stems.

In the eastern United States, *A. quadrimaculatus* is primarily a pond breeder, although it may be found in other places. *A. crucians* also is found mainly in ponds, one race in the pools in coastal salt-marshes, the other in the fresh-water ponds of the interior. *A. punctipennis* frequently breeds in ponds and marshes, but also breeds abundantly in springs, streams and ditches. *A. barberi* is found only in tree holes. Two other rarer species occur in this area, *A. atropos* breeding in brackish water along the Gulf Coast and *A. walkeri* found locally all over the area, usually breeding in the flood-pools near rivers.

IV. *Determination of the Dangerous Vectors of the Locality*

There are three ways in which one may get an idea as to which species of *Anopheles* are the really important vectors of malaria in any locality.

I. EPIDEMIOLOGICAL "INDEX"

Sometimes it is possible to correlate the occurrence of severe malaria with the presence of a particular species of *Anopheles.* If, for example, surveys are made of two localities, one with severe

malaria, the other with little or none, and it is found that the only
difference between the anopheline faunas of the two localities is
that a certain species of *Anopheles* is abundant in the malarious
region and rare or absent from the non-malarious region, it creates
a strong presumption that this species is the vector of the disease.
Such clear-cut cases are not often encountered, however, so that it
is usually necessary to resort to more laborious measures.

2. EXPERIMENTAL INDEX OF INFECTION

If hospital facilities are available, so that several patients who
are good gamete carriers (see page 539) can be kept at hand, information regarding the potentialities of the different species of
Anopheles as malaria-vectors may be obtained by breeding out large
numbers of female *Anopheles* from pupæ, allowing them to feed on
the gamete carriers, and dissecting them from four to ten days later
to see if the malaria parasites have developed in them. Under these
circumstances it is not unusual to find from 25 per cent to 50 per
cent of the specimens of a good vector infected, so that it is not
necessary to dissect very large numbers of mosquitoes. One is never
quite certain, however, that laboratory conditions and natural conditions are the same. It is conceivable that a species of *Anopheles*
which is potentially a dangerous vector may in nature have habits
which make it feed on human beings so seldom that it is not, in
fact, of any sanitary importance.

3. NATURAL INDEX OF INFECTION

This is obtained by collecting adult female anophelines, particularly in houses, and dissecting them in search of the malaria
parasites after they have been kept alive in the laboratory for a few
days to give them time to digest their latest blood-meal. This is the
most reliable of the three methods, but since the natural rate of
infection may be as low as 1 per cent and is usually below 10 per
cent, even in a good vector, large numbers of mosquitoes must be
dissected before accurate conclusions can be reached. In comparing
natural infection rates secured in different places or at different
times it must be remembered, also, that the percentage of the individuals of any species of *Anopheles* which are infected with malaria
parasites must obviously depend on many other factors besides its
capacity to act as a host for these parasites. Some of these factors
are, in all probability, the percentage of good gamete carriers in the
human population, the comparative abundance of human and animal

sources of blood, and the climatic conditions of temperature, humidity and so on.

4. COMBINED METHODS

In view of the deficiencies in any of the foregoing indices, it would seem advisable to use a combination of methods, each of which yields definite information on some particular characteristic of the mosquito responsible for making it a good vector. If, for example, the experimental index, which gives us a measure of the susceptibility of the species to malaria, is combined with a study of preferential feeding or a survey of the kinds of mosquitoes found in dwellings housing malarious patients, it is probable that a better idea of the importance of the species in transmission of malaria can be thus obtained than by the natural index. Information on the preferences of mosquitoes for certain types of animals can be obtained through the establishment of traps into which various types of animals are placed at night and the collection the following morning of all mosquitoes found within these traps. It is also possible to determine the percentage of a given species feeding on man and other animals by the collection in nature of engorged females and the determination by precipitin tests of the type of blood contained within the mosquitoes.

V. *Dissection of Anopheline Mosquitoes*

The so-called "dissection" of anopheline mosquitoes is not so difficult as it sounds. A dissecting lens or binocular microscope should be used for the actual dissection and the high power (4 mm. objective, $\times$ 10 ocular) of the compound microscope is needed in the examination for malaria parasites.

As has been described in Section I of this book, the malaria parasites may be found in two parts of the mosquito, as oöcysts in the stomach-wall or as sporozoites in the cells of the salivary glands. In dissecting mosquitoes we aim only at extracting these two organs for examination. The tools needed are dissecting forceps with fine points, Hagedorn needles fixed in handles, ordinary one by three inch microscopic slides, cover glasses of No. 2 thickness, and some physiological saline.

After being lightly chloroformed, the mosquitoes are placed on the stage of the dissecting microscope, and the legs and heads are cut off with the needle blades. A drop of the physiological saline is placed on the right of the mosquito and the mosquito arranged with the thorax directed toward the drop. The mosquito is steadied by a needle held in the left hand and inserted in the dorsal aspect of the thorax. A small bit of cover slip, six millimeters square, is held by the forceps in the right hand by allowing one blade of the forceps to hold the cover slip on either side of the square. The cover glass is now sloped down on the thorax so as to rest upon its anterior edge and while in this position the forceps are released. With the tips of the forceps on top of the cover glass, the latter is now pressed down gently while the mosquito is moved to the left with the left hand. In this manner the glands are pressed out and left under the cover glass. The preparation can now be examined directly or fixed and stained and then examined.

After removal of the salivary glands, the stomach can be removed as follows. A small opening is made in the dorsal wall of the abdomen and while holding the thorax with the needle, the tip of the abdomen is grasped with the forceps and the stomach slowly drawn out to the drop of fluid. The Malpighian tubules are carefully brushed back away from the stomach, and the latter is mounted in a drop of saline under another cover slip. Preparations should now be examined under the low power of the microscope for the presence of oöcysts and then carefully gone over with the high dry objective to make sure that no oöcysts have been overlooked. (The method here described is the one recommended by Barber and Rice, 1936. Their paper should be read for further directions upon the preparation of permanent mounts of stomachs and salivary glands.)

CHAPTER XXXVII

EPIDEMIOLOGY AND CONTROL OF MALARIA

A. EPIDEMIOLOGY

Attempts to control malaria in various parts of the world have not met with the success which was expected after the discovery of the means of the transmission of the disease by Ronald Ross in 1898. This rather general failure to control malaria in the wide areas where it takes its yearly toll of millions of human lives has not been due to apathy on the part of medical and public health officials nor to lack of investigations upon these problems. To understand this failure we need to look to the extremely complex problems involved. The life-cycle of the malarial parasite involving both man and mosquito, as outlined in Section I of this book, is in itself a very complicated life-cycle. However, these complications are increased by a great many factors which we shall briefly examine at this time.

First, let us realize that we are not dealing with one disease but with at least three, since we know that the three species of parasites vary widely in their effects upon man, and that none of them gives immunity to the others. All three of them are usually present in any region of the world where malaria is found at all. Hence, we not only have three diseases with which to contend, but we have the possibilities of mixed infections and also the chance that these three species are not homogeneous but are probably made up of a number of varieties which behave differently, both in the mosquito and in man. When we turn to the mosquitoes which transmit the diseases, we meet a much greater degree of complication. We now have to deal with a large number of species capable of transmitting malaria and differing very widely in their habits and abilities to transmit the diseases. Their predilection for particular types of breeding-places, their preferences for certain types of blood, their natural hiding places, and their susceptibilities to the various species of malaria parasites are so widely different that information gained in the study in attempts to control one, has seldom been directly helpful in understanding and controlling another. It is now a well proved fact that at least some of the species of *Anopheles* consist of some two to several varieties very similar to each other morphologically but differing so widely from each other in certain biological ways as to make their respective parts in the transmission of malaria quite different. There are also very significant variables on the human side of this problem. These have to do with the social conditions, the economic status of the population and racial differences. Hypothetically, at least, the problems of epidemiology of human malaria differ also from those of most other diseases by the possibility that the interrelationships between any two members of this triumvirate are further complicated by the possibilities of greater variability due to sexual reproduction. Since man, the parasites, and the mosquitoes are all bisexual organisms, the possibilities of variation due to inheritance are thus greatly increased. While there has been no experimental proof of the occurrence of genetic change in the parasites because of sexual reproduction, the possibility does exist. On the other hand, the mosquitoes are undergoing sexual reproduction several times a year and hence may be changing genetically in every characteristic with which successful malaria transmission is concerned. While this has not yet been proved to be true with human malaria in anopheline mosquitoes, it has been shown to exist with avian malaria in culicine mosquitoes (Huff, 1929, 1932, 1935). In the case of *Plasmodium cathemerium* in *Culex pipiens* it has been shown that the susceptibility of the mosquito to this parasite behaves as a recessive Mendelian characteristic. The part played by heredity in the natural immunity and susceptibility of the human host to malaria parasites has not yet been worked out, but in view of the wide demonstration of the importance of heredity in a large number of vertebrate hosts as a factor in determining the degree of susceptibility of these hosts to a wide variety of infectious agents, we must at least admit the possibility that malaria in man will be no exception to these findings.

In addition to all of the variables in each of the members of this triumvirate and in their interrelations, we must not neglect consideration of the influence of physical factors on each of these members. Chief amongst these are the climatic conditions and the topography of the country. Their effects are primarily upon the mosquitoes and upon man. For the growth of *Anopheles* mosquitoes suitable bodies of water must be present. These are determined in a large degree by the topography. Climatic conditions must also be favorable. The amount and distribution of rainfall will determine in a large number of cases whether malaria exists at all, exists to only a limited degree, or is a serious public health problem in a given locality. In addition, temperature is of great importance, inasmuch as each species and variety of mosquito has its own optimum requirement of temperature. And furthermore, the development of the parasites within the mosquito occurs only within certain temperature limits, the optimum being different for the three species of parasites. Climatic and topographical conditions greatly influence those economic and social conditions of man which relate to the malarial problem. A consideration of the foregoing principles of the epidemiology of malaria demonstrates the absolute need for preliminary studies upon each of these factors before successful control can be effected.

B. CONTROL

Although some of them do not belong strictly to the entomological section of this book, we may, for the sake of completeness, briefly notice the various methods of dealing with malaria.

I. *Measures of Defense*

1. CHEMOPROPHYLAXIS

Quinine has been very widely used in the past as a prophylactic drug. However, since the introduction of therapeutic malaria into the treatment of general paralysis, it has been possible to test very thoroughly the prophylactic value of quinine and other drugs. Experiments have clearly demonstrated that none of the chemotherapeutic agents known to be of value in the treatment of malaria is a complete prophylactic drug in the sense that it prevents an infection. Some of these drugs behave as a prophylactic against malaria when parasites are injected from another patient, but they are ineffective against the sporozoites introduced by mosquitoes. Therefore, we should probably apply the words, *abortive treatment,* rather than prophylaxis to the administration of such drugs previous to exposure to malaria. Under certain circumstances this abortive treatment will be advisable, but the persons using it are subject to relapse when the drug is discontinued.

2. SEGREGATION

Since the natives and especially the native children are the main reservoirs from which mosquitoes become infected in the tropics, it is possible to protect a small foreign colony by locating it far enough away from the native habitations so that few or no female *Anopheles* will fly from one to the other. This method has only a limited usefulness and of course cannot be applied in regions where a large group of people is to be protected.

3. SCREENING

While the screening of houses or sleeping rooms and the use of bed-nets or head-veils by individuals are more often prompted by a desire to be free from the annoyance of mosquito bites than undertaken as an antimalarial measure, they are nevertheless valuable for the latter purpose. As an antimalarial measure, screening both prevents mosquitoes from biting gamete carriers and thus becoming infected and protects healthy individuals from the bites of infected mosquitoes. Ordinary fly-screens are of no value against mosquitoes. The mesh must be at least sixteen to the inch (eighteen is better) and metal screening should be of copper or a resistant alloy, particularly in the tropics or near the seacoast. The screening should be thorough, and in barracks or houses whose doors are frequently opened at dusk there should be a supplementary routine of capturing or killing any mosquitoes which get inside.

Under this same heading should be mentioned the possibility of painting the walls of unscreened houses with substances which repel mosquitoes. Creosote has been used for this purpose.

II. *Measures of Attack*

I. STERILIZATION OF HUMAN CARRIERS OF MALARIA PARASITES

In the cases where it has been possible to carry out careful field experiments comparing the cost and efficacy of control by the administration of drugs to people as against control by mosquito reduction, it has been clearly demonstrated that the mosquitoes can be controlled at much less cost than is required for the treatment of malarious patients. This test has further shown that the most thorough quininization has been of negligible value in the reduction of incidence of malaria.

The new drug, plasmochin, offers greater promise in this respect. When given in sub-therapeutic doses this drug is capable of rendering the gametocytes in the blood of the malarious patient incapable of further development. To be effective, however, this drug would need to be administered continuously as long as gametocytes appeared in the blood during the mosquito season. It is possible that such a drug may prove to be of value if it can ever be given in such a way as to reach those people who are furnishing most of the infections for mosquitoes.

2. MOSQUITO REDUCTION

The method of controlling malaria by reducing the numbers of the mosquito vectors to a point where they can no longer carry the disease effectively is the best-known and most widely used malaria-control measure. As has already been suggested, it is advisable to find out what species of *Anopheles* are the really important vectors and restrict control-measures to these species, so far as is possible. This keeps down the cost of the work, which is the real problem nowadays. The work of Gorgas in Panama showed that malaria could be controlled under the most unfavorable conditions, provided expense was a secondary matter. The goal we must aim for now is to devise methods which will enable us to control malaria in any community *at a cost which that community is able and willing to bear.*

Killing adult mosquitoes. No satisfactory way of attacking the adult stage has yet been devised. Hand-catching has been used to a certain extent in the Canal Zone as a supplementary measure. Traps of various sorts have been tried out, but neither a satisfactory model for a trap nor an efficient bait has yet been developed. Fumigation with sulphur dioxide, fumes of insect-powder or hydrocyanic acid gas has occasionally proved useful, particularly when resting or hibernating adults were found in large numbers in houses. Various insects, animals and birds, including dragon-flies, swallows, swifts, goatsuckers and bats, are known to feed on mosquitoes to some extent, but no one has found a way to increase their numbers to a point where the mosquitoes will be decidedly reduced.

Killing larval mosquitoes. The larval stages, which are always found in water, offer the easiest point of attack if we want actually to kill mosquitoes. Use is made both of poisons of various sorts and of natural enemies. Poisonous chemicals used to kill mosquito larvæ are often called "larvicides" and are of two types, *contact poisons* which kill when they touch the larva, and *stomach poisons* which have no effect until they are eaten by the larva.

Oiling. The petroleum oils are the most generally used contact larvicides. Freeborn and Atsatt (1918) have shown that an oil film does not kill mosquito larvæ by plugging the tracheæ and thus asphyxiating them, as most people suppose, but is actually toxic to them. A volatile oil like gasoline is more toxic than a heavier oil like kerosene or crude oil. However, the heavier oils are more generally used because they are cheaper and form a more permanent film. Fuel oil and crude oil are so heavy that they must be either heated or mixed with a certain amount of kerosene before they can be used in a sprayer. The addition of a small percentage of castor oil or pine oil will make the resulting film spread farther and more rapidly.

The most generally useful implement for applying oil is the knapsack sprayer. Oil-soaked sawdust is useful for broadcasting over water with thick vegetation, such as rice-fields, and for treating water-soaked pastures full of hoof prints. Mops dipped in oil may also be used in the last-named type of breeding-place. Oil-soaked sawdust or cotton-waste may be packed into bags or cages and anchored in streams or ponds. A great variety of "drip-cans" and "bubblers" have also been devised to keep up a continual application of oil to streams or ponds.

A single application of oil will kill all mosquito eggs, larvæ and pupæ in the water at that time, and prevent egg-laying until the film begins to break up. Another application must be made in time to kill the larvæ which hatch from the first eggs laid before they reach the adult stage. In practice it has been found advisable to repeat the oiling once a week throughout the breeding season. In the interest of economy, it is best to have an inspector go over the area each week and mark for oiling only those breeding-places where large larvæ or pupæ are actually present. Oil applied to breeding-places where there are no larvæ is absolutely wasted.

Other contact larvicides. Many other contact poisons besides oil have been used against mosquito larvæ. The best known mixture is the "Panama larvicide," a soap of caustic soda and resin containing crude phenol. This mixes with the water and kills larvæ and the algæ on which they feed in dilutions up to 1-10,000. It also kills fish and should not be used in water which may be used for drinking or cooking. Creosote, nitre cake and borax have also been used for poisoning water in abandoned cisterns, fire buckets and barrels.

Paris Green. The stomach poison most generally used against *Anopheles* larvæ is Paris green. This arsenical is in the form of a very fine powder, relatively insoluble in water. The small particles remain floating on the water, where they are eaten by the surface-feeding larvæ of *Anopheles* but not by the larvæ of culicine mosquitoes, which feed below the surface. Since the Paris green must be eaten to have any effect, it does not kill eggs or pupæ, nor does it prevent oviposition. Paris green is so deadly to *Anopheles* larvæ that it may be diluted with some fine inert powder, such as ordinary road dust, before applying it. One part of Paris green to 100 parts of the inert dust is enough. This mixture may be applied by tossing handfuls of it into the air to form dust-clouds which will drift with the wind over the pond or marsh to be treated or by means of "dust-guns" or "blowers." It is preferable to make the application on a sunny day with gentle wind, after the dew has disappeared from the vegetation. It must be repeated every week or ten days. Russell (1934) has made some progress in the development of an automatic dusting machine for Paris green useful for species of mosquitoes breeding in running streams. There is need for further exploitation of this idea, in which the natural forces of wind and water power are utilized to make the dusting automatic.

Paris green is extremely effective in killing *Anopheles* larvæ, even when the water is thickly covered with aquatic vegetation. It is used in such small amounts that there is no danger of poisoning fish or animals which may drink the water on which it has been used. A possible exception is the continued use of Paris green on bodies of water used for urban water supply until a sufficient quantity of the chemical has accumulated to be detrimental to man. Unless the person who applies it is very careless about inhaling the dust or not cleansing his hands after handling the Paris green mixture, he runs very little risk of arsenical poisoning.

Roubaud (1920, 1926) has shown that powdered paraform, trioxymethylene and calcium arsenate may be used in the same way as Paris green. He also points out that these chemicals, particularly trioxymethylene, may be made to sink below the surface by mechanical agitation of the water and are then effective against culicine larvæ.

Natural enemies of mosquito larvæ. Although there are many aquatic insects and insect larvæ which feed more or less on mosquito larvæ, these are not of practical value in control work. Use may often be made, however, of small, surface-feeding fish. The best types for use in control work are the viviparous top-minnows, like *Gambusia affinis* of the southern United States. Besides being surface-feeders, which eat mosquito larvæ whenever they can get at them, this particular type of fish has the additional advantage of giving birth to living young, so that they are able to breed anywhere, even in tanks and wells.

In nature it often happens that we find top-minnows and *Anopheles* larvæ very abundant in the same body of water. Study of such areas always shows that the existence of the larvæ is dependent on the presence of aquatic vegetation thick enough to shelter them from the fish. To obtain effective fish control, then, it is necessary either to remove the sheltering vegetation or to use such large numbers of minnows that they will be driven by hunger to penetrate into the vegetation, where they would not attempt to go if sufficient food were available elsewhere.

Many larger fish feed on the little top-minnows, so that it is necessary either to use them only in bodies of water which do not contain other fish or to make sure that there are shallow areas around the edges where the larger fish cannot follow them.

Various species of top-minnows and other small, larva-eating fish are found in many different parts of the world. Before attempting to introduce some foreign species, therefore, it is advisable to study the local fish fauna, to see if there is not some native species which could be used just as effectively.

3. DESTROYING MOSQUITO BREEDING-PLACES

Since mosquito larvæ can live only in water, it is obvious that if the water is removed the mosquitoes can no longer breed there.

Surface drainage. In most cases, the easiest way to destroy a pond or marsh is to dig a ditch which will drain off the water. Drainage ditches should be as straight as possible, with gradual curves, if necessary, rather than sharp bends. The sides should slope steeply and the bottom be narrow, and both should be kept free of vegetation or other obstructions which would impede the free flow of water and make the ditch itself a possible breeding-place. In drainage work which is intended to be permanent, it may be cheaper in the long run to give the ditches a lining of concrete or asphalt. Ditches are usually dug by hand, but in large operations ditching machines or a series of charges of dynamite may be used. If dangerous anophelines are breeding along the edges of streams, the stream-bed must be made ditch-like so as to destroy such breeding-places.

Sub-soil drainage. Underground drains of tile or pipe have the advantage of lowering the ground water level and of doing away with all possibility of breeding in the drainage ditches. They are often used to intercept seepage outcrops and must be used to a considerable extent in regions where the principal vectors of malaria breed in rapid streams and ditches.

Vertical drainage. In limestone regions, where pervious strata of rock occur near the surface, ponds or marshes can sometimes be drained by boring a well through the impervious surface strata in the center of the area and draining all the water into this well so that it is carried off underground.

Filling. Small pools or marshes which cannot be economically drained may be filled in with earth or rock. Near large cities, rubbish, ashes and the like may be used. Care should be taken, of course, to avoid making new breeding-places in "borrow-pits" from which earth is taken.

Ponding. If confronted with a large marsh which can be neither drained nor filled in at a reasonable cost, one solution is to dig a pond in the center and concentrate all the water in it, thus reducing the surface area. Breeding in such a pond can then be controlled by the introduction of top-minnows or the use of larvicides.

Clearing and cleaning up. When a dangerous species of *Anopheles* breeds only in shaded pools, its breeding-places may be destroyed by clearing away the trees and shrubs about these pools. More often, however, it will be found that the dangerous vectors are not shade-breeders, so that clearing the ground around a jungle pool may convert an innocuous into a dangerous breeding-place.

It is also obvious that if a dangerous anopheline should be found breeding in artificial containers or in water-holding plants these must be removed, screened or destroyed. Cleaning up artificial containers about houses will, in any case, greatly reduce the numbers of the domestic culicines, and is often undertaken for that purpose.

4. GENERAL CONSIDERATIONS

Area to be controlled. One of the most important questions for decision in any malaria-control campaign is as to the size of the area to which control measures are to be applied. In theory one should control a zone surrounding the area to be protected and wide enough that the dangerous anophelines cannot fly across it. If heavy breeding were found the zone would need to be wider than if the breeding were light. Flights of over one mile for *A. quadrimaculatus* and over two miles for *A. albimanus* have been reported, and the control of zones as wide as this is quite expensive. In practice, then, the width of the control zone surrounding the area will depend to a considerable extent on the amount of money available. Fortunately experience has shown that even partial control of anopheline breeding may give a decided reduction in malaria, so that it is worth while to do control work even if the width of the surrounding zone must be reduced to one-half or even one-quarter of a mile.

Comparative advantages of drainage and larvicidal measures. The destruction of mosquito larvæ by the use of oil, Paris green and so on is a control measure the first cost of which is very low. But since it must be repeated many times during each breeding season, year after year, it becomes very expensive if continued long enough. The destruction of breeding-places by drainage, on the other hand, is a control measure with a high first cost but a much smaller expenditure for upkeep, which makes it much cheaper than larvicidal measures over a term of years.

If, then, one wishes to control malaria for a year or two only, little drainage should be done and oil and Paris green used freely. However, if a permanent control program is in view, drainage should be used as much as possible and larvicidal measures given a very subordinate place. If the money for a complete drainage program is not immediately available, as much new drainage as possible should be put in each year, after reserving funds for the upkeep of previously constructed drainage and for larvicidal control of all undrained breeding-places. In this way the program will ultimately be completed and control continuously maintained. It is probably needless to point out that anti-malarial drainage is an engineering problem, and should be supervised by a trained Sanitary Engineer, if possible.

"Trap breeding-places." It is not always advisable to destroy certain breeding-places, even though they could be easily abolished. If the destruction of an easily controllable, preferred breeding-place might force the mosquitoes to breed in another potential breeding-place which could not be easily controlled but is not of importance so long as the preferred breeding-place remains available, it would be best not to destroy the first breeding-place but to leave it to act as a trap. The mosquitoes could be allowed to lay their eggs there and the resulting larvæ prevented from reaching maturity by the use of fish or larvicides. This principle is not usually of great importance in malaria-control work, but is occasionally of use, and it becomes of considerable importance in the control of the yellow-fever mosquito.

CHAPTER XXXVIII

CULICINE MOSQUITOES

The name "culicine mosquitoes" is often used to apply to all mosquitoes except the anophelines, although, strictly speaking, it should be used only for those which belong to the tribe CULICINI. Keys have already been given (page 514) to the tribes of CULICINÆ by adult and larval characters. One of these tribes may be dismissed very briefly, since it includes no species of importance to parasitology.

I. *Tribe Megarhinini*

Includes only a single genus, *Megarhinus*. The adults are large mosquitoes with brilliant metallic coloration. They may be differentiated from all other mosquitoes by the form of the proboscis, which is very long, curved, and tapering in both sexes. In this genus even the females are unable to bite, and feed only on nectar and other plant juices. The larvæ are large, dark-colored, and feed on other mosquito larvæ. They usually breed in tree-holes, Bromeliads and other collections of water held by plants, but occasionally occur in artificial containers. Only about fifty species are known, and *M. septentrionalis* is the only species which is at all abundant in the United States.

II. *Tribe Culicini*

The genera listed by some other writers under the tribes URANO-TÆNINI and SABETHINI are reduced here to groups under the tribe CULICINI. This large tribe includes all the common wild and domestic non-anopheline mosquitoes which are pests of man and animals and vectors of disease. It consists of five groups as follows:

1. *Sabethes* GROUP

Includes a considerable number of genera, some of which are found only in the New World, while others are peculiar to the Old World. The adults may be large or small, brilliantly metallic or dull in coloration. Some species bite man readily, others do not, but since all of them breed in collections of water held by plants they seldom are abundant enough to constitute real pests. The larvæ and pupæ are usually whitish or yellowish in color. Most of the larvæ feed on minute organisms or fragments of dead insects, but the larvæ of some of the larger species eat other mosquito larvæ. Most of the species are tropical. The only generally distributed form in the eastern United States is *Wyeomyia smithi,* which breeds in the leaves of the pitcher-plant, *Sarracenia purpurea.*

2. *Uranotænia* GROUP

Includes only a single genus, *Uranotænia.* The adults are small mosquitoes, which almost always have lines or patches of brilliant blue scales on the dorsal or lateral surface of the thorax and sometimes on the basal portion of certain wing-veins. The larvæ of many species may easily be mistaken at first glance for small *Anopheles* larvæ, since they lie horizontally in the water and have an oval head. The short air-tube is not obvious in looking down upon the larvæ as they rest at the surface, although it is readily seen in a side view. They usually breed in permanent ponds and marshes but are also found in pitcher-plants in the Orient. *U. sapphirinus* is the only species found in the eastern United States.

3. *Theobaldia-Mansonia* GROUP

This group includes the genera *Theobaldia, Orthopodomyia, Mansonia, Aëdeomyia* (and *Ficalbia* which does not occur in the Western Hemisphere). These forms constitute a rather loosely related group which are, perhaps, most closely related to the primitive stock from which modern culicine mosquitoes descended (Edwards, 1932).

4. *Aëdes* GROUP

The genera *Aëdes, Psorophora, Hæmagogus, Eretmopodites, Armigeres, Heizmannia,* and *Opifex* constitute this group. The last four of these do not occur in the Western Hemisphere. These mosquitoes usually breed in temporary pools, laying their eggs singly in the débris at the bottom of depressions which will later be filled with water.

5. *Culex* GROUP

The large genus *Culex* with many subgenera (among them, *Lutzia*), together with a nearly related genus *Deinocerites,* make up this last group. For the most part these mosquitoes breed in permanent bodies of water and lay their eggs in rafts on the surface of the water.

The following keys (modified from Edwards, 1932) are for the differentiation of the American species.

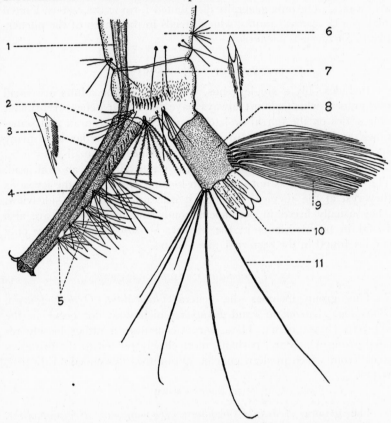

FIG. 260.—Posterior end of larva of *Culex* showing the parts most used for identification of culicine larvæ. (Original. Huff)

1—Tracheæ
2—Plumose tuft
3—Pecten of tube
4—Air-tube
5—Hair-tufts of tube
6—Abdominal segment, 7

7—Comb scale of 8th segment
8—Anal segment
9—Ventral brush of anal segment
10—Anal gills
11—Dorsal anal tuft

KEYS TO THE AMERICAN GENERA OF TRIBE CULICINI

By Adult Characters (See Figs. 260 and 261.)

1. Squama fringed (usually completely); 6th vein reaching well beyond fork of 5th vein 2

Squama bare or rarely with 1-4 short hairs 13

2. Pulvilli present; pleural hairs well developed, but spiracular and post-spiracular bristles absent 3
Pulvilli absent or rudimentary 4

3. Second antennal segment short in both sexes; antennæ of ♂ nearly always plumose .... *Culex.*
Second antennal segment elongate in both sexes; antennæ of ♂ not plumose .... *Deinocerites.*

4. Post-spiracular bristles absent; claws of ♀ simple (except in *Hæmagogus*) 5
Post-spiracular bristles present (even if only one or two); claws of ♀ usually toothed, dorsocentral and upper sternopleural bristles nearly always well developed 11

5. Spiracular bristles present (sometimes only one or two)....... 6
Spiracular bristles absent 8

6. Several upper sternopleural bristles; subcostal vein basal to humeral cross-vein usually hairy beneath .... *Theobaldia.*
At most one or two upper sternopleural bristles; subcostal vein basal to humeral cross-vein bare beneath 7

7. Clypeus with setæ .... *Trichoprosopon (Joblotia).*
Clypeus bare .... *Goeldia.*

8. Dorsocentral and prescutellar bristles absent; pronotal lobes approximated .... *Hæmagogus.*
Dorsocentral and prescutellar bristles well developed; pronotal lobes well separated 9

9. All segments of ♀ antenna, and last two of ♂ antenna short and thick; middle femora with scale-tuft .... *Aëdeomyia.*
Antennæ normal, slender; middle femora without scale-tuft.... 10

10. First segment of front tarsi longer than the last four together, fourth very short in both sexes .... *Orthopodomyia.*
First segment of front tarsi not longer than last four together; fourth not shortened in ♀ .... *Mansonia.*

11. Spiracular bristles present, even if few .... *Psorophora.*
Spiracular bristles absent 12

12. Wing-scales generally mostly narrow (or if all broad, ♀ claws toothed); usually a few hairs on upper surface of subcostal stem basal to humeral cross-vein (stem vein) .... *Aëdes.*
Wing-scales all very broad; ♀ claws simple, subcostal stem basal to humeral cross-vein (stem vein) bare .... *Mansonia.*

13. Wing-membrane without microtrichia (or only visible at high magnification); second marginal cell (R₂) shorter than its stem; 6th vein ends basal to fork of 5th vein.... *Uranotænia.*
Wing-membrane with distinct microtrichia 14

14. Middle legs with "paddles" formed of very long erect scales ....*Sabethes.*
Middle legs without "paddles" 15

15. Clypeus with hairs; large species, with long palpi in male ....*Trichoprosopon (Joblotia).*
Clypeus bare, or with scales only 16

16. Hind tarsi with long suberect scales; large species, with long palpi in male .... *Goeldia.*

Hind tarsi with appressed scales only; smaller species, with short
palpi in male 17
17. No bristles on sub-alar knob; pronotal lobes large and almost in
contact; mesonotal scales all metallic ....*Sabethoides.*
Bristles present on sub-alar knob; pronotal lobes more widely
separated; mesonotal scales rarely metallic 18
18. Spiracular area with scales only; hind tarsus with one claw
....*Limatus.*
Spiracular area with 1-4 bristles; hind tarsus with two claws
....*Wyeomyia.*

By Larval Characters (See Fig. 261.)

1. Anal segment with ventral brush of at least four separate hairs 2
Anal segment with one pair of ventral hairs 13
Anal segment without ventral hairs ....*Culex.*
2. Eighth segment with lateral chitinous plates, with one row of
comb-teeth on its margin; mouthbrushes normal
................................*Uranotænia, Aëdeomyia.*
Eighth segment without lateral plates (except sometimes in
Psorophora) 3
3. Air-tube with pecten, teeth usually denticulate (pecten rarely
reduced) 4
Air-tube without pecten or rarely with a few simple teeth...... 10
4. Air-tube with several pairs of hair-tufts, or else very long and
slender 5
Air-tube with one pair of hair-tufts, and never very long 7
5. Mouthbrushes forming matted prehensile tufts..*Culex (Lutzia).*
Mouthbrushes normal 6
6. Mandibles with hairy projection at base ....*Deinocerites.*
Mandibles without such projection
..................*Culex, Theobaldia (Culicella, Climacura).*
7. Hair-tuft on air-tube basal ....*Theobaldia.*
Hair-tuft on air-tube near middle, often beyond ....;.. 8
8. Mouthbrushes forming matted prehensile tufts
....*Psorophora, Aëdes.*
Mouthbrushes normal 9
9. Anal segment with ring complete......*Psorophora, Uranotænia.*
Anal segment (except rarely) with ring incomplete
....................................*Aëdes, Hæmagogus.*
10. Valves of air-tube highly modified for piercing......*Mansonia.*
Valves of air-tube not modified 11
11. Abdominal segments 6-8 normally with dorsal chitinous plates
....*Orthopodomyia.*
Abdomen without plates on segments 6-8 12
12. Antennæ very large and flattened ....*Aëdeomyia.*
Antennæ nearly round 13
13. Eighth abdominal segment without comb, but with small lateral
plate bearing a simple bristle......*Trichoprosopon (Joblotia).*
Eighth abdominal segment with lateral comb as usual.......... 14
14. Eighth segment with a pair of dorsal chitinous hooks
....*Sabethoides.*

Eighth segment without dorsal hooks 15
15. Maxilla large, ending in two strong articulated horns...*Goeldia.*
    Maxilla without such horns................................ 16
16. Maxilla with a slender spine or tooth at its tip........*Sabethes.*
    Maxilla hairy at tip 17
17. Lateral comb of eighth abdominal segment consisting of a few
    separate scales ....*Limatus.*
    Comb scales numerous, sometimes attached to a lateral plate
    ....*Wyeomyia.*

III. *Comments on Some of the Genera of the Tribe Culcini*

Aëdes. A very large genus including small or medium-sized mosquitoes, which often have white-banded legs and a thorax marked with stripes or patches of silver or golden scales. It has been divided into many subgenera, mainly on hypopygial characters. The apparently more primitive subgenera, such as *Howardina, Stegomyia* and *Finlaya,* usually breed in tree-holes, Bromeliads or other collections of water held by plants, while the more typical subgenera (*Ochlerotatus* and *Aëdiomorphus*) are found in temporary pools produced by rain, melting snow, flooded streams or high tides. The yellow-fever mosquito, *Aëdes* (*Stegomyia*) *ægypti* Linn., is a member of the former group which has become domestic. The common "wood-mosquitoes" of spring and the "salt-marsh mosquitoes" of New Jersey and other coastal regions are examples of the latter group. Some species of *Aëdes* will be found to be common and troublesome in nearly every region of the world. In all species of *Aëdes* and *Psorophora* the female abdomen tapers toward the tip and the terminal *cerci* are prominent and easily seen.

Psorophora. This genus is found only in America. The species all breed in temporary pools, and most of them are vicious biters. It is divided into three groups which are sometimes treated as subgenera. The subgenus *Psorophora* includes very large mosquitoes whose larvæ feed on other mosquito larvæ. The "gallinipper" (*Ps. ciliata*), which ranges from the United States to Argentina, belongs to this group. In the subgenus *Janthinosoma* we find fairly large mosquitoes with dark metallic blue or purplish coloration. The legs are not regularly banded, but some species have one or more of the terminal hind tarsal joints all white. *Ps. posticatus* (including *sayi*) and *Ps. lutzi* are widely distributed species with the last two hind tarsals all white. *Ps. cyanescens* is another species which is troublesome in many regions, but has no white on the hind legs. The larvæ of species of this group never feed on other mosquito larvæ and usually have long antennæ. In the third group, often called the subgenus *Grabhamia,* are found medium-sized or small mosquitoes with much-banded legs and brown or dark gray coloration. Some species have a mixture of dark and light scales on their wings and bear a superficial resemblance to *Mansonia.* The larvæ do not feed on other

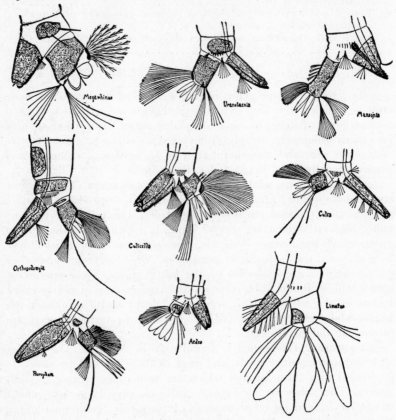

FIG. 261.—Lateral views of the terminal abdominal segments of the mature larvæ of some common genera of culicine mosquitoes. *Culicella* is replaced by *Theobaldia* in the text. (Original. Root)

mosquito larvæ and usually have short antennæ. The species most abundant in the eastern United States is *Ps. columbiæ.*

Hæmagogus. A small genus of tropical American mosquitoes which breed in tree-holes and bamboo. The larvæ are indistinguishable from those of *Aëdes,* but the adults have taken on brilliant metallic blue or purple colors which make them closely resemble certain species of *Sabethes* (subgenus *Sabethoides*).

Theobaldia. A genus of fairly large mosquitoes which breed in more or less permanent pools. Most of the species lay their eggs in rafts like *Culex,* but have only one pair of hair-tufts on the larval air-tube, as in *Aëdes.* Many species have indistinct dark spots on the wings, such as in *Anopheles quadrimaculatus.* The species of *Theobaldia* are found almost exclusively in the north-temperate regions of both the Old and the New Worlds. *T. inornata* is the commonest species of the eastern United States.

Orthopodomyia. A small genus of medium-sized mosquitoes which breed in tree-holes and other collections of water held by plants. Most of them have the legs banded and the thorax striped with white, so that they resemble some species of *Aëdes. O. signifera,* the only species which is found in the United States, has a slight resemblance to the yellow-fever mosquito, and is sometimes mistaken for it. Species of *Orthopodomyia* are found in most parts of the world, but are usually rare on account of their specialized breeding-places.

Aëdeomyia. This genus includes three species which are widely distributed in the tropics of America, Africa and the Orient, respectively. The adults look like miniature *Mansonia,* but the larvæ are very different. They breed in permanent bodies of water with much surface vegetation, particularly among masses of water-lettuce (*Pistia*) or water-hyacinth (*Eichornia*).

Mansonia. Species of this genus are found all over the world. The adults have white-banded legs and usually a mixture of black and white scales on the wings. The larvæ and pupæ have their air-tubes or breathing-trumpets ending in sharp points, which they thrust into the air-containing tissues of aquatic plants, thus obtaining oxygen without coming to the surface of the water. *M. titillans* is a species which is widely distributed in the American tropics, and whose larvæ and pupæ attach themselves to the roots of the floating water-lettuce (*Pistia*). The only species which is found in the United States (except in Florida) is *M. perturbans,* whose larvæ and pupæ are attached to the roots of sedges.

Culex. A very large genus of small or medium-sized mosquitoes, most of which do not have banded legs nor a distinctly marked thorax. The species of *Culex* and *Mansonia* all lay their eggs in rafts or clumps and the abdomen of the female does not taper toward the tip, which is abruptly truncate, with the cerci hidden. The majority of the species breed in permanent bodies of water, but a few breed in temporary pools and others in Bromeliads and tree-holes. The genus has been divided into many subgenera on hypopygial characters. The subgenus *Culex* includes most of the brownish or grayish, medium-sized species which are annoying to man or animals, while the sub-genera *Melanoconion* and *Mochlostyrax* contain small black species, which are often found breeding in company with *Anopheles,* but seem rarely to attack man or domestic animals. Some of the tropical American subgenera (*Carrollia, Isostomyia, Microculex*) breed only in tree-holes, Bromeliads and other water-holding plants.

Two species of the subgenus *Culex* have become domestic mos-quitoes, breeding both in ground pools and in all sorts of artificial containers, particularly where the water is more or less polluted. *Culex pipiens* is found in temperate regions all over the world and *C. fatigans* (or *quinquefasciatus*) throughout the tropics and sub-tropics. In most parts of the world there will also be found other species of this same subgenus which have adopted similar habits to a greater or less extent. In the eastern United States, for example, *C. territans* and *C. salinarius* are often found breeding in rain-barrels and other containers, as well as in pools. The subgenus *Lutzia* in-cludes very large mosquitoes with larvæ which prey on other mosquito larvæ. All the species are tropical. The American species have wing-veins with alternating areas of dark and pale scales, much as in *Anopheles*. Other species are found in Africa and the Orient. The larvæ occur either in ground pools or in tanks and other containers, usually feeding on *Culex* larvæ.

Deinocerites. This genus includes a few tropical American mos-quitoes which breed only in crab-holes. They do not bite man, but the crab-holes are also inhabited by species of *Culex* and *Aëdes,* some of which do bite human beings.

CHAPTER XXXIX

CULICINE MOSQUITOES IN RELATION TO DISEASE

Several diseases of man and of animals are transmitted by culicine mosquitoes. Among those caused by filterable viruses are: yellow fever, dengue fever, equine encephalomyelitis, herpes-encephalomyelitis, and epithelioma contagiosum (of fowls). The avian malarias caused by species of *Plasmodium* are transmitted by these mosquitoes, as are also the diseases, filariasis of man, and heartworm of dogs.

I. *Yellow Fever*

Yellow fever is an acute, non-contagious, febrile disease, accompanied by albuminuria, hemorrhages and jaundice, and with a high death-rate. Children and negroes usually have the disease in a much milder form than other people. The causative agent is a filter-passing organism. The disease is transmitted in nature by the bite of certain mosquitoes. To become infected, the mosquito must bite a yellow-fever patient during the first three or four days of illness and it only becomes infective for other persons after the lapse of a period of from twelve to fourteen days.

The original home of yellow fever and of *Aëdes aegypti,* its chief vector, was probably on the west coast of Africa. This mosquito has spread all over the tropical and subtropical portions of the world (from about 38° North Latitude to about 38° South Latitude) but the disease has remained confined mainly to the tropical coastal regions bordering on the Atlantic Ocean, although it did spread also to the Pacific Coast of Central and South America. The endemic centers were large cities of the tropics, such as Habana, Cuba; Vera Cruz, Mexico; Colon and Panama City, Panama; Rio de Janeiro, Brazil; Guayaquil, Ecuador,—cities in which the mosquito could breed the year around and where non-immune people were continually supplied by immigration. From these cities the disease tended to spread to surrounding areas and to temperate regions where the mosquitoes became established and survived only during the summer. In the days when yellow fever mosquitoes were carried on sailing ships, summer epidemics of yellow fever occurred in such cities as Baltimore, Philadelphia, New York and Quebec. In 1878 there occurred 4046 deaths in New Orleans as the result of one epidemic; and such epidemics were frequent in the cities of Southern United States. The control of the disease was made possible in these urban areas by the discoveries of Finlay (1886) and later by the American Commission headed by Reed (1900) that *Aëdes ægypti* is the chief agent of transmission. Thus the mosquito control work of Gorgas in Habana eliminated the disease from that city, and the successful control of mosquitoes in the Canal Zone made possible the building of the Panama Canal.

For a period of almost 30 years it was generally believed that *Aëdes ægypti* was uniquely the transmitting host and that the disease could not last long in any locality in the absence of this species of mosquito. However, Bauer (1928) showed that other African mosquitoes were able to transmit the disease experimentally to animals, and Philip (1929) added still other African species to the list of possible vectors. Davis and Shannon (1929) made similar findings on South American species of mosquitoes; and one Oriental mosquito, *Aëdes albopictus,* has been proved to be a carrier by Dinger, Schüffner, Snijders and Swellengrebel (1929). A list of these mosquitoes is given below:

Mosquito vectors of experimental yellow fever

Aëdes (Stegomyia) africanus	African
Aëdes (Stegomyia) albopictus	Oriental
Aëdes (Stegomyia) luteocephalus	African
Aëdes (Stegomyia) simpsoni	African
Aëdes (Stegomyia) vittatus	African
Aëdes (Ædiomorphus) stokesi	African
Aëdes (Ochlerotatus) scapularis	South American
Aëdes (Finlaya) fluviatilis	South American
Eretmopodites chrysogaster	African
Mansonia africana	African

Numerous other species of culicine mosquitoes have been shown to be capable of harboring the virus of yellow fever without transmitting it through their bite. Others can transmit the disease but do so very poorly. Among the latter is the very ubiquitous and domestic species, *Culex fatigans* (Davis, 1933). Very little is known about the habits of any of these species or their importance in the natural transmission of the disease. In a survey of four cities in Northern and Southern Nigeria, Beeuwkes, Kerr, Weathersbee, and Taylor (1933) concluded that none of the experimental vectors plays any important part in the natural transmission of yellow fever except *Aëdes ægypti* and in northern Nigeria possibly *Mansonia africana*.

II. *Dengue Fever*

Dengue fever is an epidemic disease which begins abruptly and is accompanied by intense aches and pains in the head, eyes, muscles and joints, and sometimes by vomiting. It lasts from 3 to 8 days and is seldom fatal. The causative agent is a filterable virus resembling very closely the yellow fever virus except in pathogenicity. The insect vectors are *Aëdes ægypti* and *Aëdes albopictus. Culex fatigans* has definitely been shown not to transmit the disease. To become infected, mosquitoes must bite the patient during the first three days of symptoms. They become infective by bite in about eleven days after feeding and probably remain infective for the remainder of their lives.

Epidemics of dengue fever have occurred at some time or other in nearly every part of the tropics and subtropics. It is likely to be met with wherever its vectors are abundant. Since it is carried chiefly by the same mosquitoes as yellow fever, the control of these two diseases can be discussed together.

III. *Relation of Mosquitoes to Some Other Filterable Virus Diseases*

Recent work by Kelser (1933) and Merrill, Lacaillade, and Ten Broeck (1934) has indicated that equine encephalomyelitis may be transmitted by mosquitoes. The former showed that *Aëdes ægypti* could transmit the western type from infected guinea pigs to horses. The latter workers incriminated the salt-marsh mosquito, *Aëdes sollicitans,* in the transmission of both western and eastern strains of this disease. Attempts to transmit the western type of the disease by means of *Aëdes dorsalis* and *Anopheles maculipennis* have been, however, unsuccessful (Herms, Wheeler and Herms, 1934). The western type has recently been transmitted experimentally by *Aëdes albopictus* (Simmons, Reynolds, Cornell, 1936).

While the final proof has not been furnished, preliminary experiments by Simmons, Kelser and Cornell (1933) indicate that the virus of herpesencephalomyelitis may be transmissible by *Aëdes ægypti*. This resembles equine encephalomyelitis in that it is a neurotropic virus.

A disease of chickens and pigeons called fowl-pox (epithelioma contagiosum) is transmissible by *Culex pipiens, C. fatigans, Aëdes ægypti* and *A. vexans*. The virus is known to live for at least 38 days and probably indefinitely in the infected mosquito. (Kligler, Muckenfuss, and Rivers, 1929; Oliveira Castro, 1930; Blanc and Caminopetros, 1930; Matheson, Brunett, and Brody, 1931).

IV. *Avian Malaria*

Culicine mosquitoes undoubtedly play an important part in the transmission of the various species of malarial parasites of the genus *Plasmodium* in birds. A wide variety of these species exists and they are distributed widely geographically and systematically in birds. Complete mosquito transmissions have been effected experimentally of *Plasmodium cathemerium, P. relictum, P. gallinaceum* and *P. capistrani,* and development to the oöcyst or sporozoite stage has been demonstrated in mosquitoes for the species *P. elongatum, P. rouxi* and *P. circumflexum.* The following mosquitoes have been infected with one or more of the known species of avian malaria:

> *Culex (Culex) fatigans*
> *Culex (Culex) pipiens*
> *Culex (Culex) hortensis*
> *Culex (Culex) territans*
> *Culex (Culex) salinarius*
> *Culex (Culex) tarsalis*
> *Culex (Lutzia) fuscana*
> *Theobaldia longeareolata*
> *Theobaldia annulata*
> *Aëdes (Ochlerotatus) communis*
> *Aëdes (Ochlerotatus) mariæ*
> *Aëdes (Finlaya) triseriatus*
> *Aëdes (Stegomyia) ægypti*
> *Aëdes (Stegomyia) albopictus*
> *Anopheles (Myzomyia) subpictus*

(For experiments upon the above species see the review by Huff, 1932, and the articles by Nono, 1932; Reichenow, 1932; Russell, 1932; and Brumpt, 1936).

V. *Filarial Diseases*

Filariasis is the infection by nematode worms of the family FILARIIDÆ (see Section II of this book). It is of interest to medical men chiefly because of the probable connection between *Wuchereria bancrofti* and elephantiasis.

I. WUCHERERIA BANCROFTI

This species is of especial interest historically because Manson's discovery (1878) that it was a mosquito which was responsible for its transmission is one of the great landmarks in the history of Medical Entomology. Cases of infection with *W. bancrofti* have been found in nearly all tropical and subtropical regions. Endemic filariasis occurs in the United States only in Charleston, South Carolina.

The adult worms live in the lymphatics, and the female sheds the embryos or microfilariæ into the blood. In most cases of filariasis due to *W. bancrofti* the microfilariæ are found in the peripheral circulation in great numbers at night, but retreat to the heart, lungs and larger arteries during the day. This periodicity is very interesting and difficult to explain. It has been shown that the periodicity may be reversed by making a patient sleep by day and work at night for several days. It has also been shown that filarial periodicity is more or less correlated with the habits of the intermediate host. Most strains of *W. bancrofti* exhibit a nocturnal periodicity and are carried by night-biting mosquitoes, particularly *Culex fatigans*. But in the Pacific Islands there is a strain which exhibits no periodicity and is carried mainly by a mosquito, *Aëdes (Stegomyia) variegatus,* which bites only by day. It should also be noted that microfilariæ of a related filarial worm, *Loa loa,* exhibit a definite diurnal periodicity and are carried by day-biting tabanid flies of the genus *Chrysops.*

The development of the microfilariæ in the mosquito has already been treated in Section II of this book. It will be remembered that the microfilariæ undergo a period of development in the thoracic muscles of the mosquito and then migrate into the proboscis sheath or labium. While comparatively little is known about mosquitoes as intermediate hosts of filarial worms, it has been shown that the microfilariæ are not able to develop equally well in all mosquitoes. In the work of Bahr (1912) in the Fiji Islands, for example, he found that when microfilariæ were taken in by *Aëdes (Stegomyia) variegatus* they developed rapidly, and practically all of them reached maturity and migrated into the proboscis. In *Culex fatigans,* development was slower and only two or three microfilariæ completed their development in each mosquito, while in *Culex annulirostris* and *Aëdes (Stegomyia) ægypti* the microfilariæ developed very slowly for a time and then degenerated in the thoracic muscles of the mosquito without ever attaining maturity.

Although *Culex fatigans* and *Aëdes variegatus* are probably the most important intermediate hosts of *W. bancrofti,* the development of the microfilariæ has been recorded in a number of other mosquitoes, and there must be many more species which are capable of acting as intermediate hosts, but have never been experimentally tested. The following is a list of species in which complete development or transmission of *W. bancrofti* has been observed:

> *Anopheles (Anopheles) algeriensis*
> *Anopheles (Anopheles) hyrcanus*
> *Anopheles (Nyssorhynchus) albitarsis*
> *Anopheles (Nyssorhynchus) tarsimaculatus*
> *Anopheles (Myzomyia) funestus*
> *Anopheles (Myzomyia) gambiæ*
> *Anopheles (Myzomyia) subpictus*
> *Mansonia annulata*
> *Mansonia longipalpis*
> *Aëdes (Stegomyia) ægypti*
> *Aëdes (Stegomyia) scutellaris*
> *Aëdes (Finlaya) koreicus*
> *Aëdes (Finlaya) togoi*
> *Culex (Culex) fatigans*

2. DIROFILARIA IMMITIS

Heartworm, an important disease of dogs in tropical and subtropical countries, is caused by a filarial worm, *Dirofilaria immitis,* with a life-cycle somewhat similar to that of *Wuchereria.* This worm is known to be transmitted by several species of *Anopheles, Aëdes,* and *Culex.* Instead of developing in the thoracic muscles of the mosquito, as with *Wuchereria, Dirofilaria immitis* migrates to the malpighian tubules and undergoes its development there.

VI. *Nuisance Mosquitoes*

Entirely aside from questions of disease transmission, mosquitoes play an important part as pests of man and animals. The more voracious species can make a region practically uninhabitable if present in sufficient numbers. The less severe biters contribute also to the discomfort, annoyance, and distress felt by the majority of people when they are attacked by them. Particularly in areas of large urban population, real estate values may be greatly reduced by the presence of these pests. However, with a great increase in travel by summer vacationists, this loss to real estate owners may now reach into any part of the country which is frequented by the vacationists. Agricultural regions may also suffer from the presence of mosquitoes in other ways. Many regions otherwise well suited to dairying are rendered unprofitable to dairy farmers by the attacks of mosquitoes upon the cows, with a consequent reduction in milk yield. In other places crops cannot be harvested because laborers refuse to work in the fields where mosquitoes are particularly abundant.

The salt-marsh mosquitoes are notorious as pests. *Aëdes sollicitans* and *Aëdes tæniorhynchus* breed in brackish waters along the Atlantic coast and may migrate inland as much as 40 miles. They are voracious biters, and a few dozen bites may cause nausea and acute discomfort in their victim. *Aëdes dorsalis* and *A. squamiger* are most troublesome on the Pacific coast, and *A. aldrichi* in British Columbia. Of the fresh-water breeders, *Aëdes vexans* is, perhaps, the most notorious and ubiquitous biter in the United States. No attempt will be made here to discuss the great number of other nuisance mosquitoes.

VII. *Biology and Control of Important Culicine Mosquitoes*

I. AËDES ÆGYPTI

Aëdes ægypti, often popularly referred to simply as the Stegomyia mosquito, is a small, dark mosquito with conspicuously white-banded legs and a pattern of narrow silvery lines somewhat resembling a lyre on the mesonotum (Figure 262). It is the only species of the subgenus *Stegomyia* which is found in America, but in Africa and the Orient there are many other species. It bites both at night and in the daytime, but avoids direct sunlight. It is often very annoying in houses and offices, where it hides under tables or desks and bites people on the ankles or the under sides of the wrists.

The yellow-fever mosquito is the most domestic mosquito known, and breeds almost exclusively in and near houses. It is supposed to have been a tree-hole breeder originally and is still sometimes found in such places, but more often occurs in roof-gutters, wells, tanks, jars and other receptacles in which clean water is stored. It does not usually breed in polluted water and never in ordinary ground pools. Like most tree-hole breeders, the yellow-fever mosquito usually lays her eggs not on the water surface but on the wall of the container, just above the water surface. The eggs are able to withstand drying for several months and hatch only after the water rises and submerges them, which assures the larvæ of a good supply of water at

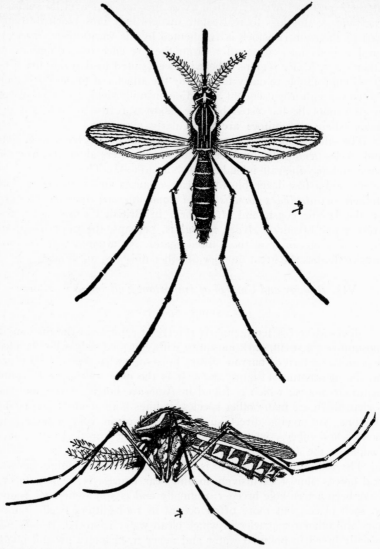

FIG. 262.—Dorsal and lateral views of the female yellow-fever mosquito, *Aëdes ægypti.*
(After Howard)

least when they begin their larval life. The larvæ (Figure 263) may
be distinguished from those of other American species of *Aëdes* by
the "sole-shaped" comb-scales, but are very difficult to differentiate

from larvæ of some of the other Old World species of the subgenus *Stegomyia.*

The larvæ are very shy, so that when they are resting at the surface of the water a passing shadow or a slight jar is sufficient to make them hastily retire to the bottom of the container, where they press themselves closely against the bottom or sides. This enables

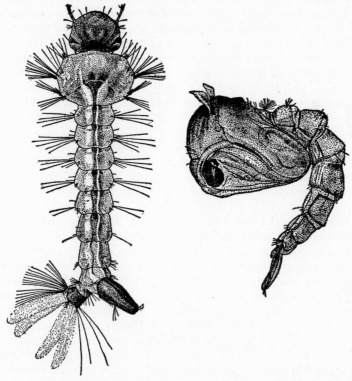

FIG. 263.—Larva and pupa of the yellow-fever mosquito, *Aëdes ægypti.* (After Howard)

them to breed in containers of drinking-water which are periodically emptied and refilled, since most of them escape being dipped or poured out because of this reaction. This habit also makes the detection of their presence by inspection more difficult.

In the tropics the yellow-fever mosquito continues to breed throughout the year. Since it breeds mainly in water stored for domestic uses, it is often found in abundance even in arid regions where most other mosquitoes are rare or absent. In the subtropics breeding occurs only in warm weather, and the species may survive the winter either as dry eggs or by means of hibernating females. The flight of the adult Stegomyia is not strong, and it probably rarely flies more than 100 yards from its breeding-place. They may be carried for long distances, however, on ships or trains.

Control. Since mosquitoes must become infected from yellow-fever patients and then must bite healthy persons in order to transmit the disease, it is obvious that careful screening of both patients and the general population is a measure of value. Since unfavorable breeding-places often produce a crop of very small yellow-fever mosquitoes, the mesh must be fine, not less than eighteen to the inch.

Fumigation of houses in or near which a case of yellow fever has developed, with the idea of destroying mosquitoes which have bitten the patient before they have time to become infective, has also been used and should, theoretically at least, be of value, because of the weak flight of this species.

As in the case of malaria, however, our main reliance on the control of yellow fever is placed in a campaign against the larvæ and breeding-places of the mosquito. This work must be carried on by a definite organization of laborers and inspectors who cover the entire city each week. All water containers near houses, whether natural or artificial, should be removed or destroyed. Tin cans, broken bottles and jars must be removed. Tree-holes should be filled up or the trees cut down. Roof-gutters may be entirely removed or repaired so that they drain completely. The greatest effort must be devoted to control of breeding in receptacles used for water-storage inside the houses. Large tanks, wells or cisterns can be covered or screened so that mosquitoes can neither get in nor out. Smaller containers can be emptied and dried in the sun once a week. In arid regions it may be necessary to strain the larvæ out of the water when containers are emptied, in order to save the water. Recently there has been a considerable use of fish control in tanks, cisterns, wells and even in jars and other small containers. Small fish which will eat mosquito larvæ under such conditions may be found in almost any region. Top-minnows are probably one of the best types, since they not only feed voraciously on the larvæ, but also their viviparous reproduction enables them to breed in tanks and cisterns. One great advantage of fish control is the fact that it makes the work of the inspectors much easier and more efficient. Inspectors can detect the presence of fish much more easily than the presence of larvæ, and are justified in assuming that if the fish are still present, larvæ are absent. Another advantage of fish control or the emptying of containers instead of screening or destroying them is that it leaves these favored containers to act as "trap-breeding-places." It must be remembered, also, that the yellow-fever mosquito will breed in almost any sort of collection of reasonably clean water, so that vases of cut flowers, baptismal fonts, tins of water placed under table-legs to keep out ants, and other similar places must be carefully watched, and emptied or oiled when it is necessary.

It is neither possible nor necessary, in practice, to exterminate the yellow-fever mosquito in any locality. What must be done is to reduce the numbers of mosquitoes to a point where they can no longer carry the disease effectively. It is usually considered that reduction is sufficient when the "Stegomyia index" (the percentage of houses examined in which breeding is found) is reduced to about 1 per cent. This strict control work must be continued for twelve months after the discovery of the last case of yellow fever.

The successful transference of the virus of yellow fever to monkeys and the production of a neurotropic strain in mice has made possible, through mouse protection tests, much more accurate mapping of the distribution of endemic areas of the disease. These studies have yielded hitherto unsuspected results, including a much wider distribution of the disease in Africa and the existence in Brazil of rural yellow fever without *Aëdes ægypti,* and jungle yellow fever, a disease which may possibly exist as an epizoötic in some animal reservoir and only occasionally be transferred to man. (Soper *et al.,* 1933, Soper, 1935). These findings have caused public health workers to resolve their old hope for the extermination of yellow fever into a more modest desire to understand it sufficiently to keep it under control.

2. CULEX FATIGANS AND OTHER VECTORS OF FILARIASIS

Control of *Wuchereria bancrofti* is to be based, evidently, on the control of the mosquito intermediate host, and the same general principles already brought out in regard to the control of malarial and yellow fever mosquitoes will apply. In any given region the principal mosquito vector or vectors must be determined and their habits and breeding places studied before efficient control work can be undertaken. Where the domestic species of *Culex* are the main carriers, control would be much like yellow fever control, but with special attention to breeding-places containing polluted or foul water. In the Oceanic Islands, on the other hand, where *Aëdes variegatus* is the most important vector, attention must be centered on coconut shells, cacao pods, natural and artificial cavities in trees and artificial containers with clean water. On theoretical grounds, it ought to be possible to bring about control of filariasis by a much smaller reduction in the mosquito population than is necessary for the control of malaria and yellow fever. Not only is there no multiplication of the worms within the mosquito, but the presence of a large number of the former is detrimental or even fatal, to the mosquito. This fact in itself probably accounts for the endemic character of the infection.

3. NUISANCE MOSQUITOES

It is difficult to formulate any general rules for the control of the many species of nuisance mosquitoes not discussed under the above headings. The methods used against vectors of malaria and yellow fever will often be applicable, to a certain extent, to the nuisance mosquitoes. However, it is more likely that the latter will present new problems in control which will need to be solved through a study of the habits of the species in question.

CHAPTER XL

OTHER BLOOD-SUCKING NEMATOCERA (FAMILIES CERATOPOGONIDÆ, PSYCHODIDÆ, SIMULIIDÆ)

Besides the CULICIDÆ, three other families of the NEMATOCERA include species which feed on vertebrate blood. These forms are all considerably smaller than mosquitoes and are often lumped together by those whom they annoy under the general name of "sand-flies." All three groups include species which are vicious biters and often extremely troublesome. Species belonging to all of the groups have been definitely implicated in the transmission of human diseases.

Family CERATOPOGONIDÆ ("punkies" or "sand-flies"). This family was formerly considered a subfamily of the CHIRONOMIDÆ but was raised to familial status by Malloch (1917), a change with which Edwards (1926) concurred. The adults of the two families may be separated on the following differences:

I. *Ceratopogonidæ*

	CERATOPOGONIDÆ	CHIRONOMIDÆ
Head:	rounded behind.	flattened behind
Mouthparts:	complete; mandibles usually well developed in both sexes and toothed; 2nd segment of palpus with sensory organ.	reduced; mandibles absent in both sexes; blade of maxilla wanting; 2nd segment of palpus without sensory organ.
Media (of wing):	forked (except in *Leptoconops* and *Brachypogon*).	always simple.
Thorax:	with few exceptions not projecting over head; sternopleura not enlarged and not extending to tips of fore coxæ.	projecting over head; sternopleura enlarged, extending below tips of fore coxæ.
Wings:	almost invariably superimposed over back during rest.	never superimposed over back during rest.

Only three of the fairly numerous genera comprising this family are known to bite man or domestic animals: *Lasiohelea, Leptoconops* (including *Acanthoconops*), and *Culicoides.*

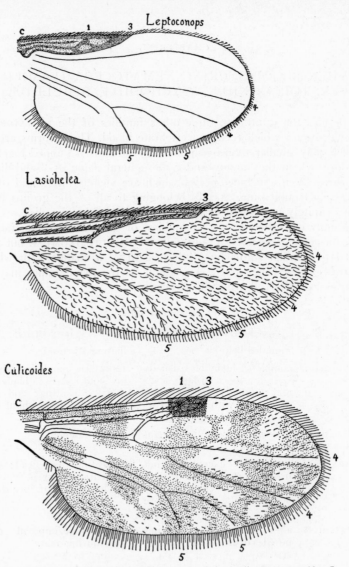

FIG. 264.—Wings of the three blood-sucking genera of the family Ceratopogonidæ. C., costa; 1, first vein; 3, third vein; 4, 4, fourth vein; 5, 5, fifth vein. (Original. Root)

The following key will enable one to identify these blood-sucking genera and also a few of the commoner non-blood-sucking genera with certainty.

KEY TO THE GENERA OF CERATOPOGONIDÆ *

1. Empodium as long as claws 2
   Empodium very short or absent 3
2. Costa extending to about middle of wing; wings with dense macrotrichia all over (*Euforcipomyia* Malloch, *Lasiohelea* Kieffer) (3) ....*Forcipomyia* Meigen.
   Costa extending well beyond middle of wing; macrotrichia sparser, sometimes absent (4) ....*Atrichopogon* Kieffer.
3. Cross-vein (anterior or radio-median) absent; a fold looking like a simple vein between third and fourth veins; first and third veins indistinct, more or less fused. (*Tersesthes* Townsend) .... *Leptoconops* Skuse.
   Cross-vein absent; no vein-like fold between third and fourth veins 4
4. Costa extending to about middle of wing; second radial cell short and square-ended, first radial cell obliterated; macrotrichia usually dense (*Pseudoculicoides* Malloch, *Isoecacta* Garrett) (5) ....*Alluaudomyia* Kieffer.
   Costa extending well beyond middle of wing; radial cells usually otherwise 5
5. Humeral pits present and conspicuous; microtrichia of wings distinct; claws of female small and equal; at least some macrotrichia present. (*Æcacta* Poey) (9, 10)..*Culicoides* Latreille.
   Humeral pits absent or else microtrichia absent or else claws of female very unequal 6
6. The two radial cells small and equal or one or both of them obliterated; wings finely punctate but without distinct microtrichia; legs not thickened 7
   Either second radial cell much longer than broad or else wings with distinct microtrichia or else legs modified 8
7. Wings with at least one dark spot and with some macrotrichia; female claws unequal (*Neoceratopogon* Malloch) ....*Alluaudomyia* Kieffer.
   Wings whitish, without dark markings, and without macrotrichia; female claws equal (8) ....*Ceratopogon* Meigen.
8. Hind femora noticeably thicker than the others 9
   Hind femora not thickened 10
9. Hind femora much thickened and spinose beneath; hind tibiæ not thickened (*Ceratolophus* Kieffer) (1).*Serromyia* Meigen.
   Hind femora not spinose; both hind femora and hind tibiæ moderately thickened (7) ....*Monohelea* Kieffer.
10. First and third veins connected by a cross-vein, 2 radial cells 11
    First and third veins not connected, one long radial cell 15
11. Front femora spinose beneath 12
    Front femora not spinose beneath 13

* Slightly modified from Curran (1934).

12. Front femora conspicuously swollen ....*Heteromyia* Say.
  Front femora not conspicuously swollen ....*Palpomyia* Meigen.
13. The branches of the fourth vein petiolate basally (*Hartomyia* Malloch) ....*Stilobezzia* Kieffer.
  The branches of the fourth vein arise at or before the cross-vein 14
14. Last segment of front tarsi much swollen (2).*Clinohelea* Kieffer.
  Last segment of front tarsi not swollen (6)
  ....*Johannsenomyia* Malloch.
15. Branches of fourth vein petiolate basally 16
  Branches of fourth vein arise at or before the cross-vein 17
16. At least one pair of femora with spines beneath
  .... *Pseudobezzia* Malloch.
  Femora without spines beneath ....*Parabezzia* Malloch.
17. Posterior branch of the fourth vein elbowed basally in the female
  (12) .... *Stenoxemus* Coquillett.
  Posterior branch of fourth vein not elbowed 18
18. At least one pair of femora with spines beneath (11)
  ....*Bezzia* Kieffer.
  Femora without spines beneath ....*Probezzia* Kieffer.

I. BLOOD-SUCKING GENERA

Lasiohelea. Several species of this genus, chiefly tropical forms, are known for their biting propensity. Available evidence suggests that the majority probably feed from the veins of larger insects, as do a number of species of *Forcipomyia*. The larvæ are terrestrial, occurring in moist decomposing vegetable matter.

Leptoconops. The species of *Leptoconops* are uniformly colored with unspotted wings in which R_{2+3} (2nd longitudinal vein) cannot be recognized (see Figure 264). The majority are tropical or subtropical in distribution. All seem to be vicious biters. Very little is known of the early stages of *Leptoconops*. Painter reared *L. bequærti* in Honduras from wet sand above the tidal line. *L. torrens, L. carteri* (*torrens?*) and *L. americanus* occur in the Western States.

Culicoides. This genus includes several hundred described species, the majority of which appear to be vicious biters, and is by far the most important genus of the CERATOPOGONIDÆ from a parasitological standpoint. It is nearly world-wide in distribution, being a scourge to man even in Greenland. No species are known from Patagonia or New Zealand. Some species such as *C. obsoletus* (*sanguisuga*) are widely distributed both in Europe and North America. The genus is best characterized by the presence of inconspicuous humeral pits. These occur, though less conspicuously, in a few other genera but the latter can be differentiated by other salient characters from *Culicoides*. Several examples of parasitism of *Anopheles* mosquitoes by species of *Culicoides* are reported by Galliard and Gaschen (1937).

The immature stages are passed chiefly in aquatic environments such as tree-holes, water of bromeliaceous plants, bottoms of shallow water deposits, crab holes and algal growths. Some species possess considerable power of adaptation, for though normally aquatic they may occur in exposed vegetation which retains some moisture. Others occur in modified terrestrial habitats such as exuded tree sap and manure. Several live in brackish or salty water, *C. furens,* a notorious species of the Caribbean littoral, being an example. Their development is very slow, probably requiring from 6 to 12 months to be completed.

As a result of the biting habits of the above genera the development of many areas has been retarded, some regions have been almost deserted, and the inhabitants of others endure their misery as best they can. At times fever has been recorded in the wake of the attacks of numbers of these insects. These records have come from such widely separated areas as Japan, Mexico, the West Indies, and West Africa. Whether this effect is due to a specific etiological agent or the salivary secretion is not known.

Several species of *Culicoides* have been demonstrated as intermediate hosts of Filaroidea. In British Cameroon Sharp (1927) discovered the development of *Acanthocheilonema perstans* in *Culicoides austeni. C. grahami* may also serve as host to this nematode. The development of *Mansonella ozzardi* has been recorded as occurring in *C. furens* on the island of St. Vincent, British West Indies. The various stages of *Onchocerca cervicalis* of the horse in England have been traced in *C. nubeculosus.* Unidentified microfilariæ have been found in *Leptoconops mediterraneus,* a North African form. Dampf (1936) recovered developing microfilariæ from a number of examples of an undescribed *Culicoides* in the region of Southwest Mexico where onchocerciasis occurs. George has traced the development of *Tetrapetalonema marmosetæ* in *Culicoides furens* in Panama. This species is a parasite of the marmoset and the yellow titi.

2. CONTROL

Any attempt at control of *Culicoides* or other CERATOPOGONIDÆ requires consideration of the type of habitat utilized by the immature stages of the species concerned. The life histories and biological requirements of most of the important species have not yet been worked out. Encouraging results have been obtained by the Bureau of Entomology of the United States Department of Agriculture, in the states bordering the Gulf of Mexico by the use of tide gates across small streams near which the sand flies are breeding. These gates are constructed so as to permit fresh water streams to flow during low tide, but to close automatically during the rise of tidal waters. They have also found that a mixture of 1 part of crude carbolic acid to 90 parts of creosoted pine sap is effective in dilutions up to 10,000 in salt water against larvæ of sand-flies when it is sprayed upon the soil near the edges of the water in regions where salt marsh sand-flies are breeding. In some instances filling in of water deposits eliminates local breeding areas. Such an operation in the case of two brackish ponds adjacent to one of the most beautiful beaches in the West Indies could change it from a deserted shore to a resort of considerable usefulness. The use of traps consisting of electric lights and exposed metal carrying a current of electricity may aid in reducing the numbers of biting gnats attracted to individual dwellings, since a number of species of the group are attracted to light. Just as in the case of control of mosquitoes, it is likely that proper control of sand flies will depend upon the careful study of the species involved and the special requirements of the locality.

II. *Psychodidæ*

Family PSYCHODIDÆ ("moth-flies") genus *Phlebotomus* ("sand-flies"). The family PSYCHODIDÆ contains a number of genera, some of which, *Psychoda,* for example, include a very large number of species from all parts of the world. In the United States one form, *Psychoda alternata* Say, has come into considerable prominence because of the tremendous numbers of this species which often breed in sprinkling filter beds used for the purification of sewage.

In this family the wing-veins are thickly fringed with long hairs and the body and legs are covered with hairs or scales. The wings have six or sometimes seven longitudinal veins, of which the second is usually three-branched and the fourth forked. Cross-veins are present only at the extreme base of the wing. The only blood-sucking genus is *Phlebotomus,* which may be distinguished from the other genera by the fact that the first forking of the second vein is near the middle of the wing instead of near the base (see Figure 265). The anterior one of the two branches formed by this first bifurcation forks again before reaching the wing margin. The species of *Phlebotomus* also have longer and more slender bodies, wings and legs than the typical Psychodids, and usually hold their wings flat together and erect in repose, while the more typical members of the family hold them roof-like over the abdomen.

I. PHLEBOTOMUS

This genus includes a considerable number of species, found in all of the warmer parts of the world. All the species are of small size and some of them are the most minute blood-sucking Diptera known. Identification of the males of the different species depends very largely on the hypopygia, especially on the number and arrangement

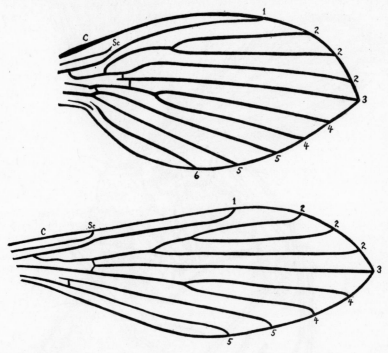

Fig. 265.—Wing venation of *Psychoda* (above) and *Phlebotomus* (below). C, costa; Sc, subcosta; 1, first vein, 2, 2, 2, second vein; 3, third vein; 4, 4, fourth vein; 5, 5, fifth vein; 6, sixth vein. (Original. Root)

of the strong spines on the terminal segment of the most dorsal of the three pairs of clasper-like appendages. Females are identified by the following characters: the spermathecæ, and the armature of the buccal cavity and of the pharynx. In the sand-flies of the Western Hemisphere, examination of the buccal cavity is essential for specific determination. The relative lengths of palpal segments is a character of secondary importance.

The larvæ and pupæ of *Phlebotomus* are very minute and difficult

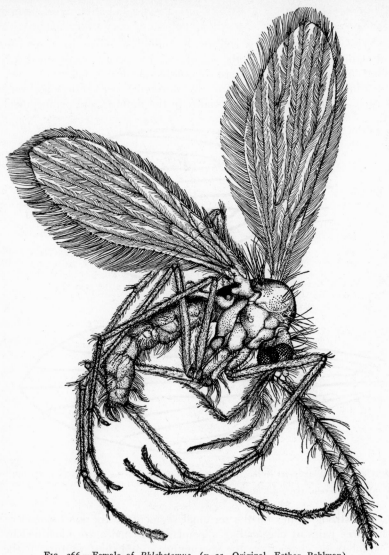

Fig. 266.—Female of *Phlebotomus*. (x 25. Original. Esther Bohlman)

to find. They occur in situations which have a solid substratum of stone, concrete or hard earth, which is kept dark and damp. Such places are the interior of stone walls or piles of rock, the walls of caves and cesspools or deep cracks in the earth. In attempting to locate the breeding-places of *Phlebotomus* it is not advisable to search for larvæ and pupæ. A better plan is to cover over a small portion of a suspected area with a cage of fine-meshed gauze or cloth and examine the cage each morning to see whether any adults have bred out.

The adults of *Phlebotomus* are so minute that they are able to pass through most screens and bed-nets without difficulty, but they cannot fly against even a light wind and ordinarily appear only on windless nights. Recent studies indicate that their range of flight is very limited indeed. Some authors believe that they never fly more than a few yards from their breeding-places.

2. PHLEBOTOMUS AS DISEASE-CARRIERS

Papataci fever (sand-fly fever, three-day fever) is transmitted by *P. papatasii* Scopoli and probably by other species as well. The disease is very much like dengue, but usually of shorter duration. The causative agent is a filter-passing organism. The disease is prevalent in the Mediterranean and Oriental regions and may be more widely· distributed.

Considerable controversy still exists over the relation of *Phlebotomus* to Oriental Sore and Kala Azar which are diseases caused by protozoa of the genus *Leishmania* (see Section I of this book). While the proof may not be as convincing as it is in the case of some other insects and disease the following statements seem to be fairly well proved. Oriental Sore in the Eastern Hemisphere is carried by *Phlebotomus sergenti* and *P. papatasii*, the former being the better carrier. Mediterranean visceral leishmaniasis is carried by *P. major* in Greece, and by *P. perniciosus* in Italy, Malta, France, Tunis, and Algeria. In India, Kala Azar is transmitted by *P. argentipes*, and in China by *P. chinensis*. The vectors of cutaneous leishmaniasis and of the newly discovered visceral leishmaniasis in South America have not yet been determined, although *P. intermedius* has been suspected of transmitting the former.

Harara is a skin disease caused by sand-flies and consists of an intense reaction in sensitive people to the bites of sand-flies of this genus.

There has also been much controversy over the nature of Carrion's disease and the possibility of its transmission by insects. By some it is considered that the Peruvian physician, Dr. Carrion, suffered from a combination of two diseases, Oroya fever and Verruga peruana. Others believe that these two names have been applied to manifestations of the same disease. There is some evidence to indicate that this disease-complex is transmitted by *Phlebotomus verrucarum*, but because of the controversy which still exists upon this point further work is needed before the question can be settled conclusively.

3. CONTROL

Although it is possible to avoid the bites of *Phlebotomus* by the use of very fine-meshed screens or bed-nets, electric fans and repel-

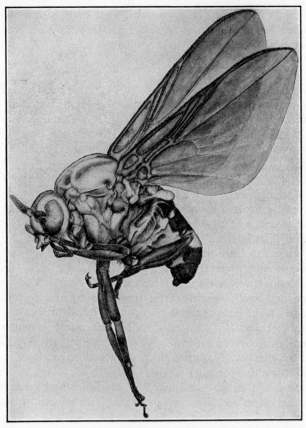

FIG. 267.—Female of *Simulium*. (x 16. Original. Esther Bohlman)

lent ointments, the destruction of breeding-places is probably the most satisfactory control measure. The area that must be controlled is comparatively small, due to the weak flight of these flies. Stone walls and the like may be faced with mortar or cement, earth-cracks filled and tamped and walls of cesspools periodically sprayed with kerosene or some other larvicide.

III. *Simuliidæ*

These flies are rather small and of robust build, with short, strong legs and short, broad wings. In the wings (Figure 269), the costa does not extend to the tip of the wing. The second and third veins may both be present, but usually are fused together to form a single vein. The costa, subcosta, first, second, and third veins and the base of the fourth vein are prominent and concentrated near the anterior margin of the wing. The other veins are weak and difficult to distinguish from the folds which are also present. The antennæ are short and bare; the compound eyes are separated in females but larger and meeting in the mid-line in males. The thoracic color pattern of males and females of the same species is often very different. The females often attack man and animals in swarms. Frequently the bite itself is entirely painless, but an itching ulcer-like sore appears later at the seat of each bite.

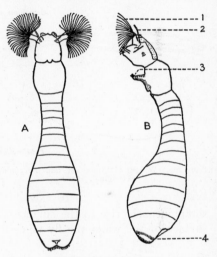

The larvæ and pupæ live in swift running streams, attached to leaves or stones. The larvæ are elongate and somewhat swollen posteriorly (Figure 268). They usually stand upright, attached to the substratum by a large sucker armed with rows of hooklets

Fig. 268.—Dorsal (A) and lateral (B) views of larva of *Simulium*. (Original. Huff)
1—Oral fans
2—Antenna
3—Proleg of thorax
4—Caudal sucker

which is at the extreme posterior end of the body. Ventrally, just behind the head is a short *proleg* tipped by a smaller sucker. The head bears, in addition to the usual mouth parts, a pair of large fan-like processes which bear a close resemblance in structure and function to the mouth brushes of mosquito larvæ.

The larva contains a pair of long silk glands, and is able to spin silken threads, which it uses in attaching itself during its larval life and out of which it constructs a *cocoon* shaped like a "wall-pocket," before pupation. The pupa is attached to the cocoon only by rows of hooklets on the abdominal segments, which become entangled in the threads of the cocoon. From the sides of the thorax of the pupa arise

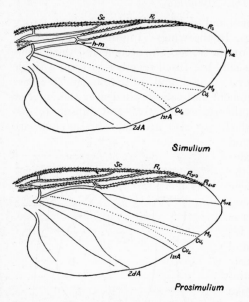

the long, chitinized respiratory filaments, each of which is usually branched. The number of branches and mode of branching of these filaments is usually characteristically different in different species.

The i m a g o emerges from the pupal case in a manner which reflects a nice adaptation to the conditions of rapidly running water. Just previous to emergence t h e r e is an accumulation of gas inside the pupal case. As the volume of this gas increases, the pupal skin is split in the dorsal thoracic region and through the slit thus formed the fly and a bubble of gas emerge and simultaneously rise to the surface of the water. Upon reaching the surface of the water the fly takes flight immediately.

Fig. 269.—Wings of *Simulium* and *Prosimulium*. (Original. Root)

I. CLASSIFICATION

While many authors still consider that the family SIMULIIDÆ includes only the single genus *Simulium,* the revision of the North American SIMULIIDÆ by Dyar and Shannon (1927) recognizes the four genera mentioned in the following key, adapted from their paper.

KEY TO THE NORTH AMERICAN GENERA OF SIMULIIDÆ

1. First vein hairy dorsally throughout its length   2
   First vein hairy dorsally at base and tip, but bare between humeral cross-vein and cross-vein connecting the third and fourth veins ....*Simulium.*
2. First vein joining costa at middle of the length of the latter
   ....*Parasimulium.*

First vein joining costa near its tip 3
3. Both second and third veins present ....*Prosimulium.*
Second and third veins fused into one ....*Eusimulium.*

2. SIMULIIDÆ AS DISEASE-CARRIERS

Black flies have been known and dreaded for many years because of the effects of their bites. It is said that during the American Civil War cattle, horses, and mules died in large numbers as the result of their attacks. Large outbreaks of these flies still occur in the lower Mississippi valley and bring about through their bites the loss of considerable numbers of farm animals, particularly mules. In one famous outbreak in 1923 in Roumania it is said that over 16,000 domestic animals died as the result of the bites of *Simulium reptans.* The mouth parts are in the form of a piercing stylet composed of a labrum-epipharynx, the hypopharynx and the mandibles, the latter being inserted between the first two parts. The bite is itself sometimes painless, but the injection of the salivary toxin at the time of the bite produces rather large lesions with exudate and extensive œdema. Some of the most attractive spots for vacationing are rendered uninhabitable by these flies during their season. Trout fishermen, particularly, suffer from their attacks because the larvæ breed in just the kind of streams in which trout are found.

Blacklock (1926) has shown that *S. damnosum* is the intermediate host of the *Onchocerca volvulus* of man in Africa (see Section II of this book). Three species of *Simulium* in Guatemala (*S. avidum, S. ochraceum,* and *S. mooseri*) have been shown to be concerned in the transmission of Central American onchocerciasis (Strong, Sandground, Bequaert, Ochoa, 1934).

O'Roke (1930) demonstrated that *Simulium venustum* transmits a disease of ducks caused by the protozoon *Leucocytozoon anatis.* The disease is highly fatal to ducklings and less so to adult ducks. A similar parasite of turkeys, *L. smithi* has been shown to be transmitted by *Simulium occidentale.*

CHAPTER XLI

SUBORDER ORTHORRHAPHA, SECTION BRACHYCERA, FAMILY TABANIDÆ

In contrast to the Section NEMATOCERA, most of whose members are small flies, the Section BRACHYCERA includes a number of families of comparatively large flies, many species being over an inch in length. The only family of medical importance is the family TABAN-IDÆ, whose species are commonly called "horse-flies," "deer-flies," "mangrove-flies" and "Seroots."

I. *Characteristics*

Some species of the family are as small as an ordinary house-fly, but the majority of them are larger, some much larger. The females of many species are vicious biters, but the males are incapable of biting, as is the case in blood-sucking NEMATOCERA. As a rule, it is only the smaller genera and species which attack human beings habitually. The larger forms usually obtain blood from the larger domestic and wild animals.

The head is large, usually as wide as the thorax, with very large compound eyes which meet in the mid-line in males but are separated in females. In life the eyes are often brilliantly colored or patterned, but these colors usually disappear completely in dried specimens. The antennæ are usually described as three-segmented, but the third joint is made up of a large basal portion and from three to seven smaller *annuli* or *rings* (Figure 270) which probably really represent antennal segments. The number of annuli of which the third segment is composed and the comparative lengths of the first and second segments are valuable in distinguishing the different genera. The *proboscis* or mouth part complex is usually rather short, but may be longer than the whole body in certain species.

The mouth parts of the larger species of the family are excellent objects for the study of the different portions of the piercing and sucking mechanism. The blade-like *mandibles* work like scissors in piercing the skin, and the protrusion and retraction of the rod-like, toothed *maxillæ* serve further to lacerate the tissues. The blood is sucked up through a tube formed by the apposition of the grooved *epipharynx* and the flat *hypopharynx,* within the latter of which the salivary duct may be seen. All these structures lie in the dorsal groove of the proboscis sheath or *labium,* which has at its tip a pair of large *labellæ* whose inner surfaces bear a system of *pseudo-tracheal tubules* for sucking up water and other liquids, similar to those which are found in the non-biting flies of the house-fly type. To the bases of the maxillæ are attached a pair of two-segmented *maxillary palpi.*

The wings have the same general type of venation as in the other members of the Section BRACHYCERA (Figure 271). They may be perfectly clear, entirely suffused with dark pigment, or else spotted or marbled with pigment to produce more or less definite patterns, which are sometimes characteristic of certain genera or species.

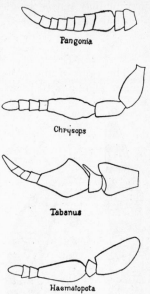

Pangonia

Chrysops

Tabanus

Haematopota

Fig. 270.—Antennæ of some common genera of Tabanidæ. (Original. Root)

The thorax and abdomen are stout and usually hairy, often black, brown or yellowish in color, sometimes with definite whitish or dark

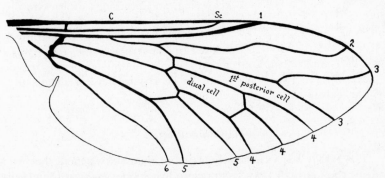

Fig. 271.—Wing venation of a Tabanid fly. C, costa; Sc, subcosta; 1 to 6, first to sixth veins. (Original. Root)

markings on the abdomen. The legs are strong and the *empodium* between the claws at their tips is a hairy pad like the pulvilli. There

may or may not be long, spine-like *spurs* at the tips of the tibiæ of
the hind legs.

II. *Life History*

The eggs of the TABANIDÆ are usually laid in large masses on
aquatic plants or rocks which overhang water. When the larvæ hatch
they drop into the water and soon bur-
row into the mud at the bottom. The
larvæ are elongate, tapering toward both
ends and usually have each of their segments more or less completely encircled
by a series of protuberances armed with
hooklets (Figure 272). They feed voraciously on all sorts of small, soft-bodied
insect larvæ and other similar organisms, and will destroy each other if two
larvæ are kept in the same receptacle.
Some may have as many as six moults.
As they grow older they wander into
drier and drier situations, finally pupating just below the surface of the ground,
often some distance away from the pond
or stream where they began their larval
life. The pupa is much like the chrysalis
of a butterfly, with a hard, chitinous
covering, and has rings of backwardly-
pointing spines on its abdominal segments. Development is comparatively
slow. In the tropics, the entire cycle
may be completed in four months or so, but in temperate regions
a year or even two years seems to be required. (For details of a
typical Tabanid life-cycle see Cameron, 1934.)

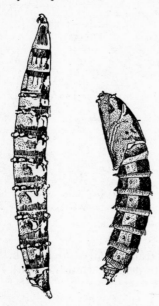

FIG. 272.—Larva and pupa of *Tabanus*. (After Neave)

III. *Classification*

The family TABANIDÆ includes more than sixty genera, but over
half of these include only from one to five species and are found only
in one particular part of the world. The following key, adapted from
a larger one given by Surcouf (1921), includes all the widely distributed and important genera, as well as some others which are often
met with in America.

KEY TO SOME OF THE GENERA OF THE FAMILY TABANIDÆ

1. Hind tibiæ without spurs; ocelli rudimentary or absent
.... (subfamily TABANINÆ) 2
Hind tibiæ with spurs; three ocelli usually present
.... (subfamily PANGONINÆ) 6
2. Third joint of antenna with a basal portion and three annuli
.... *Hæmatopota.*
Third joint of antenna with a basal portion and four annuli.... 3
3. Basal portion of third antennal joint with a dorsal tooth or
process 4
Basal portion of third antennal joint without any dorsal projection 5
4. Basal portion of third antennal joint with a slender dorsal
process; body rather slender .... *Dichelacera.*
Basal portion of third antennal joint with a massive dorsal tooth;
body stout .... *Tabanus.*
5. Thorax and abdomen dark, with iridescent green tomentum
.... *Lepidoselaga.*
Thorax and abdomen yellowish, without any green tomentum
.... *Diachlorus.*
6. Third joint of antenna with a long basal portion and four annuli 7
Third joint of antenna with a short basal portion and seven
annuli 8
7. First and second joints of antenna both long and of about equal
length .... *Chrysops.*
Second joint of antenna short, about half as long as first joint
.... *Silvius.*
8. Upper corner of eye acutely angled in female.......... *Goniops.*
Upper corner of eye not acutely angled in female 9
9. Proboscis not longer than palpi .... *Apatolestes.*
Proboscis longer than palpi, often much longer 10
10. Tips of second branch of third vein and first branch of fourth
vein fused together for a short distance
.... *Pangonia, Esenbeckia, Erephopsis,* etc.
Tips of these veins not fused together 11
11. Eyes hairy .... *Diatomineura.*
Eyes bare .... *Corizoneura.*

IV. *Notes on Some Genera of Tabanidæ*

Although the large genus *Hæmatopota* has a world-wide distribution, species and individuals are most numerous in Africa and the
Orient, less so in Europe and comparatively rare in America. The
species are fairly large and usually have the wings delicately mottled
with gray.

Tabanus is the largest genus of the family, including over a thousand species, occurring in every part of the world. It includes some
small species which attack man, but most of the species are large and

feed mainly on domestic animals. The wings are most often clear, but many species show a small amount of dark spotting and a few have the wings mostly or entirely dark.

Two smaller genera, *Diachlorus* and *Dichelacera,* are almost entirely confined to the American tropics. Both have a generally yellowish or brownish coloration. In *Diachlorus* the wings are mainly clear, with indistinct infuscated areas along the anterior margin and at the tip. The species are small and often attack man. In *Dichelacera,* the species average somewhat larger and the wings are usually extensively mottled with brown and yellow.

Lepidoselaga is a small genus (four species) found in tropical America. The species are very small and frequently bite man. The wings are mainly dark on their basal two-thirds, with the terminal third clear.

Chrysops is a large genus, found all over the world, the species being particularly numerous in temperate as well as tropical America. The species are all fairly small. Usually the wings are clear, with a narrow dark area along the anterior margin and a broad dark bar across the wing at the level of the discal cell or just beyond it. The tip of the wing may be clear or more or less completely dark. These "deer-flies" bite man readily and have been shown to be the vectors of two human diseases.

The genus, *Silvius,* is smaller but very widely distributed. Species are particularly numerous in the Australian region. Many of them have a superficial resemblance to the smaller species of *Tabanus.*

The genera *Pangonia* and *Corizoneura* have a world-wide distribution, while *Esenbeckia* is found only in South America and *Erephopsis* and *Diatomineura* occur mainly in South America and Australia. All these species are of fairly large size and have unusually long proboscides. In many species the proboscis is longer than the body. It has sometimes been stated that these "long-beaked" Tabanids bite while hovering on the wing, but this is probably erroneous. Several species have been observed to settle on the bodies of domestic animals and insert the long proboscis into the skin at an acute angle. The wings may be clear but are often somewhat infuscated throughout their extent.

V. *Tabanids as Disease-Carriers*

I. LOAIASIS

The filarial worm *Loa loa* is not infrequently found in man on the west coast of Africa. The adult parasite wanders about through the connective tissues and may produce "Calabar swellings" or cause trouble by entering the conjunctiva. The microfilariæ or embryos occur in the blood, as do those of *Wuchereria bancrofti,* but are present in the peripheral circulation only by day instead of only at night. Leiper (1912) and the Connals (1922) have shown that the microfilariæ develop normally in *Chrysops silacea* and *C. dimidiata,* undergo partial development in *Hæmatopota,* and do not develop at all in *Tabanus, Stomoxys* and *Glossina.* Apparently normal development of the microfilariæ of *Loa loa* has also been reported in *Chrysops centurionis.*

2. TULARÆMIA OR DEER-FLY FEVER

Tularæmia is a plague-like disease of rodents, caused by *Pasteurella tularense,* and readily transmissible to man. It was originally found affecting ground-squirrels in California and is apparently present among rabbits in many different parts of the United States. In laboratory experiments it is readily transmitted from one animal to another by various biting flies, lice, fleas, bedbugs and ticks. Human beings may become infected by skinning or handling infected rodents. In Utah and Idaho, Francis (1922) has shown that the disease is carried from jackrabbits to man by *Chrysops discalis.* Since the disease is so widely distributed among rabbits and is so easily transmissible to man (it is said that every one who has worked with the disease in the laboratory for any length of time has ultimately contracted it), it seems peculiar that more human cases are not reported.

3. DISEASES OF DOMESTIC ANIMALS

Since the larger Tabanid flies feed mainly on domestic animals, and are frequently shaken off by one animal and forced to complete their interrupted meal from another member of the herd, it is natural to find that they may transmit mechanically various diseases whose causative agents occur in the blood, such as anthrax and trypanosomiasis. Most of the cattle trypanosomes of tropical Africa are normally carried by tsetse flies (*Glossina*), but they are sometimes transmitted by Tabanids, especially in regions where the tsetse flies are not found. *Trypanosoma evansi* (causative agent of "Surra") seems to be ordinarily transmitted by Tabanids, and is found only in areas where *Glossina* is absent. It is not improbable that other trypanosome diseases of horses and cattle, which occur in tropical America and the Orient, are transmitted in a similar manner.

4. CONTROL

Nets, smudges and repellent dips or sprays have been used to protect domestic animals from the attacks of Tabanids and other biting flies, but no serious control of Tabanids seems to have been attempted. Portchinski pointed out that newly-emerged Tabanids promptly seek out certain pools for the purpose of drinking, and claimed that considerable numbers of the flies could be destroyed by oiling the surface of these pools with kerosene.

CHAPTER XLII

THE HIGHER DIPTERA; STRUCTURE, LIFE HISTORY AND CLASSIFICATION

The insects most commonly called "flies" belong, for the most part, to the Suborder CYCLORRHAPHA or Higher Diptera. They differ from the ORTHORRHAPHA (Lower Diptera) in that the larvæ do not possess a distinct head and in the method of emergence of the adult from the pupal case. The name Cyclorrhapha is derived from the fact that the adult emerges through a circular opening in the pupal case whereas the adult of Orthorrhaphous diptera emerges through a T-shaped opening.

This Suborder includes a large variety of flies, most of which are non-blood-sucking forms. Several of the groups into which it is divided may be discussed very briefly, while others are of considerable importance to the parasitologist.

While systematists usually divide this group of flies into the sections *Aschiza* and *Schizophora,* the characteristics upon which such a division is made are often difficult to distinguish in the adult. It is likewise true that further subdivisions of these flies according to their zoölogical relationships is often of less value to the parasitologist than the groupings which can be made on basis of their similarities in habits. There are wide differences of opinion amongst dipterologists even about the separation of families of these flies. Therefore, we shall employ here only those systematic groupings upon which there is a fair degree of agreement, and shall supplement this with groupings based upon biological similarities. Most of the higher diptera of interest to parasitology fall into two large Tribes, ACALYPTRATÆ and CALYPTRATÆ.

I. *Tribe Acalyptratæ*

The Acalyptrate muscoid flies, as they are often called, have the little *squamæ* or calyptræ at the bases of the wings very small and almost imperceptible. The subcosta is sometimes well developed, but often reduced or practically absent. The majority of the flies in this tribe are small, decidedly smaller than an ordinary house-fly.

Many of the flies of this tribe may be lumped together under the two categories of "dung-flies," which breed in fecal matter, and "fruit-flies," which breed in decaying fruit. A few genera of dung-flies, such as *Sepsis* (Family SEPSIDÆ) and *Borborus* (Family BORBORIDÆ) are sometimes found in houses. The fruit-flies of the genus *Drosophila* (Family DROSOPHILIDÆ) are often found about fruit, especially bananas, in stores and houses. Some species of this genus frequent fecal matter as well as fruit, and might perhaps carry intestinal diseases. The tiny "eye-flies" of the Family OSCINIDÆ are often extremely annoying because of their habit of crawling on the skin or darting into the eye in search of perspiration and other liquids. Their relations to transmission of disease will be discussed in Chapter XLIV.

II. *Tribe Calyptratæ*

The Calyptrate muscoid flies have well developed squamæ and the subcosta is never reduced. The majority of the species are about the size of the house-fly or larger. Many of the forms included in this tribe are of great parasitological importance and must be treated in more detail in the chapters to follow. They may affect the health of man and animals in three ways. First, there is a group of blood-sucking genera (Family MUSCIDÆ, *Stomoxys* group, and the Family HIPPOBOSCIDÆ, etc.) which includes the tsetse-flies, vectors of African sleeping sickness and the ectoparasitic flies commonly placed in the Section Pupipara. Second, there are many non-biting domestic flies (belonging to the Families MUSCIDÆ, ANTHOMYIDÆ, CALLIPHORIDÆ and SARCOPHAGIDÆ) which frequent both feces and human food, and may therefore carry intestinal diseases of many kinds. And, in the third place, there are many species whose larvæ either must or may live as parasites in the natural cavities or the tissues of men and animals, sometimes producing severe symptoms. This condition is called *myiasis*. In the Family ŒSTRIDÆ, the larvæ of all the species are parasitic, mainly in wild and domestic animals. Larvæ of various species belonging to the Families SARCOPHAGIDÆ, CALLIPHORIDÆ, MUSCIDÆ and ANTHOMYIDÆ have also been found in the bodies of man and animals.

I. STRUCTURE

The following discussion of the adult anatomy is by no means exhaustive, and is intended primarily to serve as a glossary of terms used in the keys.

1. The Head

The head bears the large *compound eyes* laterally, the three *ocelli* or simple eyes dorsally, the proboscis ventrally and the antennæ anteriorly. Various regions of the head, particularly on its anterior surface, have been given names, although they are not definitely delimited from each other (see Figure 273).

The dorsal region of the head, between the eyes, is called the *vertex* and bears two pairs of large *vertical bristles*. The *ocelli* lie in a triangular *ocellar plate,* from which arise the *ocellar bristles.* Anteriorly, the region between the eyes, extending from the ocellar plate above to the *frontal lunule,* just above the bases of the antennæ, is called the *frons* or *front.* It is subdivided into a central region, the *frontalia,* extending laterally almost to the *frontal bristles* and two narrow lateral regions, the *parafrontals,* between the frontalia and the eyes. The parafrontals bear the *fronto-orbital bristles.*

The rest of the anterior surface of the head, from the frontal lunule to the *oral margin,* that is, the edge of the opening through which the proboscis protrudes, is called the *face.* From the ends of the frontal lunule there extend downward and outward the *frontal sutures.* The whole arched scar formed by the frontal lunule and the frontal sutures is sometimes called the *ptilinal suture.* It is, of course, the scar left after the withdrawal within the head of the protrusible sac called the *ptilinum,* which the fly used in breaking its way out of the puparium. Within the area enclosed by the ptilinal suture are the *antennal grooves,* in which the antennæ lie. Between the antennal grooves and the suture there is, on either side, a well-

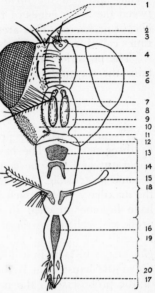

Fig. 273.—Front view of head of freshly emerged muscoid fly (*Calliphora erythrocephala*). (Redrawn, from Graham-Smith, 1930)

1—Verticals
2—Fronto-orbital
3—Ocellar
4—Compound eye
5—Frontal
6—Lower fronto-orbital
7—Arista
8—Antenna
9—Facial plate
10—Gena (cheek)
11—Vibrissa
12—Epistome
13—Trapezoidal plate
14—Anterior arch of fulcrum
15—Maxillary palp
16—Labrum-epipharynx
17—Lateral fold
18—Rostrum
19—Haustellum
20—Oral disc

developed *facial ridge,* bearing the *facial bristles.* At their lower ends the facial ridges bend inwardly to form the *vibrissal angles* from which arise a pair of very strong bristles, the *vibrissæ.* The narrow regions between the eyes and the frontal sutures are called the *para-facials* and bear the *facio-orbital bristles.* Ventrally, the regions between the lower edges of the eyes and the oral margin are called the *cheeks* or *buccas.* This area is often hairy and these hairs are sometimes called, collectively, the *beard.*

The posterior surface of the head is called the *occiput* and contains the *occipital foramen* or neck opening.

2. The Proboscis

The mouth parts or proboscis of the muscoid flies are made up of three portions. The basal joint or *rostrum* contains the sucking apparatus and may be considered a portion of the head which has become protrusible. Although the *maxillæ* have entirely disappeared, the maxillary *palpi,* which in these flies consist of only a single joint, have become attached to the rostrum. The middle portion of the proboscis, called the *haustellum,* corresponds to the *labium* of the horse-fly, minus the labellæ but plus the *epipharynx* and *hypopharynx,* which lie in a dorsal groove and form a food-canal. At the tip of the haustellum is the *oral disc,* forming the terminal portion of the proboscis. In the non-blood-sucking forms the labellæ, when opened out, form a large, spongy mass whose heart-shaped terminal surface is covered with rows of *pseudo-tracheal tubules* into each of which liquid food may be sucked through a double row of tiny perforations. From the pseudo-tracheal tubules the food passes into larger collecting ducts which lead to the *mouth* or *stoma* in the center of the labellæ. Around the mouth lies a V-shaped *discal sclerite* from which arise a few small, weak *prestomal teeth.*

In the blood-sucking muscoid flies the labellæ become much smaller and the pseudo-tracheal tubules ultimately disappear, while the prestomal teeth become much stronger and more numerous, so that they are capable of scarifying and finally even of piercing the skin of man and animals. In these forms, also, the haustellum becomes more heavily chitinized and usually elongate and slender. What really amount to stages in the evolution of such a specialized proboscis as that of *Glossina* may be seen by studying first the proboscis of the house-fly, *Musca,* then that of the Oriental *Philæmatomyia,* and then that of our common biting stable-fly, *Stomoxys* (compare Figure 276).

3. The Antennæ

In all the muscoid flies, the antennæ are of essentially the same type, consisting of two short basal joints and an elongate third joint which bears a dorsal *arista* near its base. The differences between the antennæ of different groups are in minor details, especially in the vestiture of the arista, which may be *bare, pubescent* (covered with short hairs), *pectinate* (Figure 278) (with a single row of bristles dorsally), or *plumose* (Figure 247) (with rows of bristles both dorsally and ventrally).

4. The Thorax

As in all DIPTERA, the

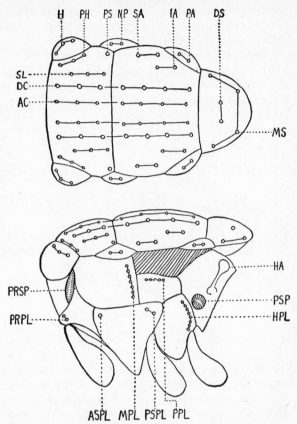

FIG. 274.—Dorsal (above) and lateral (below) views of the thorax of a Muscoid fly, to show the locations of the various bristles. AC, acrostichal row of bristles, divided into anterior (or pre-sutural) acrostichals and posterior (or post-sutural) acrostichals; ASPL, anterior sternopleural bristles; DC, dorsocentral row of bristles, divided into anterior (or pre-sutural) dorsocentrals and posterior (or post-sutural) dorsocentrals; DS, discal scutellar bristles; H, humeral bristles (on the humeral callus); HA, haltere; HPL, hypopleural bristles (on the hypopleura); IA, intra-alar bristles; MPL, mesopleural bristles (on the mesopleura); MS, marginal scutellar bristles; NP, notopleural bristles (on the notopleural callus); PA, post-alar bristles (on the post-alar callus); PH, post-humeral bristles; PPL, pteropleural bristles (on the pteropleura); PRPL, propleural bristles; PRSP, prothoracic spiracle; PS, pre-sutural bristle; PSP, postthoracic spiracle; PSPL, posterior sternopleural bristles; SA, supra-alar bristles; SL, sublateral row of bristles. (Original. Root)

mesothorax is greatly enlarged and makes up the greater part of the thorax. Dorsally a *transverse suture* separates the *prescutum* from the *scutum*. Posterior to the scutum is a smaller *scutellum*. On each

side of the *mesonotum* there are three indistinctly separated promi-
nences called the *humeral callus,* the *prealar callus* and the *postalar
callus* (see Figure 274).

Laterally, the thorax shows four main sclerites, the *mesopleura,
sternopleura, pteropleura* and *hypopleura.* The thoracic openings of
the respiratory system, the *prothoracic spiracle* (between the propleura and mesopleura) and the *post-thoracic spiracle* (posterior to

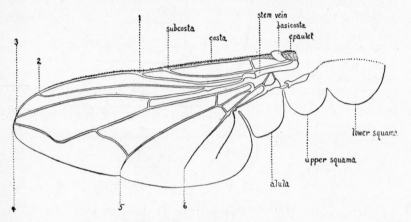

FIG. 275.—Wing of *Musca domestica.* (Original. Root)

the hypopleura) are also laterally situated. From the taxonomic
viewpoint, the greatest significance of these thoracic sclerites comes
from the use in classification of the number of bristles in the various
groups, which often bear the names of the sclerite or callus upon
which they are located. Figure 274 gives a diagrammatic representation of the thoracic sclerites and bristles of one of these flies, and
will serve much better than a description to indicate their positions.

5. The Wings

The wing venation of a muscoid fly is shown in Figure 275.
There is comparatively little variation in the venation of different
genera. The most important point to note, probably, is the form
of the tip of the first posterior cell which is determined by the
degree of curvature or angling of the terminal section of the fourth
vein. The presence or absence of a row of hairs on the base of the
first and third veins is also a valuable character. The base of the
first vein, from the base of the wing to about the level of the *humeral
cross-vein* (connecting costa and subcosta) is sometimes called the

stem vein. On the under side of the base of the wing may be seen a small, triangular *subcostal sclerite,* extending from the subepaulet to the first vein. At the base of the costa there are sometimes two little overlapping scale-like structures. The one nearer the body is called the *epaulet* and the other the *subepaulet* or *basicosta.* The color and vestiture of these little structures are sometimes important. If the wing is stretched forward to its full extent (as in Figure 275), one can see that its posterior border is continued basally beyond the wing proper in the form of three membranous lobes. The one nearest the wing is the largest and resembles the wing-membrane in appearance. It is called the *alula.* The other two are usually opaque, often whitish in color, and are called the *squamæ* or *calyptræ.* The upper *squama* (nearest to the alula) is usually smaller than the *lower squama.* When the wing is laid back along the abdomen, the upper squama is folded back so that it lies upside down just above the lower squama, the dorsal surfaces of both being in apposition with each other. The margins of the squamæ are usually hairy but the presence or absence of hairs on the upper or lower surfaces may be a characteristic of value.

6. The Abdomen

The number of visible segments in the abdomen varies considerably; often there are only four or five. In the females of some species, the ordinary house-fly for example, the four terminal abdominal segments form a long slender *pseudo-ovipositor,* and lie, telescoped together, inside of the abdomen and entirely out of sight except while the fly is depositing its eggs. In some other species no such structure is present. In male muscoid flies the terminal segments of the abdomen are modified to form the hypopygium, or external genitalia. The form of these structures is often of great importance for identification. In fact, in certain genera which include a very large number of similar species, *Sarcophaga* for example, it may be practically impossible to identify the species by any other characters. Those interested may consult Aldrich (1916) and Shannon (1923, 1924) for figures of male hypopygia and further details.

2. LIFE HISTORY

The majority of the muscoid flies lay eggs. In some few species or groups the eggs hatch within the body of the female and larvæ are deposited instead of eggs. Sometimes the larvæ do not increase in size while in the uterus of the female fly. In the genus *Sarcophaga,* for example, all the species which have been studied deposit a large number of first-stage or newly-hatched larvæ. In some other flies the larvæ undergo a certain amount of growth in the uterus. Some species deposit a small number of second-stage larvæ, and in the HIPPOBOSCIDÆ and *Glossina,* only a single larva develops at a time and it is retained within the body of the female fly until it has reached the third stage and is ready to pupate.

The larvæ of the muscoid flies (see Figure 284) are legless, worm-like "maggots," with very small and unchitinized heads. Normally the posterior end of the body is large and truncate while the anterior end is tapering. Each segment of the body may show *spinose areas,* which sometimes form a complete ring around the body. The second segment from the anterior end bears, in second-stage and third-stage larvæ, a pair of small hand-like *anterior spiracles.* The truncate posterior end of the larva bears the *anus,* with its *anal tubercles,* ventrally, and the pair of darkly-chitinized *posterior spiracles* dorsally. The posterior spiracles lie in an area called the *stigmal field,* which is sometimes depressed to form a slight pit or even invaginated, forming a pocket. When the stigmal field is depressed it is bounded by a ridge which usually bears several pairs of tubercles.

The larvæ of the muscoid flies nearly always live under conditions which surround them with a supply of food which they can obtain with very little effort on their own part. Many breed in masses of decaying plant or animal matter or in fecal material. Others have become adapted for a parasitic existence in the bodies of snails, insects or mammals. The various species of *Sarcophaga* show a particularly wide range in their choice of larval habitats.

In the case of the typical filth-breeding and carrion-breeding flies, which include all the common domestic species, the mature larvæ tend to migrate when they are full-fed, probably because the optimum conditions for their larval life are not suited to pupation and pupal existence. At any rate, when the larvæ are ready to pupate they tend to leave the manure or carrion in which they have been feeding and burrow into the earth or sand to pupate. As will be pointed out later, this habit must be taken into account in planning control measures for the domestic flies.

The pupa of the muscoid flies is of the *coarctate* type. That is, it has no heavy chitinous covering of its own, but is enveloped and protected by the last larval skin, contracted and hardened to form what we call a *puparium.* This puparium is usually elongate-ovoid in shape and yellow to dark brown or black in color. It is absolutely motionless, resembling a seed. Most of the larval structures, such as anterior and posterior spiracles, spinose areas and tubercles, can be seen more or less distinctly in the puparium. When the adult fly is ready to emerge, it breaks off a circular cap at the anterior end of the puparium by the repeated expansion and contraction of its *ptilinum* (see page 503).

3. CLASSIFICATION

In the key to the families of the DIPTERA (page 506) are given the diagnostic characteristics of the families MUSCIDÆ, ANTHOMYIDÆ, CALLIPHORIDÆ, SARCOPHAGIDÆ, TACHINIDÆ, DEXIIDÆ and ŒSTRIDÆ. But it should be emphasized that the dividing lines between these families are not always clearly marked, so that some genera have been shifted from one family to another and then back again, perhaps. An entirely satisfactory arrangement has not yet been reached.

In order to get a general view of the possible relationships of these Calyptrate muscoid flies, it is convenient to think of them as centering about the *Musca* group of the family MUSCIDÆ. From this group, which includes such genera as *Musca, Morellia, Cryptolucilia, Pyrellia* and *Myiospila,* we may think of the lines of evolution as radiating out in several directions. The most obvious connection is with the blood-sucking *Stomoxys* group, through the genus *Philæmatomyia.* This line may be considered as culminating in *Glossina* and the HIPPOBOSCIDÆ. In another direction, the genera of the *Muscina* group provide a transition to the ANTHOMYIDÆ. And, passing over to the CALLIPHORIDÆ, which until recently were considered to be a group of the family MUSCIDÆ, we find the genera of true blow-flies such as *Calliphora, Lucilia, Phormia* and *Cochliomyia* trending toward the SARCOPHAGIDÆ, while *Pollenia* shows some affinities with the TACHINIDÆ and DEXIIDÆ and the African *Cordylobia* and its allies resemble the ŒSTRIDÆ particularly in their larval structure and habits.

The key given earlier in this section (page 506) will serve for the allocation of specimens to families. The following keys to the genera of MUSCIDÆ, CALLIPHORIDÆ and ŒSTRIDÆ will aid in the identification of adults belonging to the more common and important genera. For the identification of genera and species of SARCOPHAGIDÆ, the student is referred to the monograph by Aldrich (1916). Keys to the species of North American CALLIPHORIDÆ are given by Shannon (1923, 1924) and will be found very useful for this region.

KEY TO IMPORTANT GENERA OF THE FAMILY MUSCIDÆ

1. Haustellum of proboscis long, slender, chitinized; labellæ small. 2
   Haustellum of proboscis shorter, stout, usually not well chitinized; labellæ large, with a well developed system of pseudo-
   tracheal tubules 8
2. Antennal arista with plumose bristles above; three sternopleural
   bristles present; base of fourth vein deeply curved..*Glossina.*
   Antennal arista with simple bristles above and sometimes below
   also; only one or two sternopleural bristles; base of fourth
   vein nearly straight 3
3. Antennal arista pectinate, with bristles above only 4
   Antennal arista plumose, with bristles both above and below... 6
4. Palpi much shorter than proboscis; bases of first and third veins
   hairy .... *Stomoxys.*
   Palpi as long as proboscis 5
5. First posterior cell narrowed at wing-margin; base of first vein
   bare; base of third vein hairy ....*Stygeromyia.*
   First posterior cell widely open; bases of first and third veins
   both bare .... *Hæmatobia.*
6. Bases of first and third veins hairy.*Lyperosiops* (*Bdellolarynx*).
   Bases of first and third veins bare 7
7. First posterior cell narrowed at wing-margin; palpi slightly
   spatulate ....*Hæmatobosca.*
   First posterior cell widely open; palpi strongly spatulate
   ....*Bdellolarynx.*
8. Antennal arista bare (*Synthesiomyia*) or pectinate (*Hemichlora*).
   Antennal arista plumose 9
9. Middle tibiæ with one or more prominent bristles on inner side
   beyond middle 15
   Middle tibiæ without prominent bristles on inner side beyond
   middle 10
10. Tip of fourth vein with a more or less rounded angle 11
    Tip of fourth vein gently curved 12
11. Haustellum of proboscis well chitinized; prestomal teeth rather
    large and prominent ....*Philæmatomyia.*
    Haustellum of proboscis weakly chitinized; prestomal teeth very
    small .... *Musca.*
12. Eyes hairy 13
    Eyes bare 14
13. Sternopleural bristles none in front, two behind....*Graphomyia.*
    Sternopleural bristles two in front and two behind....*Myiospila.*
14. One or more pairs of anterior acrostichal bristles and bristles on
    outer side of hind tibia present ....*Muscina.*
    Anterior acrostichal bristles and bristles on outer side of hind
    tibia absent ....*Morellia.*
15. First vein extending beyond the level of the cross-vein connect-
    ing the fourth and fifth veins ....*Mesembrina.*
    First vein ending before the level of the cross-vein connecting
    the fourth and fifth veins 16

16. Sternopleural bristles one in front and two behind
    ....*Cryptolucilia.*
    Sternopleural bristles one in front and three behind....*Pyrellia.*

KEY TO IMPORTANT GENERA OF THE FAMILY CALLIPHORIDÆ

1. Eyes hairy ....*Somalia, Neocalliphora, Tyreomma.*
   Eyes bare 2
2. Vibrissal angle well above oral margin 3
   Vibrissal angle at about same level as oral margin 7
3. Sternopleural bristles one in front and one behind 4
   Sternopleural bristles two in front and one behind 5
4. Body grayish, with yellow, woolly hairs among the bristles
   ....*Pollenia.*
   Body metallic, without yellow, woolly hairs........*Chrysomyia.*
5. Body metallic green or blue; parafacials hairy throughout...... 6
   Body black or dark metallic gray; parafacials bare or hairy
   only above ....*Neopollenia.*
6. Post-thoracic spiracle light colored; palpi large..*Compsomyiops.*
   Post-thoracic spiracle dark; palpi small...........*Cochliomyia.*
7. Species wholly metallic blackish, bluish or greenish in color..... 8
   Species brownish or yellowish in color...................... 13
8. Base of first vein hairy above; subcostal sclerite with small
   black bristles 9
   Base of first vein bare above; subcostal sclerite with minute
   hairs only 11
9. Disc of upper squama bare; anterior acrostichal bristles distinct 10
   Disc of upper squama thinly hairy; anterior acrostichal bristles
   not distinct; prothoracic spiracle black.........*Protophormia.*
10. Four intra-alar bristles; prothoracic spiracle dark or black
    .... *Protocalliphora.*
    Two intra-alar bristles; prothoracic spiracle light orange
    .... *Phormia.*
11. Upper side of lower squama bare ....*Lucilia.*
    Upper side of lower squama distinctly hairy 12
12. One sublateral bristle ....*Cynomyia.*
    Three sublateral bristles ....*Calliphora.*
13. Large robust flies; abdomen elongate; parafacials with several
    rows of hairs; abdomen with well developed bristles; eyes of
    males widely separated 14
    Not fitting the above description 15
14. Pteropleural bristles distinct ....*Auchmeromyia.*
    No pteropleural bristles ....*Bengalia.*
15. Parafacials with several rows of hairs..............*Cordylobia.*
    Parafacials bare ....*Mesembrinella,* etc.

KEY TO IMPORTANT GENERA OF THE FAMILY ŒSTRIDÆ

1. Fourth vein of wing straight, not extending to the margin of
   the wing ....*Gasterophilus.*
   Fourth vein of wing curved forward at tip, narrowing or closing the first posterior cell 2

2. Tips of third and fourth veins fused together, closing the first
   posterior cell .... *Œstrus.*
   Tips of third and fourth veins not fused, leaving the first posterior cell narrowly open 3
3. Antennal arista bare 4
   Antennal arista pectinate 5
4. Proboscis reduced; palpi absent .... *Hypoderma.*
   Proboscis well developed; palpi present .... *Bogeria.*
5. Tarsal joints of legs broad, flat and hairy; alula of wing large
   .... *Cuterebra.*
   Tarsal joints of legs slender, not very hairy; alula of wing
   moderate .... *Dermatobia.*

CHAPTER XLIII

BLOOD-SUCKING MUSCIDÆ AND HIPPOBOSCIDÆ

The blood-sucking genera of the family MUSCIDÆ form a compact group, beginning with the genus *Philæmatomyia,* which can hardly be distinguished from *Musca* and leading up to such specialized forms as the tsetse flies of the genus *Glossina,* which show many resemblances to the Pupiparous flies of the family HIPPOBOSCIDÆ.

The blood-sucking MUSCIDÆ are particularly characteristic of the Oriental and African regions, where a great variety of genera and species are to be found. Except for the genus *Glossina,* most of them breed in horse or cow dung and feed on animals much more often than on man. Two species of this group, *Stomoxys calcitrans* and *Hæmatobia irritans,* although probably originally Oriental, have become distributed all over the world, wherever domestic horses and cattle are present. These are the only common blood-sucking MUSCIDÆ of the Americas.

With the exception of the notorious tsetse flies of the genus *Glossina,* none of the blood-sucking MUSCIDÆ has been definitely incriminated as a vector of human disease. It is believed, however, that some of them do serve, at times, as vectors of certain parasites and diseases of domestic animals.

I. *Stomoxys calcitrans.* The Biting Stable-Fly

This species is of much the same size and general appearance as the ordinary house-fly (*Musca domestica*), but may readily be distinguished from it by its piercing proboscis (Figure 276) and curved (not angled) fourth vein. It is abundant nearly everywhere and bites man as well as animals freely. Its preferred breeding-place seems to be decaying vegetable matter, such as rotting hay or straw, but it will breed in stable manure if there is a decided admixture of straw or other bedding material. Severe outbreaks of this fly have usually been traced to the presence of large piles of rotting straw. Control, of course, centers on the destruction of such breeding-places by scattering or burning the straw. It is advisable, also, to take measures to prevent breeding in horse manure.

Although *Stomoxys* was once suggested as a possible carrier of pellagra (Jennings and King, 1913) and two cases are on record where poliomyelitis was transmitted from monkey to monkey by this fly (Rosenau and Brues, 1912, Anderson and Frost, 1912), the species is not believed at present to be concerned in the transmission

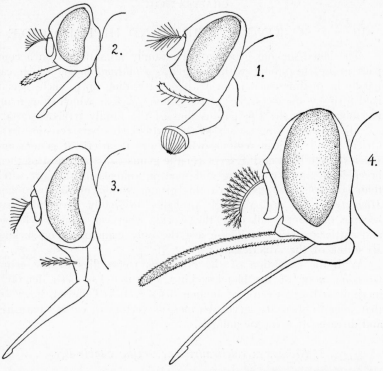

FIG. 276.—Profile views of the heads of some blood-sucking Muscoid flies. 1, *Philæmatomyia crassirostris;* 2, *Hæmatobia irritans;* 3, *Stomoxys calcitrans;* 4, *Glossina palpalis.* (Original. Root)

of any disease of human beings. As regards domestic animals, however, it has been shown to be capable of transmitting anthrax (Mitzmain, 1914) and infectious anemia of horses (Scott, 1922), so that it may be of considerable importance to the veterinary entomologist.

II. *Hæmatobia irritans.* The Horn-Fly

The horn-fly is only about half as large as a house-fly or stable-fly and also differs from the latter species by having the palpi longer

than the proboscis (Figure 276). It was introduced into the United
States at Philadelphia about 1885, and spread rapidly, so that in
1892 it was found all over the country east of the Rocky Mountains.
Two years later it reached California. This species feeds almost
exclusively on cattle and breeds only in cow manure. It is not known
to transmit disease.

III. *Genus Glossina. The Tsetse Flies*

The genus *Glossina* includes about twenty species, all inhabiting
tropical Africa, south of the Sahara, except that one species (*G.
tachinoides*), which has a wide range in Africa, is also found in
the southern tip of the Arabian peninsula. The important species of
the genus are not much larger than a house-fly, but some of the
rarer and less important ones are considerably larger. Flies of this

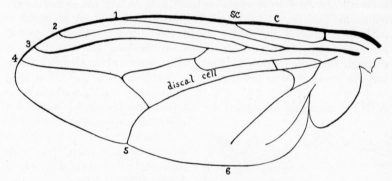

FIG. 277.—Wing venation of *Glossina*. (Original. Root)

genus may be easily identified by noting the slender proboscis with
its bulbous base and ensheathing palpi (Figure 276) ; the *branched*
dorsal bristles of the antennal arista (Figure 278) ; and the decided
curvature of the base of the fourth vein of the wing (Figure 277),
which makes the discal cell have a shape something like a butcher's
cleaver. The wings are long and in life are laid flat, one above the
other, when the fly is at rest. They project considerably beyond
the tip of the abdomen. The species are very similar to each other
and not easy to identify. For full details, consult the monographs
by Austen (1911) and Newstead (1924).

Several species of *Glossina,* particularly *G. morsitans* Westwood,
are known to be the usual vectors of Nagana and other trypanosome
diseases of domestic animals. *G. morsitans* and the closely related
G. swynnertoni are the vectors of Rhodesian sleeping sickness of

man (caused by *Trypanosoma rhodesiense*) and *G. palpalis* and perhaps *G. tachinoides* are vectors of Gambian sleeping sickness (caused by *Trypanosoma gambiense*).

Glossina palpalis is rather generally distributed in the wet jungle country of West and Central Africa, ranging from Senegal to Angola on the west coast and extending into the interior to Lake Victoria and Lake Albert. It is found only in the immediate neighborhood of water and where the undergrowth is dense. It seems to be especially abundant at fords and boat-landings or along native paths, where human blood is readily accessible. The female selects sandy beaches or loose soil for larviposition, places which have suitable soil and are densely shaded and near water being preferred. It bites by day, but not at night.

Glossina morsitans was the original tsetse fly and its bite was known to be fatal to domestic animals long before the causative trypanosome had been discovered. It inhabits the belt of savannah or park land around the edges of the wet jungles wherein *palpalis* flourishes. Its range extends south to Rhodesia and Zululand, up through the lake region to the Anglo-Egyptian Sudan and thence west to Senegal. It is not uniformly distributed, but occurs in localized areas, or "fly-belts," which expand and contract their limits with the changing seasons. Like *palpalis,* it bites by day but not at night. The females select loose soil under fallen trees or limbs which do not quite touch the ground as their favorite place of larviposition.

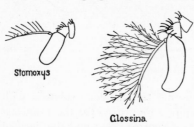

Stomoxys

Glossina.

Fig. 278.—Antennæ of *Stomoxys* and *Glossina*. (Original. Root)

The control of tsetse flies is particularly difficult because of their mode of reproduction. In other DIPTERA, the easiest method of control is to kill the larvæ or abolish the breeding-place. In the case of *Glossina,* the adult female carries the larva in her body, so that it cannot be reached. Measures for destroying adults have been tried. On the island of Principe (DaCosta, 1916) success was attained by the use of men carrying fly-paper on their backs, but elsewhere this method has not been successful. Specially trained "fly-boys" are able to catch large numbers of adults, but not, apparently, to exterminate the flies in this way. The question of whether it is possible to drive out the flies by destroying the game animals on which they feed is still a hotly-debated one. In the case of *G. palpalis,* local elimination of the fly is possible by clearing away the undergrowth which provides the dense shade that it seems to require. A promising line of investigation at present is the construction of artificial trap breeding-places, where pupæ can be regularly collected and destroyed, and the study of the effect of large-scale clearing and grass-burning operations on the distribution of the flies. But, in general, the control of *Glossina* is a problem that has not yet been satisfactorily solved.

In Zululand, South Africa, Harris (1931, 1932) has had astonishing success in trapping tsetse flies (*Glossina pallidipes*) by means of a trap of his own invention. The trap resembles a quadruped in bulk and shape, and its efficacy depends upon the visual impression made upon the fly. The flies attack on the lower side of the trap which is in shadow and thence fly upward into a cage above. Reduction in

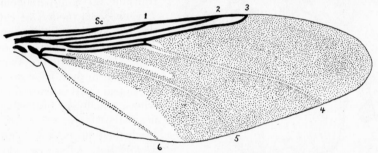

Fig. 279.—Wing of *Pseudolynchia*, illustrating the type of wing venation found in the family Hippoboscidæ. (Original. Root)

the fly population is shown by the fact that in September, 1931, 983 of these traps captured over two million tsetses, while in February, 1937, 6,525 traps captured only 1,296. Dr. Harris writes that "the scarcity of the tsetse today is proved by the fact that we now keep milch cows in safety without treatment where formerly a dog could not live a month."

IV. *Pupiparous Flies—Especially the Family Hippoboscidæ*

These flies are practically all ectoparasitic, in the adult stage, on birds and mammals. Two families (STREBLIDÆ and NYCTERIBIIDÆ) are exclusively parasitic on bats.

The "tick-flies" or "louse-flies" included in the family HIPPOBOSCIDÆ are parasitic on mammals and birds and have much the same method of reproduction as *Glossina*, producing only one larva at a time, and retaining it within the body of the female fly until it is ready to pupate. These flies rarely attack man but some of them act as vectors of blood-inhabiting protozoa of animals. A key to the genera of HIPPOBOSCIDÆ has been published by Aldrich (1923). Some of the more common genera and species are noted below.

The genus *Hippobosca* includes a number of Old World species with well-developed wings, all parasitic on mammals except *H.*

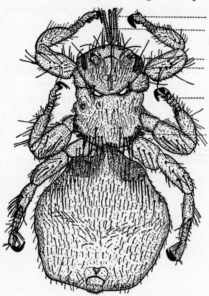

FIG. 280.—The sheep ked *Melophagus ovinus.*
(x 7. Original. Huff)

1—Maxillary palp	4—Compound eye
2—Proboscis	5—Tarsal claw
3—Antenna	6—Haltere

struthionis which is found on the ostrich. *H. equina* occurs on horses, *H. capensis* on dogs, *H. maculata* and *H. rufipes* on cattle, and *H. camelina* on camels. Theiler (1903) showed that *H. rufipes* and *H. maculata* could transmit the non-pathogenic *Trypanosoma theileri* of cattle. The species of the genus *Lipoptena* are parasitic on deer. Upon emergence from the puparia they have well-developed and functional wings, which are broken off near the body after they reach their hosts. The genus *Melophagus* (Figure 280) contains the entirely wingless form, *Melophagus ovinus,* parasitic on sheep. This common "sheep-tick" or "ked" is the vector of the non-pathogenic trypanosome of sheep, *Trypanosoma melophagium.* The genus *Pseudolynchia* (Figure 279) contains a number of species parasitic on birds. The winged *Pseudolynchia maura* and its varieties are found on nestling pigeons in the tropics and subtropics. It is the vector of "pigeon malaria" caused by species of *Hæmoproteus. H. columbæ* has been shown to be transmitted by *Pseudolynchia maura, P. brunnea, P. capensis,* and *Microlynchia pussilla. Hæmoproteus lophortyx* of the California Valley quail is also transmitted by *Lynchia hirsuta* (O'Roke, 1930) and *H. sacharovi* of mourning doves by *P. maura* (Huff, 1932).

CHAPTER XLIV

NON-BLOODSUCKING-FLIES CONCERNED IN THE TRANSMISSION OF DISEASE

I. *"Eye-flies" or Frit flies*

The small flies belonging to the family CHLOROPIDÆ (OSCINIDÆ) have attracted considerable attention because some of them attack the eyes of people and others swarm around open sores and in this way may be concerned in the transmission of disease. They are very small flies, found almost everywhere, and ordinarily live on plants. The forms which attack man have mouth-parts modified in such a way that the tips of the pseudo-tracheal rings of the labellæ act as cutting edges capable of injuring the epithelium of the conjunctiva or of cutting into granulation tissue of wounds. The Eye Gnat *Hippelates pusio* (Figure 283) occurs in great abundance in the Coachella Valley, California, where it is a vector of a catarrhal conjunctivitis or "pink eye" (Herms, 1926). Species of this genus are also thought to play some part in the spread of pink eye in Florida where they are found in abundance (Bengtson, 1933). In India, *Siphunculina funicola* is particularly abundant and attacks open sores, cuts, and the corners of the eyes of both man and animals. *Hippelates pallipes* has for some time been suspected of transmitting the spirochæte of yaws in the West Indies by attacking infected persons about the lesions caused by these spirochætes. Recently Kumm and Turner (1936) have succeeded in transmitting yaws from man to rabbits by means of this fly. While not much is known about the breeding habits of this group of flies, they apparently breed in decaying vegetable matter and feces, and their life-cycle requires from one to two weeks.

II. *Domestic Flies*

The domestic flies, particularly the common house-fly, *Musca domestica* Linn., are often accused of carrying the causative organisms of intestinal diseases, such as typhoid fever, Asiatic cholera, and dysentery, from human feces to human food. It is very difficult to determine how important such carriage is, although the possibility of its occurrence is undoubted.

In the case of typhoid fever, for example, the causative bacilli occur in the feces of typhoid patients or carriers. In order to cause new cases of the disease these bacilli must reach human food or drink and be swallowed by non-immune individuals. Most large epidemics of typhoid fever can be traced back to a polluted water or milk supply. In such cases, evidently, flies do not play an important rôle. Small outbreaks of typhoid fever can often be connected with the presence of a typhoid carrier. If the region is well sanitated and the carrier is a food-handler, it seems obvious that the disease has been spread by direct contamination of food. If sanitary conditions are not good, however, and no typhoid-carriers can be found among those in charge of the preparation of food, the fly-transmission theory becomes more probable. In the army camps during the Boer War and the Spanish-American War, when large bodies of men were assembled under poor sanitary conditions, it seems probable that flies had a considerable part in the carriage of typhoid fever.

The flies which may be of importance in such transmission of intestinal diseases are evidently those domestic species which feed extensively and indiscriminately on both human fecal material and human food. Their breeding-places are probably of little importance. The internal changes which take place during the pupal stage are so extensive that it is unlikely that many of the bacteria or other disease-producing organisms taken up by the larva are passed on to the adult fly. Such flies as the green-bottles (genus *Lucilia*) which breed in decaying meat, are probably just as dangerous in proportion to their numbers as is the house-fly (*Musca domestica*) which often breeds in human fecal material, since both of them, in the adult stage, visit both excrement and food materials for feeding purposes. Conversely, such flies as *Morellia micans* and certain species of *Sarcophaga,* which often breed in human excrement in large numbers, are of practically no importance, since they are rarely, if ever, found in houses or around human food.

From this viewpoint, the domestic species of *Musca* (which in America means the species *Musca domestica*) are by far the most dangerous forms, since they are the most abundant flies in kitchens and dining-rooms and are also very numerous about fecal matter. Other flies which have somewhat the same habits and are also dangerous when present in houses and about food include the non-biting stable-fly (*Muscina*) the lesser house-flies (*Fannia,* family ANTHO-MYIDÆ), certain of the flesh-flies (*Sarcophaga*) and a number of genera of the blow-flies (CALLIPHORIDÆ), particularly *Calliphora, Lucilia, Cochliomyia* and *Chrysomyia.*

The main diseases which these flies are accused of carrying include typhoid and paratyphoid fevers, cholera, dysentery (both bacillary and amœbic) and summer diarrhea. There have been a good many records of finding the eggs of various helminth parasites of man in the alimentary canal or fecal droplets of flies, but such findings are of little importance. The eggs of most human helminths must undergo a definite period of development outside the human body before they become infective, and the chance of their being deposited by the fly in a favorable environment for this development is extremely small. Flies might perhaps, however, function in the transmission of two helminth parasites; one of these, *Hymenolepis nana,* utilizes the same individual as both intermediate and final host; the other, *Echinococcus granulosus,* has the dog as its final host and may utilize man as an intermediate host.

Flies are also believed to play a part in the transmission of certain diseases whose causative organisms occur in discharges from the eyes or from open sores and wounds. The domestic species of *Musca* feed readily on such discharges and have been suspected of carrying ophthalmia in Egypt and Greece, and yaws (caused by *Treponema pertenue*) in the tropics. In Panama, Darling (1911) proved that a disease of horses and mules caused by *Trypanosoma hippicum* was being transmitted by *Musca domestica* in this manner. Certain nematodes responsible for "summer sores" in horses undergo their development in flies. *Habronema megastoma* and *H. muscæ* are two such parasites. The eggs of these worms are ingested by the fly larvæ which live in horse manure. The infection in the maggot is passed through the pupal stage to the adult and thence back to horses at the time the adult feeds upon the open sores of the horse. (See Section II.)

III. *The Control of Domestic Flies*

In attempting to control the domestic flies, especially the housefly, two points should be kept in mind. In the first place, it is much easier and better to eliminate the breeding-places or kill the larvæ than to attack the fly in its adult stage. Second, the domestic flies seem to have an innate tendency to wander about. At Miles City, Montana, Parker (1916) released over 300,000 marked flies and captured some of them two miles away a day later. In Texas, Bishop and Laake (1921) released 60,000 marked flies and caught one thirteen miles away after a few days. So fly control must be a community measure, not an individual matter. An individual can protect his house from flies fairly effectually by careful screening or continual trapping of adults, but in order to really get rid of flies the whole community must coöperate. A single neglected manure pile can produce flies enough for a whole village.

The favorite breeding-place of the house-fly is fresh horse manure, but it will also breed in excrement of almost any animals except cattle, and in garbage or decaying vegetable matter. The blow-flies breed mainly in decaying meat, either in garbage or in dead carcasses. To eliminate fly breeding-places, all such material should be buried, burned, enclosed or screened in such a way that flies cannot get at it to lay their eggs. Manure may also be rendered useless as a breeding-place for flies if it is spread on fields in a thin layer, so that it dries out quickly. If manure or garbage is removed periodically, it must be remembered that although, even in hot weather, it usually takes at least ten to twelve days for the fly to develop from egg to adult, the larva may reach the migratory stage and leave its breeding place in five or six days.

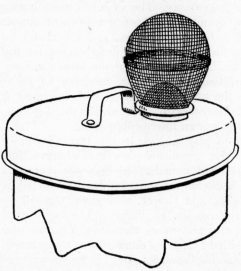

Fig. 281.—Top of garbage-can with small balloon fly-trap attached. (After Bishopp)

Many ingenious schemes have been devised to kill fly larvæ in manure before 'they are able to pupate. The most obvious measure, the use of chemicals which will kill the larvae, is not very satisfactory, most chemicals either injuring the fertilizing properties of the manure or else being too expensive for large-scale use. The United States Department of Agriculture recommends the use of 0.62 pound of borax or 0.75 pound crude calcium borate to each eight bushels of manure. In China, Woodworth (1924) has reported success in using sodium cyanide solution to kill fly larvæ in the "kongs" in which human manure is stored.

Several different "maggot traps" have been developed to catch and kill the larvæ during the migratory period. The manure is stored on an elevated platform or bin with a perforated floor and kept moist enough so that the larvæ will not pupate in it. They migrate downward when full-fed, pass through the perforated floor and drop into a concrete basin filled with water, where they drown. Other sanitarians have taken advantage of the fact that the heat of fermentation in a large manure pile is sufficient to kill any larvæ in its interior. Patton (1920) has adopted the plan of digging a hole in the center

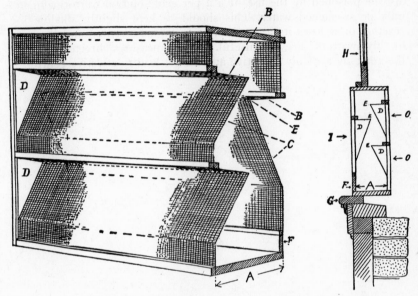

Fig. 282.—Hodge type window fly-trap. At left, trap with one end removed to show construction; at right, cross-section of trap in place in a window. (After Bishopp)

of the pile every day and shoveling into it all the superficial manure in which fly-breeding is going on. Others have suggested keeping in the heat of fermentation by packing a tight layer of earth over the manure pile or covering it with a tarpaulin.

Adult flies may be destroyed in large numbers by the use of fly-traps, sticky fly-paper and poison. The fly-traps (Figures 281 and 282) are of many different designs but all depend on the fact that although flies will crawl into a dark place in search of food or for the purpose of laying eggs, when they leave they always fly upward and toward the light, and the fact that when flies alight on a window-screen or other surface they crawl upward rather than down. Sticky fly-paper may be used in the usual sheets. It is said, however, that hanging wires or spirals smeared with the sticky mixture are more effective. A sticky mixture of this sort may be prepared by heating twenty pounds of clear resin in five quarts of castor oil and stirring until a clear solution is obtained.

When flies are troublesome in houses, they can be destroyed by a crude sort of fumigation, using the fumes of burning insect-powder, or by spraying one of the commercial preparations. They can also be poisoned by the use of a 2 per cent solution of formalin in milk or sweetened water. This should be kept slightly alkaline in reaction or it loses its attractiveness to flies. Screening and the use of "fly-swatters" are also useful. But all measures directed against the adult fly are only palliative and do not lead to effective control.

CHAPTER XLV

MYIASIS AND THE IDENTIFICATION OF FLY LARVÆ

I. *Myiasis*

Myiasis is the name applied to the diseases or symptoms produced by fly larvæ when they live parasitically in the bodies of man and other mammals. Clinically, myiases may be classified according to the part of the body invaded by the larvæ into:

Cutaneous myiasis—in which the larvæ live in or under the skin.
Intestinal myiasis—in which the larvæ are in the stomach or intestine.
Cavity and wound myiases—in which the larvæ invade natural (nasopharynx, frontal sinuses, vulva) or artificial (wound) cavities in the body.
Perhaps another category, that of external myiasis, should be added in order to include the case of blood-sucking maggots.

Although the larvæ of a great variety of flies have been reported as living parasitically in the human body, especially in the intestinal tract, the flies whose larvæ are of real importance in human and veterinary medicine belong very largely to the families ŒSTRIDÆ, CALLIPHORIDÆ and SARCOPHAGIDÆ.

A very satisfactory classification of the flies which produce myiasis has been made by Patton. It is based primarily upon the ovipositing habits of the female flies. It is in no sense a systematic classification.

GROUP I. SPECIFIC MYIASIS-PRODUCING DIPTERA (OBLIGATORY SARCOBIOTS)

These flies oviposit (or larviposit) in or near living tissues. They are further subdivided into:

Subgroup 1. The flies in this group are not attracted directly to the animals which are to serve as host for their larvæ but may larviposit in the places frequented by these hosts. The larvæ, therefore, have to penetrate the unbroken skin. *Cordylobia anthropoph-*

aga, the Thumbu Fly of Africa, is an example of this kind of fly. It is probably attracted to places frequented by rats by the feces of the latter, and larviposits on the moist soil. The first-stage larvæ then attack the rats, or quite often dogs or man. The presence of the larva in the skin of man leads to irritation and pain and the lesion may resemble a small boil. A very remarkable immunity to this parasite is established in experimentally infested rats as shown by Blacklock and Gordon (1927).

Instead of depositing larvæ in the environment of the animal to be parasitized, *Dermatobia hominis* lays its eggs on the body of some arthropod which visits animals or man. In tropical America, larvæ of *Dermatobia hominis* Linn. are not infrequently found in the skin of human beings, although they are much more abundant in cattle. The occurrence of these larvæ in their normal location in an un-usual host is bound up with the extremely interesting mode of oviposition of this species. Instead of laying her eggs on the body of the host of the larvæ, the female *Dermatobia* catches mosquitoes and other flies which visit cattle and lays her eggs in two packets on the sides of the abdomens of her captives. In Central America and northern South America, *Dermatobia* eggs are found almost ex-clusively on the mosquitoes, *Psorophora lutzii* and *Psorophora ferox,* but in Brazil they have been found both on these mosquitoes and also on the biting flies, *Stomoxys* and *Hæmatobia,* and even on non-biting flies such as *Musca domestica.* When the larvæ are ready to hatch from the egg, the body heat of a warm-blooded animal seems to stimulate them to leave the egg-shell and crawl onto the skin while their vector is feeding. They then burrow into the skin and form a swelling similar to those produced by *Hypoderma* larvæ. When full-grown they emerge and drop to the ground to pupate.

Certain blood-sucking larvæ belonging to the family CALLI-PHORIDÆ may also be included in this group although strictly speaking they do not produce myiasis. The larvæ of *Auchmeromyia luteola,* called the "Congo floor-maggots" are commonly found on the floor of native huts in Africa where they attack the natives at night and suck blood. The larvæ of *Protocalliphora* feed on nestling birds in America and Europe in the same manner, and are known to bring about the death of many nestling bluebirds, song sparrows, and other birds.

Subgroup 2. The female flies of this group are attracted to ani-mals by the odor of blood or of necrotic tissue. The eggs or larvæ are deposited in or near the wound or diseased tissue and the larvæ do not enter unbroken skin. Consequently they cause cutaneous, cavity, and wound myiases but are not involved in intestinal myiasis. Infection usually consists of the presence of many larvæ whereas the infections with maggots of Subgroup 1 are usually from single larvæ. The species of the genus *Wohlfahrtia* (family SARCOPHAGIDÆ) are examples of these flies. *W. magnifica* has been found breeding in wounds of animals and the nose, ears, and skin of man, in Europe and Africa. In America *Wohlfahrtia vigil* and *W. meigeni* have been bred from larvæ in the skin of infants and in rabbits. There is usually very considerable destruction of tissues by these larvæ unless they are promptly removed.

The larvæ of *Chrysomyia bezziana* (Old World Screw Worm) are important in the production of myiasis in animals in Africa and the Philippine Islands, and in India frequently attack man producing myiasis of wounds and sores in almost every part of the body.

Subgroup 3. Most of the bot and warble flies of animals fall into this group (family ŒSTRIDÆ). The female flies lay their eggs or larvæ on hair or other parts of the body of an animal and the larvæ then either attack the tissues directly or undergo a migration before reaching the tissue to be attacked. These larvæ can only live upon tissues of living animals.

The family ŒSTRIDÆ is a rather heterogeneous assemblage of genera, almost certainly of multiple origin, but until we know more about the relationships of the different forms it does not seem worth while to subdivide it. All the genera agree in having larvæ which can only live as parasites of mammals, and in having the mouth parts of the adult flies more or less reduced and rudimentary. The larvæ are found, for the most part, in three locations in their hosts, the stomach, the nasal passages or the skin. They are usually found in wild or domestic animals and only occasionally and accidentally in man.

Genera whose larvæ occur in the stomach. This group includes the common "stomach-bots" of horses. (*Gasterophilus*) and related forms from the rhinoceros (*Gyrostigma*) and elephant (*Cobboldia*). In *Gasterophilus* the eggs are laid attached to hairs on the horse. They hatch under the influence of friction and moisture when the horse is licking its own body or that of another horse and the larvæ cling to the tongue and are swallowed. They attach themselves to the stomach-wall and remain attached until full-grown, when they pass out with the excrement and pupate in the earth.

Genera whose larvæ occur in the nasal passages. This group includes a considerable number of genera. The best known are *Œstrus* from sheep and various antelopes and *Rhinœstrus,* species of which occur in horses, in the African river-hog and in the hippopotamus. Representatives of other genera are found in various African antelopes (*Kirkiœstrus, Gedœlstia*), camels (*Cephalopsis*) and deer (*Cephenomyia*). In *Œstrus* and *Rhinœstrus* the female flies deposit newly hatched larvæ in the nose of the host. The larvæ work their way into the sinuses where they become attached to the mucous membrane. When fully grown they make their way out of the nostrils and drop to the ground to pupate.

Genera whose larvæ occur in the skin. This group includes the "warbles" of cattle (*Hypoderma*) and of the reindeer (*Œdama-*

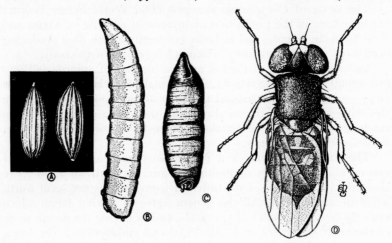

FIG. 283.—Stages of the eye gnat *Hippelates pusio* Loew. A, Eggs; B, Larva; C, Puparium; D, Adult. (After Hall, 1932)

gena), the "gusano del monte" of tropical America (*Dermatobia*), which occurs normally in cattle and not infrequently in man, and several genera (especially *Cuterebra* and *Bogeria*) whose larvæ usually occur in rodents and other small mammals. In *Hypoderma*, the eggs are laid on the skins of cattle, attached to the hairs. When the larvæ hatch it is thought that they burrow into the skin and migrate through the body for some time, later appearing on the back, where they produce subcutaneous swellings. When full-grown they emerge through a small opening which they have made in the skin and drop to the ground to pupate.

Except in the case of *Dermatobia,* human cases of myiasis due to Œstrid larvæ are comparatively rare. Cases in which young larvæ of *Hypoderma* and *Gasterophilus* have been found migrating under

the skin of human beings, producing one form of "creeping eruption," have been reported. In some parts of Europe females of
Rhinœstrus purpureus Brauer occasionally deposit their larvæ in the
nose or eyes of human beings. *Œstrus ovis* Linn. is said to have the
same habit in some parts of the world. The presence of these larvæ
in the eyes produces severe conjunctivitis and may cause the loss of
sight if the larvæ are not promptly removed.

GROUP II. SEMI-SPECIFIC MYIASIS-PRODUCING DIPTERA

The females of this group ordinarily oviposit on dead animals,
the larvæ feeding upon the decaying tissues of the carcasses and
being called Blow-flies (families CALLIPHORIDÆ and SARCOPHAGIDÆ).
The larvæ of many different blow-flies are occasionally found in the
neglected wounds of man and animals; there are some species whose
larvæ very frequently occur in such situations; and a very few in
which the parasitic habit of life has become essential. Myiases caused
by these larvæ are more dangerous to man than any other type and
are also very important in connection with domestic animals, particularly cattle, horses and sheep, because of the extensive tissue
destruction which results. Larvæ of *Calliphora, Cynomyia, Lucilia,
Phormia* and some species of *Chrysomyia* are occasionally found in
wounds, in the soiled wool of sheep, and so on. "Screw-worms," the
larvæ of *Cochliomyia macellaria* Linn., frequently infest the wounds
of animals and sometimes the nose of human beings in tropical and
sub-tropical America. This fly will still breed in decaying meat, but
the larvæ are frequently parasitic. Many species of the genus *Sarcophaga* breed in decaying meat and are occasionally found infesting
neglected wounds of man or animals.

GROUP III. ACCIDENTAL MYIASIS-PRODUCING DIPTERA

This group contains flies of widely different habits which normally oviposit in excrement or in vegetable matter but occasionally
are accidentally ingested by man. They may produce intestinal or
urinary myiasis. It is probable that most of the eggs or larvæ so
ingested are killed by the digestive juices and it is usually considered
that most intestinal myiases are transient and unimportant. In some
cases, however, there is good evidence that the presence of various
species of fly larvæ in the stomach or intestine has given definite
symptoms of irritation. Hall and Muir (1913) reported on a case of
gastric myiasis in a five-year-old boy caused by rat-tailed maggots,
Eristalis (SYRPHIDÆ). He had been suffering from indigestion,
vomiting, and chronic constipation for ten weeks before treatment.

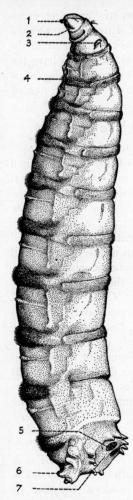

Fig. 284.—Mature larva of a muscoid fly. (Original. Esther Bohlman)

1—Head papillæ
2—Mouth hooks
3—Anterior spiracle
4—Ventral spinose area
5—Posterior spiracle
6—Anal tubercle
7—Stigmal plate

Numerous other cases of myiasis from syrphid larvæ are on record. A remarkable case has been noted by Patton and Evans (1929) in which larvæ of *Aphiochæta scalaris* (PHORIDÆ) were passed over an interval of a year by a European living in Burma. Other observations tend to support the view that this fly can in certain cases undergo its entire life cycle within the intestine of man. Meleney and Harwood (1935) have recorded a case of intestinal myiasis caused by larvæ of the Soldier-Fly, *Hermetia illucens* (STRATIOMYIDÆ). The Cheese-Skipper, *Piophila casei* is another fly frequently found in the human intestine.

II. *Identification of Fly Larvæ*

The identification of first and second stage larvæ of the muscoid flies is a matter of considerable difficulty, in most cases. This is in part because the young larvæ do not have such easily recognizable characteristics as the mature larvæ and in part because the young larvæ have not been sufficiently studied. The papers by Miss Tao (1927) and by Knipling (1936) may be consulted. In the third stage or mature larvæ, the most important structures can usually be made out fairly well if living or preserved larvæ are examined with the binocular microscope, although the details can be seen much better if a small portion of the integument, including the spiracles, is cut off, treated with caustic potash and mounted in balsam for examination with the compound microscope. In some larvæ, so much chitin is deposited in the posterior spiracles just before pupation that they must be bleached before the structure can be made out clearly.

Each of the posterior spiracles usually consist of three parts (compare Figure 285). Surrounding the whole spiracle there is often a complete or almost complete chitinous *ring*.

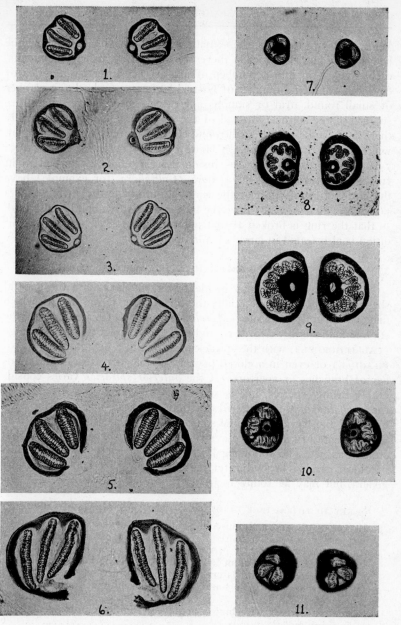

FIG. 285.—Posterior spiracles of third-stage larvæ of some common genera of Muscoid flies. 1, *Calliphora erythrocephala*; 2, *Cynomyia cadaverina*; 3, *Lucilia sericata*; 4, *Phormia regina*; 5, *Cochliomyia macellaria*; 6, *Sarcophaga bullata*; 7, *Stomoxys calcitrans*; 8, *Musca domestica*; 9, *Cryptolucilia cornicina*; 10, *Morellia micans*; 11, *Muscina stabulans*. (Original. Root)

Within this are the *slits,* the actual apertures by which air enters the body of the larvæ. Typically there are three straight or sinuous slits, each divided up into a number of smaller apertures by a series of chitinous bars. In a number of Œstrid larvæ, we find a large number of small round, oval or sinuous apertures scattered over the entire surface of the spiracle, instead of the usual three large slits. Usually there can also be seen a small round chitinized area, often perforated, which is called the *button.* In larvæ of the MUSCIDÆ (Figure 285: 7-11) the button usually lies inside the ring and is attached to it. In the CALLIPHORIDÆ, some genera (*Calliphora,* for example) have the button forming part of the ring (Figure 285: 1-3), while others (*Cochliomyia, Phormia*) have the button area very slightly chitinized, so that the ring is broken at that point (Figure 285: 4-5). This condition is also found in larvæ of *Sarcophaga.*

FLY LARVÆ: IDENTIFICATION

Other features of value in identifying fly larvæ are the general shape of the body and especially the form of the posterior end, which may be abruptly truncate (*Morellia*), rounded (*Musca*), with the stigmal field slightly depressed and surrounded by a tuberculate ridge (CALLIPHORIDÆ), with the spiracles situated in a definite pit (SARCOPHAGIDÆ) or even in a closed pocket (certain ŒSTRIDÆ). The number of branches or apertures of the *anterior spiracles* varies considerably in any species, but is sometimes of value. The structure of the *cephalopharyngeal sclerites* within the head and anterior segments of the larvæ also show some very characteristic modifications in different larvæ, but these structures have not been thoroughly studied as yet. The following key is by no means complete and has not been carried beyond referring the larvæ to certain groups of genera, but may be found to be useful.

KEY TO THIRD-STAGE LARVÆ OF SOME OF THE MUSCOID FLIES

1. Larvæ of the normal muscoid shape, i.e., slender, cylindrical, tapering anteriorly, more or less truncate posteriorly, without lateral or posterior processes 2

   Larvæ either large, stout and more or less flattened dorso-ventrally or else with lateral or posterior processes 7

2. Posterior spiracles with button area well chitinized and ring complete 3

   Posterior spiracles with button area very slightly chitinized and ring incomplete 6

3. Button area a part of the ring; slits nearly straight
   ....*Calliphora, Lucilia, Anastellorhina, Neopollenia.*

   Button area within ring 4

4. Slits only slightly bent ....*Muscina.*
   Slits sinuous, much curved 5
5. Posterior spiracle D-shaped; each slit thrown into several loops
   Musca, Philæmatomyia, Hæmatobia, Cryptolucilia, Morellia,
   etc. ....
   Posterior spiracle triangular with rounded corners; each slit
   S-shaped ....*Stomoxys, Bdellolarynx, Hæmatobosca.*
6. Inner slits sloping downward and outward; middle slits nearly
   vertical; outer slits sloping downward and inward
   ....*Sarcophaga, Wohlfahrtia,* etc.
   All of the slits sloping downward and inward
   ....*Cochliomyia, Chrysomyia, Phormia, Protophormia.*
7. Larvæ large, stout, more or less flattened dorso-ventrally, usually
   without processes ....(ŒSTRIDÆ). 9
   Larvæ short, stout, cylindrical, with a very long, tubular process
   posteriorly ....*Eristalis* (SYRPHIDÆ).
   Larvæ with fleshy or spinose lateral processes 8
8. Posterior spiracles placed in a depressed stigmal field
   ....*Chrysomyia albiceps, varipes* and *villeneuvii.*
   Posterior spiracles elevated on short tubercles..........*Fannia.*
9. Posterior spiracles each with three distinct slits 10
   Posterior spiracles each with a large number of small apertures. 13
10. Slits of posterior spiracles nearly straight
    .... *Dermatobia, Cobboldia.*
    Slits of posterior spiracles decidedly curved or sinuous 11
11. Each slit bent at its middle ....*Gasterophilus.*
    Each slit thrown into several loops 12
12. Slits separate and not parallel to each other
    ....*Cordylobia* (CALLIPHORIDÆ).
    Slits close together and parallel to each other......*Gyrostigma.*
13. Each posterior spiracle a single solid plate; its apertures without
    obvious cross-bars 14
    Each posterior spiracle more or less distinctly divided into sev-
    eral plates; its apertures small, curved, cross-barred slits
    ....*Cuterebra.*
14. Button area a part of the spiracular plate
    ....*Œstrus, Rhinœstrus, Gedœlstia,* etc.
    Button area separate, lying in an indentation of the spiracular
    plate 15
15. Button area strongly chitinized, lying in a deep indentation of
    the spiracular plate ....*Hypoderma.*
    Button area weakly chitinized, lying in a shallow indentation
    .... *Cephalopsis.*

III. *The Use of Maggots in Surgery*

There are many very early references to the beneficial effects of
maggots upon the healing of deep wounds. It would seem that a large
number of careful observers throughout recorded history have made
note of the aid to healing which is given by certain fly larvæ in the
wound. Paré, in the sixteenth century, observed unusually rapid

healing of wounds which were suppurating and in which blow flies
had oviposited. Napoleon's famous surgeon, Dr. Larrey, also noted
that larvæ in the wounds of soldiers during the Syrian campaign
expedited the healing of these wounds. Dr. W. S. Baer was with
the American Expeditionary Forces during the World War, and saw
soldiers brought in from the battle-field who had been lying as much
as seven days without attention and who were suffering from compound fractures. He found the wounds filled with maggots, but
much to his surprise these wounds consisted of healthy pink granulation tissue instead of pus. Upon his return to the United States he
instituted a scientific study of the effect of maggots upon chronic
infections, and in 1929 introduced maggots into the treatment of
osteomyelitis. He treated over 300 cases of osteomyelitis and recorded recovery in all of the children treated and in several of the
adults. Since that time the treatment has been given by numerous
surgeons in every state in the United States and in most of the other
countries of the world. The beneficial effects of the larvæ are ascribed
to their ingestion of necrotic tissue and to their predigestion of such
tissue by the tryptase present in the excreta, which becomes active in
the presence of calcium carbonate exuded through the body wall and
in the alkaline reaction caused by the ammonia in the excreta. Robinson has also shown (1935) that the substance allantoin, which is a
constituent of the urinary secretions of the maggots, has a very
beneficial effect in that it stimulates healing in slowly healing suppurative wounds. He has shown that allantoin from other sources has
this stimulating action in the absence of maggots. This action of
allantoin had been observed earlier by Macalister (1912) who believed the effectiveness of camfrey in aiding healing of ulcers was
due to the high concentration of allantoin in its tissues. The flies
most commonly used are the common blow-flies, *Lucilia sericata* and
Phormia regina. It is important in the use of maggots to employ
only such species as commonly feed upon necrotic tissue. It must
be remembered that even with these species there is some danger that
they will attack the normal tissues. Stewart (1934) showed this to be
true of *Lucilia sericata*.

Considerable study has been devoted to the best technique for
rearing maggots for surgical use. The essential requisites of such a
technique are that the maggots must be grown under sterile conditions and must be readily obtainable at any time of the year. A
student interested in the details of this technique should consult the
excellent article by White (1937). Attention is also called to the
review of literature relating to the use of maggots, by Robinson
(1934).

CHAPTER XLVI

ORDER SIPHONAPTERA—FLEAS

I. *Characteristics*

Fleas may be readily recognized as such by their complete lack of wings, their compressed or laterally flattened form and their remarkable jumping ability. Their life history includes a complete metamorphosis, with egg, larval, and adult stages. The adult fleas are ectoparasites of birds and mammals and feed only on blood, although they may spend considerable time in the nest or burrow of their host instead of on its body. As a rule, each species of flea shows a tendency to infest a particular host species or group of species but fleas are much more apt to straggle on to unusual hosts than lice, for example, because of their much smaller host specificity and their greater motility. The larvæ of fleas are not parasitic, although they usually live in the nest of the host of the adult species. However, Faust and Maxwell (1930) have reported finding larvæ of the chigœ (*Tunga penetrans*) full of blood in skin scrapings from an individual who had been infested with adult chigoes.

II. *Structure of Adult Flea*

On the sides of the head there may be a pair of *ocelli* or simple eyes. These are vestigial or absent in some fleas. Just behind the eyes are a pair of *antennal grooves,* in which the antennæ lie when at rest. The antennal grooves divide the head more or less completely, into an anterior *frons* and a posterior *occiput.* The ventral edge of the *frons* is called the *gena* and bears a *genal comb* or *genal ctenidium* of stout spines in some genera. The antennæ are much like those of the TABANIDÆ, consisting of three segments of which the terminal one or *club* is more or less completely divided into about nine smaller divisions. The mouthparts project ventrally or ventro-anteriorly from the lower anterior corner of the head. The *maxillæ* and the *labium* are both short and reduced, but bear prominent, jointed *maxillary* and *labial palpi.* The piercing organs are the two *mandibles,* with serrated edges. There is also a slender rod-like *epipharynx.* In use, the mandibles and epipharynx lock together, forming a food canal and a salivary duct.

Since wings are entirely absent and each of the three thoracic segments bears a pair of legs, they are all of about the same size and of comparatively simple structure, each consisting of a dorsal *tergite* and a ventral *sternite.* The sternites of the mesothorax and metathorax bear internal rod-like thickenings (Figure 286) which

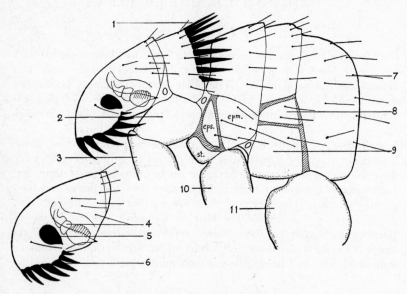

FIG. 286.—Head and thorax of female *Ctenocephalides felis,* with head of female *C. canis* below, for comparison. (Original. Root)

1—Pronotal comb	6—Genal comb
2—Prothoracic sternite	7—Epimeron
3—First coxa	8—Episternum
4—Antenna	9—Metathoracic sternite
5—Eye	10—Second coxa

11—Third coxa

mark out the limits of areas which are called *episternum, epimeron* and *sternum.* The *epimeron* of the metathorax is large and overlaps the abdomen, taking the place of the sternite of the first abdominal segment. The tergite of the prothorax may bear a *pronotal ctenidium* of spines similar to that on the gena.

The legs are strong, particularly the hind pair which is used for jumping. Each leg is made up of coxa, trochanter, femur, tibia and five tarsal segments. The last tarsal segment bears a pair of long claws. The arrangement of the spines and bristles on the various segments of the legs is often of importance in distinguishing genera and species.

The abdomen consists of ten segments, of which the last two are considerably modified for sexual purposes. Each segment has a dorsal *tergite* and a ventral *sternite*. Both tergite and sternite usually have one or more rows of backwardly pointing bristles. Dorsally, near its posterior margin, the seventh tergite bears a pair of very strong *antepygidial bristles*. Just posterior to these bristles is a hairy pad, probably sensory in function, known as the *pygidium*. In male fleas the abdomen ends with the clasping apparatus, and in cleared specimens a complicated internal genital apparatus may also be seen. In female fleas the external genitalia are less complex and all that can be seen of the internal structures in specimens treated with caustic potash is the chitinized *spermatheca* or *receptaculum seminis* and the *bursa copulatrix*. The details of form of the male claspers and *manubrium* and of the spermatheca of the female are often of great importance in identifying fleas (see Fox, 1914).

III. *Life History of Fleas*

The female flea lays her small oval or elongate eggs either in the nest of the host or among its hairs or feathers. In the latter case they are not attached to the host and normally drop off before hatching. The larva (Figure 287) is a slender, legless, worm-like organism with a distinct head, looking not unlike the larvæ of some of the DIPTERA NEMATOCERA. Flea larvæ feed on any nourishing particles in the débris in which they live, particularly on the fecal pellets of the adult fleas and particles of dried blood. After moulting or casting its skin three times the larva is mature and spins a thin silken cocoon, to which adhere dust and other débris. Within this cocoon pupation occurs. Usually, in any brood of flea larvæ, some will pupate at once after making their cocoons, while others will lie quiescent within the cocoon for a longer or shorter time before pupating. Consequently the fleas proceeding from a single batch of eggs do not all emerge at once but come out of their cocoons at intervals over some little period of time. The length of the entire life history may be as short as four weeks for some individuals in hot, moist climates, but may be much longer, even in other individuals of the same brood.

IV. *Classification*

The Order SIPHONAPTERA is divided into two suborders, the FRACTICIPITA, in which the antennal grooves divide the head completely and the frons and occiput are capable of independent movement, and the INTEGRICIPITA, in which the frons and occiput are fused together dorsally, the division of the head by the antennal grooves being incomplete. Each of these suborders is further divided into a number of families, of which the most important to us are, in the FRACTICIPITA, the family HYSTRICHOPSYLLIDÆ and in the INTEGRICIPITA, the families HECTOPSYLLIDÆ, PULICIDÆ, and DILI-CHOPSYLLIDÆ.

A fairly complete key to the genera of fleas of the world, with the notable exception of the new genera separated from the old genus *Ceratophyllus,* will be found in Fox (1925). From the parasitological viewpoint, the fleas of interest are those which are commonly found on rats and other rodents which are subject to plague and endemic typhus, and those which may attack man or become pests in houses. The following simple key includes only those genera which come under these categories.

KEY TO THE GENERA OF SIPHONAPTERA WHICH ARE OF KNOWN
MEDICAL IMPORTANCE

1. The three thoracic tergites together shorter than the first abdominal tergite 2
   The three thoracic tergites together longer than the first abdominal tergite 3
2. Hind coxa with a patch of small spinules on its inner side
   .... *Echidnophaga.*
   Hind coxa without a patch of spinules on its inner surface
   ....*Tunga.*
3. Eyes well developed 4
   Eyes vestigial or absent; both pronotal and genal combs present 9
4. Neither pronotal nor genal combs present 5
   Pronotal comb, at least, present 6
5. Mesosternite with only one internal rod-like thickening, which extends from the insertion of the coxa forward to the anterior border .... *Pulex.*
   Mesosternite with two internal rod-like thickenings, one extending forward and the other upward............... *Xenopsylla.*
6. Both pronotal and genal combs present 7
   Pronotal comb present but genal comb absent 8
7. Genal comb running horizontally along lower border of gena
   ....*Ctenocephalides.*
   Genal comb running obliquely across gena ....*Cediopsylla.*
8. With but one row of bristles on the second to seventh abdominal tergites .... *Hoplopsyllus.*
   With at least two rows of bristles on the second to seventh abdominal tergites 10
9. Some of the bristles on the posterior margin of the tibiæ forming a comb ....*Ctenopsyllus.*

None of the bristles on the posterior margin of the tibiæ forms a comb .... *Ctenophthalmus.*
10. One or no lateral bristles on outer surface of front femur; no long, thin bristles on inner surface of mid- and hind coxæ ....*Orchopeas.*
Long, thin bristles present on inner surface of mid- and hind coxæ 11
11. Long, thin bristles extending from base to apex of inner surface of mid- and hind coxæ 12
Long, thin bristles present at most on apical half of inner surface of mid- and hind coxæ 13
12. Eighth sternite of male small; female with 2 antepygidial bristles .... *Diamanus.*
Eighth sternite of male narrow and horizontal with apical bristles; female with 3 or more antepygidial bristles .... *Oropsylla.*
13. Twenty-four or more spines in pronotal comb....*Ceratophyllus.*
Less than twenty-four spines in pronotal comb............... 14
14. Eighth sternite of male vestigial and without apical bristles; apex of bursa copulatrix of female coiled up in a spiral .... *Nosopsyllus.*
Eighth sternite of male a narrow horizontal sclerite with bristles and an apical membranous flap; apex of bursa copulatrix of female not coiled up in a spiral .... *Monopsyllus.*

V. *Family Hectopsyllidæ*

The fleas belonging to this family are sometimes called the "burrowing fleas," because the pregnant female attaches herself firmly to the skin of her host, causing such irritation that the skin swells up around her, partly or completely enclosing her body.

Tunga penetrans Linn.: This is the "chigoe" of tropical America, which has also been introduced into Africa. The pregnant female attaches herself to the skin of man, dogs and pigs and becomes almost completely enclosed by the resultant swelling. Within this enclosure the abdomen of the flea swells up to the size of a pea because of the numerous eggs developed. The eggs pass out through a small aperture and drop to the ground. When all the eggs are laid the flea dies and the swelling in which she lived often becomes secondarily infected, sometimes with serious results. In man, the skin of the foot, particularly between the toes, is the most usual site of infestation.

Echidnophaga gallinacea Westwood (Figure 288): The "sticktight flea" of chickens, which usually attaches itself about the head of chickens and other birds, is also frequently found on rats, dogs, and cats and sometimes on man. It was probably originally an inhabitant of Asia, but it is now found throughout the warmer portions of the world and occasionally extends well up into the temperate zone.

VI. *Family Pulicidæ*

Pulex irritans Linn. (Figure 288) : This species is usually referred to as the "human flea," and is the species most frequently found in houses and on human beings in most parts of the world. In the eastern and southeastern United

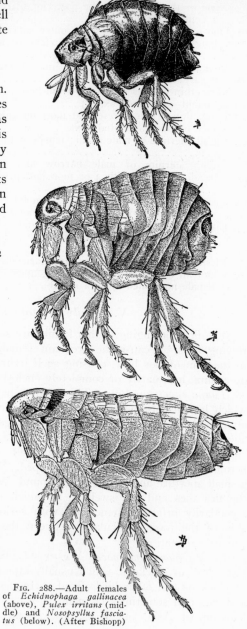

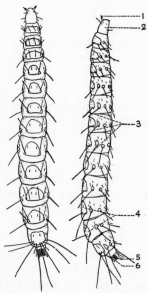

FIG. 287—Larva of *Xenopsylla cheopis.* Dorsal view (right), lateral view (left). (x 10. Redrawn from Bacot and Ridewood, 1914)

1—Antenna
2—Head
3—Setæ
4—Somites
5—Anal strut
6—Hairs of anal comb

FIG. 288.—Adult females of *Echidnophaga gallinacea* (above), *Pulex irritans* (middle) and *Nosopsyllus fasciatus* (below). (After Bishopp)

States, curiously enough flea infestation of houses is almost invariably due to dog and cat fleas, although the "human flea" is sometimes found in these regions in enormous numbers on hogs. It sometimes occurs on rats, dogs, and other small mammals.

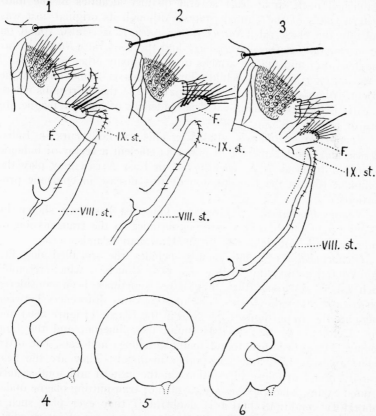

Fig. 289.—Differential characters of three species of *Xenopsylla*. 1, modified abdominal segments of male *X. brasiliensis;* 2, same of *X. cheopis;* 3, same of *X. astia;* 4, seminal receptacle of female *X. brasiliensis;* 5, same of *X. cheopis;* 6, same of *X. astia.* F., outer flap of clasper; VIII. st., and IX. st., eighth and ninth sternites. (Redrawn after Rothschild)

Xenopsylla: This genus includes a number of species, mainly Old World forms infesting various rodents. Five species are commonly found on rats. They may be differentiated by the differences in the male claspers and the female spermathecæ. (Figure 289).

Xenopsylla cheopis (Rothschild) : This is the Indian rat flea, and is probably of more importance than any other species in the transmission of bubonic plague from rat to human. It is now the most abundant rat flea in nearly all parts of the tropics and subtropics, and is frequently encountered in ports which are in the temperate zone but have considerable trade with tropical countries. Also it has established itself in at least several distinct localities in the midwestern states of the United States. Although its original host was probably the black rat (*Rattus rattus rattus*), it is also found on the brown rat (*Rattus norvegicus*) and the roof rat (*Rattus rattus alexandrinus*) and readily attacks man and many other mammals.

Xenopsylla astia Rothschild: This rat flea is found only in the Orient. It has been shown (Cragg, 1921, 1923) that in regions where *X. astia* is the predominant rat flea, epidemics of bubonic plague are rare or absent.

Xenopsylla brasiliensis (Baker): This rat flea ocurs in India, Africa, and South America. It is not as efficient a vector of bubonic plague in India as is *X. cheopis* but in East Africa may play the dominant rôle in the transmission of this disease in epidemic proportions.

Xenopsylla hawaiiensis Jordan: This flea has been shown by Eskey (1934) to be of primary importance in the transmission of endemic plague of field rats in the Hawaiian Islands.

Ctenocephalides *: This genus includes the so-called dog flea (*Ct. canis* Curtis) and cat-flea (*Ct. felis* Bouché), which resemble each other so closely that they have sometimes been considered varieties of a single species. The most obvious differences between them are the proportions of the head in the female (Figure 286) and the chætotaxy of the metepisternum, metepimeron, and the hind femur. These fleas are found mainly on dogs and cats, but often occur on man, rats, and many other mammals. They are the fleas usually found in house infestations in the eastern and southeastern United States. These species are capable of transmitting plague under laboratory conditions but it is doubtful if they ever play such a rôle under natural conditions. These fleas may serve as intermediate hosts of the tapeworms *Dipylidium caninum* and *Hymenolepis diminuta*. The dog flea has been suspected to be a vector of infantile kala-azar but all investigational findings have been negative.

Cediopsylla: This genus contains some of the rabbit fleas which are not of known medical importance, but are mentioned because of their superficial resemblance to the dog and cat fleas and also be-

---

* New genus erected by Stiles and Collins (1930) to replace the preoccupied genus *Ctenocephalus*.

cause they may be of importance in transmitting among rabbits diseases which are communicable to man.

Hoplopsyllus anomalus Baker: This species is one of the common fleas of the Beechey ground squirrel (*Citellus beecheyi* subsp.) and other related rodents and may be regarded as one of the possible, efficient vectors of sylvatic plague as found in the western United States.

VII. Family *Dolichopsyllidæ*

Ceratophyllus: This genus formerly included a great many species of fleas infesting both birds and small mammals but Jordan (1933) made the badly needed revision and the present genus *Ceratophyllus* includes only bird fleas.

Nosopsyllus (= *Ceratophyllus*) *fasciatus* (Bosc.) (Figure 288): The common rat flea of Europe and North America. It is probably originally the flea of the brown rat (*Rattus norvegicus*). Although this flea is considered to be a relatively inefficient vector of plague it is, however, an efficient vector of endemic typhus.

Monopsyllus (= *Cerotophyllus* in part) *anisus* (Roths.): Replaces *Nosopsyllus fasciatus* as the common rat flea of North China and Japan.

Diamanus (= *Ceratophyllus*) *montanus* (Bak.) (= *C. acutus*): This is a very common flea of the rodents of the western United States susceptible to sylvatic plague and has been somewhat indefinitely implicated in its transmission.

Oropsylla (= *Ceratophyllus*) *silantiewi* (Wagner): The flea of Manchurian marmot or "tarbagan" (*Arctomys bobac*), which is an important rodent host of plague is capable of transmitting the infection.

Oropsylla (= *Ceratophyllus*) *idahœnsis* (Bak.): This is another rodent flea of the western United States which has been somewhat indefinitely implicated in the transmission of sylvatic plague.

VIII. Family *Hystrichopsyllidæ*

Ctenopsyllus segnis Schön (= *Leptopsylla musculi* Duges): This species is the common flea of the house mouse (*Mus musculus*) in Europe. In America it is commonly found on the house mouse, the rat, and other small rodents.

IX. Fleas as Disease-Carriers

Fleas are of interest to parasitologists mainly because of their connection with the transmission of plague from rats and other rodents to human beings and from rodent to rodent, and also because of their ability to transmit endemic typhus from rat to man and from rat to rat.

Bubonic plague is primarily a disease of rats, transmissible to ground-squirrels, marmots, and other rodents and also, unfortunately, to human beings. While the pneumonic type of plague is transmitted from man to man by droplets of saliva expelled during respiration, the bubonic and septicæmic types are transmitted from rat to rat and rat to man by fleas and are apparently almost never transmitted from man to man.

There are two ways in which fleas may transmit plague. When the plague bacilli (*Pasteurella pestis*) are taken into the alimentary tract of the flea with its blood meal they undergo considerable multiplication there, but do not penetrate into other parts of the body; the salivary glands, for example, remaining free from them. Large numbers of plague bacilli pass out in the fecal droplets deposited by an infected flea and it is probable that human infections may result from rubbing these fecal drops into the bite when it is scratched. Bacot and Martin (1914) have also shown that in some infected fleas the multiplication of the plague bacilli is so rapid that they actually obstruct the small spherical proventriculus to such an extent that little or no blood can pass into the stomach. Such fleas make violent and persistent efforts to feed, in the course of which some of the plague bacilli are mixed with the blood and regurgitated into the wound made by the bite, thus bringing about infection. This latter appears to be the most common mechanism of transmission, at least in India. Experiments have proved that most species of fleas found on rats and other plague-infected rodents will readily bite human beings. On the other hand, however, some fleas such as the European field mouse flea (*Ctenophthalmus agrytes*) and *Synopsylla fouquernii* of rats of Madagascar rarely if ever can be induced to bite man although they may, as is the case with the latter species, become infected with plague bacilli after feeding upon infected rats. Such fleas play an important part in the transmission of plague from rodent to rodent and thus maintain a reservoir of infection, even though they do not transmit plague to man.

In Manchuria, South Africa, and the western United States where plague is primarily a disease of wild rodents, rather than of rats and mice living in or close to human habitations, the disease is known as "sylvatic plague."

Endemic typhus is a mild form of typhus which is not epidemic and is a *Rickettsia* infection. It is primarily a disease of rats and may be transmitted among them and from them to man by fleas, *Xenop-sylla cheopis* and *Nosopsyllus fasciatus*. It is thought that fleas effect transmission through the medium of infective feces rather than by bites. In infected fleas the *Rickettsia* are found in the epithelial cells of the stomach.

Since plague and endemic typhus are primarily diseases of rodents and man is infected only by accident, it is usual to find the diseases widely prevalent among the rodent population when the first human cases are recognized.

To control these diseases, it is necessary to prevent contact between rodents (or rather their fleas) and human beings or else to eradicate the disease among the rodents.

Rat-proof construction. The most valuable measure in keeping rat-fleas from coming in contact with man is the rat-proofing of all buildings and other structures where rats can obtain food and shelter. In dealing with the ordinary brown rat, reinforced concrete or cement construction in cellars, basement, and ground floors is particularly necessary, since this species is a terrestrial, burrowing rodent which is rarely found in the upper portions of buildings. The black rat was originally an arboreal, climbing species, and may be found in the upper stories of even tall buildings. It is often found on ships. Proper screening of all inlets and outlets of buildings is also essential in rat-proofing.

If plague among the rats is confined to a definite area, contact between rat fleas and man may be prevented by the temporary depopulation of the district while an intensive effort to destroy all the rats in it is being made.

Killing rats. When killing rats to combat plague or endemic typhus, it is of the greatest importance that as many dead rats as possible be brought into the laboratory and examined so that the degree of infection in the rat population and the location of foci can be determined. Rats sent in for examination should have been first dipped in kerosene to kill all of their fleas and should always be labelled with the locality from which they came, and the date.

When a plague or endemic typhus focus has been found, an intensive campaign of rat-killing and rat-proofing should be carried on all around it, in an attempt to isolate it and eradicate the disease within it.

In actually killing rats, the main reliance is placed on traps and poisons. But the older rats, particularly, are very wary, and before they can be successfully trapped or poisoned it is necessary to cut off their food supply, so that they will be desperate with hunger.

This requires the placing of all garbage and refuse in rat-proof receptacles pending collection and incineration, and the protection of stored food-stuffs and animal feeds from rats. Special attention must be given to the rat-proofing of stables, yards, and wharves where carelessness may make food available for the rats.

Trapping is done either with snap-traps or cage-traps. The former are usually more effective, but a certain number of rats should be trapped alive in cage-traps to obtain data on the kind of fleas present and their numbers. In general the type of trap used is of much less importance in determining success than is the skill and experience of the trapper.

The use against rats of stomach poisons if they contain arsenic, phosphorus, or strychnine, for example, is rather dangerous since these substances are also fatal to human beings. However, red squills and barium carbonate can be used safely and they are more readily acceptable to rats. Red squills is considered specifically toxic to rats, and barium carbonate acts as an emetic when ingested by man. Whatever poison is employed, pre-baiting is desirable so that the suspicions of the rats may be allayed and they may become accustomed to finding food in given places. The use of various pathogenic viruses against rats is of little value and is generally considered hazardous from the public health viewpoint. In the case of ships, warehouses, and buildings known or suspected to harbor infected rats, fumigation with hydrocyanic acid gas, or some similar compound, is very effective in destroying the rats, but must be cautiously done, since the gas is also very highly poisonous to man.

When plague infection spreads from the city rats to wild rodents such as ground-squirrels and sylvatic plague is thus established, their suppression must be undertaken. Such control measures may best be effected by a combination of poison baits and fumigation of burrows. These activities are efficient only when they are based upon a sound and detailed knowledge of the ecology of the rodents being controlled. Where poison baits are employed it is necessary to change the baits in accordance with seasonal feeding habits and repletion of restricted appetites. Furthermore, it is necessary to produce rodent-free belts about urban centers to prevent sylvatic plague from becoming established in domestic rodents and leading to human epidemics. In the suppression of sylvatic plague it also seems desirable, if not actually necessary, to attempt to control fleas in rodent burrows, by means of suitable fumigation, as well as the rodents themselves since these parasites are capable of serving as pseudo-reservoirs of the infection.

In anti-plague and anti-endemic-typhus campaigns it has, perhaps unwisely, not been usual to lay any particular stress on the control of fleas. When homes become heavily infested with fleas, however, it is necessary to take measures to eradicate them and prevent their reintroduction. To eradicate fleas and other insect pests in houses, fumigation with hydrocyanic acid gas is very effective, but so dangerous that it cannot always be attempted and if so only by men thoroughly trained in its use. Simpler measures, which are often efficacious, are mopping the floors with kerosene, sprinkling them with powdered naphthalene, or spraying floors, rugs, and furniture with cresol compounds. These measures must be repeated several times at short intervals to insure success. In the eastern and southern United States, flea infestation of houses is practically always due to the multiplication of fleas from dogs or cats, and these pets should be regularly bathed with dilute creolin (3 per cent) or dusted with insect powder to keep them comparatively free of fleas. Their bedding should be burned or their kennels treated with cresol solution weekly to prevent flea breeding.

CHAPTER XLVII

ORDER ANOPLURA—LICE

The lice, like the fleas, are wingless, ectoparasitic insects. They differ decidedly from the fleas in two respects. First, their bodies are flattened dorsoventrally instead of laterally, and second, they are ectoparasitic throughout their entire life-cycle, even their eggs being firmly attached to the hairs or feathers of their hosts. The larval stages have exactly the same habit of life as the adults and resemble them closely in form, so that there is practically no metamorphosis in their life history.

The Order ANOPLURA is now considered as including two sub-orders, the MALLOPHAGA (biting lice or "bird lice") and the SIPHUN-CULATA (sucking lice or true lice).

I. *Mallophaga*

The "bird lice" have mouth parts of the chewing type, not unlike those of a grasshopper or beetle, and most of them, at least, are believed to feed on bits of dead skin, feathers or hair. The thorax shows a division into at least two distinct segments. The last of the two tarsal joints bears one or two claws, and only rarely is the tip of the tibia so formed that it is apposable to the claw. There is a great variety of species of MALLOPHAGA, most of which are ecto-parasites of birds, but there are several genera which are ectopara-sitic on mammals only. None of them attacks man, so that they are of very little interest from the medical viewpoint. They are, how-ever, of great interest to the student of evolution and zoogeography, (see papers by Kellogg, 1913, 1914). The following brief summary of their classification will be adequate for our needs.

Order ANOPLURA, Suborder MALLOPHAGA.
> Superfamily ISCHNOCERA (antennæ slender, three-jointed or five-jointed).
>> Family TRICHODECTIDÆ (antennæ three-jointed, feet with 1 claw, parasitic on mammals).
>>> Genus *Trichodectes*, etc.
>> Family PHILOPTERIDÆ (antennæ five-jointed, feet with 2 claws, parasitic on birds).
>>> Genera *Philopterus, Lipeurus, Goniodes, Degeeriella*, etc.

Superfamily AMBLYCERA (antennæ clubbed, four-jointed).
Family MENOPONIDÆ (feet with 2 claws, parasitic on birds).
Genera *Menopon, Colpocephalum, Trinoton,* etc.
Family BOOPIDÆ (feet with 2 claws, parasitic on mammals, especially marsupials).
Genera *Boopia, Trimenopon,* etc.
Family GYROPIDÆ (feet with 1 claw, parasitic on mammals).
Genera *Gyropus, Gliricola,* etc.

II. *Siphunculata*

The true lice have mouth parts of the sucking type, adapted to pierce the skin of their hosts and suck out blood. The three thoracic segments are fused together, without any clear dividing line between them. The single tarsal joint bears only one claw and in most species the tip of the tibia is widened and drawn out into a "thumb-like process" apposable to the claw. All of the true lice are ectoparasites of mammals.

I. STRUCTURE OF THE SIPHUNCULATA

The head may or may not bear a pair of simple eyes or *ocelli.* The short *antennæ,* which may consist of from three to five joints, are laterally placed, just in front of the eyes, if the latter are present. The oral opening is at the anterior end of the head, surrounded by a ring of *prestomal hooklets,* which grip the skin of the host firmly when the louse is feeding. From the oral opening can be protruded the piercing *proboscis,* which is made up of three slender stylets whose exact homologies are not well understood.

The thorax may show traces of segmentation, but is never completely segmented. A chitinous *sternal plate* may be present in the middle of the ventral surface. The middle thoracic segment has a pair of large *spiracles* or respiratory openings.

The legs are short and strong, with only one tarsal joint, as a rule. The tip of the tibia usually has a "thumb-like process," apposable to the single tarsal *claw.*

The abdomen usually shows nine segments, of which the first may be much reduced and the last two modified for sexual purposes. There are usually six pairs of abdominal spiracles, on segments 3-8 inclusive. Each of the abdominal segments has typically both a dorsal *tergite,* a ventral *sternite* and a pair of lateral *pleural plates.* The size and form of the pleural plates are often useful in identification.

2. CLASSIFICATION

The suborder SIPHUNCULATA is divided into four families. Two of these are of no particular interest to us, since the family ECHINOP-

THIRIIDÆ includes only the lice infesting seals, sea-lions and walruses and the family HÆMATOMYZIDÆ contains the single genus *Hæma-tomyzus,* parasitic on elephants. From the medical viewpoint the family of greatest importance is the PEDICULIDÆ, distinguished by the presence of well-pigmented eyes. It is divided into two sub-families, of which the PEDICININÆ contains the lice of the Old World monkeys, while the PEDICULINÆ includes lice from lemurs, anthro-poid apes, New World spider-monkeys and man. The family HÆMATOPINIDÆ is of importance to veterinarians, since it includes the great majority of the lice found on wild and domestic mammals. It includes several subfamilies, but the two main types of lice con-tained in the family are well typified by the large species of *Hæma-topinus* and *Linognathus,* usually found on ungulates, and the smaller forms belonging to *Polyplax, Hæmodipsus,* and many other genera, which are parasitic on rodents and other small mammals.

The following condensed key includes all the genera of the PEDICULIDÆ and will also enable the student to get a general idea of the generic identity of the common lice of domestic animals. To this is added a brief tabulation of the species of SIPHUNCULATA and MALLOPHAGA which are ordinarily encountered on the usual domestic and laboratory animals and birds. For further details re-garding the lice encountered on wild mammals; see the papers by Kellogg and Ferris (1915) and by Ferris (1920, 1921, 1922, 1923).

KEY TO SOME OF THE GENERA OF THE SUBORDER SIPHUNCULATA

1. Body with spines or hairs in definite rows, never with scales...   2
   Body thickly covered with short stout spines or with spines
      and scales .... (Family ECHINOPTHIRIIDÆ).
2. Head not elongated; tibia with thumb-like process   3
   Head tubularly produced anteriorly; tibia without a thumb-like
      process .... (Family HÆMATOMYZIDÆ).
3. Eyes rudimentary or absent .... (Family HÆMATOPINIDÆ).   4
   Eyes present, usually well pigmented .... (Family PEDICULIDÆ).   8
4. Antennæ three-jointed... (EUHÆMATOPININÆ) *Euhæmatopinus.*
   Antennæ five-jointed   5
5. All legs and claws of the same size
      .... (HÆMATOPININÆ) *Hæmatopinus,* etc.
   Anterior legs and claws smaller than the posterior ones
      .... (LINOGNATHINÆ)   6
6. Abdomen entirely without pleural plates.......*Linognathus,* etc.
   Abdomen with well developed pleural plates...................   7
7. Abdominal tergites and sternites mostly with only one trans-
      verse row of hairs or bristles
      ....*Hæmodipsus, Enderleinellus,* etc.
   Abdominal tergites and sternites mostly with more than one
      transverse row of hairs or bristles.*Polyplax, Hoplopleura,* etc.

8. Antennæ of adult three-jointed ....(PEDICININÆ)   9
   Antennæ of adult five-jointed ....(PEDICULINÆ)   10
9. Anterior legs smaller than middle and posterior pairs
   ....,.....................*Phthirpedicinus.*
   All legs of about same size ....*Pedicinus.*
10. Anterior legs smaller than middle and posterior pairs   11
    All legs of about same size ....*Pediculus.*
11. Abdomen long ....*Phthirpediculus.*
    Abdomen short and stout ....*Phthirus.*

Lice Commonly Encountered on Domestic and Laboratory Animals

Host	MALLOPHAGA	SIPHUNCULATA
Rhesus	.........................*Pedicinus rhesi* Fahr.	
monkey		*Phthirpedicinus micropilosus* Fahr.
Dog	*Trichodectes canis* DeGeer *Heterodoxus longitarsus*	*Linognathus setosus* Olfers
Cat	*Felicola subrostrata*	...............♦............
Horse	*Bovicola equi* Linn. *Trichodectes pilosus*	*Hæmatopinus asini* Linn.
Pig	.........................*Hæmatopinus suis* Linn.	
Cow	*Bovicola bovis* Linn.	*Hæmatopinus eurysternus* *Linognathus vituli*
Sheep	*Bovicola ovis* Linn.	*Linognathus pedalis*
Goat	*Bovicola capræ* Gurlt *Trichodectes hermsi* Kell. & Nak.	*Linognathus stenopsis* Burm.
Rabbit	.........................*Hæmodipsus ventricosus* Denny	
Guinea-pig	*Gyropus ovalis* Nitzsch *Gliricola porcelli* Schrank	....
Rat	.........................*Polyplax spinulosa* Burm.	
Chicken	*Menopon gallinæ* Linn. *Eomenacanthus stramineum* Nitzsch *Lipeurus heterographus* Nitzsch *Lipeurus caponis* Linn.	....
Turkey	*Goniodes meleagridis* Linn. *Lipeurus gallipavonis* Geoffroy *Eomenacanthus stramineum* Nitzsch	....
Duck	*Philopterus dentatus* Scopoli *Esthiopterum crassicorne* Scopoli	....
Pigeon	*Columbicola columbæ* Linn. *Goniocotes bidentatus* Scopoli	....

III. *Species of Lice Found on Man*

Man is parasitized by two species of lice, the pubic or crab louse (*Phthirus pubis* Linn. Figure 291) and the human louse (*Pediculus humanus* Linn. Figure 290). Authorities seem to agree that the latter species may be divided into two hybridizing subspecies, the head louse (*P. humanus humanus* Linn.) and the body louse or clothes louse (*P. humanis corporis* DeGeer). Some students of the group believe that these two subspecies are characteristic of the Caucasian race, and that there are other subspecies of *P. humanus* which were originally confined to Negroes, Chinese, and American Indians respectively (see Ewing, 1926). They admit, however, that all forms of *P. humanus* interbreed and that many of the lice encountered in civilized lands are of hybrid type. Other authorities deny the existence of varieties of lice characteristic of the different races of mankind.

The species and varieties of lice found on man differ somewhat in their habitats and habits. The head louse inhabits the head, attaching its eggs to the hair, while the body louse inhabits the clothing, usually attaching its eggs to the fibers of the cloth (Figure 292). The crab louse is usually found among the hairs of the pubic region, but in badly-infested individuals it may spread to the body and even to the head. It attaches its eggs to the hairs.

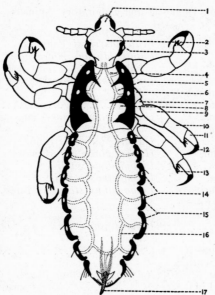

Fig. 290.—Male of *Pediculus humanus*. (Original. Root)

1—Clypeus	9—Femur
2—Frons	10—Tibia
3—Eye	11—Tarsus
4—Prothorax	12—Tarsal claw
5—Mesothorax	13—Tibial thumb
6—Coxa	14—Spiracles
7—Trochanter	15—Pleural plates
8—Metathorax	16—Trachea
	17—Dilator

The eggs of lice hatch in from five to nine days, depending on the temperature to which they are exposed. Eggs of the body louse attached to clothing which is not being worn may lie dormant, without hatching, for as long as thirty-five days, if exposed to cold.

The larval forms closely resemble the adults except for their smaller size. There are three larval stages, and the adult stage is reached about twelve or fourteen days after hatching of the egg, if the larvæ are able to feed on blood regularly.

IV. *Lice as Disease-Carriers*

While all human lice are irritating, they are not equally important as disease carriers. The crab louse has not been incriminated as a carrier of any disease and the head l o u s e is thought to be much less important than the body louse as a transmitter. Lice have been proved

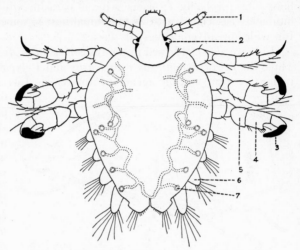

FIG. 291—Female of *Phthirus pubis.* (Original. Root)
1—Antennæ   4—Tibia
2—Eye   5—Femur
3—Tarsal claw   6—Tubercle
7—Spiracle

to be the vectors of typhus fever, trench fever, and the so-called European or epidemic types of relapsing fever.

Trench and typhus fevers are caused by rickettsiæ which are taken up by lice from infected patients and passed on through the bite or the feces of the lice. *Rickettsia prowazeki* which causes typhus fever lives within the cells of the gut epithelium and causes the death of many lice. *R. pediculi* (of trench fever) lives only in the lumen of the gut of the louse. It seems likely that *R. prowazeki* has become adapted relatively recently to transmission by the louse. (See Huff, 1938.)

Epidemic relapsing fever is probably also a disease recently adapted to man and his body lice, since it is very similar to the endemic type which is well adapted to and transmitted by ticks. The spirochætes invade the blood of the louse and are not transmitted to another host either by the bite of the louse or by fecal contamination. The louse must be crushed on the skin before transmission is effected.

It has been shown that body lice are very delicately adapted to the normal temperature of the human body and tend to become very active and to migrate if the temperature is raised even a few degrees, so that when their host is in a febrile condition they tend to leave him. This probably explains why a parasite which is usually so intimately associated with its individual host is sometimes responsible for wide-spread epidemics of disease.

Lice are also concerned in the transmission of diseases of animals. Thus, the lice, *Hæmodipsus ventricosus* and *Polyplax serrata,* of the rabbit are transmitting agents of tularemia. Lice of the marmots of western Montana have been shown to be naturally infected with plague bacilli (Eskey, 1936). *Polyplax spinulosa* of the rat transmits *Bartonella muris,* an ubiquitous blood parasite of wild and laboratory rats (Cannon and McClelland, 1928; Eliot and Ford,

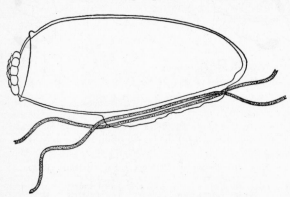

FIG. 292.—Egg of *Pediculus humanus corporis,* attached to fibers of cloth. (Original. Root)

1929). A somewhat similar blood parasite of mice, *Eperythrozoon coccoides,* is transmitted by *Polyplax serrata* (Eliot, 1936). The dog louse, *Trichodectes canis,* may serve as the intermediate host of the tapeworm, *Dipylidium caninum.* When the diseases of animals have been more thoroughly studied it is very probable that others of them will be shown to be transmitted by lice living on these animals.

In ordinary civil life, louse control is a comparatively simple matter, except when one has to deal with a population with little or no idea of cleanliness and sanitation. The ordinary laundry and dry-cleaning processes are both effective in destroying lice and their much more resistant eggs or "nits" on clothing, and a bath with a kerosene or cresol soap will kill body lice on the person. Head lice may be eradicated by rubbing into the hair thoroughly a mixture of equal parts of kerosene and vinegar, covering tightly with a towel for half an hour, and then washing the hair with soap and warm water.

In armies under war conditions, and in the case of immigrants and unsanitary populations who are suffering from epidemics of typhus fever, it is necessary to apply "delousing" measures to large bodies of people. This involves bathing the individuals with an insecticidal soap, together with hair-clipping or other measures when head lice are present, and the treatment of all clothing and blankets to kill body lice and their eggs. The lice and "nits" can be destroyed by the action of heat (baking, boiling or steaming), by fumigation with hydrocyanic acid gas, or by immersing garments in gasoline, benzene, kerosene, turpentine, or the like. In actual practice it is usual to treat most garments and bedding with steam sterilization, and to use hot-air sterilizers or cyanide gas for leather and rubber goods, furs, varnished articles and such fabrics as are injured by steam.

Conditions vary so much that it is not worth while to give any detailed account of the many different types of buildings or installations that have been devised for delousing purposes. All of them include, of course, a bath with insecticidal soap and hair-clipping, if necessary, for the individuals, together with the appropriate measures for sterilizing clothing and bedding. The two important principles to keep in mind in devising an installation to fit the conditions met with are that there should be a complete separation of the "clean" and the "infested" portions of the plant and that there should be a most meticulous inspection at the point where the individuals pass from the infested to the clean side. A "horse-shoe" arrangement, with check-rooms and sterilizers in the center, is often the most convenient plan.

When a delousing plant is not available, individuals may be protected by wearing overall suits of oiled silk or rubber, fastened tightly at wrists, neck and ankles. The use of repellent substances, such as oil of birch tar or oil of eucalyptus, and the various palliative measures, such as the use of powders, sachets, or ointments containing naphthalene, iodoform, and the like, are not very satisfactory, since although these measures may kill or stupefy the lice they have no effect on the eggs.

CHAPTER XLVIII

ORDER HEMIPTERA—TRUE BUGS

The insects belonging to the two closely related Orders HEMIP-TERA and HOMOPTERA are, for the most part, adapted to feeding upon the juices of plants or are predacious upon smaller inverte-brates. Consequently they are of great importance in agriculture through their injury to crops, both by direct injury to the plants and by the transmission of diseases from plant to plant. A few of the groups of the HEMIPTERA have become adapted to feeding upon the blood of vertebrates. A consideration of those forms concerns us here. The HEMIPTERA and HOMOPTERA share the peculiarity of having their piercing and sucking mouth parts enclosed in a *jointed* sheath formed by the labium. Within this sheath lie four slender stylets: a pair of barbed, piercing *maxillœ* and a pair of doubly-grooved *mandibles* which lock together to form a food canal and a salivary duct. The two orders differ primarily in the structure of the wings. In the HOMOPTERA both pairs of wings are membranous, while in the HEMIPTERA the basal half or two-thirds of the fore wing is thickened while the terminal half or one-third remains mem-branous. At rest, the fore wings form a protective covering for the membranous hind wings, the thickened basal portions of the two fore wings lying side by side, while the membranous terminal por-tions overlap, one above the other, covering the tips of the hind wings. In both orders, metamorphosis is incomplete, the larvæ resembling their parents in mode of life and in structure, except for their smaller size and the absence of functional wings and sex organs.

The few genera which have any direct interest to parasitologists occur in the two families, CIMICIDÆ (bedbugs) and REDUVIIDÆ ("assassin-bugs"). It should be noted, however, that all of the HEMIPTERA and HOMOPTERA have mouth parts of essentially the same structure as the blood-sucking forms, and that a number of them will occasionally bite man.

I. Family Cimicidæ—Bedbugs

In this family the wings are vestigial, the hind wings being entirely absent while the fore wings are reduced to little pads. Two species of the genus *Cimex* have become "habitat parasites" of man, living and breeding in houses and feeding on blood. Other species of this and related genera, closely resembling bedbugs in their general appearance, are parasitic on poultry, pigeons, swallows and bats. They may attack man, but usually do not continue their attacks.

The two species which are found in houses are *Cimex lectularius* Linn. (the bedbug) and *Cimex hemipterus* Fabr. (the Oriental bedbug). The main difference between them is in the form of the prothorax (compare Figure 293), which in *C. lectularius* is deeply

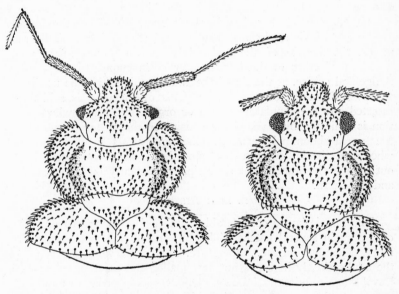

Fig. 293.—Head and thorax of *Cimex lectularius* (left) and of *Cimex hemipterus* (right). (Original. Root)

sinuate anteriorly, with the middle of the dorsum convex and the sides flattened, while in *C. hemipterus* the convexity of the dorsum extends to the margins and the anterior edge is less deeply excavated. *Cimex lectularius* is found all over the world, although it is largely replaced by *C. hemipterus* in the Old World tropics. In the American tropics the latter species seems to be comparatively rare.

I. ADULT ANATOMY

The body of the bedbug is decidedly flattened dorsoventrally, as in the lice. The head bears laterally the compound eyes and the slender, four-jointed antennæ. The mouth parts forming the proboscis are attached to the anterior end of the head, but when at rest are folded back against the ventral surface of the head and prothorax. The proboscis-sheath (labium) is four-jointed.

In the thorax, the prothorax is large and conspicuous, with its anterior border more or less concave. The mesothorax is smaller, visible dorsally as the triangular mesonotum, to which are attached the pair of pad-like fore wings or elytra. The metanotum is somewhat larger, but is largely concealed by the overlying elytra. Each of the thoracic segments bears a pair of well-developed legs with only three tarsal joints.

The abdomen is broad and rounded, particularly in the female. It consists of eight obvious segments and two more genitalic segments. At the tip of the male abdomen the asymmetrical penis sheath, projecting to the left, is very conspicuous. In the female, the genital orifice, at the tip of the abdomen, is said to be used only for oviposition. In copulation, the penis of the male is said to be inserted into the copulatory pouch or organ of Berlese, whose location is indicated by a triangular incision in the posterior margin of the fourth abdominal sternite, to the right of the median line. The whole body is clothed with short stout hairs, which are often frayed out or slightly branched at their tips, particularly on the pronotum and the elytra.

2. LIFE HISTORY

The female lays a considerable number (150 or more) of white, oval eggs in several batches. The eggs hatch in about ten days or more, depending on the temperature. The five larval stages resemble the adults closely in form, but are smaller and paler in color. Each larval stage requires at least one blood meal in order to moult and pass on to the next stage, and the female needs a blood meal before she can develop her eggs. Bedbugs are able to live for several months, perhaps even a year, without feeding, and feed readily on rats and other animals if human beings are not available.

3. BEDBUGS AND DISEASE

Bedbugs have not been definitely incriminated as important vectors of any disease. It was long believed that the Oriental bedbug

(*Cimex hemipterus*) was the probable carrier of kala azar (see page 585) and this idea has not yet been absolutely disproved. In laboratory experiments bedbugs have been shown to be capable of transmitting relapsing fever, bubonic plague and tularemia, but it is not probable that they are of any great importance in the natural transmission of any of these diseases.

4. CONTROL

Bedbugs are easily killed by most insecticides which actually come into contact with them, but their habit of lurking in all sorts

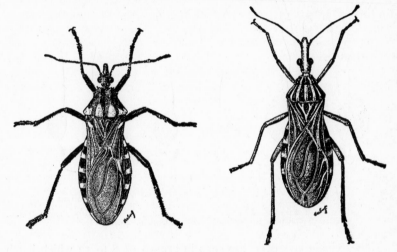

FIG. 294.—Adult males of *Triatoma megista* (left) and *Rhodnius prolixus* (right). (After Brumpt)

of deep cracks and crevices often makes them very difficult to exterminate. Barracks and similar buildings may be fumigated with cyanide gas or sulphur or heated to about 140° Fahrenheit for six hours. Kerosene, gasoline and various cresol and phenol mixtures are effective, but must be applied to beds, floors and walls with a small brush, a feather or a spray syringe to be sure of getting the insecticide into the crevices where the bedbugs hide.

A very efficacious measure for the control of bedbugs in the animal quarters of laboratories is the weekly sterilization of all animal cages by live steam. The bugs which are attracted each night to the animals usually hide in the crevices of the cages by day, where they are destroyed by the heat when the cages are steamed.

II. Family Reduviidæ—"Assassin-Bugs"

The bugs of this family have long narrow heads, bearing prominent compound eyes, long, four-jointed antennæ and usually two small ocelli. The proboscis is three-segmented, folded back under the head when at rest, and is usually long, slender and straight in blood-sucking genera; shorter, stouter and arched or bent in genera that feed on other insects. The prothorax is provided with functional wings and the legs are long, with three-jointed tarsi.

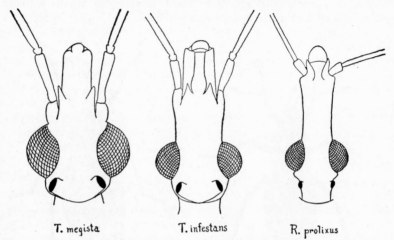

T. megista T. infestans R. prolixus

Fig. 295.—Heads of *Triatoma megista* and *infestans* and of *Rhodnius prolixus*, showing where the antennæ arise. (Original. Root)

The female lays over 200 eggs in groups of 8 to 12 which hatch within 20 to 30 days. The larvæ feed for the first time in about 5 days, and as in the case of bedbugs, secrete themselves in dark crevices and other hiding places during the day. A blood meal is necessary before each moult, and the length of time spent in each stage is about 40 to 50 days. The entire life-cycle usually requires a year or more.

Most reduviids feed on other insects, piercing their chitinous integument and sucking out the internal soft parts. Many of these species will occasionally bite man if carelessly handled. But in certain genera (*Triatoma* and *Rhodnius*) all the species whose habits have been studied live as habitat parasites in houses or in the nests of animals. These genera (Figure 295) are of parasitological interest because they include the vectors of South American trypanosomiasis caused by *Trypanosoma cruzi*.

The genera, *Triatoma* and *Rhodnius* are often called cone-nosed bugs because of the great extension of the head in front of the eyes. In Brazil they are known as "barbeiros" (barbers) because they frequently bite the faces of sleepers. In Spanish America they are often called "vinchucas" or "chinchas voladoras" (flying bedbugs). The species are mostly either brownish without any striking markings, or else dark, almost black, with regularly arranged red or yellow markings on prothorax, wings or the borders of the abdomen. A number of species frequent houses, especially the rude dirt huts of the poorer natives, and feed on human blood. Others are sometimes found in houses, but occur more often in chicken-houses or in the burrows of armadillos and rodents, and a few species have only been taken in this last habitat. It seems probable that all the species are able to transmit *Trypanosoma cruzi*, for laboratory experiments with many different species of *Triatoma* and *Rhodnius* and species of the related genera *Eratyrus* and *Panstrongylus* have been successful. The species which are of most importance in transmitting the disease to man are probably *T. megista* and *T. sordida* in Brazil, *T. infestans* in Argentina and Paraguay, and *Rh. prolixus* in Venezuela. *T. geniculata* and *Rh. pallescens* have been incriminated as vectors in Panama. Kofoid and Donat (1933) discovered *Trypanosoma cruzi* in *Triatoma protracta* in California and were able to infect a large number of species of rats and mice with it. Natural infections have also been found in *Triatoma uhleri* (Kofoid and Whitaker, 1936) in western United States and in *T. pallidipennis* and *T. phyllosoma* in Mexico (Whitaker, 1937). So far, no human case of the disease has been reported.

The three genera mentioned above may be distinguished by the characters given in the following synopsis (compare Figure 295):

SYNOPSIS OF THE GENERA OF BLOOD-SUCKING REDUVIIDÆ

Ocelli present; anterior coxæ short; thorax constricted anteriorly; apex of scutellum with one spine or none; ocelli behind and as far apart as compound eyes; antennæ inserted laterally..........
    Mesonotum with lateral spines ....*Eratyrus*.
    Mesonotum without lateral spines ....
        Abdomen very broad, extending far beyond folded wings on the sides ....*Meccus*.
        Abdomen more slender, most of it concealed by the wings when they are folded ....
            Antennæ inserted near the anterior end of the head .... *Rhodnius*.
            Antennæ inserted near compound eyes or else about midway between compound eyes and anterior end of head .... *Triatoma*.

CHAPTER XLIX

THE CLASS ARACHNIDA AND THE ORDER ACARINA

The Class ARACHNIDA is a very large group of arthropods and includes many parasites of man and animals which either produce disease directly or are responsible for the transmission of serious diseases. The spiders, scorpions, ticks, mites, and other related groups are included in the ARACHNIDA.

The main structural characteristics which differentiate the Class ARACHNIDA from the Class INSECTA are the absence of wings and antennæ, the presence of four pairs of legs, and the fact that the head and thorax are always fused together, forming a *cephalothorax*. In the Order ACARINA, in which we are particularly interested, this fusion has advanced even farther, and usually head, thorax and abdomen are all fused together so that the whole body is a single, unsegmented sack.

The Class ARACHNIDA is divided into about eleven orders. Of these, five include the true spiders (Order ARANEIDA) and other creatures of similar appearance, with small, compact bodies and long legs. Three other orders include the scorpions and their allies, with large bodies, short, stout legs, and slender, elongate abdomens, which bears a sting at its tip in the true scorpions (Order SCORPIONIDA). The other three orders are the king or horseshoe crabs, the "water-bears," and the ticks and mites (Order ACARINA). Only the last-named order is of great parasitological interest, although some spiders by their bites, and scorpions, by their stings, are occasionally troublesome to man. The scorpions found in the United States are too small to be dangerous, and the only spider found in this country whose bite is really serious is the black, red-spotted species sometimes called the "Black Widow" (*Latrodectus mactans*).

The Order ACARINA includes the ticks and mites, most of which are of small size. In this order the head, thorax and abdomen are all fused together forming an unsegmented body. At the anterior end of this body, a small part of the head region is usually segmented off and hinged to the body proper to serve as a movable base for the mouth parts. This base, together with the mouth parts, bears the name of *capitulum,* and the base itself is termed the *basis capituli.* The mouth parts of the ACARINA include a pair of *chelicerœ* or *mandibles,* which sometimes bear chitinized teeth or claws at their tips; a pair of palp-like structures, the *pedipalps,* consisting of five joints or less; and a median *hypostome,* which can sometimes be seen to consist of two fused halves. This hypostome is a prominent structure covered with small backwardly-pointing teeth in the ticks, but is usually inconspicuous and unarmed in the other mites. One or more pairs of simple eyes or *ocelli* may be present, but are always placed on the anterior part of the body proper, never on the capitulum.

In some mites the chitinous integument is membranous throughout, in others some portions of the integument are thickened into protective plates or shields. Often there is a dorsal shield or *scutum,* covering either the entire back or the anterior portion of it. Sometimes ventral plates are present also, often around or near the anal and genital apertures. The *anus* is placed ventrally, near the posterior end of the body, in most forms. The *genital aperture* is also ventral and always anterior to the anus, sometimes so far forward that it is near the capitulum. The body and legs of mites usually bear regularly arranged hairs or bristles.

The legs are usually attached to the ventral surface of the body, the basal joints or *coxœ* sometimes resembling additional ventral plates. Usually each leg consists of about six similar joints, which are called *coxa, trochanter, femur, tibia, protarsus* and *tarsus.* The last joint or tarsus may bear *claws,* a pad or *pulvillus,* a *sucker* or merely some long *bristles.* In some mites the two posterior pairs of legs are far separated from the two anterior pairs.

Some mites have no obvious *spiracles* or respiratory apertures. In others there are spiracles on the cephalothoracic portion of the body. In the ticks and some related forms, there is a pair of *spiracles* or *stigmal plates* laterally near the coxæ of the third or fourth pair of legs.

The ACARINA differ in their internal anatomy rather markedly from the insects. The following brief description of the internal anatomy of ticks will serve to demonstrate these differences (see Figure 296). The alimentary canal consists of fore-gut, mid-gut, and hind-gut. The fore-gut consists of the *buccal cavity,* a single pair of *salivary glands* with their ducts, the *pharynx* which serves as a pumping organ, and an S-shaped *esophagus* which passes through the brain. The mid-gut is made up of the *stomach, rectum, rectal sac* and a pair of *Malpighian tubules.* The stomach is the

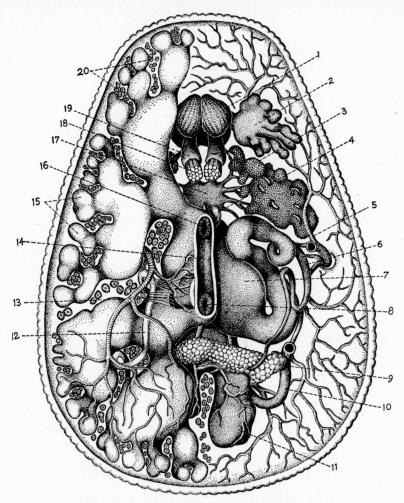

FIG. 296.—Internal anatomy of tick. (Redrawn from Robinson and Davidson by Esther Bohlman)

1—Gené's organ
2—Glandular portion, Gené's organ
3—Salivary gland
4—Accessory genital gland
5—Trachea
6—Oviduct
7—Uterus
8—Rectum
9—Ovary
10—Malpighian tubule

11—Rectal sac
12—Malpighian tubule
13—Heart
14—Stomach
15—Alimentary ceca
16—Esophagus
17—Brain
18—Muscles of chelicera
19—Chelicera
20—Dorso-ventral body muscles

largest organ of the body and consists of four large lobes or ceca which fill in the spaces left by the other organs. The rectal sac is a large vesicle into which the rectum and Malpighian tubules open and from which a short canal communicates with the anus. The two Malpighian tubules pass forward and upward and may be coiled or convoluted. They end blindly near the base of the capitulum. An opaque white substance is excreted by them into the rectal sac. Dorsal to the stomach is the heart, a single-chambered vessel which exhibits rapid, regular pulsations. The *cephalic aorta* runs forward from the heart to the dorsal surface of the brain, where it opens into the *periganglionic sinus* which envelops the central nervous system. Four arterial trunks leaving this sinus on either side supply blood to the legs. Corresponding nerves lie within these arteries. The anterior portion of the sinus encloses the esophagus and pharynx and supplies the chelicerae. The blood finds its way back through the lacunar spaces between the organs of the body. Contractions of the dorso-ventral body muscles effect a circulation of the blood in the middle and hind parts of the body. The respiratory system consists of a pair of external *spiracles* and a highly developed system of tracheae which divide and subdivide until all of the organs are supplied by their branches. Excretion is accomplished by the Malpighian tubules and the *coxal glands* which lie above and between Coxa I and Coxa II and are known to secrete copiously during and after engorgement. An olfactory organ (*Haller's organ*) is located on the tarsi of the first pair of legs and *tactile* hairs are distributed over most of the body, but conspicuously on the ends of the pedipalps. *Eyes* are present in some species on the lateral, anterior margins of the body. The genital organs of the female consist of a single *ovary, oviducts,* a *uterus, vagina,* and *Gené's organ.* There is no seminal receptacle, the uterus serving in this capacity. The *accessory glands* open into the vagina and are probably concerned with oviposition. All ticks are oviparous. Gené's organ is a large paired organ (see Figure 296) in the anterior portion of the body which probably prevents premature drying of the eggs at oviposition by its secretions. The male genital organs consist of a single *testis,* a pair of *vasa deferentia,* a *seminal vesicle,* a *ductus ejaculatorius* and *accessory glands.* There is no intromittent organ. The spermatozoa are introduced into the female genital tract in the form of *spermatophores* by the capitulum of the male.

In their life histories, ACARINA usually pass through four stages, egg, larva, nymph and adult. The larva has only three pairs of legs (see Figure 297). When it moults to become a nymph it acquires a fourth pair of legs but still lacks a genital aperture. The nymph, in turn, moults and becomes an adult, with four pairs of legs and a genital aperture. Where there are sexual differences between male and female adults, as in the hard ticks, the nymphs all resemble the females in these respects.

Mites are extremely numerous both in species and in individuals and are found in all sorts of habitats. Some are ectoparasitic, others

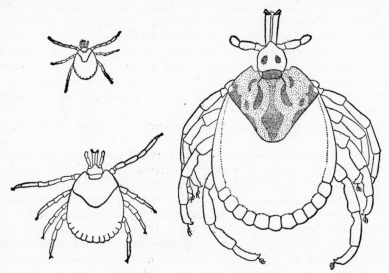

FIG. 297.—Unfed larva, nymph and adult female of *Amblyomma cajennense,* drawn to the same scale. (Original. Root)

endoparasitic on or in all sorts of animals and plants. Some are terrestrial, others live in fresh or salt water. Some feed on decaying animal or vegetable matter, others on stored foods, others on plants, others on minute animals, and the parasitic forms on blood. The following keys to the superfamilies and families of mites are adapted from those given by Ewing (1929). Names in parentheses indicate groups which contain no forms of importance in the transmission or causation of disease.

KEYS TO THE SUBORDERS, SUPERFAMILIES AND FAMILIES OF ACARINA

I. *Key to the Suborders and Superfamilies of* ACARINA

1. Tracheæ opening through a pair of spiracles situated laterally
   on the sides of the body .................MESOSTIGMATA   (5)
   Tracheæ, when present, not opening on the sides of the body.   (2)

2. Tracheæ usually present and opening at or near the bases of the cheliceræ; adults free-living; larvæ frequently parasitic .... PROSTIGMATA (6)
Tracheæ, when present, never opening at or near bases of the chelickeræ .... (3)

3. Tracheæ present; abdomen showing evidences of segmentation; females frequently with a pair of clavate sensory organs between the bases of the first and second legs .... HETEROSTIGMATA (8)
Tracheæ wanting; abdomen without true segmentation; females never provided with clavate sensory organs between first and second legs .... (4)

4. Body stout, not vermiform, legs composed of more than three segments .... ASTIGMATA (9)
Body vermiform, legs rudimentary and apparently composed of but three segments; parasitic in hair follicles of mammals .... BRACHYPODA (10)

5. Hypostome small or absent, never with recurved teeth; tracheæ each opening through a chitinous plate; sternal plate seldom absent .... PARASITOIDEA (see Key II)
Hypostome large and provided with recurved teeth; tracheæ each opening through a chitinous plate; sternal plate nearly always wanting; skin always leathery... IXODOIDEA (Ticks).

6. Last palpal segment never forming a thumb to the preceding; legs without swollen tarsi .... (EUPODOIDEA).
Last palpal segment forming a thumb to the preceding, which ends in a claw; tarsi frequently swollen .... (7)

7. Legs not adapted for swimming. Land mites .... TROMBIDOIDEA (see Key III)
Legs adapted for swimming. Water mites.. (HYDRACHNOIDEA).

8. The single superfamily ...... TARSONEMOIDEA (see Key IV)

9. Skin without fine parallel folds; tarsi without stalked suckers; adults never true parasites on vertebrates.. TYROGLYPHOIDEA.
Skin with fine parallel folds; tarsi frequently provided with stalked suckers; parasitic in all stages and chiefly on vertebrates .... SARCOPTOIDEA (see Key V)

10. Single superfamily and family .... DEMODICOIDEA.

II. *Key to the Families of* PARASITOIDEA

1. First pair of legs usually inclosed with the mouthparts in a body opening; genital apertures of both sexes entirely surrounded by the sternal plate; nymphs frequently attached to arthropods by means of a gluelike pedicel for purposes of transportation .... (UROPODIDÆ).
First pair of legs not so inclosed, genital opening of female never completely surrounded by sternal plate; nymphs never attached by pedicel to arthropods 2

2. Cheliceræ of a generalized type with incurved tips and with teeth, the fixed arm usually bearing a seta near its tip; body usually well covered with chitinous plates; anal plate in both sexes, if present, usually united with ventral plate. Chiefly

free or associated with arthropods ....PARASITIDÆ.
Cheliceræ modified, usually without teeth and fixed arm always
without seta; body usually only partly covered both above
and below with chitinous plates; anal plate nearly always
present and distinct from ventral plate in females. Parasitic
on vertebrates ....DERMANYSSIDÆ.

III. *Key to the Families of* TROMBIDOIDEA

1. Cheliceræ sickle-shaped, not needle-like   2
   Cheliceræ usually styletiform or needle-like   4
2. First and second legs provided with processes bearing large
   spines, integument with large chitinous shields. (CÆCULIDÆ).
   First and second legs without processes bearing spines; integument without large chitinous shields   3
3. Cephalothorax without any rod-like structure nor median dorsal groove, legs more slender and tarsi never swollen
   .... (ANYSTIDÆ).
   Cephalothorax with a rod-like structure at the bottom of a
   median dorsal groove, legs stouter and usually with swollen
   tarsi .... TROMBIDIIDÆ.
4. Cephalothorax with rod-like structure in a dorsal median
   groove; tarsi usually somewhat swollen, never attenuated;
   body well clothed with short setæ .... (ERYTHÆIDÆ).
   Cephalothorax without rod-like structure nor dorsal groove;
   tarsi attenuated; body sparsely clothed with setæ of varying lengths   5
5. Each tarsus provided with either comb-shaped distal appendage or clinging hairs or both; palpi moderate or small.
   Plant-feeding mites .... (TETRANYCHIDÆ).
   Tarsi usually without comb-shaped appendage and always without clinging hairs; palpi usually large; predaceous or parasitic species ....CHEYLETIDÆ.

IV. *Key to the Families of* TARSONEMOIDEA

1. Females with elongate bodies; capitulum and first pairs of legs
   not hidden by any projecting cephalothoracic shield   2
   Females usually with subdiscoidal bodies; capitulum and first
   two pairs of legs hidden by the projecting cephalothoracic
   shield .... (DISPARIPEDIDÆ).
2. Females with four pairs of legs and the last pair ending in two
   claws and caruncle. Usually ovoviviparous...PEDICULOIDIDÆ.
   Fourth pair of legs of female, if present, devoid of claws and
   usually of caruncles. Usually oviparous......TARSONEMIDÆ.

V. *Key to the Families of* SARCOPTOIDEA

1. Either maxillæ or some of the legs modified into hair-clasping
   organs. Parasitic on mammals ...........LISTROPHORIDÆ.
   Without any specialized apparatus for clasping the hairs of
   mammals. Parasitic on insects, birds or mammals.........   2

2. Body strongly depressed; sexual dimorphism sometimes very
    pronounced. Live among feathers of birds..... ANALGESIDÆ.
    Body seldom strongly depressed. Not found on or in feathers.
    Soft-bodied mites   3
3. Inhabit living tissues of vertebrates   4
    Parasitic exclusively upon insects .... (CANESTRINIIDÆ).
4. Vulva longitudinal. Parasitic in tissues of birds. CYTOLEICHIDÆ.
    Vulva transverse; mouth-parts free. Parasitic on or in the
    skins of birds and mammals .... SARCOPTIDÆ.

CHAPTER L

THE TICKS (SUPERFAMILY IXODOIDEA)

The ticks are distinguished from the other mites by their toothed or armed hypostome and by the presence of a pair of definite spiracles placed just behind the third or fourth pair of coxæ. They are also decidedly larger than most mites, the newly hatched larvæ of the ticks being about the same size as the adult stage of the larger

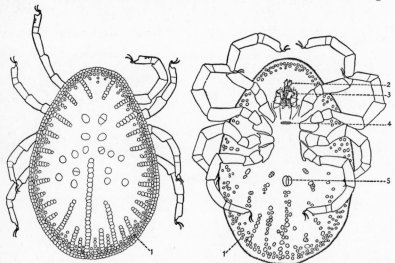

Fig. 298.—Dorsal (left) and ventral (right) views of *Argas persicus*. (x 24. Original. Root; Huff)

1—Integumental discs	3—Pedipalp	5—Anus
2—Chelicera	4—Genital opening	

species of mites. Ticks are usually regarded as blood-sucking ectoparasites of vertebrates, although it is worth pointing out that many of them do not remain on the host after engorgement is completed and are, strictly speaking, free-living organisms during the periods when they moult and lay eggs. Most ticks are normally parasitic on certain mammals, birds, reptiles or amphibians, but nearly all species will bite man if they have the opportunity and certain species are known to be the usual carriers of human diseases. Other ticks are vectors of important diseases of domestic birds and mammals.

The superfamily IXODOIDEA is divided into two families, the ARGASIDÆ and IXODIDÆ. In the soft ticks, constituting the family ARGASIDÆ, the two sexes are much alike (Figure 298). Neither sex has a hard dorsal scutum, the capitulum is ventrally located, the spiracles are behind the third pair of coxæ, the coxæ are not spurred and the tarsi bear no pads or pulvilli. The ticks of this family have much the same habits as bedbugs, hiding in cracks or crevices in houses or in the nests of their hosts and coming out at night to feed on the blood of the host for a short period, usually less than half an hour. The larvæ and nymphs usually feed several times

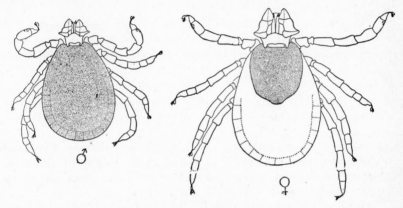

FIG. 299.—Dorsal views of male and female hard ticks, *Hæmaphysalis leporis-palustris*. (Original. Root)

before moulting and the adult female usually feeds a number of times, laying a small batch of eggs after each feed.

In the hard ticks (family IXODIDÆ) the two sexes are often very dissimilar in appearance (Figure 299), because the hard dorsal scutum, which both sexes possess, covers the entire dorsal surface in the male but extends over only a small part of the anterior portion of the dorsum of the female. The capitulum is placed at the anterior end of the body, the spiracles are behind the fourth pair of coxæ, the coxæ are generally armed with spurs and the tarsi always have pads or pulvilli as well as claws. The ticks of this family attach themselves firmly to their hosts and remain upon them, sucking blood, for days or even weeks. The larvæ and nymphs take only one blood meal in each stage and the adult female takes only a single enormous blood meal before dropping off the host to digest the blood and lay a single large batch of eggs.

I. Family Argasidæ—Soft ticks

This family includes only two genera, *Argas* and *Ornithodorus*. The typical species of the two genera are distinct enough, but there are some intergrading forms which are difficult to place. *Nuttalleilla* has been proposed as a new genus to contain some of these species. The principal characteristics of the two genera are as follows:

> *Argas:* Body thin and flat, with a sharp-edged lateral margin which is distinct even when the tick has fed; integument minutely wrinkled, with many oval or rounded discs, arranged in radiating lines.
>
> *Ornithodorus:* Body thicker, with the margin thick, rounded and poorly defined, even in unfed ticks; integument covered with rounded protuberances or mammillæ, and usually without discs.

I. SOFT TICKS CONCERNED IN THE TRANSMISSION OF DISEASE

Argas persicus Oken: this species is common in many parts of the tropics and subtropics. It is ordinarily parasitic on fowls, but will occasionally bite man. It is the vector of fowl spirochætosis (*Spironema gallinarum*), and of *Ægyptianella pullorum,* a parasite of unknown affinities which is found in the blood of the fowl (Bedford and Coles, 1933). In Europe there are other species of *Argas* which parasitize pigeons and bats.

Ornithodorus moubata Murray: the fever tick of tropical Africa. This species has adopted exactly the mode of life of a bedbug. It lives in cracks of walls or floors of the native huts, coming out at night to feed. The life history is unusual in that the larval stage is passed in the egg, without a blood meal, a nymph emerging from the egg about twenty days after the egg was laid. This species is the vector of the tropical African or endemic type of relapsing fever (often called tick fever) caused by *Spirochæta duttoni*. As is often true in tick-borne diseases, a female *O. moubata* infected with the relapsing fever spirochæte normally produces infected offspring, also capable of transmitting the disease. In the laboratory the infection has thus been passed on from a single infected female to three generations of her progeny (Möllers, 1907) without any further contact with the spirochætes. Another similar and closely related species, *Ornithodorus savignyi* Audouin, transmits relapsing fever (*Sp. persica*) in Abyssinia, Persia and India.

Ornithodorus talaje Guerin-Meneville; *Ornithodorus turicata* Duges: these two species are the vectors of the relapsing fever of tropical America (*Sp. novyi*). They are sometimes found in large numbers in crude bunks or bedsteads made of bamboo and other materials which afford them numerous crevices to hide in.

A new species, *Ornithodorus hermsi,* has been shown to be a vector of relapsing fever in California (Herms and Wheeler, 1936), and *O. turicata* has been incriminated in Texas by Kemp, Moursund, and Wright (1934).

Ornithodorus megnini Duges: this species rarely attacks man, but is worth mentioning because of its aberrant life history. The larvæ and nymphs are usually found in the ears of cattle and horses and are known as "spinose ear-ticks." When the nymph is full-grown it drops to the ground and moults to become an adult. The adults do not attempt to find a host, but climb up fence-posts and walls and hide in the crevices, where copulation and egg-laying occur.

The American species of argasid ticks may be identified by the following key.

KEY TO THE AMERICAN SPECIES OF THE FAMILY ARGASIDÆ

1. Margin of body flattened, sharp-edged ....*Argas*   2
   Margin of body thick, rounded, not clearly defined
   .... *Ornithodorus*   3
2. Margin of body with quadrangular "cells" ....*A. persicus.*
   Margin of body striate; body narrowed anteriorly
   ....*A. reflexus* var. *magnus.*
3. Integument pitted ....*O. megnini.*
   Integument mammillated or granular   4
4. Fourth tarsus smooth above, without spurs or humps..........   5
   Fourth tarsus with a prominent subapical spur or hump dorsally   7
5. First tarsus without humps dorsally; a lateral flap on each side
   of capitulum ....*talaje.*
   First tarsus with three or four dorsal humps; no lateral flaps
   near capitulum   6
6. Mammillæ of mid-dorsal region about 10 per linear millimeter;
   three humps on tarsus I ....*turicata.*
   Mammillæ of mid-dorsal region about 18 per linear millimeter;
   four humps on tarsus I ....*parkeri.*
7. Eyes present; first tarsus with medial and subapical spurs
   .... *coriaceus.*
   Eyes absent   8
8. First tarsus with subapical hump; without spurs..*venezuelensis.*
   First tarsus with spurs   9
9. First tarsus with basal and subapical spurs ....*rostratus.*
   First tarsus with subapical spur only ....*hermsi.*

The species described by Matheson (1935) from Central American bats (*O. dunni, O. azteci, O. brodyi*) are not included in the above key. Likewise, *O. brasiliensis* Aragão and *O. nicollei* Mooser have not been included because of lack of opportunity for examining specimens of them. The former would seem to be related to *rostratus* and the latter to *venezuelensis*. McIvor has (1937) described a new species, *Ornithodorus wheeleri*, from California which according to her description is closely related to *turicata* and differs from this species in having longer club-shaped hairs, in the thickenings of the anterior margins of the transverse post-anal groove, in having a more pointed capitulum, in the distinctive arrangement of the hypostomal teeth, and in the number and arrangement of protuberances on tarsi I and IV. Tarsus I of *O. wheeleri* has five of these protuberances, well-defined, with a club-shaped hair between the basal two; tarsus IV has one well-defined protuberance above the claws and six long spines surrounding the claws.

II. *Family Ixodidæ—Hard Ticks*

This family includes a number of genera and a very large number of species. The relatively small and inconspicuous males can be readily assigned to genera, since in many of them there are characteristically located thickened plates or shields on the ventral surface. The females lack these ventral shields and are often difficult to identify, particularly when fully engorged. The following brief summary of the characters used in identifying the genera of the IXODIDÆ will enable the student to use the key to the genera more readily.

Capitulum (Figure 300). The basis capituli may appear rounded, rectangular or hexagonal in dorsal view. The mouth parts, consisting of hypostome, cheliceræ and pedipalps, may be either short (about the same length as the basis capituli) or long (much longer than the basis capituli). In the pedipalps, the elongation, when present, affects especially the second joint. The pedipalps consist of four joints the first and third being always short, while the fourth is always reduced to a small spherical structure, usually placed in a depression near the tip of the third joint. In most genera the pedipalps ensheath the other mouth parts and the entire mouth part complex is narrower than the basis capituli, but in *Hæmaphysalis* the second joints of the pedipalps are laterally produced so that they extend beyond the edges of the basis capituli.

Body. Dorsally there is a shield or *scutum* which is comparatively small in the female but covers the entire dorsal surface in the male. When *eyes* are present, they are placed on or near the lateral margins of the scutum. In some ticks the scutum is *ornate*, that is, it has a more or less brilliant, enamel-like coloration, often white, yellow, or red, which makes it stand out clearly in the female against the dark or brownish body-color. Around the posterior edge of the body there is sometimes a submarginal furrow or groove, connected with the margin by a number of shorter grooves, w h i c h break up the margin into little rectangular areas called *festoons*.

Ventrally all adult ixodid ticks have the *genital opening* a little behind the capitulum and the *anus* posteriorly, near the tip of the body. The four pairs of *coxæ* form shield-like plates on the ventral surface. In most of these ticks, certain grooves are readily seen ventrally. The pair of *genital grooves* begin anteriorly at the sides of the genital opening and run posteriorly and then somewhat outwardly to the posterior margin of the body. The single *anal groove* usually connects the two genital grooves, being arched posteriorly so that it runs behind the anus, but in *Ixodes* the anal groove runs in front of the anus and both

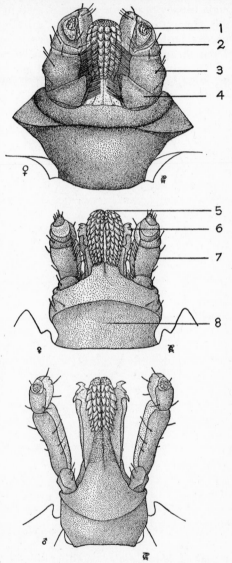

FIG. 300.—Ventral views of capitula of *Rhipicephalus* (above), *Dermacentor* (middle) and *Amblyomma* (below). (After Hunter and Hooker)

1—4th pedipalp joint	5—Hypostome
2—3rd pedipalp joint	6—Chelicera
3—2nd pedipalp joint	7—Pedipalp
4—1st pedipalp joint	8—Basis capituli

ends usually reach the posterior margin of the body, without having any connection with the genital grooves. In species having the anal groove posterior to the anus there is sometimes a *post-anal groove,* from the middle of the anal groove toward the posterior margin.

In the males of certain ixodid genera, *ventral plates* are present. In *Rhipicephalus, Hyalomma* and *Boophilus* (Figure 303) there is

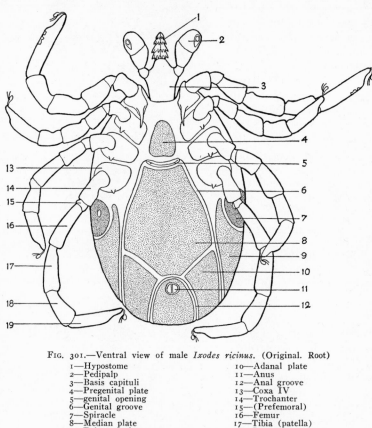

FIG. 301.—Ventral view of male *Ixodes ricinus.* (Original. Root)

1—Hypostome	10—Adanal plate
2—Pedipalp	11—Anus
3—Basis capituli	12—Anal groove
4—Pregenital plate	13—Coxa IV
5—genital opening	14—Trochanter
6—Genital groove	15—(Prefemoral)
7—Spiracle	16—Femur
8—Median plate	17—Tibia (patella)
9—Epimeral plate	18—Protarsus

19—Tarsus

a pair of *adanal plates* on either side of the anus and a pair of *accessory plates* lateral to the *adanal plates* and separated from them by the genital grooves. In *Margaropus* there is a posteriorly forked *preanal plate,* which may correspond to fused adanal plates. In the male of *Ixodes* (Figure 301), the greater part of the ventral surface is covered with plates, consisting of a pair of *adanal plates,* a pair of *epimeral plates* outside the genital grooves, an *anal plate* which bears the anus, a large *median plate* between the anus and the genital opening, and a small *pregenital plate* between the genital opening and the capitulum.

Behind and above the fourth pair of coxæ are the *spiracles,* which are sometimes round or oval but often more or less comma-shaped. As has been pointed out by Stiles (1910) the shape and minute structure of the spiracles are often useful in differentiating closely-related species of ticks.

KEY TO THE GENERA OF THE FAMILY IXODIDÆ

1. Anal groove running in front of anus; pedipalps usually spatulate in form; male with numerous ventral plates..........*Ixodes.*
   Anal groove either running behind anus or so indistinct that it cannot be seen clearly 2
2. Mouth parts about as long as basis capituli; second joint of pedipalps not much longer than wide 3
   Mouth parts much longer than basis capituli; second joint of pedipalps much longer than wide 8
3. Anal groove plainly visible; festoons usually present 4
   Anal groove absent or indistinct; festoons absent 7
4. Second joint of pedipalps laterally produced, so that it extends beyond the edges of the basis capituli; eyes absent
   ....*Hæmaphysalis.*
   Second joint of pedipalps not laterally produced; eyes present.. 5
5. Basis capituli rectangular in dorsal view; scutum usually ornate; male without ventral plates; fourth coxa of male much larger than the others ....*Dermacentor.*
   Basis capituli hexagonal in dorsal view; scutum usually not ornate 6
6. Male without ventral plates and with fourth coxa much larger than the others ....*Rhipicentor.*
   Male with ventral plates and with fourth coxa not much larger than the others ....*Rhipicephalus.*
7. Male with forked pre-anal plate; joints of fourth pair of legs greatly swollen ....*Margaropus.*
   Male with paired adanal and accessory plates; joints of fourth pair of legs normal ....*Boophilus.*
8. Eyes absent; males without ventral plates..........*Aponomma.*
   Eyes present 9
9. Eyes submarginal; males with ventral plates........*Hyalomma.*
   Eyes marginal; males without ventral plates.......*Amblyomma.*

I. LIFE HISTORY OF IXODID TICKS

The majority of ixodid ticks whose life history is known have what is called the "three-host" type of life-cycle. In such a tick as

Dermacentor andersoni, the spotted fever tick, for example, the larval tick after hatching from the egg climbs to a blade of grass or a bush and waits for a host to come within its reach. When it gets on a host it attaches itself, engorges with blood and drops off again, digesting the blood meal and moulting to become a nymph on the ground. The nymph repeats this procedure on a second host and

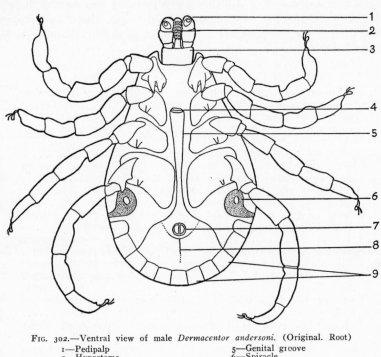

FIG. 302.—Ventral view of male *Dermacentor andersoni.* (Original. Root)

1—Pedipalp
2—Hypostome
3—Basis capituli
4—Genital opening
5—Genital groove
6—Spiracle
7—Anus
8—Post-anal groove
9—Festoons

again drops off to digest its meal and transform to the adult stage. The adult female is fertilized by the male either before or after she becomes attached to a third host. When fully engorged, the female drops from the host, digests the blood meal and lays a very large batch of eggs before dying. Not infrequently, ixodid ticks have different species of hosts in their different stages. In the case of *Dermacentor andersoni,* for example, the larvæ and nymphs are found in the greatest numbers on ground-squirrels and other rodents, while the adults are most numerous on cattle, horses and other large mammals.

It is obvious that this "three-host" type of life-cycle is a rather

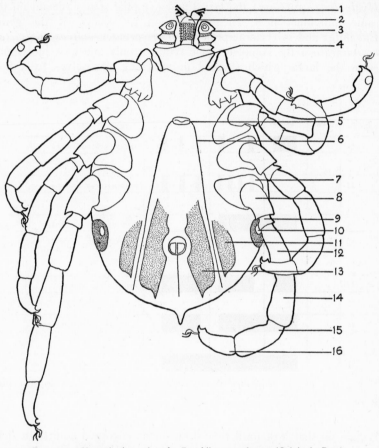

FIG. 303.—Ventral view of male *Boophilus annulatus*. (Original. Root)

1—Chelicera	9—(Prefemoral)
2—Hypostome	10—Spiracle
3—Pedipalp	11—Accessory plate
4—Basis capituli	12—Femur
5—Genital opening	13—Adanal plate
6—Genital groove	14—Tibia (patella)
7—Coxa	15—Protarsus
8—Trochanter	16—Tarsus

wasteful one, since each tick has to be lucky enough to have a host come within its reach three separate times in order to attain the adult condition and reproduce. A few species of ixodid ticks are known which have adopted the more efficient plan of remaining on a single host individual during two or even during all three stages of their life-cycle. In three species (*Rhipicephalus evertsi* and *bursa* and *Hyalomma ægyptium*) the larval and nymphal stages remain on the same individual host. In the common cattle-ticks of the genus *Boophilus* and in certain species of *Dermacentor* (*nitens, albipictus, nigrolineatus*) the complete cycle requires only one host individual, since the larvæ which succeed in attaching themselves to a host

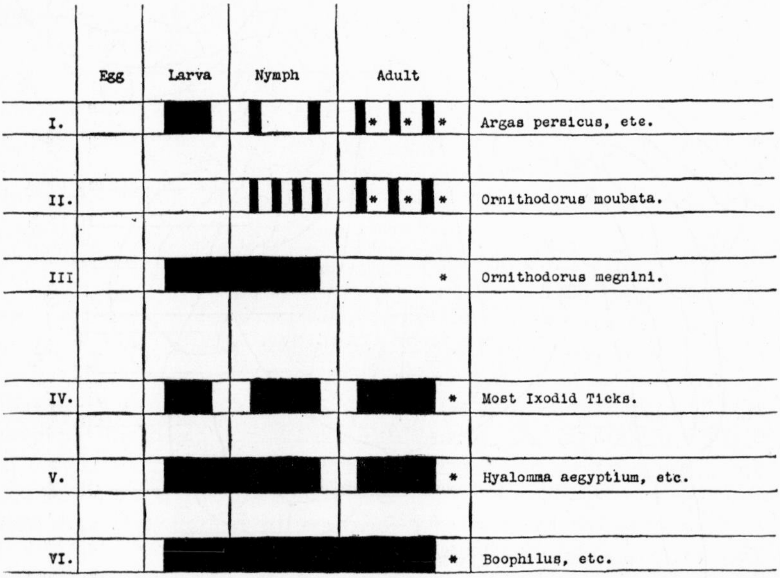

	Egg	Larva	Nymph	Adult	
I.		■	▮	* * *	Argas persicus, etc.
II.		▮▮▮▮		* * *	Ornithodorus moubata.
III		▬▬▬		*	Ornithodorus megnini.
IV.		■ ▮	▬▬	*	Most Ixodid Ticks.
V.		▬▬▬	▬	*	Hyalomma aegyptium, etc.
VI.		▬▬▬▬		*	Boophilus, etc.

Fig. 304.—Diagram illustrating the different types of life-cycles of various ticks. Black areas indicate periods of attachment to host; asterisks indicate ovipositions. (Original. Root)

remain on that host until they drop off as engorged adults. In ticks with this type of life-cycle, the passing on of a disease-producing organism from an infected female to her progeny, which is the rule in all tick-borne disease, is absolutely essential to the transmission of the disease in nature, since each tick feeds on only a single host individual.

The table (Figure 304) illustrates graphically the various types of life-cycles found in ticks. The black rectangles in the columns headed "larva," "nymph" and "adult" indicate approximately the periods during which the ticks are attached to their host. The asterisks in the column headed "adult" show the time of oviposition by the female.

2. NOTES ON SOME OF THE GENERA OF IXODID TICKS

Ixodes Latreille: the ticks of this genus are sharply separated from the other ixodid ticks by the position of the anal groove and the number of ventral plates present in the male. The spatulate pedipalps are also very characteristic. Two small groups of species which parasitize marine birds and bats, respectively, are separated generically from the other forms by some authors. The more typical species are mainly parasites of large and small mammals. The best-known species is *I. ricinus* (Figure 301), which is found on sheep, cattle and various wild mammals in Europe, North Africa, Asia and North America. *I. hexagonus* is found on many small mammals in Europe and *I. hexagonus* var. *cookei* has been taken from a number of small mammals in the United States. *I. holocyclus* is an Australian species which causes tick paralysis of human beings and domestic animals. Many other species are described and illustrated by Nuttall *et al.* (1911).

Hæmaphysalis Koch: the lateral projection of the second joints of the pedipalps is especially characteristic of this genus. In the United States the most abundant species is *H. leporis-palustris* of rabbits (Figure 299). *H. leachi* is a common dog tick in Africa and also occurs in Asia and Australia. *H. cinnabarina* has been frequently found on birds in the United States, but the variety *punctata* of Europe has usually been taken from the larger domestic animals. Other species are described and illustrated by Nuttall and Warburton (1915).

Dermacentor Koch: this genus includes a number of very similar species. Stiles (1910) has pointed out the value of the form and structure of the spiracles for distinguishing the species of this genus. It includes the common "wood-ticks" and "dog-ticks" of the United States, *D. variabilis* in the Eastern States, *D. andersoni* (Figure 302) in the Rocky Mountain region and *D. occidentalis* on the Pacific coast. In Europe, Asia and Africa *D. reticulatus* is found on many of the larger mammals. *D. nitens* is found in the ears of horses in the American tropics.

Rhipicephalus Koch (Figure 300): this genus is connected with *Dermacentor* through the small and unimportant genus *Rhipicentor* Nuttall and Warburton, in which the male resembles *Rhipicephalus* dorsally and *Dermacentor* ventrally. *Rhipicephalus* includes a number of species, most of which are African. *R. sanguineus* is widely distributed in warm regions, including the southern United States, occurring especially on dogs. *R. bursa* is found on sheep and cattle in Africa and southern Europe. *R. evertsi, R. appendiculatus, R. simus,* and *R. capensis* are tropical African species found on cattle and horses.

Boophilus Curtice: this genus and the closely related *Margaropus* Karsch differ from all other ixodid ticks in lacking an anal groove. It includes the common "cattle-tick" of the southern United States, *B. annulatus* (Figure 303). Very similar species or varieties occur in other parts of the world, for example, *australis* in Australia, South America; *decoloratus* in Africa, and so forth. In all these forms the male is exceedingly small as compared with the enormous size attained by engorged females.

Hyalomma Koch: this genus includes only a few species, of which *H. ægyptium* is the most important. It is found on cattle and other large mammals in Africa, Asia and southern Europe. The male has ventral plates and also two protrusions from the tip of the abdomen which are capped with chitinous points.

Amblyomma Koch: this includes more species than any other genus of ticks. About half the species are American, the rest are distributed in Africa, Asia and Australia. Many species are parasitic on large mammals, many others on reptiles or amphibians, fewer on small mammals and very few on birds. In all the species the scutum is ornate, in some very brilliantly colored. *A. americanum* is found on cattle in the southern United States and tropical America. It is sometimes called the "lone star tick," because of the silvery spot at the tip of the female scutum. *A. maculatum* also occurs on these hosts in the same general region. *A. cajennense* (Figure 297) is very abundant in many parts of tropical and subtropical America. It is found on many of the larger mammals, including man, and the larvæ or "seed-ticks" sometimes attack human beings in large numbers, causing great annoyance. *A. hebræum,* the "bont tick" of South Africa, is found on many large mammals, both wild and domestic. *A. dissimile* is common on snakes, lizards and toads in the American tropics. For the numerous other species see Robinson (1926). The closely related genus or subgenus *Aponomma* differs from *Amblyomma* in the more rounded body form and the absence of eyes. The species of *Aponomma* occur on reptiles, especially snakes, in the Old World tropics.

3. IXODID TICKS AS VECTORS OF DISEASE

The most important group of diseases of man transmitted by ixodid ticks is Rocky Mountain spotted fever and its close relatives. The true Rocky Mountain spotted fever is found chiefly in Montana and Idaho, although it has been reported from practically all of the western United States. It is a disease of wild rodents and is transmissible to man and to laboratory animals. The causative organism is a rickettsia, *Dermacentroxenus rickettsi,* which lives intracellularly in both the ixodid and the vertebrate hosts and is regularly passed on from infected female ticks to their progenies through the eggs. For this reason, the ticks acquire their infections as larvæ or nymphs and carry the disease organisms over the winter in the nymphal stage. When the adults emerge in the spring shortly after the melting of the snow they may attack man and transmit the disease to him. The ticks most responsible for transmitting the disease are *Dermacentor andersoni* and *Hæmaphysalis leporispalustris.* In laboratory experiments *D. variabilis, D. marginatus,* and *Amblyomma americanum* have also been shown to be able to transmit the infection (Mayer, 1911).

Diseases similar to Rocky Mountain spotted fever are now known to exist in other parts of the country and the world. Eastern spotted fever, a much milder form than the Rocky Mountain type, is found widely distributed over the eastern United States but occurs chiefly in the Allegheny mountains. It is transmitted by the common wood tick, *Dermacentor variabilis.* Boutonneuse fever is found in the Mediterranean region where it is transmitted by the dog tick, *Rhipicephalus sanguineus.* In South Africa this tick and also *Hyalomma ægyptium* are the vectors. São Paulo fever is a similar disease in Brazil and is known to be transmitted by *Amblyomma cajennense.*

In nature only a very small percentage of ticks are infective and human cases are not very common except in certain restricted localities. By way of control, measures for reducing the number of ticks have been used, such as dipping domestic animals in an arsenical solution, burning over the infected areas or grazing sheep on them so that they will pick up the ticks, which soon die in their wool. Tourists, campers and hikers should be careful not to allow ticks to become attached to their bodies when they are in a region where Rocky Mountain spotted fever is known to occur. A fairly effective vaccine has been made from infected ticks which reduces the mortality very considerably in persons receiving it as a prophylaxis. It is worthy of note that it represents the first successful vaccine to be prepared from the arthropod vectors of a disease.

Tularemia is transmitted from rodent to rodent by *Hæmaphysalis leporis-palustris* and ticks of the genera, *Rhipicephalus* and *Amblyomma*. The transmission can be made from rabbit to man by *Dermacentor andersoni* and possibly *D. variabilis*.

In several different parts of the world there occurs a progressive paralysis of man or animals, apparently as a direct result of the bites of certain species of ticks. This tick paralysis may result in death if neglected, but the removal of the engorging tick is said to result in speedy recovery without any injurious sequelæ. In the Rocky Mountain region of North America, tick paralysis of children and of sheep is caused by the bites of *Dermacentor andersoni*. In Australia a similar disease of human beings and domestic animals is produced by *Ixodes holocyclus*. In Africa *Ixodes pilosus* causes a similar disease of sheep.

The ixodid ticks are of far greater importance in the transmission of diseases of animals than they are in the transmission of human disease. The piroplasmas of animals cause serious disease in various parts of the world. In all cases they are transmitted by ticks, and, as in the case of Rocky Mountain spotted fever, the causative organisms are passed through the egg stage. There are, however, many variations as to the stage in the life of the tick at which the infection is acquired and also at which it is transmitted. Other important diseases of animals caused by Anaplasmas, Rickettsiæ, and related organisms are also transmitted by ticks, and recently a number of filterable viruses of animals have also been found to be transmitted by ticks.

Vectors of bovine and ovine piroplasmoses. *Babesia bigemina* which causes Texas cattle or redwater fever is transmitted by *Boophilus annulatus* and its varieties, and by *Rhipicephalus appendiculatus* and *Hæmaphysalis punctata* (in northern Europe). *Babesia bovis* which also produces a hæmoglobinuric fever is transmitted by *Ixodes ricinus* and *Hæmaphysalis punctata,* while *Babesia mutans* which causes a benign infection is transmitted by *Rhipicephalus evertsi* and *R. appendiculatus*. In the case of *B. mutans* the parasite is not transmitted through the egg stage. Another serious disease of cattle, East Coast fever, is caused by *Theileria parva* and occurs chiefly in Africa. It is transmitted by *Rhipicephalus appendiculatus, R. capensis, R. evertsi, R. simus, Dermacentor reticulatus, D. nitens,* and *Hyalomma ægyptium.*

Babesia motasi causes a hæmoglobinuric fever in sheep and goats and *B. ovis* causes a disease called carceag in the same animals. They are transmitted by *Rhipicephalus bursa. Theileria recondita* of sheep is transmitted by *Dermacentor silvarum.*

Vectors of equine piroplasmoses. A hæmoglobinuric fever of horses in southern Europe is caused by *Babesia caballi* and is transmitted by *Dermacentor reticulatus. Babesia equi* causes a similar disease in Africa, South America, southern Europe and Transcaucasia. It is transmitted by *Rhipicephalus evertsi* in South Africa and by *R. bursa* in Italy.

Vectors of canine piroplasmoses. Malignant jaundice of dogs (*Babesia canis*) is transmitted by *Hæmaphysalis leachi* in S. Africa, by *Rhipicephalus sanguineus* in Asia, Europe, and North Africa and by *Dermacentor reticulatus* in Europe. It has been experimentally transmitted by *Dermacentor andersoni. Babesia gibsoni* is transmitted by *Hæmaphysalis bispinosum* in India, and *Rhipicephalus simus* which is found on jackals is suspected of transmitting this disease to them.

A hæmogregarine, *Hepatzoon canis,* is transmitted by *Rhipicephalus appendiculatus.*

Vectors of Anaplasmoses. Gallsickness of cattle is caused by *Anaplasma marginale* and is transmitted by a large number of ticks: *Boophilus decoloratus, B. annulatus,* and *B. microplus; Rhipicephalus bursa, R. simus,* and *R. sanguineus; Dermacentor andersoni, D. variabilis, D. occidentalis; Ixodes ricinus,* and *Hyalomma lusitanicum.* There is a difference of opinion as to whether this organism can be carried through the egg stage of the tick. *Anaplasma ovis* is transmitted by *Dermacentor silvarum.*

Vectors of various other animal diseases: heartwater, a disease of sheep, goats, and cattle in South Africa is caused by *Rickettsia ruminantium* and is transmitted by *Amblyomma hebræum* and *A. variegatum. Eperythrozoon wenyoni* of cattle is transmitted by a species of *Hyalomma.*

The filterable viruses of animals which are known to be transmitted by ticks are: louping ill of sheep, Nairobi sheep disease, tick fever (of sheep), and equine encephalomyelitis (western strain). Louping ill is a disease of high mortality transmitted by *Ixodes ricinus* and *Rhipicephalus appendiculatus.* Nairobi sheep disease is transmitted by *Rhipicephalus appendiculatus* and *Amblyomma variegatum.* Tick fever is transmitted by *Ixodes ricinus.* The virus of the western strain of equine encephalomyelitis has been experimentally transmitted by *Dermacentor andersoni* (Syverton and Berry, 1936).

CHAPTER LI

PARASITIC MITES

The term, *mite,* is applied to all of the ACARINA excepting the superfamily Ixodoidea (the ticks). They are among the smallest of the arthropods and are known to live in about every type of habitat and climate. A large percentage of them are free-living. Among the parasitic ones there is every degree of parasitism from incidental parasitism to obligate parasitism. They attack plants and animals— vertebrate and invertebrate, aquatic and terrestrial. They do not constitute a natural or systematic group but are thought to have arisen from many different stems. Some produce disease, others transmit disease among higher animals and man. This chapter will be devoted to the more important of the parasitic forms.

I. *Superfamily Parasitoidea*

The gamasid mites include many parasitic forms. The families can be separated by means of Key II, page 663. Most of the species of UROPODIDÆ are free-living, although some parasitize arthropods. The PARASITIDÆ includes both free-living species and species parasitic on vertebrates and invertebrates. The DERMANYSSIDÆ are all parasitic and are found on reptiles, birds, and mammals.

Keys for the genera of PARASITIDÆ and DERMANYSSIDÆ are given by Ewing (1929). The PARASITIDÆ contains the genera, *Lælaps, Echinolælaps,* and *Hæmogamasus* which are parasites of rodents and moles. *Echinolælaps echidninus* is the vector of the hæmogregarine of rats, *Hepatozoon muris,* the life-cycle of which was carefully studied by Miller (1908).

In the family DERMANYSSIDÆ the genera, *Dermanyssus, Liponyssus,* and *Pneumonyssus* are of particular interest to us. *Dermanyssus gallinæ,* the chicken mite, is blood-sucking but does not ordinarily remain long upon its host after feeding. Its biting habits resemble those of argasid ticks and bedbugs. This mite may also attack man and cause a dermatitis. *Liponyssus bursa,* the Tropical Fowl Mite, and *L. sylviarum,* the Northern Fowl Mite, are both

682

injurious to poultry. *Liponyssus saurarum* is the vector of the coc-cidian, *Schellackia bolivari,* of lizards. The Tropical Rat Mite, *Liponyssus bacoti* (see Figure 305), is known to attack man not infrequently, and Dove and Shelmire (1932) have shown that this

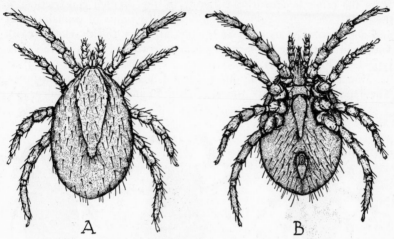

FIG. 305.—Dorsal (A) and ventral (B) views of female *Liponyssus bacoti,* the tropical rat mite. (x 50. After Dove and Shelmire)

mite can transmit endemic typhus from rat to rat. Their finding that the Rickettsiæ of this disease pass through the egg stage to the next generation of mites indicates that typhus may have originated from mites (see Huff, 1938).

II. *Superfamily Trombidoidea*

All of the mites of this group are free-living in the adult stage. Their larvæ may be free-living or parasitic. The family CÆCULIDÆ consists of free-living mites and the family ERYTHRÆIDÆ consists of species parasitic on invertebrates only. The TETRANYCHIDÆ, or Spinning Mites, are not parasitic but one of the species, *Tetranychus telarius,* (Spider Mite) often crawls onto man, although it does not bite him. Some species of the family CHYLETIDÆ are parasitic, though none of them is of much importance. Some species of the genus, *Harpyrynchus,* infest the skins of birds and produce large tumors about the feather follicles.

The family TROMBIDIIDÆ includes, among other forms, the "harvest mites," "chiggers" or "red-bugs," which are often so annoying to human beings. These very minute, red mites which attack man in many different parts of the world, are the six-legged larval stage of mites of the genus *Trombicula*. The nymphal and adult stages of these mites, which are not parasitic but feed on arthropod excreta, decaying vegetable matter, and the like, may be easily differentiated from the other genera of the family by the decided constriction of the body (see Figure 306), which defines the limits of cephalothorax and abdomen. The nymphs and adults are very thickly clothed with feathered hairs, but the larvæ have only scattered hairs of the same type (see Figure 306).

Man is apparently only an accidental host for these larval mites. The Japanese species are found in large numbers on field mice, par-

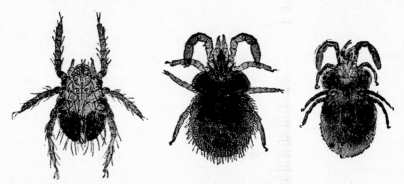

FIG. 306.—Larva (left), nymph (center) and adult (right) of *Trombicula akamushi*. Not to the same scale. (After Nagayo *et al.*)

ticularly on the ears. According to Ewing (1921, 1926) turtles and perhaps snakes are important hosts of the common American species. Ewing (1923) states that the species which occurs in the eastern and southern United States is *Trombicula tlalzahuatl* Murray, originally described from Mexico.

In Japan, the larvæ of *Trombicula akamushi* (Figure 306) have been proved to be the vectors of Tsutsugamushi disease, also called Japanese river (or flood) fever. This disease is a typhus-like fever caused by a rickettsia. It occurs in certain limited areas, near rivers, in Japan. The same or similar diseases, believed also to be carried by *Trombicula* larvæ, are reported from Formosa, China and Sumatra. In the last-named region the disease is known as "pseudo-typhus." In Tsutsugamushi disease the infection is acquired by the larvæ of one generation and is passed on through the nymphal, adult, and egg stages to the next generation of larvæ which can then transmit it to rodents and man. The adults and nymphs cannot transmit the disease directly to vertebrates because they are not parasitic. In Japanese localities where Tsutsugamushi disease has been studied, Nagayo and others (1921) have found larvæ of five species of *Trombicula* on field mice, but find that only one of these species (*T. akamushi*) attacks man.

The larvæ of *Trombicula autumnalis* and *T. irritans* * are respectively the Autumnal Chigger of Europe and the North American Chigger. The latter are also referred to as "Red Bugs." They attack a large variety of animals and man. Unless they are killed or removed shortly after they attack man they cause a small lesion which is very annoying. *Neoschöngastia americana* is very injurious to chickens in the southern United States.

There are a number of other genera of TROMBIDIIDÆ, but not much is known of their habits and life-histories. In some genera, the larvæ are parasitic on house-flies, grasshoppers and other insects, but apparently do not attack vertebrates.

III. *Superfamily Hydrachnoidea*

The Water Mites are parasitic in the larval stage upon aquatic invertebrates. They resemble harvest mites very much, but, unlike them, are adapted to swimming. They are of little importance to parasitology.

IV. *Superfamily Tarsonemoidea*

Many of the mites of this family are destructive to cultivated plants, and are therefore of considerable economic importance. Others are beneficial, since they are predaceous on certain insect pests of crops. One of these species, *Pediculoides ventricosus,* is often predaceous on the larvæ of several minute insects which infest grain and straw. Threshing crews, grain-handlers and people sleeping on mattresses stuffed with unsterilized straws are sometimes attacked by large numbers of these mites, which produce a severe and annoying skin eruption (see Webster, 1910).

The Tracheal Mite of the Honey Bee, *Acarapis woodi,* causes "Isle of Wight" disease in adult bees. These mites live within the thoracic tracheæ of the bee and bring about paralysis of the muscles of flight. Another species is of interest because of its extreme degeneracy. *Podapolipus reconditus* is found only under the elytra of

---

* Ewing (1938) points out that the name *irritans* is preoccupied and the species must, therefore, be designated *Trombicula alfreddugèsi* Oudemans.

certain species of beetles in the Old World, and the female is reduced to little more than a sac containing eggs.

V. *Superfamily Tyroglyphoidea*

Many species of these "cheese mites" live and feed upon stored food products of various kinds, and some of them will attack man at times. Species of *Glyciphagus,* for example, are found in sugar and may produce a dermatitis known as "grocer's itch." Diseases known as "copra itch," "coolie itch," and the like are also produced by mites of this family. Since these mites occur in all sorts of food, they are frequently swallowed by human beings, and the mites and their eggs are often encountered when making fecal examinations to detect the presence of protozoa or the eggs of helminths.

VI. *Superfamily Sarcoptoidea*

These mites are well adapted to the parasitic habit. Besides the forms causing itch and mange which are placed in the SARCOPTIDÆ, there are four other families (see Key V, page 664). The LISTRO-PHORIDÆ are the "hair-clasping" mites which cling to the hairs of small mammals and feed upon them. The ANALGESIDÆ or Feather Mites consist of a large number of genera and species some of which parasitize the flight feathers, others are found on other feathers of birds, while still others live next to the skin. The CYTOLEICHIDÆ occur within the tissues of birds, particularly in the air passages. One species, *Cytoleichus nudus,* occurs in gallinaceous birds. The CANES-TRINIIDÆ are parasitic on insects.

The family SARCOPTIDÆ includes the itch and mange mites of man, mammals and birds, and is of great medical and veterinary interest. Most of the species are small, with striated integument and the two anterior pairs of legs widely separated from the two posterior pairs at their origin. Some of the legs usually end in stalked suckers, others in long bristles. There are often sexual differences in this respect. The following key to the genera of SARCOPTIDÆ is from Ewing (1929).

KEY TO THE GENERA OF SARCOPTIDÆ

1. Tarsal suckers with unsegmented pedicels 2
   Tarsal suckers with segmented pedicels; males with rudimentary posterior legs and with anal suckers..............*Psoroptes.*
2. Both sexes provided with tarsal suckers on all legs....*Psoralges.*
   One or both of the sexes with at least one pair of legs without tarsal suckers 3

3. Males with all the legs provided with a tarsal sucker 4
   Some of the legs of the males without tarsal suckers 9
4. Females with some of the legs provided with tarsal suckers.... 5
   Females without tarsal suckers on legs 8
5. Females with tarsal suckers on first, second and fourth pairs of
   legs ....*Chorioptes.*
   Females with tarsal suckers on first and second pairs of legs only 6
6. Male with abdomen two-lobed behind and provided with anal
   suckers .... *Caparina.*
   Male with abdomen not bilobed, or very slightly so 7
7. In the female each leg of the last two pairs ending in a single
   long seta ....*Prosopodectes.*
   In the female each leg of the last two pairs ending in two long
   setæ .... *Otodectes.*
8. Females with a pair of dorsal, longitudinal bars and with long
   terminal setæ; anal opening terminal ....*Cnemidocoptes.*
   Females without such bars and terminal setæ; anal opening dorsal .... *Nycteridocoptes.*
9. Some of the legs of females provided with tarsal suckers...... 10
   All of the legs of females without tarsal suckers....*Teinocoptes.*
10. Anal opening dorsal; dorsal surface of body with only short,
   sharp setæ .... *Notoedres.*
   Anal opening not dorsal, but terminal; dorsal surface of body
   studded with sharp, pointed scales and small, stubby spines
   .... *Sarcoptes.*

The genera *Sarcoptes* and *Notœdres* include the "itch mites" of
man and other mammals. The species found on man is *Sarcoptes
scabiei.* In these itch mites, the pregnant female burrows into the
skin, laying eggs along the burrow as she progresses. An intolerable
itching is produced, followed by inflammation and pustule formation.
As with most forms of acarine dermatitis, sulphur ointment is the
standard remedy. The skin should be repeatedly washed with soap
and water before applying the ointment. Success in ridding an individual of the infestation can only be attained by persistent repeti-
tion of the treatment semi-weekly until all of the parasites have
been killed. Other species or varieties of *Sarcoptes* cause similar
conditions known as itch or mange in various wild and domestic
animals. Mites of the genus *Notœdres* produce similar diseases in
cats and other small mammals.

Most of the other genera of SARCOPTIDÆ may be lumped together
as "scab mites." These mites do not burrow into the skin, but remain
on the surface, often producing such irritation that a many-layered
scab is produced. Beneath this scab and between the layers the mites
may be present in very large numbers. The species *Psoroptes ovis*
(Figure 307) has several varieties which cause sheep scab, Texas itch

of cattle and mange in horses and dogs. *Psoroptes cuniculi* often causes extensive scab-formation in the ears of laboratory rabbits. Species of *Chorioptes* and *Otodectes* also produce similar diseases in horses, sheep and cattle. *Otodectes cynotus* may invade the inner ear

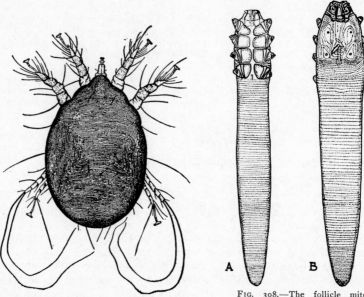

FIG. 307.—Adult female of *Psoroptes ovis* as an example of a sarcoptid mite. (After Salmon and Stiles)

FIG. 308.—The follicle mite *Demodex folliculorum.* (A) ventral view of female, (B) dorsal view of male. (Redrawn from Patton and Evans. After Hirst)

of the dog and cause deafness and convulsions. In the genus *Cnemidocoptes,* parasitic on birds, *C. mutans* causes the "scaly leg" disease of poultry while *C. gallinæ* is called the "depluming mite" of fowls because it irritates the skin so much that the hens pluck out their feathers. *Notœdres cati* causes head mange in cats which is a severe type of scabies.

VII. *Superfamily Demodicoidea*

This superfamily consists of the single family DEMODICIDÆ, which has but one genus, *Demodex*. *Demodex folliculorum* (Figure 308) is said to be parasitic in the sebaceous glands and hair follicles of a large proportion of the human race. It appears to do no particular damage to its host, whereas related species or varieties of *Demodex* cause severe mange in dogs and damage the skins of swine and cattle.

CHAPTER LII

MISCELLANEOUS ARTHROPODS OF PARASITOLOGICAL INTEREST

In the foregoing chapters of this text we have discussed the most important arthropods concerned in the causation and transmission of disease in man and animals. A large number of other arthropods, some of them belonging to groups not already mentioned, may also assume considerable interest by becoming incidental parasites or by producing symptoms in man or animals by their toxic secretions. Many of the most important arthropods from the standpoint of their transmission of disease attract very little interest by their direct parasitism of man. Thus a yellow fever mosquito might transmit yellow fever which might be fatal to man and yet the direct and immediate effect of the bite itself might even go unnoticed. The arthropods under consideration in this chapter usually do not produce serious disease; on the other hand, they may at times become very annoying and therefore attract considerable attention.

A second group of arthropods contains many species which serve as intermediate hosts for other parasites of man and animals. This group is so large and complex that it cannot be given detailed consideration in this book. A brief summary, however, will be given at the end of this chapter.

I. *Arthropods Which Produce Symptoms by their Direct Action on the Host*

Some of the most important of these forms have already been discussed in the foregoing chapters. Thus the action of fly larvæ in producing myiasis is discussed in Chapter XLV. There are also discussions of the action of ticks in producing tick paralysis in man and animals, of the harmful effect of parasitic mites, including the one which produces scabies, and some mention is made of the bites of spiders and scorpions. We shall here discuss some of the orders of arthropods which have not received consideration so far, and in addition will give further consideration to forms only casually mentioned in the preceding chapters.

I. COLEOPTERA

The COLEOPTERA, or beetles, are well known insects, and are easily distinguished by the greatly thickened first pair of wings which serve as wing covers for the membranous hind wings. These wing covers, or *elytra,* meet in a straight line over the abdomen.

Beetles may act as facultative parasites or incidental parasites. They are also of interest in the production of blisters by the vesicating principle found in some of them. Beetles or their larvæ sometimes set up a parasitism in man or animals the effect of which is referred to as Canthariasis. This is rather an uncommon happening and probably usually results from ingestion of the beetles or their eggs or larvæ along with food of the host, or by the crawling of the insects into some natural cavity of the body. The churchyard beetle, *Blaps mortisaga,* has on several occasions been found to act as an accidental parasite. This species and several closely related forms have been described from the intestine and very probably had been ingested along with food. Some of the forms which are thought to attack directly by crawling into wounds or cavities are scarabæid beetles, which in Ceylon are known to produce intense diarrhea in children. Others have been recorded from the urinary tract, from the conjunctiva of the eye, and from discharges from the sphenoid sinuses. In the latter case the black carpet beetle, *Attagenus piceus,* was incriminated.

The Blister Beetles receive their name from the action of a vesicating principle, known pharmacally as *cantharidin,* in producing blisters on the skin. Most of them belong to the family MELOIDÆ although one genus of rove beetles, *Pæderus,* possesses the vesicating property. The best known species as a source of cantharidin is the so-called Spanish Fly, *Meloë vesicatoria,* although species of the genus *Mylarbris* give a larger yield of the substance. Curiously enough most of the cantharidin is found in the elytra. While the extract is still used externally as a vesicant its action internally as a diuretic and aphrodisiac is extremely dangerous.

The general subject of the insects used in medicine is reviewed by Hinman (1933).

2. HEMIPTERA

The bugs which act as true parasites of vertebrates have already been discussed in Chapter XLVIII. In addition, a large number of these insects which normally feed upon plant juices or are predaceous on small animals occasionally attack man and animals. The NOTONECTIDÆ or back swimmers inflict a painful bite, as also do some of the giant water bugs (BELOSTOMIDÆ: *Lethocercus* and *Benacus*). The latter are popularly known as electric light bugs because of the attraction which electric street lights have for them.

The families MIRIDÆ, ANTHOCORIDÆ, and LYGÆIDÆ contain species which may occasionally suck blood or at least by attempting to do so, cause an irritation to result on the skin at the site of the bite. The tarnished plant bug, *Lygus pratensis,* and the insidious flower bug, *Triphleps insidiosus,* are two of these incidental parasites. Many others have been reported but none is known to be of importance as a parasite.

Hoffman (1927) recorded an irritation of the skin resulting from the secretion from *Loxa flavicollis,* one of the PENTATOMIDÆ.

3. LEPIDOPTERA

Cases of direct parasitism by moths or butterflies are very rare. However, a large number of caterpillars and a smaller number of adult moths possess poisonous spines which have an urticating action on the human skin. Some of these are: *Megalopyge opercularis* and *Lagoa crispata,* flannel-moths, the caterpillars of which are called "puss" caterpillars (Family MEGALOPYGIDÆ); *Sibine stimulea,* the saddle-backed caterpillar, and *Parasa chloris* (Family EUCLEIDÆ); *Automeris io,* the most generally known moth in the eastern and central states with urticating hairs (Family SATURNIIDÆ); and the brown-tail moth (*Euproctis chrysorrhœa*) and the tussock moth (*Hemerocampa leucostigma*) of the family LYMANTRIIDÆ. Tyzzer (1907) described the pathology of the brown-tail moth dermatitis and Kephart (1914) described the histology of the hypodermis of the brown-tail moth caterpillar and reviewed the literature up to that date on the properties of the substance responsible for the urticaria.

4. HYMENOPTERA

None of the insects of this order is parasitic on higher animals, but many are provided with an ovipositor modified into a stinging apparatus. The poison used in stinging is secreted by glands which have connections with the modified ovipositor. Although considerable study has been given to the poison, the chemical composition of the active principle has not yet been determined. Many species of bees, wasps and hornets and some species of ants are capable of stinging. The effect of the sting varies greatly with the species of animal attacked and, in man, with the individual susceptibility. To some individuals a bee sting is a very serious matter requiring the attention of a physician. Bee keepers have learned some very helpful rules for avoiding the attacks of bees, the most effective of which is that the person should be entirely clothed in white garments. Bee stings are usually fatal to ducklings which attempt to eat the bee and are stung on the tongue.

5. POISONOUS ARACHNIDA

Order Scorpionida. The scorpions are arachnida in which the pedipalps are developed into strong claws or chelæ and which have an abdomen divided into two portions. The first seven segments are broad, whereas the five terminal ones are narrow, giving the appearance of a tail. This "tail" is often turned forward over the head and is provided on the last segment with a sharp spine curved ventrally and provided with a pair of poison glands. These animals have a very bad reputation and some of the tropical species are now known to be so poisonous as to bring death to individuals stung by them. There are, however, no dangerous species known in the United States.

Order Araneida. The spiders have a cephalothorax and the fusion of segments of the abdomen is usually complete. The eight legs are all attached to the cephalothorax. A pair of cheliceræ serve as mandibles and the pedipalps resemble legs. The spiders which are poisonous owe this characteristic to the presence of poison glands which connect by a small duct to the tips of the claws on the cheliceræ. Like the scorpions, the spiders are very much feared and the effects of their bites have been much exaggerated. It is rather generally agreed now that the bites of most species of spiders are relatively harmless, but that the species of the genus *Latrodectus* deserve much of their evil reputation. The Black Widow spider (*L. mactans*) is, perhaps, the only poisonous spider in the United States. Several other species of the genus in other parts of the world are known to be poisonous and some to produce death. The female, which is responsible for the bites inflicted, is one-half to two inches in length and glossy black with red or yellow markings. The bright red patch on the ventral surface of the abdomen is the most characteristic marking. The shape of this spot has given the spider the name, the Hour-glass Spider. While the effects of the bite of this species may be severe—depending somewhat upon the site of the bite—it is not definitely known to be fatal to normal individuals but might be so to individuals with badly diseased hearts and other ailments of a serious nature. The literature on this spider was reviewed by Bogen (1926).

II. *Arthropods Serving as Intermediate Hosts*
of Miscellaneous Helminths

Although many of the important helminth parasites which utilize arthropods as intermediate hosts have already been discussed in the preceding chapters, many of the arthropods which serve as intermediate hosts of less important helminths have received scant or no consideration. Hall (1929) collected a list of arthropod hosts of worms and arranged them according to the natural relationships of the worms and also according to groups of arthropods. He listed a total of 271 species of arthropods which serve as intermediate hosts of worms. The number of species of worms involved was 143.

There were 49 species of crustacea which act as intermediate hosts for cestodes, 22 for trematodes, and 12 for nematodes. Twenty-five species of insects serve as intermediate hosts for cestodes, 46 for trematodes, 122 for nematodes and 15 for acanthocephala. Two species of myriopods serve as hosts for cestodes and six species of arachnids are intermediate hosts for nematodes. The following list by Hall shows the distribution of the arthropods by orders, serving as intermediate hosts for cestodes, trematodes, nematodes, and acan-

Arthropod group	Cestoda	Trematoda	Nematoda	*Acantho-* cephala
Amphipoda	+	+	+	+
Branchiopoda	−	+	−	−
Cladocera	+	−	+	−
Copepoda	+	+	+	−
Decapoda	+	+	−	+
Isopoda	−	−	+	+
Ostracoda	+	−	−	−
Anoplura	−	−	+	−
Coleoptera	+	+	+	+
Dermaptera	+	−	−	−
Diptera	+	+	+	−
Ephemerida	−	+	+	−
Isoptera	−	−	+	−
Lepidoptera	+	+	−	−
Mallophaga	+	−	+	−
Neuroptera	−	+	−	+
Odonata	+	+	+	−
Orthoptera	−	−	+	+
Plecoptera	−	+	−	−
Siphonaptera	+	−	+	−
Trichoptera	−	+	−	−
Insecta; unplaced	−	+	−	−
Myriapoda	+	−	−	−
Arachnida	−	−	+	−

thocephala. The plus marks indicate known cases of intermediate hosts in the group in which it occurs, the minus signs the lack of any such cases.

Summarizing further from Hall's paper, the outstanding groups of intermediate hosts for the four orders of parasites are:

For Cestoda: Copepoda and Ostracoda; Coleoptera.

For Trematoda: Decapoda; Diptera, Trichoptera, Odonata, Ephemerida.

For Nematoda: Copepoda; Diptera and Coleoptera.

For Acanthocephala: Amphipoda; Coleoptera.

A few of the more interesting and important parasites and their hosts not already discussed are given in Table V.

TABLE V

Scientific name	Group	Vertebrate hosts	Invertebrate hosts	Group
Hymenolepis diminuta	Cestoda	Man, rat, mouse	*Tenebrio molitor*, *Akis spinosa*, *Scaurus striatus*	Coleoptera
			Tinea granella, *Asopia farinalis*, *Pyralis farinalis*	Lepidoptera
			Anisolabis annulipes	Dermaptera
			Nosopsyllus fasciatus, *Xenopsylla cheopis*, etc.	Siphonaptera
			Fontaria virginiensis	Myriapoda
Prosthogonimus macrorchis	Trematoda	Domestic fowl; ducks	*Leucorrhinia* spp., *Tetragoneuria*, spp., *Epicordulina* spp.	Odonata
Gongylonema scutatum	Nematoda	Sheep, cattle, horse	*Blatella germanica*	Orthoptera
			Species of *Blaps*, *Aphodius*, *Onthophagus*, etc.	Coleoptera
Macracanthorhynchus hirudinaceus	Acanthocephala	Swine, man	Species of *Melolontha*, *Diloboderus*, *Phyllophaga*, etc.	Coleoptera
Moniliformis moniliformis	Acanthocephala	Rodents, man	*Blaps gigas*, *Blaps mucronata*, *Periplaneta americana*	Coleoptera
			Blatta orientalis	Orthoptera

NOTES ON COLLECTING, PRESERVING, AND REARING ARTHROPODS OF PARASITOLOGICAL IMPORTANCE

I. *Collecting*

The arthropods of parasitological interest may be roughly divided into three groups, the blood-sucking flies, the flies whose larvæ live in feces or carcasses or parasitize living mammals and the ectoparasitic insects and ACARINA.

The adults of the blood-sucking flies can be captured while feeding on man or on a horse or cow used as bait. This method will secure only the females of those groups in which this sex alone feeds on blood. Males of mosquitoes and tabanids can be secured in numbers only by breeding out specimens from the larvæ. This has the added advantage of procuring perfect and undamaged specimens.

Similarly the adults of the muscoid flies whose larvæ live in filth or carrion or are parasitic, may usually be collected on appropriate baits or around the animals their larvæ parasitize. But in this case also, better specimens are usually obtained by breeding out adults from eggs laid by captive females or from captured larvæ.

The ectoparasitic forms are usually collected from the bodies of their hosts or in the nests of the hosts. Fleas may also be bred from the nests of animals and birds by enclosing the nest in a box or other container, with moist blotting-paper added to maintain a humid atmosphere. When fleas, lice and ticks are collected, the host species should be accurately identified and recorded.

Most of the smaller blood-sucking flies can be captured in test-tubes or in a chloroform tube, prepared by placing rubber bands or a slice of a rubber stopper in the bottom of a large tube and allowing the rubber to soak up all the chloroform it will absorb. The rubber should then be prevented from coming in contact with the insects by pushing a piece of blotting paper or a wad of cotton tied up in gauze down upon it. Such killing tubes may be used for some time without the addition of any more chloroform, if they are kept tightly corked when not in use. For capturing the larger flies, such as tabanids and muscoid flies, an insect net is often necessary. The bag should be made of bobbinet or fine-meshed gauze, so that the net may be used to capture mosquitoes and black-flies occasionally.

Parasitic insects may be stupefied by chloroform and then picked from their hosts with fine forceps or combed out from the fur with a fine-toothed comb. They are usually placed directly into vials of alcohol to kill and preserve them. If captured alive, lice, mites and ticks may be killed by pouring over them water which is not quite boiling hot. This tends to make them die with legs well extended. This is also the best method of killing larvæ of the muscoid flies. All material killed in hot water should be transferred to alcohol for preservation.

II. *Preserving*

Adult insects and ticks will keep indefinitely if they are simply allowed to become dry and then are preserved from breakage, insect pests and molds. In permanent collections, insects are usually trans-fixed with special insect-pins and pinned in rows into cork-lined boxes or cabinets. Large flies, like tabanids and the muscoid flies, may be pinned with No. 3 pins. Smaller flies, like mosquitoes, are usually impaled upon the points of very fine, short pins (called "minuten pins") which have been previously thrust through a small strip of cork or a rectangular bit of cardboard or celluloid. The other end of the cork or celluloid is then transfixed by a large insect pin (No. 5 is very convenient for this purpose) by which it may be handled and pinned into the cabinet. When traveling, it is often most convenient to preserve mosquitoes and other small flies in pill-boxes partly filled with cotton. If a number of such pill-boxes are kept in a tin can with tight-fitting cover, they can be conveniently fumigated at intervals, with a few drops of carbon disulphide, to destroy the minute insect pests which would otherwise eat the specimens. Speci-mens preserved in this way may later be glued to the tips of wedge-shaped bits of cardboard with a tiny drop of shellac and pinned into the insect box or cabinet with other specimens.

The larvæ and larval and pupal skins of mosquitoes and other small flies may be mounted in balsam on microscopic slides for study and permanent preservation without any special treatment. In select-ing *Anopheles* larvæ for total amounts, the least pigmented and most transparent larvæ should be picked out, in order to obtain the best results. In mounting culicine larvæ, it is often advisable to cut the larva in two at the seventh abdominal segment, mounting the anterior portion to give a dorsal view and the posterior portion to give a lateral view.

In making balsam mounts of larger fly larvæ and of small adult flies, fleas, lice and ticks the usual method is to soak the insects in 10 per cent solution of sodium or potassium hydroxide until the soft parts are destroyed, leaving only the chitinous integument. This method is also used in preparing the male terminalia of mosquitoes, and the like, for mounting. The process should be carefully watched, the object being to destroy the internal structures as completely as is possible without bleaching or damaging the external chitinous parts. The process can be speeded up by warming the liquid and even boiling temperatures are sometimes used, but the cold process, while much slower, usually yields better preparations. After treatment with caustic soda or potash, the insects must be thoroughly washed in water before putting them into alcohol.

Before insects and their larvæ and larval skins, either treated with caustic potash or not, can be mounted in Canada balsam under the cover-glass, they must be dehydrated and cleared. This is most easily accomplished by soaking them for some minutes, first in 95 per cent ethyl alcohol and then in carbol-xylol (carbolic acid crystals— 1 part and xylol—3 parts). In the tropics, especially, carbol-xylol is essential, on account of the extreme difficulty of keeping absolute alcohol water-free in a humid atmosphere. Sometimes weak-skinned larvæ tend to collapse when passed directly from carbol-xylol into balsam. This may be avoided by passing them from carbol-xylol into cedar oil (the kind prepared for use as a clearing agent, not the thickened cedar oil used with oil-immersion lenses) and then into balsam. Cedar oil also has the useful property of absorbing small air-bubbles which sometimes get inside the specimens and are difficult to remove in any other way.

Some authorities prefer to stain caustic potash preparations before mounting them, particularly lice and the male hypopygia of small flies. Acid Fuchsin or Magenta Red are used, after the caustic potash treatment and thorough washing, but before the preparations are placed in alcohol.

It is difficult to overemphasize the importance of careful labeling of all specimens collected. The label should include place and date of collection and, in the case of parasitic forms, the name of the host. The name of the specimen and of the collector are usually added, also. Pinned insects should bear a small paper label on the pin. Specimens preserved in alcohol should have a paper label, written in waterproof India ink, inside the vial, with the specimens. Pill-boxes may be labeled, of course, by writing on the cover. Specimens mounted on slides may have labels pasted on at one or both ends of the slide.

Slide mounts will, of course, be studied under the compound microscope by transmitted light. For studying mosquitoes and other small flies, also unmounted fleas, lice and ticks, a binocular microscope is almost indispensable, although much may be accomplished with a dissecting microscope or a good hend-lens.

III. *Rearing*

Often the greatest obstacle to the laboratory study of the arthropods of parasitological importance is the difficulty of learning their peculiar breeding requirements. Years of study may be spent in learning these requirements and applying them successfully to the laboratory breeding of a species. Then when the attempt is made to breed even a closely related species it is often found that none of the techniques already worked out applies to the species to be grown. Since these techniques are so highly specialized no attempt will be made here to go into the details of the methods for growing any of the forms treated in this section. Students interested in breeding any of these parasitic arthropods would do well to go first to Galtsoff, Lutz, Welch, and Needham (1937) where techniques for breeding of the following forms are described: cockroaches, lice (of, hogs), bedbugs, anopheline and culicine mosquitoes, *Psychoda,* Ceratopogonidæ, *Simulium,* horseflies, blowflies (including the special technique for growing them for surgical use), *Stomoxys, Musca, Muscina,* Hippoboscidæ, spiders, ticks, and parasitic water mites. Much of the original literature referred to in the foregoing chapters will contain descriptions of the technique of rearing and breeding arthropods. Wolbach, Todd, and Palfrey (1922) give a good description of the methods used in the rearing of *Pediculus.* Bacot (1914) gives an excellent account of the methods employed in rearing rat fleas.

BIBLIOGRAPHY

The literature of Parasitology is contained principally in textbooks and reference books on the subject, textbooks and reference books on tropical medicine, and in journals of parasitology, tropical medicine, zoölogy and general biology. The authors list below what they believe to be the more important of the comprehensive books and monographs and also a list of the journals that include, from time to time, papers on parasitology. Titles are abbreviated in a few cases to save space, and the names of journals are in almost all cases abbreviated according to the system now prevalent among scientific writers. The method used is to give the name of the author followed by the date of publication, then the title of the paper, the journal in which it appeared, the volume of that journal and finally the first and last pages of the paper separated from the volume number by a colon.

I. PROTOZOÖLOGY

1. BOOKS AND JOURNALS

a. Books on Protozoölogy (in whole or in part)

BECKER (E. R.). 1934. *Coccidia and Coccidiosis*. 147 pp. Ames, Iowa.

BLACKLOCK (D. B.) and SOUTHWELL (T.). 1931. *A Guide to Human Parasitology*. 271 pp. London.

BRUMPT (E.). 1922. *Précis de Parasitologie*. 5th ed. 2139 pp. Paris.

BÜTSCHLI (O.). 1880-1889. Protozoa. *Bronn's Klassen und Ordnungen des Thier-Reichs*. I. 2035 pp. Leipzig and Heidelberg.

BYAM (W.) and ARCHIBALD (R. G.) (Editors). 1921-1923. *The Practice of Medicine in the Tropics*. Vol. I, 1921, 856 pp. Vol. 2, 1922, pp. 857-1683. Vol. 3, 1923, pp. 1685-2550. London.

CALKINS (G. N.). 1901. *The Protozoa*. 347 pp. New York.

CALKINS (G. N.). 1933. *The Biology of the Protozoa*. 2d ed. 607 pp. Philadelphia.

CASTELLANI (A.) and CHALMERS (A. J.). 1919. *Manual of Tropical Medicine*. 3d ed. 2436 pp. London.

CRAIG (C. F.). 1926. *Parasitic Protozoa of Man.* 569 pp. Philadelphia.

CRAIG (C. F.). 1934. *Amebiasis and Amebic Dysentery.* 315 pp. Springfield, Ill.

CRAIG (C. F.) and FAUST (E. C.). 1937. *Clinical Parasitology.* 733 pp. Philadelphia.

DOBELL (C.). 1919. *The Amœbœ Living in Man: a Zoölogical Monograph.* 155 pp. London.

DOBELL (C.) and O'CONNOR (F. W.). 1921. *The Intestinal Protozoa of Man.* 211 pp. London.

DOFLEIN (F.) and REICHENOW (E.). 1928. *Lehrbuch der Protozoenkunde.* Jena.

FLETCHER (W.) and JEPPS (M. W.). 1924. *Dysentery in the Federated Malay States.* 82 pp. London.

GEDOELST (L.). 1911. *Synopsis de Parasitologie de l'Homme et des Animaux Domestiques.* 325 pp. Lierre.

HALL (M. C.). 1936. *Control of Animal Parasites.* 162 pp. Evanston, Ill.

HARTMANN (M.) and SCHILLING (C.). 1917. *Die Pathogenen Protozoen.* 462 pp. Berlin.

HEGNER (R. W.), CORT (W. W.) and ROOT (F. M.). 1923. *Outlines of Medical Zoölogy.* 275 pp. New York.

HEGNER (R. W.) and TALIAFERRO (W. H.). 1924. *Human Protozoölogy.* 597 pp. New York.

HEGNER (ROBERT). 1927. *Host-Parasite Relations between Man and His Intestinal Protozoa.* 231 pp. New York.

HEGNER (R.) and ANDREWS (J.). 1930. *Problems and Methods of Research in Protozoölogy.* 532 pp. New York.

KNOWLES (ROBERT). 1928. *An Introduction to Medical Protozoölogy.* 887 pp. Calcutta.

KUDO (R. R.). 1931. *Handbook of Protozoölogy.* 451 pp. Springfield, Ill.

LAVERAN (A.). 1917. *Leishmanioses.* 521 pp. Paris.

LAVERAN (A.) and MESNIL (F.). 1912. *Trypanosomes et Trypanosomiases.* 1000 pp. Paris.

LYNCH (K. M.). 1930. *Protozoan Parasitism of the Alimentary Tract.* 258 pp. New York.

MANSON-BAHR (P.). 1936. *Manson's Tropical Diseases.* 10th ed. 1003 pp. Baltimore.

MINCHIN (E. A.). 1912. *Introduction to the Study of the Protozoa.* 520 pp. London.

PROWAZEK (S. v.) and others. 1911. *Handbuch der Pathogenen Protozoen*. Leipzig.
ROGERS (L.). 1919. *Fevers in the Tropics*. 3d ed. 404 pp. London.
ROSS (SIR RONALD). 1911. *The Prevention of Malaria*. 2d ed. 711 pp. London.
RUDOLF (G. DE M.). 1927. *Therapeutic Malaria*. 223 pp. Oxford.
SMITH (T.). 1934. *Parasitism and Disease*. 196 pp. Princeton, N. J.
STITT (E. R.). 1927. *Practical Bacteriology, Blood Work and Animal Parasitology*. 8th ed. 837 pp. Philadelphia.
TALIAFERRO (W. H.). 1929. *Immunology of Parasitic Infections*. 414 pp. New York.
THOMSON (J. G.) and ROBERTSON (A.). 1929. *Protozoölogy*. 376 pp. London.
WENYON (C. M.). 1926. *Protozoölogy*. 2 vols. 1563 pp. London.
WENYON (C. M.) and O'CONNOR (F. W.) 1917. *Human Intestinal Protozoa in the Near East*. 218 pp. London.
ZIEMANN (H.). 1924. *Malaria und Schwarzwasserfieber*. 592 pp. Leipzig.

b. Journals that Contain Contributions on Protozoa

American Journal of Hygiene. Baltimore. Vol. I. 1921.
American Journal of Tropical Diseases and Preventive Medicine. New Orleans. Vol. I. 1913.
American Journal of Tropical Medicine. Baltimore. Vol. I. 1921.
Annales de l'Institut Pasteur. Paris. Vol. I. 1887.
Annales de Parasitologie. Paris. Vol. I. 1923.
Annals of Tropical Medicine and Parasitology. Liverpool. Vol. I. 1907.
Archiv für Protistenkunde. Jena. Vol. I. 1902.
Archiv für Schiffs-und Tropenhygiene. Leipzig. Vol. I. 1897.
Archives de l'Institut Pasteur de Tunis. Tunis. Vol. I. 1906.
Biological Bulletin. Woods Hole, Mass. Vol. I. 1899.
Bulletin de la Société de Pathologie Exotique. Paris. Vol. I. 1908.
Bulletin de l'Institut Pasteur. Paris. Vol. I. 1903.
Centralblatt für Bakteriologie, Parasitenkunde, und Infectionskrankheiten. Jena. Vol. I. 1887.
Comptes Rendus hebdomadaires des séances de la Société de Biologie. Paris. Vol. I. 1849.
Illinois Biological Monographs. Urbana. Vol. I. 1914.
Indian Journal of Medical Research. Calcutta. Vol. I. 1913.
Indian Medical Gazette. Calcutta. Vol. I. 1866.
Journal of Experimental Medicine. Baltimore. Vol. I. 1896.

Journal of Experimental Zoölogy. Baltimore. Vol. I. 1904.
Journal of the London School of Tropical Medicine. London. Vol. I. 1911. Vol. 2, 1913.
Journal of Parasitology. Lancaster, Pa. Vol. I. 1914.
Journal of the Royal Army Medical Corps. London. Vol. I. 1903.
Journal of Tropical Medicine and Hygiene. London. Vol. I. 1898.
Memorias do Instituto Oswaldo Cruz. Rio de Janeiro. Vol. I. 1909.
Parasitology. Cambridge. Vol. I. 1908.
Proceedings of the Society for Experimental Biology and Medicine. New York. Vol. I. 1903.
Quarterly Journal of Microscopical Science. London. Vol. I. 1853. n. s. Vol. I. 1861.
Rivista di Malariologia. Rome. Vol. I. 1922.
Rivista di Parassitologia. Rome. Vol. I. 1937.
Transactions of the Royal Society of Tropical Medicine and Hygiene. London. Vol. I. 1907.
Tropical Diseases Bulletin. London. Vol. I. 1912.
Tropical Veterinary Bulletin. London. Vol. I. 1912.
University of California Publications in Zoölogy. Berkeley. Vol. I. 1902.
Zentralblatt für Bakteriologie und Parasitenkunde. Jena. Vol. I. 1887.

2. ARTICLES ON PROTOZOÖLOGY IN JOURNALS

ADIE (H. A.). 1924. The sporogony of *Hæmoproteus columbæ. Bull. Soc. Path. Exot.,* 17 : 605-613.
ANDREWS (J. M.). 1925. The cultivation of *Endamœba histolytica* by Boeck's method. *Amer. Journ. Hyg.,* 5 : 556-557.
ANDREWS (J. M.). 1926. Coccidiosis in mammals. *Amer. Journ. Hyg.,* 6 : 784-798.
ANDREWS (J. M.). 1927. Host-parasite specificity in the coccidia of mammals. *Journ. Parasit.,* 13 : 183-194.
ANDREWS (J.). 1932. Host-specificity in *Balantidium coli. Trans. 8th Cong. Far E. Assoc. Trop. Med.,* 194-214.
ANDREWS (J.). 1934. The diagnosis of intestinal protozoa from purged and normally passed stools. *Jour. Parasit.,* 20 : 253-254.
ATCHLEY (F.). 1935. Effects of environmental changes on growth and multiplication in populations of *Balantidium. Amer. Journ. Hyg.,* 21 : 151-166.
BAETJER (W. A.) and SELLARDS (A. W.). 1914. The behavior of amœbic dysentery in lower animals, etc. *Bull. Johns Hopkins Hosp.,* 25 : 237-241.

BARRET (H. P.) and SMITH (M. M.). 1923. The cultivation of an *Endamœba* from the intestine of a turtle. In Proc. Soc. Hygiene. *Amer. Journ. Hyg.*, 3: 205-207.

BARRET (H. P.) and YARBROUGH (N.). 1921. A method for the cultivation of *Balantidium coli*. *Amer. Journ. Trop. Med.*, 1: 161-164.

BASS (C. C.). 1911. On the development of malarial parasites in vitro, etc. *Journ. Trop. Med.*, 25: 341.

BASS (C. C.). 1919. Studies on malarial control. *South. Med. Journ.*, 12: 460-462.

BASS (C. C.). 1922. Studies on inoculation of experimental animals with malaria. *Trans. Amer. Soc. Trop. Med.* (Nov. 1921): 107-114.

BASS (C. C.) and JOHNS (F. M.). 1912. The cultivation of malarial plasmodia (*Plasmodium vivax* and *Plasmodium falciparum*) in vitro. *Journ. Exp. Med.*, 16: 567-579.

BASS (C. C.) and JOHNS (F. M.). 1915. Pyorrhea dentalis and alveolaris. Specific cause and treatment. *Journ. Amer. Med. Assoc.*, 64: 553-558.

BECKER (E. R.). 1923. Observations on the morphology and life cycle of *Crithidia gerridis* Patton in the water-strider, *Gerris remigis* Say. *Journ. Parasit.*, 9: 141-152.

BECKER (E. R.). 1923. Studies on the relationship between insect flagellates and Leishmania. *Amer. Journ. Hyg.*, 3: 462-468.

BECKER (E. R.). 1923. Transmission experiments on the specificity of *Herpetomonas muscæ-domesticæ* in muscoid flies. *Journ. Parasit.*, 10: 25-34.

BECKER (E. R.). 1925. The morphology of *Mastigina hylæ* (Frenzel) from the intestine of the tadpole. *Journ. Parasit.*, 11: 213-216.

BECKER (E. R.) and TALBOTT (M.). 1927. The protozoan fauna of the rumen and reticulum of American cattle. *Iowa State College Journ. Sci.*, 1: 345-373.

BENTLEY (C. A.). 1904. A short note on the parasite of kala-azar. *Indian Med. Gaz.*, 39: 81.

BERCOVITZ (N.). 1924. Viability of cysts of human intestinal amœbas, etc. *Univ. Cal. Pub. Zoöl.*, 26: 249-261.

BISHOP (A.). Further observations upon a *Trichomonas* from pond water. *Parasit.*, 28: 443-445.

BISHOP (A.) and BAYON (H. P.). 1937. Cultivation of *Histomonas meleagridis* from the liver lesions of a hen. *Nature*, 139: 370.

BLACKLOCK (B.) and ADLER (S.). 1922. A parasite resembling

Plasmodium falciparum in a chimpanzee. *Ann. Trop. Med. and Parasit.,* 16:99-106.

BLACKLOCK (B.) and ADLER (S.). 1924. A malaria parasite of the chimpanzee. *Ann. Trop. Med. and Parasit.,* 18: 1-2.

BLAND (P. B.), GOLDSTEIN (L.), WENRICH (D. H.) and WEINER (E.). 1932. Studies on the biology of *Trichomonas vaginalis. Amer. Journ. Hyg.,* 16:492-512.

BLAND (P. B.) and RAKOFF (A. E.). 1936. The investigation of a new pentavalent arsenical, aldarsone, in the treatment of trichomonas vaginitis. *Amer. Journ. Obst. and Gynec.,* 32:835-844.

BOECK (W. C.). 1921. On the longevity of human intestinal protozoan cysts. *Amer. Journ. Hyg.,* 1: 527-540.

BOECK (W. C.). 1921. The thermal death-point of the human intestinal protozoan cysts. *Amer. Journ. Hyg.,* 1: 365-387.

BOECK (W. C.) and DRBOHLAV (J.). 1925. The cultivation of *Endamœba histolytica. Amer. Journ. Hyg.,* 5: 371-407.

BOECK (W. C.) and STILES (C. W.). 1923. Studies on various intestinal parasites (especially amœba) of man. *Bull. No. 133, Hyg. Lab., Washington,* 202 pp. (Contains extensive discussion of the nomenclature of the intestinal protozoa.)

BOYERS (L. M.), KOFOID (C. A.) and SWEZY (O.). 1925. Chronic human amebiasis. *Journ. Amer. Med. Assoc.,* 85: 1441-1447.

BRANDT (B. B.) 1936. Parasites of certain North Carolina *Salientia. Ecological Monog.,* 6: 491-532.

BRUCE (D.). 1895. Preliminary report on the tsetse fly disease or nagana in Zululand. Umbobo, December, 1895.

BRUCE (D) and NABARRO (D). 1903. Progress report on sleeping sickness in Uganda. *Rep. Sleep. Sickn. Comm., Roy. Soc.,* 1 : 11-88.

BRUG (S. L.). 1918. *Entamœba cuniculi* n. sp. *Geneesk. Tijdschr. v. Ned. Indië,* 1918.

BRUG (S. L.). 1919. De entamœben van de rat. *Jaarversl. Cent. Milit. Geneesk. Lab.,* 1918, pp. 127-141.

BRUG (S. L.). 1919. *Endolimax williamsi:* the amœboid form of the iodine-cysts. *Indian Journ. Med. Res.,* 6: 386-392.

BRUMPT (E.). 1909. Démonstration du rôle pathogène du *Balantidium coli.,* etc. *C. R. Soc. Biol.,* 67: 103.

BRUMPT (E.). 1925. Étude sommaire de l' *"Entamœba dispar"* n. sp. Amibe à kystes quadrinucléés, parasite de l'homme. *Bull. Acad. Sci.,* 154: 1-9.

BRUMPT (E.). 1925. Recherches morphologiques et expérimentales sur le *Trichomonas felis* da Cunha et Muniz, 1922, parasite du chat et du chien. *Ann. Parasit.*, 3 : 239-251.

BRUMPT (E.). 1928. Differentiation of the human intestinal amœbæ with four nucleated cysts. *Trans. Roy. Soc. Trop. Med. and Hyg.*, 22 : 101-124.

BRUMPT (E.) and JOYEUX (C.). 1912. Sur un infusoire nouveau, parasite du chimpanzé, *Troglodytella abrassarti* n. g., n. sp. *Bull. Soc. Path. Exot.*, 5 : 499-503.

BRUMPT (E.) and LAVIER (G.). 1924. Un nouvel euglénien poly-flagellé parasite du têtard de *Leptodactylus ocellatus* au Brésil. *Ann. Parasit.*, 2 : 248-252.

BUISSON (J.). 1923. Les infusoires ciliés du tube digestif de l'homme et des mammifères. *Trav. Lab. Parasit. Fac. Méd.*, 200 pp. Paris.

BUNDESEN (H. N.). 1935. Plumbing in relation to infectious diseases. *Amer. Jour. Trop. Med.*, 15 : 455-466.

CASTELLANI (A.). 1903. Trypanosoma in sleeping sickness. *Brit. Med. Journ.*, 1 : 1218.

CASTELLANI (A.). 1905. Observations on some protozoa found in human fæces. *Centralbl. f. Bakt.* 1 Abt. Orig., 38 : 66-69.

CHAGAS (C.). 1909. Ueber eine neue Trypanosomiasis des Menschen. *Mem. Inst. Oswaldo Cruz.*, 1 : 159-218.

CHATTON (E.). 1918. L'amibiase intestinale expérimentale du cobaye à *Entamœba dysenteriæ*. *Arch. Inst. Pasteur Tunis*, 10 : 137-156.

CHIANG (S. F.). 1925. The rat as a possible carrier of the dysentery amœba. *Proc. Nat. Acad. Sci.*, 11 : 239-246.

CHRISTOPHERS (S. R.). 1907. Preliminary note on the development of the *Piroplasma canis* in the tick. *Brit. Med. Journ.*, 1 : 76.

CLARK (J. H.). 1866. The anatomy and physiology of the vorticellidan parasite (*Trichodina pediculus*, Ehr.) of *Hydra. Mem. Boston Soc. Nat. Hist.*, 1 : 114-130.

CLARK (H. C.). 1924. The distribution and complications of amœbic lesions found in 186 postmortem examinations. *Proc. Internat. Conference on Health Problems in Trop. Amer.*, 1924 : 365-379. (United Fruit Co., Boston.)

CLEVELAND (L. R.). 1923. Correlation between the food and morphology of termites and the presence of intestinal protozoa. *Amer. Journ. Hyg.*, 3 : 444-461.

CLEVELAND (L. R.). 1924. The physiological and symbiotic relationships between the intestinal protozoa of termites and their host, with special reference to *Reticulitermes flavipes* Kollar. *Biol. Bull.*, 46 : 177-225.

CLEVELAND (L. R.). 1925. The effects of oxygenation and starvation on the symbiosis between the termite, *Termopsis*, and its intestinal flagellates. *Biol. Bull.*, 48: 309-326.

CLEVELAND (L. R.). 1925. The feeding habit of termite castes and its relation to their intestinal flagellates. *Biol. Bull.*, 48: 295-308.

CLEVELAND (L. R.). 1928. The suitability of various bacteria, etc., as food for the flagellate *Tritrichomonas fecalis*, etc. *Amer. Journ. Hyg.*, 8: 990-1013.

CLEVELAND (L. R.) and SANDERS (E. P.). 1930. Excystation, etc. of *Entamœba histolytica. Arch. Protist.*, 70: 223-266.

COATNEY (G. R.). 1936. A check-list and host-index of the genus *Hæmoproteus. Journ. Parasit.*, 22: 88-105.

COATNEY (G. R.). 1937. A catalog and host-index of the genus *Leucocytozoon. Journ. Parasit.*, 23: 202-212.

CONNAL (A.). 1922. Observations on the pathogenicity of *Isospora hominis*, Rivolta, emend Dobell. *Trans. Roy. Soc. Trop. Med. and Hyg.*, 16: 223-245.

COUNCILMAN (W. T.) and LAFLEUR (H. A.). 1891. Amœbic dysentery. *Johns Hopkins Hosp. Rept.*, 2: 393-548.

COVENTRY (F. A.). 1925. The reaction product which inhibits reproduction of the trypanosomes in infections with *Trypanosoma lewisi*, with special reference to its changes in titer throughout the course of the infection. *Amer. Journ. Hyg.*, 5: 127-144.

COWDRY (E. V.) and DANKS (W. B. C.). 1933. Studies on East Coast fever. *Parasit.*, 25: 1-63.

CRAIG (C. F.). 1921. The classification and differential diagnosis of the æstivo-autumnal malarial plasmodia. *Amer. Journ. Trop. Med.*, 1: 57-96.

CRAIG (C. F.). 1926. A simplified method for the cultivation of *Endamœba histolytica. Amer. Journ. Trop. Med.*, 6: 333-339.

CRAIG (C. F.). 1926. Observations upon the cultivation of *Endamœba histolytica. Amer. Journ. Trop. Med.*, 6: 461-464.

CRAIG (C. F.). 1927. The symptomatology of infection with *Endamœba histolytica* in carriers. *Journ. Amer. Med. Assoc.*, 88: 19-21.

CRAIG (C. F.). 1927. Observations upon the hemolytic, cytolytic and complement-binding properties of extracts of *Endamœba histolytica. Amer. Journ. Trop. Med.*, 7: 225-240.

CRAIG (C. F.). 1928. Complement fixation in the diagnosis of infections with *Endamœba histolytica. Amer. Journ. Trop. Med.*, 8: 29-38.

CRAIG (C. F.) and ST. JOHN (J. H.). 1927. The value of cultural methods in surveys for parasitic amebæ of man. *Amer. Journ. Trop. Med.*, 7: 39-48.

CUNHA (A. M. DA) and MUNIZ (J.). 1927. Sobre os ciliados do genero *Balantidium* parasitos dos Macacos. *Boletim Biol.*, Fasc. 5: 6-15.

CUNNINGHAM (D. D.). 1871. A report on cholera. Calcutta. From: *Ann. Rept. of Sanitary Commissioner with Govt. of India*, pp. 141-243.

CUNNINGHAM (D. D.). 1885. On the presence of peculiar parasitic organisms in the tissue of a specimen of Delhi boil. *Sci. Mem. Med. Off. Army India*, 1 : 21.

DARLING (S. T.). 1910. Sarcosporidiosis in the opossum, etc. *Bull. Soc. Path. Exot.*, 3: 513-517.

DARLING (S. T.). 1910. Studies in relation to malaria. *Isthmian Canal Commission. Lab. Board of Health. Panama.* 38 pp. Washington, D. C.

DARLING (S. T.). 1920. Observations on the geographical and ethnological distribution of hookworms. *Parasit.*, 12: 217-233.

DASTIDAR (S. K. G.). 1925. Trichomonas infection in the urine. *Indian Med. Gaz.*, 60: 160-161.

DE BARY (A.). 1879. Die Erscheinung der Symbiose.

DeLANGEN (C. D.). 1925. Studies concerning the relation of the malarial parasite to the erythrocyte. *Trans. Sixth Cong. F. E. A. T. M.*, 2: 17-25.

DENNIS (E. W.). 1932. The life-cycle of *Bahesia bigemina*, etc. *Univ. Calif. Pub. Zool.*, 36: 263-298.

DeVOLT (H. M.) and DAVIS (C. R.). 1936. Blackhead in turkeys. Bull. 392. *Univ. Md. Agric. Exp. Sta.*: 493-567.

DOBELL (C.). 1918. Are *Entamœba histolytica* and *Entamœba ranarum* the same species? *Parasit.*, 10: 294-310.

DOBELL (C.). 1919. A revision of the coccidia parasitic in man. *Parasit.*, 11 : 147-197.

DOBELL (C.). 1921. A note on the new species of *Eimeria* found in man by Dr. E. P. Snijders. *Parasit.*, 12: 433-436.

DOBELL (C.). 1927. Further observations and experiments on the cultivation of *Entamœba histolytica* from cysts. *Parasit.*, 19: 288-313.

DOBELL (C.). 1928. Researches on the intestinal protozoa of monkeys and man. *Parasit.*, 20: 357-412.

DOBELL (C.). and LAIDLAW (P. P.). 1926. On the cultivation of

Entamœba histolytica and some other entozoic amœbæ. *Parasit.*, 18: 283-318.

DOBELL (C.) and LAIDLAW (P. P.). 1926. The action of ipecacuanha alkaloids on *Entamœba histolytica* and some other entozoic amœbæ in culture. *Parasit.*, 18: 206-223.

DOCK (G.). 1896. Trichomonas as a parasite of man. *Amer. Journ. Med. Sci.*, 111 : 1-24.

DONOVAN (C.). 1903. The ætiology of one of the heterogeneous fevers in India. *Brit. Med. Journ.*, 11 : 1401.

DRBOHLAV (J. J.). 1924. The cultivation of the protozoön of black-head. *Journ. Med. Res.*, 44: 677-678.

DRBOHLAV (J. J.). 1925. Culture *d'Entamœba gingivalis* (Gros, 1849), Brumpt 1913. *Ann. Parasit.*, 3: 361-363.

DRBOHLAV (J. J.). 1925. Studies on the relation of insect flagellates to leishmaniasis. *Amer. Journ. Hyg.*, 5: 580-621.

DUNN (L. H.). 1932. Experiments in the transmission of *Trypanosoma hippicum* Darling with the vampire bat *Desmodus rotundus murinus,* etc. *Journ. Prev. Med.*, 6: 415-424.

DUTTON (J. E.). 1902. Preliminary note upon a trypanosome occurring in the blood of man. *Thompson-Yates Lab. Repts.*, 4 : 455.

EATON (P.). 1934. *Piroplasma canis* in Florida. *Journ. Parasit.*, 20: 312-313.

ELMASSIAN (M.). 1909. Sur une nouvelle espèce amibienne chez l'homme, *Entamœba minuta* n. sp. Morphologie—Evolution—Pathogénie. *Centralbl. f. Bakt.*, 1 Abt., Orig., 52: 335-351.

ENTZ (G.). 1912. Uber eine neue Amöbe auf Süsswasser-Polypen (*Hydra oligactis* Pall.). *Arch. Protistenk.*, 27: 19-47.

ERDMANN (R.). 1910. Beiträge zur Morphologie und Entwicklungsgeschichte des Hammelsarkosporids in der Maus. *Centralbl. Bakt.*, 1 Abt., 53: 510-516.

EVANS (G.). 1880. Report on "surra" disease in the Dera Ismail Khan district. *Punjab Govt. Milit. Dept.*, No. 493-4467.

FANTHAM (H. B.). 1919-1924. Some parasitic protozoa found in South Africa. *S. African Journ. Sci.*, 16: 185-191; 17: 131-135; 18: 164-170; 19: 332-339; 20: 493-500; 21 : 435-444.

FAUST (E. C.). 1923. A new type of amœba parasitic in man observed in North China. *Journ. Parasit.*, 9: 221-226.

FONSECA (O. O. R. DA). 1915. Sobre os flagellados dos mammiferos do Brazil. Um novo parasito do homen. *Brazil-Medico.*, 29: 281.

FORDE (R. M.). 1902. Some clinical notes on a European patient in whose blood a trypanosome was observed. *Journ. Trop. Med. and Hyg.*, 5: 261.

FULTON (J. F.). 1923. *Trichodina pediculus* and a new closely related species. *Proc. Boston Soc. Nat. Hist.*, 37: 1-29.

GABALDON (A.). 1936. Carbarsone: its action on the intestinal trichomonads of rats *in vivo. Amer. Journ. Trop. Med.*, 16: 621-639.

GEIMAN (Q. M.) and RATCLIFFE (H. L.). 1936. Morphology and life-cycle of an amœba producing amœbiasis in reptiles. *Parasit.*, 28: 208-228.

GLASER (R. W.). 1922. *Herpetomonas muscæ-domesticæ*, its behavior and effect in laboratory animals. *Journ. Parasit.*, 8: 99-108.

GOLGI (C.). 1887. Sull'infezione malarica. *Arch. per le scienz. med.*, 10: 109-135.

GOODRICH (H. P.) and MOSLEY (M.). 1916. On certain parasites of the mouth in cases of pyorrhœa. *Journ. Roy. Micro. Soc.*, 1916: 513-527.

GRASSI (B.). 1879. Dei protozoi parassiti e specialmente di quelli che sono nell'uomo. *Gaz. Med. Ital. Lomb.*, 39: 445-448.

GRASSI (B.). 1888. Significato patologico dei protozoi parassiti dell' uomo. *Atti R. Accad. Lincei, Rendic.*, 4, i: 83.

GRASSI (B.), BIGNAMI (A.) and BASTIANELLI (G.). 1898. Ulteriori richerche sul ciclo dei parassiti malarici umani nel corpo del zanzarone. (Nota preliminare.) *Atti R. Accad. Lincei, Rendic*, 5 ser., 8, i: 21.

GRASSI (B.) and FELETTI (R.). 1890. Parasites malariques chez les oiseaux. *Arch. ital. de biol.*, 13: 297-300.

GRASSI (B.) and FELETTI (R.). 1890. Parassiti malarici negli uccelli. *Centralbl. f. Bakt.*, 7: 396-401.

GROS (G.). 1849. Fragments d'helminthologie et de physiologie microscopique. *Bull. Soc. Imp. Nat. Moscou.* 22 (1 partie): 549-573.

GRUBY (M.). 1843. Recherches et observations sur une nouv. espèce d'hematozoaire, *Trypanosoma sanguinis. C. R. Acad., Sci.*, 17: 1134-36.

GUNN (H.). 1922. *Councilmania lafleuri* not a new amœba. *Journ. Parasit.*, 9: 24-27.

HAKANSSON (E. G.). 1937. *Dientamœba fragilis:* some further observations. *Amer. Journ. Trop. Med.*, 17: 349-362.

HARTMAN (E.). 1927. Some notes on *Leucocytozoa* with special reference to *Leucocytozoon anatis. Journ. Parasit.*, 14: 123.

HARTMAN (E.). 1927. Three species of bird malaria, *Plasmodium præcox, P. cathemerium* n. sp., and *P. inconstans* n. sp. *Arch. Protist.*, 60: 1-7.

HAUGHWOUT (F. G.). 1921. A case of human coccidiosis, etc. *Phil. Journ. Sci.* (B), 18: 449-483.

HECKER (F.). 1916. Experimental studies with *Endamœba* Gros. *Journ. Inf. Dis.*, 19: 729-732.

HEGNER (R. W.). 1921. Measurements of *Trypanosoma diemyctyli* from different hosts and their relation to specific identification, heredity and environment. *Journ. Parasit.*, 7: 105-113.

HEGNER (R. W.). 1923. Observations and experiments on Euglenoidina in the digestive tract of frog and toad tadpoles. *Biol. Bull.*, 45: 162-180.

HEGNER (R. W.). 1924. *Cytamœba bacterifera* in the red blood cells of the frog. *Journ. Parasit.*, 7: 157-161.

HEGNER (R. W.). 1924. Infection experiments with *Trichomonas*. *Amer. Journ. Hyg.*, 4: 143-151.

HEGNER (R. W.). 1924. The relations between a carnivorous diet and mammalian infections with intestinal protozoa. *Amer. Journ. Hyg.*, 4: 393-400.

HEGNER (R. W.). 1925. The presence of the human intestinal flagellate, *Pentatrichomonas ardindelteili,* in a healthy carrier. *Amer. Journ. Hyg.*, 5: 554-555.

HEGNER (R. W.). 1925. *Trichomonas vaginalis* Donné. *Amer. Journ. Hyg.*, 5: 302-308.

HEGNER (R. W.). 1926. Animal infections with the trophozoites of intestinal protozoa and their bearing on the functions of cysts. *Amer. Journ. Hyg.*, 6: 593-601.

HEGNER (R. W.). 1926. Asexual reproduction without loss of vitality in malarial organisms. *Science,* 63: 479-480.

HEGNER (R. W.). 1926. *Endolimax caviæ* n. sp. from the guinea-pig and *Endolimax janisæ* n. sp. from the domestic fowl. *Journ. Parasit.*, 12: 146-147.

HEGNER (R. W.). 1926. Homologies and analogies between free-living and parasitic protozoa. *Amer. Nat.*, 60: 516-525.

HEGNER (R. W.). 1926. Host-parasite specificity among human protozoa. *Science Progress,* 21: 249-259.

HEGNER (R. W.). 1926. The biology of host-parasite relationships among protozoa living in man. *Quart. Review of Biology,* 1: 393-418.

HEGNER (R. W.). 1927. Excystation and infection in the rat with *Giardia lamblia* from man. *Amer. Journ. Hyg.*, 7: 433-447.

HEGNER (R. W.). 1927. Excystation *in vitro* of human intestinal protozoa. *Science,* 65: 577-578.

HEGNER (ROBERT). 1928. Experimental studies on the viability and transmission of *Trichomonas hominis. Amer. Journ. Hyg.,* 8:16-34.

HEGNER (ROBERT). 1928. Experimental transmission of trichomonads from the intestine and vagina of monkeys to the vagina of monkeys (*Macacus rhesus*). *Journ. Parasit.,* 14:261-264.

HEGNER (ROBERT). 1928. The ingestion of red blood corpuscles by trichomonad flagellates. Observations showing that it is not evidence of pathogenicity. *Journ. Amer. Med. Assoc.,* 90:741-742.

HEGNER (R.). 1928. The evolutionary significance of the protozoan parasites of monkeys and man. *Quart. Rev. Biol.,* 3:225-244.

HEGNER (R.). 1929. The infection of parasite-free chicks with intestinal protozoa from birds and other animals. *Amer. Journ. Hyg.,* 10:33-62.

HEGNER (R.). 1934. Specificity in the genus *Balantidium,* etc. *Amer. Journ. Hyg.,* 19:38-67.

HEGNER (R.). 1934. Passage of *Trichomonas hominis* in a viable condition through the stomach and small intestine of a monkey. *Journ. Parasit.,* 20:199.

HEGNER (R. W.) and BECKER (E. R.). 1922. The diagnosis of intestinal flagellates by culture methods. *Journ. Parasit.,* 9:15-23.

HEGNER (R.) and CHU (H. J.). 1930. A comparative study of the intestinal protozoa of wild monkeys and man. *Amer. Journ. Hyg.,* 12:62-109.

HEGNER (R.) and ESKRIDGE (L.). 1935. Elimination and cross-infection experiments with trichomonads from fowls, rats and man. *Amer. Journ. Hyg.,* 21:135-150.

HEGNER (R.) and HEWITT (R.). 1938. The influence of young red cells on infections of *Plasmodium cathemerium* in birds. *Amer. Journ. Hyg.,* 27:417-436.

HEGNER (R. W.) and HOLMES (F. O.). 1923. Observations on a *Balantidium* from a Brazilian monkey, *Cebus variegatus,* E. Geoffr., with special reference to chromosome-like bodies in the macronuclei. *Amer. Journ. Hyg.,* 3:252-263.

HEGNER (R.), JOHNSON (C. M.) and STABLER (R. M.). 1932. Host-parasite relations in experimental amœbiasis in monkeys in Panama. *Amer. Journ. Hyg.,* 15:394-443.

HEGNER (ROBERT) and MANWELL (R. D.). 1927. The effects of plasmochin on bird malaria. *Amer. Journ. Trop. Med.,* 7:279-285.

HEGNER (R. W.) and WU (H.-F.). 1921. An analysis of the relation between growth and nuclear division in a parasitic infusorion, *Opalina* sp. *Amer. Naturalist.,* 55 : 335-346.

HERMAN (C.). 1937. *Toxoplasma* in North American birds and attempted transmission to canaries and chickens. *Amer. Journ. Hyg.,* 25 : 303-312.

HESSE (E.). 1904. *Thelohania legeri* n. sp., microscopidie nouvelle, parasite des larves d'*Anopheles maculipennis* Meig. *C. R. Soc. Biol.,* 57 : 570.

HINSHAW (H. C.). 1926. Correlation of protozoan infections of human mouth with extent of certain lesions in pyorrhea alveolaris. *Proc. Soc. Exp. Biol. and Med.,* 24 : 71-73.

HINSHAW (H. C.). 1926. On the morphology and mitosis of *Trichomonas buccalis* (Goodey) Kofoid. *Univ. Cal. Pub. Zoöl.,* 29 : 159-174.

HINSHAW (H. C.). 1928. Experimental infection of dogs with *Endamœba gingivalis* and *Trichomonas buccalis* of human mouth. *Proc. Soc. Exp. Biol. and Med.,* 25 : 430-431.

HOARE (C. A.). 1921. Some observations and experiments on insect flagellates, with special reference to arificial infection of vertebrates. *Parasit.,* 13 : 67-85.

HOARE (C. A.). 1925. Sections of the intestine of a kitten presumably infected with *Entamœba histolytica* by rectal injection of cysts alone. *Trans. Roy. Soc. Trop. Med. and Hyg.,* 19 : 277-278.

HOGUE (M. J.). 1921. Studies on the life history of *Vahlkampfia patuxent* n. sp., parasitic in the oyster, with experiments regarding its pathogenicity. *Amer. Journ. Hyg.,* 1 : 321-345.

HOGUE (M. J.). 1926. Studies on *Trichomonas buccalis. Amer. Journ. Trop. Med.,* 6 : 75-88.

HOLMES (F. O.). 1923. Observations on the cysts of *Endamœba cobayœ. Journ. Parasit.,* 10 : 47-50.

HOLMES (F. O.). 1925. Non-pathogenicity of the milkweed flagellate in Maryland. *Phytopathology,* 15 : 294-296.

HOLMES (F. O.). 1925. Geographical distribution of the milkweed flagellate, *Herpetomonas elmassiani* (Migone). *Phytopathology,* 15 : 297-299.

HOLMES (F. O.). 1925. The relation of *Herpetomonas elmassiani* (Migone) to its plant and insect hosts. *Biol. Bull.,* 49 : 323-337.

HOWITT (B. F.). 1926. Experiments with *Endamœba gingivalis* (Gros) in mixed bacterial cultures, etc. *Univ. Cal. Pub. Zoöl.,* 28 : 183-202.

HUBER. 1909. Untersuchungen über Amöbendysenterie. *Zeitschr. Klin. Med.*, 67 : 262-271.

HUFF (C. G.). 1927. Studies on the infectivity of plasmodia of birds for mosquitoes, with special reference to the problem of immunity in the mosquito. *Amer. Journ. Hyg.*, 7 : 706-734.

JAUREGG (J. WAGNER VON). 1887. Ueber die Einwirkung fieberhafter Erkrankungen auf Psychosen. *Jahrb. Psychiat. u. Neurol.*, 7 : 94.

JAUREGG (J. WAGNER VON). 1922. Die Malariabehandlung der progressiven Paralyse. Transl. in *Journ. Nerv. and Ment. Dis.*, Albany, N. Y., 55 : 369-375.

JEPPS (M. W.) and DOBELL (C.). 1918. *Dientamœba fragilis* n. g., n. sp., a new intestinal amœba from man. *Parasit.*, 10 : 352-367.

JOHNSON (C. M.). 1935. A rapid technique for iron-hematoxylin staining requiring no microscopic control of decolorization. *Amer. Journ. Trop. Med.*, 15 : 551-553.

JOHNSTON (S. J.). 1914. Australian trematodes and cestodes; a study in zoögeography. *Med. Journ. Aust.*, 1 : 243-244.

KARTULIS (S.). 1887. Zur Aetiologie der Leberabscesse. *Centralb. Bakt.*, 2 : 745-748.

KARTULIS (S.). 1904. Gehirnabscesse nach dysenterischen Leberabscessen. *Centralb. Bakt. und Parasitol.* Orig., 37 : 527-530.

KATSUNUMA (S.). 1924. Présence de *Trichomonas vaginalis* dans l'urine d'un jeune garçon. *Bull. Soc. Path. Exot.*, 17 : 210-217.

KEILIN (D.). 1921. On a new ciliate, *Lambornella stegomyiæ*, n. g., n. sp., parasitic in the body cavity of the larvæ of *Stegomyia scutellaris* Walker. *Parasit.*, 13 : 216-224.

KESSEL (J. F.). 1923. Experimental infection of rats and mice with the common intestinal amœbæ of man. *Univ. Cal. Pub. Zoöl.*, 20 : 409-430.

KESSEL (J. F.). 1924. The distinguishing characteristics of the parasitic amœbæ of culture rats and mice. *Univ. Calif. Pub. Zoöl.*, 20 : 489-544.

KESSEL (J. F.). 1924. The experimental transfer of certain intestinal protozoa from man to monkeys. *Proc. Soc. Exp. Biol. and Med.*, 22 : 206-208.

KESSEL (J. F.). 1927. Intestinal protozoa of monkeys. *Journ. Parasit.*, 13 : 283-284.

KESSEL (J. F.). 1928. Intestinal protozoa of the domestic pig. *Amer. Journ. Trop. Med.*, 8 : 481-502.

KESSEL (J. F.). 1928. Amœbiasis in kittens, etc. *Amer. Journ. Hyg.*, 8 : 311-354.

KESSEL (J. F.). 1928. Trichomoniasis in kittens. *Trans. Roy. Soc. Trop. Med. and Hyg.*, 22:61-80.

KNOWLES (R.) and DAS GUPTA (B. M.). 1934. Latent malaria infection in monkeys. *Indian Med. Gaz.*, 269:541-545.

KOCH (R.) and GAFFKY (G.). 1887. Bericht über die Thätigkeit der zur Erforschung der Cholera im Jahre 1883 nach Egypten und Indien entsandten Kommission. *Arb. a. d. kaiserl. Gesundheitsamte*, 3:1-86.

KOFOID (C. A.). 1923. Amœba and Man. *Univ. Cal. Chron.* (1923): pp. 149-174, 291-312.

KOFOID (C. A.). 1928. Councilmania tenuis and C. dissimilis, intestinal amebas of man. *Arch. Int. Med.*, 41:558-585.

KOFOID (C. A.) and SWEZY (O.). 1921. On the free, encysted, and budding stages of *Councilmania lafleuri*, a parasitic amœba of the human intestine. *Univ. Cal. Pub. Zoöl.*, 20:169-198.

KOFOID (C. A.), SWEZY (O.) and KESSEL (J. F.). 1923. On the genus *Councilmania* budding intestinal amœbæ parasitic in man and rodents. *Univ. Calif. Pub. Zoöl.*, 20:431-445.

KOFOID (C. A.) and SWEZY (O.). 1924. *Karyamœba falcata*, a new amœba from the human intestinal tract. *Univ. Cal. Pub. Zoöl.*, 26:221-242.

KOFOID (C. A.) and SWEZY (O.). 1924. The cytology of *Endamœba gingivalis* (Gros) Brumpt, etc. *Univ. Cal. Pub. Zoöl.*, 25:165-198.

KOFOID (C. A.), WOOD (F. D.) and MCNEIL (E.). 1935. The cycle of *Trypanosoma cruzi* in tissue culture of embryonic heart muscle. *Univ. Calif. Pub. Zoöl.*, 41:23-24.

KUDO (R.). 1919. Studies on Myxosporidia. *Illinois Biol. Monographs.*, 5:265 pp.

KUDO (R.). 1921. Studies on Microsporidia, with special reference to those parasitic in mosquitoes. *Journ. Morph.*, 35:153-193.

KUDO (R.). 1924. A biologic and toxonomic study of the Microsporidia. *Illinois Biol. Monogr.*, 9:Nos. 2 & 3, 1.

KUDO (R.). 1924. Studies on Microsporidia parasitic in mosquitoes. III. On *Thelohania legeri* Hesse (= *Th. illinoisensis* Kudo). *Arch. Protist.*, 49:147-162.

KUENEN (W. A.) and SWELLENGREBEL (N. H.). 1917. Korte beschrijving van enkele minder bekende protozoën uit den menschelijken darm. *Geneesk. Tijdschr. v. Nederl.-Indië.*, 57:496-506.

KUENEN (W. A.) and SWELLENGREBEL (N. H.). 1923. Die Entamöben des Menschen und ihre praktische Bedeutung. *Centralbl. Bakt.*, 71: 378-410.

LABBÉ (A.). 1894. Recherches zoölogiques et biologiques sur les parasites endoglobulaires du sang des vertébrés. Thèses. 208 pp. Paris.

LAFONT (A.). 1909. Sur la présence d'un parasite de la classe des Flagellés dans le latex de *Euphorbia piluifera. Compt. Rend. Soc. Biol., Paris*, 66: 1011-1013.

LAMBORN (W. A.). 1921. A protozoön pathogenic to mosquito larvæ. *Parasit.*, 13: 213-215.

LARSON (M. E.), VAN EPPS (M. H.) and BROOKS (S. T.). 1925. Reaction of opalinas to various laboratory media. *Science*, 62: 289-290.

LAVERAN (A.). 1880. Note sur un nouveau parasite trouvé dans le sang de plusieurs malades atteints de fièvre palustre. *Bull. Acad. Méd.*, 9: 1235, 1268, 1346.

LAVERAN (A.). 1899. Sur le bacille parasite des hématies de *Rana esculenta. C. R. Soc. Biol.*, 51: 355.

LAVERAN and FRANCHINI. 1913. Infections expérimentales de la souris par *Herpetomonas ctenocephali. C. R. Acad. Sci.*, 157: 423-426.

LAVERAN (A.) and MESNIL (F.). 1903. Sur un protozoaire nouveau (*Piroplasma donovani* Lav. et Mesn.), parasite d'une fièvre de l'India. *C. R. Acad. Sci.*, 137: 957.

LAWSON (M. R.). 1920. Segmenting tertian malarial parasites on red corpuscles showing little or no loss of hemoglobin substance; evidence of migration. *Journ. Exp. Med.*, 32: 139-142.

LEGER (M.). 1918. Epizootie chez le cobaye paraissant due à une amibiase intestinale. *Soc. Path. Exot.*, 11: 163-166.

LEIDY (J.). 1879. On *Amœba blattæ. Proc. Acad. Nat. Sci. Philad.*, 31: 204-205.

LEISHMAN (W. B.). 1903. On the possibility of the occurrence of trypanosomiasis in India. *Brit. Med. Journ.*, 1: 1252.

LEWIS (T. R.). 1870. A report on the microscopic objects found in cholera evacuations, etc. (Appendix to *Ann. Rept. of Sanitary Commissioner with Govt. of India.*) Calcutta.

LEWIS (T. R.). 1879. Flagellated organisms in the blood of healthy rats. *Quart. Journ. Micro. Sci.*, 19: 109.

LIEBETANZ (E). 1905. Die parasitischen Protozoen des Wiederkäuermagens. *Berliner Tierärztl. Wochenschr.*, 21: 313-314.

LOESCH (F.). 1875. Massenhafte Entwickelung von Amöben im Dickdarm. *Arch. path. Anat.*, 65: 196-211.

LUCAS (C. L. T.). 1927. Two new species of amœbæ found in cock-roaches, with notes on the cysts of *Nyctotherus ovalis* Leidy. *Parasit.*, 19: 223-235.

LYNCH (K. M.). 1915. Concerning endamebiasis of the mouth. *Amer. Journ. Trop. Dis. & Prev. Med.*, 3: 231-242.

MacARTHUR (W. P.). 1922. A holotrichous ciliate pathogenic to *Theobaldia annulata* Schrank. *Journ. R. Army Med. Corps*, 38: 83.

MacCALLUM (W. G.). 1897. On the flagellated form of the malarial parasite. *Lancet*, 2: 1240-1241.

MacCALLUM (W. G.). 1898. On the hæmatozoan infections of birds. *Journ. Exp. Med.*, 3: 117-136.

MACKINNON (D. L.). 1911. On some more protozoan parasites from Trichoptera. *Parasit.*, 4: 28-38.

MACKINNON (D. L.). 1914. Observations on amœbæ from the intestine of the crane-fly larva, *Tipula* sp. *Arch. Prot.*, 32: 267-277.

MAGATH (T. B.) and WARD (C. B.). 1928. Laboratory methods of diagnosing amœbiasis. *Amer. Journ. Hyg.*, 8: 840-857.

MANSON (P.). 1894. On the nature and significance of the crescentic and flagellated bodies in malarial blood. *Brit. Med. Journ.*, 2: 1306.

MANSON (P.). 1900. Experimental proof of the mosquito malaria theory. *Brit. Med. Journ.*, 2: 949.

MANWELL (R. D.) and HERMAN (C. M.). 1935. Blood parasites of birds of the Syracuse (N. Y.) region. *Journ. Parasit.*, 21: 415-416.

MARCHIAFAVA (E.) and CELLI (A.). 1885. Nuove richerche sull'infezione malarica. *Arch. per le sc. med., Torino*, 9: 311-340.

MARTINI (E.). 1910. Ueber einen bei amöbenruhrähnlichen Dysenterien vorkommenden Ciliaten. *Zeitschr. Hyg. u. Infekt.*, 67: 387-390.

MAST (S. O.). 1926. The structure of protoplasm in amœba. *Amer. Nat.*, 60: 133-142.

McCULLOCH (I.). 1917. *Crithidia euryophthalmi*, sp. nov., from the hemipteran bug, *Euryophthalmus convivus*, Stal. *Univ. Cal. Pub. Zoöl.*, 18: 75-88.

McCULLOCH (I.). 1919. A comparison of the life cycle of Crithidia with that of Trypanosoma in the invertebrate host. *Univ. Calif. Pub. Zoöl.*, 19: 135-190.

McDONALD (J. D.). 1922. On *Balantidium coli* (Malmsten) and *Balantidium suis* (sp. nov.), with an account of their neuromotor apparatus. *Univ. Cal. Pub. Zoöl.*, 20: 243-300.

McFALL (C. M.). 1926. *Endolimax reynoldsi* nov. sp. from the intestine of the common swift. *Sceloporus undulatus. Journ. Parasit.*, 12: 191-198.

MELENEY (H. E.). 1930. Community surveys for *Endamœba histolytica* and other intestinal protozoa in Tennessee. *Journ. Parasit.*, 16: 146-153.

MELENEY (H. E.), BISHOP (E. L.) and LEATHERS (W. S.). 1932. Investigations of *Endamœba histolytica* and other intestinal protozoa in Tennessee. *Amer. Journ. Hyg.*, 16: 523-539.

MERCIER (L.). 1910. Contribution à l'étude de l'amibe de la blatte (*Entamœba blattœ* Bütschli). *Arch. Protistenk.*, 20: 143-175.

MESNIL (F.) and ROUBAUD (E.). 1920. Essais d'inoculation du paludisme au chimpanzé. *Am. Inst. Pasteur,* 34: 466.

METCALF (M. M.). 1923. The opalinid ciliate infusorians. *U. S. Nat. Mus., Bull.* 120: 1-484.

MIGONE (L. E.). 1916. Un nouveau flagellé des plantes: *Leptomonas elmassiani. Bull. Soc. Path. Exot.*, 9: 356-359.

MILLER (W. W.). 1908. *Hepatozoon pernisciosum* (n. g., n. sp.); a hæmogregarine pathogenic for white rats, etc. Bull. No. 46. Hygienic Lab. U. S. Treasury Dept., 48 pp.

MILLS (R. G.), BARTLETT (C. L.) and KESSEL (J. F.). 1925. The penetration of fruits and vegetables and other particulate matter, and the resistance of bacteria, protozoan cysts and helminth ova to common disinfection methods. *Amer. Journ. Hyg.*, 5: 559-579.

MINCHIN (E. A.) and THOMSON (J. D.). 1915. The rat-trypanosome, *Trypanosoma lewisi,* in its relation to the rat-flea, *Ceratophyllus fasciatus. Quart. Journ. Micro. Sci.*, N. S., 60: 463-692.

MORRIS (S.). 1935. Studies on *Endamœba blattœ* (Bütschli). *Journ. Morph.*, 59: 225-263.

MÜHLENS (P.). 1926. Die Behandlung der natürlichen menschlichen Malariainfektionen mit Plasmochin. *Arch. Schiffs-u. Tropen-Hyg., Beih.*, 3: 30: 25-35.

MUSGRAVE (W. E.) and CLEGG (M. T.). 1904. Amebas: their cultivation and etiologic significance. *Dept. of Interior, Bur. of Govt. Labs., Biol. Lab., Bull.* No. 18, 85 pp. (Manila).

NEGRI (A.). 1908, 1910. Beobachtungen über Sarkosporidien. *Centrlb. Bakt. Orig.*, 47: 56-61 and 612-622; 55: 435.

NELSON (E. C.). 1934. Observations and experiments on conjugation of the *Balantidium* from the chimpanzee. *Amer. Journ. Hyg.*, 20: 106-134.

NICOLLE (C.). 1908. Culture du parasite du Bouton d'Orient. *C. R. Acad. Sci.*, 146: 842-843.

NIESCHULZ (O.). 1922. Ueber Entamœben des Hausrindes. *Arch. Protist.*, 45: 410-412.

NIESCHULZ (O.). 1924. Amöben aus dem Zahnbelag von Pferden. *Arch. Tierheilk.*, 51: 41-44.

NIESCHULZ (O.). 1924. Ueber *Entamœba debliecki* Mihi, eine Darmamœbe des Schweines. *Arch. Prot.*, 48: 365-370.

NOGUCHI (H.). 1924. Action of certain biological, chemical, and physical agents upon cultures of leishmania; some observations on plant and insect herpetomonads. *Proc. Internat. Conf. Health Prob. Trop. Amer. United Fruit Company*, pp. 455-479.

NOVY (F. G.) and MACNEAL (W. J.). 1903. On the cultivation of *T. lewisi. Contributions to Medical Research Dedicated to V. C. Vaughn.* (1903) p. 549.

O'CONNOR (F. W.). 1920. A preliminary note on two intestinal parasites in pigs. *Med. Journ. Australia*, 2: 337.

O'ROKE (E. C.). 1931. The life history of *Leucocytozoon anatis* Wickware. *Journ. Parasit.*, 18: 127.

OSLER (W.). 1890. Ueber die in Dysenterie und dysenterischem Leberabscess vorhandene Amœba. *Centralb. Bakt. und Parasitol.*, 7: 736-737.

PAULSON (M.) and ANDREWS (J. M.). 1927. Detection and incidence of human intestinal protozoa by the sigmoidoscope. *Journ. Amer. Med. Assoc.*, 88: 1876-1879.

PROWAZEK (S. v.). 1911. Zur Kenntnis der Flagellaten des Darmtraktus. *Arch. Protistenk.*, 23: 96-100.

PROWAZEK (S. v.). 1912. Entamœba. *Arch. Protistenk.*, 25: 273-274.

QUINCKE (H.) and ROOS (E.). 1893. Ueber Amöben-Enteritis. *Berlin klin. Wochenschr.*, 30: 1089-1094.

RATCLIFFE (H. L.). 1927. The relation of *Plasmodium vivax* and *Plasmodium præcox* to the red blood cells of their respective hosts as determined by sections of blood cells. *Amer. Journ. Trop. Med.*, 7: 383-388.

RATCLIFFE (H. L.). 1928. The numbers of trichomonads in rats on diets of different protein content, etc. *Amer. Journ. Hyg.*, 8: 910-934.

REES (C. W.). 1927. Balantidia from pigs and guinea-pigs; their cultivation, viability and cyst production. *Science*, 66: 89-91.

REES (C. W.). 1934. Transmission of anaplasmosis by various species of ticks. *U. S. Dept. Agric., Tech. Bull.* 418. pp. 17.

REICHENOW (E.). 1910. *Hæmogregarina stepanowi. Arch. Protist.,* 20:251-350.

REICHENOW (E.). 1917. Parasitos de la sangre y del intestino de los monos antropromorfos africanos. *Bol. R. Soc. Españ. Hist. Nat.,* 17:312.

REICHENOW (E.). 1920. Den Wiederkäuer-Infusorien verwandte Formen aus Gorilla und Schimpanse. *Arch. Protistenk.,* 41 : 1-33.

REICHENOW (E.). 1920. Ueber das Vorkommen der Malaria Parasiten des Menschen bei den Afrikanischen Menschenaffen. *Centrlb. Bakt. und Parasit. Orig.,* 85 : 207-216.

REIS (VAN DER). 1923. Ueber die Bakterienflora des Darms (*Balantidium coli*) und pathologische Dünndarmbesiedlung. *Münch. Med. Woch.,* 70 : 835.

REULING (F.). 1921. Zur Morphologie von *Trichomonas vaginalis* Donné. *Arch. Protist.,* 42 : 347-363.

REYNOLDS (BRUCE D.) and LOOPER (J. B.). 1928. Infection experiments with *Hydramœba hydroxena* nov. gen. *Journ. Parasit.,* 15 : 23-30.

RIVAS (D). 1926. The effect of temperature on protozoan and metazoan parasites, etc. *Amer. Journ. Trop. Med.,* 6 : 47-73.

ROEHL (W.). 1926. Die Wirkung des Plasmochins auf die Vogelmalaria. *Arch. Schiffs-u. Tropen-Hyg.,* Beih. 3 : 30 : 11-18.

ROGERS (L.). 1904. Preliminary note on the development of *Trypanosoma* in cultures of the Cunningham-Leishman-Donovan bodies of cachexial fever and kala-azar. *Lancet,* 2 : 215-216.

ROOT (F. M.). 1921. Experiments on the carriage of intestinal protozoa of man by flies. *Amer. Journ. Hyg.,* 1 : 131-153.

ROSS (R.). 1895. The crescent-sphere-flagella metamorphosis of the malaria parasite in the mosquito. *Trans. S. Indian Branch Brit. Med. Assoc.,* 6 : 334.

ROSS (R.). 1897. On some peculiar pigmented cells found in two mosquitoes fed on malarial blood, *Brit. Med. Journ.,* 2 : 1786.

ROSS (R.). 1898. Report on the cultivation of *Proteosoma,* Labbé, in grey mosquitoes. Calcutta. *Indian Med. Gaz.,* 33 : 401, 448.

ROSS (R.). 1903. (1) Note on the bodies recently described by Leishman and Donovan. (2). Further notes on Leishman's bodies. *Brit. Med. Journ.,* 2 : 1261, 1401.

ROW (R.). 1917. On a simplified technique of Bass's method of cultivating malarial parasites in vitro, and a few observations on the malarial parasites cultured by this technique. *Indian Journ. Med. Res.,* 4 : 388-392.

SANDERS (D. A.). 1937. Observations on canine babesiasis (Piroplasmosis). *Journ. Amer. Vet. Med. Assoc.*, 90: 27-40.

SANDERS (E. P.). 1931. The life-cycle of *Endamœba ranarum* Grassi (1879). *Arch. Protist.*, 74: 365.

SCALAS (L.). 1923. L'intradermoreazione nella dissenterica amebica. *Riforma Med.*, 39: 967-969.

SCHAUDINN (F.). 1903. Untersuchungen über die Fortpflanzung einiger Rhizopoden. *Arb. kaiserl. Gesundh.-Amte.*, 19: 547-576.

SCHAUDINN (F.) and JAKOBY (M.). 1899. Ueber zwei neue Infusorien im Darm des Menschen. *Centralb. Bakt. und Parasit.*, 25: 487-494.

SCOTT (M. J.). 1927. Studies on the balantidium from the guineapig. *Journ. Morph.*, 44: 417-465.

SELLARDS (A. W.) and THIELER (M.). 1924. Investigations concerning amœbic dysentery. *Amer. Journ. Trop. Med.*, 4: 309-330.

SHORTT (H. E.). 1923. The pathogenicity of insect flagellates to vertebrates, with special reference to *Herpetomonas ctenocephali*, Fantham. *Ind. Journ. Med. Res.*, 10: 908-933.

SHORTT (H. E.). 1936. Life-history and morphology of *Babesia canis* in the dog tick *Rhipicephalus sanguineus*. *Ind. Journ. Med. Res.*, 23: 885-920.

SINTON (J. A.). 1922. A simplified method for the cultivation of *Plasmodium falciparum* in vitro. *Indian Journ. Med. Res.*, 10: 203-209 (also see pp. 210-214).

SINTON (J. A.). 1922. Situation of malarial parasite in relation to red blood corpuscle. *Indian Med. Gaz.*, 57: 367-371.

SKIDMORE (L. V.). 1932. *Leucocytozoon smithi* infection in turkeys and its transmission by *Simulium occidentale*. *Zentrl. Bakt. Orig.*, 125: 329-335.

SMITH (A. J.) and BARRETT (M. T.). 1915. The parasite of oral endamebiasis, *Endameba gingivalis*. (Gros). *Journ. Parasit.*, 1: 159-174.

SMITH (SEPTIMA C.). 1927. Excystation in *Iodamœba williamsi* in vivo and in vitro. *Science*, 65: 69-70.

SMITH (SEPTIMA C.). 1928. Host-parasite relations between *Iodamœba williamsi* and certain mammalian hosts (guinea-pigs and rats). *Amer. Journ. Hyg.*, 8: 1-15.

SMITH (T.). 1901. The production of sarcosporidiosis in the mouse by feeding infected muscular tissue. *Journ. Exp. Med.*, 6: 1-21.

SMITH (T.) and KILBOURNE (F. L.). 1893. Investigations into the nature, causation and prevention of southern cattle fever. *Report Bur. Animal Industry, U. S. Dept. Agric.* (1893), pp. 177-304.

SMYLY (H. J.) and YOUNG (C. W.). 1924. The experimental transmission of leishmaniasis to animals. *Proc. Soc. Exp. Biol. & Med.,* 21 : 354-356.

STABLER (R. M.) and CHEN (T.). 1936. Observations on an *Endamœba* parasitizing opalinid ciliates. *Biol. Bull.,* 70: 56-71.

STEPHENS (J. W. W.) and FANTHAM (H. B.). 1910. On the peculiar morphology of a trypanosome from a case of sleeping sickness and the possibility of its being a new species. *Proc. Roy. Soc. Lon.* (B) 83: 28, and (B) 85: 223.

STRONG (R. P.). 1924. Investigations upon flagellate infections. *Amer. Journ. Trop. Med.,* 4: 1-56.

SWEZEY (W. W.). 1934. Cytology of *Troglodytella abrassarti,* an intestinal ciliate of the chimpanzee. *Journ. Morph.,* 56: 621-635.

SWEZY (O.). 1922. Mitosis in the encysted stages of *Endamœba coli* (Loesch). *Univ. Cal. Pub. Zoöl.,* 20: 313-332.

TALIAFERRO (L. G.). 1925. Infection and resistance in bird malaria, with special reference to periodicity and rate of reproduction of the parasite. *Amer. Journ. Hyg.,* 5: 742-789.

TALIAFERRO (W. H.). 1924. A reaction product in infections with *Trypanosoma lewisi* which inhibits the reproduction of the trypanosomes. *Journ. Exp. Med.,* 39: 171-190.

TALIAFERRO (W. H.). 1926. Host resistance and types of infection in trypanosomiasis and malaria. *Quart. Rev. Biol.,* 1: 246-269.

TALIAFERRO (W. H.) and BECKER (E. R.). 1922. The human intestinal amœba *Iodamœba williamsi;* and its cysts (Iodine cysts). *Amer. Journ. Hyg.,* 2: 188-207.

TALIAFERRO (W. H.). and BECKER (E. R.). 1924. A note on the human intestinal amœba, *Dientamœba fragilis. Amer. Journ. Hyg.,* 4: 71-74.

TALIAFERRO (W. H.) and TALIAFERRO (L. G.). 1922. The resistance of different hosts to experimental trypanosome infections, with especial reference to a new method of measuring this resistance. *Amer. Journ. Hyg.,* 2: 264-319.

TANABE (M.) and KOMADA (K.). 1932. On the cultivation of *Balantidium coli. Keijo Journ. Med.,* 3: 385-392.

TANABE (M.). 1934. The excystation and metacystic development of *Entamœba histolytica* in the intestine of white rats. *Keijo Journ. Med.,* 5: 238-253.

THEILER (A.). 1910. *Anaplasma marginale* (gen. and spec. nov.). The marginal points in the blood of cattle suffering from a

724 PARASITOLOGY

specific disease. *Rept. Gov. Vet. Bact., Dept. Agric. Transvaal, 1908-1909,* 1.

THOMAS (H. W.). 1905. Some experiments in the treatment of trypanosomiasis. *Brit. Med. Journ.,* 1: 1140-1143.

THOMSON (J. G.) and ROBERTSON (A.). 1926. Experimental passage of the cysts of fish coccidia through the human intestine. *Brit. Med. Journ.,* 1926: pp. 420-421.

THOMSON (J. G.) and ROBERTSON (A.). 1926. Fish as the source of certain coccidia recently described as intestinal parasites of man. *Brit. Med. Journ.,* 1926: pp. 282-283.

THOMSON (M. D.). 1926. Experimental amœbiasis in the rabbit. *Univ. Cal. Pub. Zoöl.,* 29: 9-23.

TYLER (A. R.). 1926. The cultivation of *Opalina. Science,* 64: 383-384.

TYZZER (E. E.). 1920. Amœba of the cæca of the common fowl and of the turkey, *Entamœba gallinarum* sp. n. and *Pygolimax gregariniformis* gen. et. spec. nov. *Journ. Med. Res.,* 41: 199-209.

TYZZER (E. E.). 1924. The chicken as a carrier of *Histomonas meleagridis* (blackhead): the protozoön in its flagellated stage. *Journ. Med. Res.,* 44: 676-677.

TYZZER (E. E.). 1934. Studies on histomoniasis or "blackhead" infection in the chicken and the turkey. *Proc. Amer. Acad. Arts and Sc.,* 69: 189-264.

TYZZER (E. E.) and WALKER (E. L.). 1919. A comparative study of *Leishmania infantum* of infantile kala-azar and *Leptomonas (Herpetomonas) ctenocephali* parasitic in the gut of the dog flea. *Journ. Infect. Dis.,* 40: 129.

UHLEMEYER (B. L.). 1922. Some preliminary observations on *Kerona pediculus. Washington Univ. Studies. Scientific series,* 9: 237-271.

VIANNA (G.). 1911. Beitrag zum Studium der pathologischen Anatomie der Krankheit von Carlos Chagas. *Mem. Inst. Oswaldo Cruz.,* 3: 276-294.

WAGNER (E. H.). 1924. A precipitin test in experimental amœbic dysentery in cats. *Univ. Cal. Pub. Zoöl.,* 26: 15-20.

WALKER (E. L.). 1908. The parasitic amebæ of the intestinal tract of man and other animals. *Journ. Med. Res.,* 17: 379.

WALKER (E. L.). 1909. Sporulation in the parasitic ciliata. *Arch. Protist.,* 17: 297-306.

WALKER (E. L.). 1913. Experimental balantidiosis. *Phil. Journ. Sc.* (B) 8: 333-349.

WALKER (E. L.) and SELLARDS (A. W.). 1913. Experimental entamœbic dysentery. *Phil. Journ. Sci.*, (B) 8: 253-331.
WELCH (W. H.). 1897. Malaria: Definition, history, and parasitology. Loomis, *Syst. Pract. Med.*, New York, 1: 17.
WENRICH (D. H.). 1923. Variations in *Euglenamorpha hegneri*, n. g., n. sp., from the intestine of tadpoles. *Anat. Rec.*, 24: 370-371.
WENRICH (D. H.). 1936. Studies in *Dientamœba fragilis*. *Journ. Parasit.*, 22: 76-83.
WENRICH (D. H.). 1937. Studies on *Dientamœba fragilis*. *Journ. Parasit.*, 23: 183-196.
WENRICH (D. H.). 1937. Studies on *Iodamœba bütschlii* with special reference to nuclear structure. *Proc. Amer. Phil. Soc.*, 127: 183-205.
WENRICH (D. H.), STABLER (R. M.) and ARNETT (J. H.). 1935. *Endamœba histolytica* and other intestinal protozoa in 1,060 college freshmen. *Amer. Journ. Trop. Med.*, 15: 331-345.
WENRICH (D. H.) and YANOFF (J.). 1927. Results of feeding active trichomonad flagellates to rats. *Amer. Journ. Hyg.*, 7: 119-124.
WENYON (C. M.). 1915. Observations on the common intestinal protozoa of man: their diagnosis and pathogenicity. *Lancet*, 1915: pp. 1173-1183.
WENYON (C. M.). 1916. The protozoölogical findings in five hundred and fifty-six cases of intestinal disorder from the Eastern Mediterranean war area. *Journ. R. Army Med. Corps*, 26: 445.
WENYON (C. M.). 1923. "Hæmogregarines" in man with notes on some other supposed parasites. *Trop. Dis. Bull.*, 20: 527-550.
WENYON (C. M.). 1925. The genera *Councilmania, Karyamœba* and *Caudamœba*. *Trop. Dis. Bull.*, 22: 333-338.
WICHTERMAN (R.). 1936. Division and conjugation in *Nyctotherus cordiformis*, etc. *Journ. Morph.*, 60: 563-611.
WIGHT (T. H. T.) and PRINCE (L. H.). 1927. Artifacts in endamœbæ which have led to the naming of a new genus and species. *Amer. Journ. Trop. Med.*, 7: 287-308.
WILSON (C. W.). 1916. On the life-history of a soil amœba. *Univ. Calif. Pub. Zoöl.*, 16: 241-292.
WRIGHT (J. H.). 1903. Protozoa in a case of tropical ulcer ("Delhi sore"). *Journ. Med. Res.*, 10: 472.
YORKE (W.) and ADAMS (A.). 1926. Observations on *Entamœba histolytica*. I. Development of cysts, etc. *Ann. Trop. Med. and Parasit.*, 20: 279-302.

YORKE (W.) and ADAMS (A.). 1926. Observations on *Entamœba histolytica*. II. Longevity of the cysts in vitro, etc. *Ann. Trop. Med. and Parasit.*, 20: 317-326.

YORKE (W.) and ADAMS (A. R. D.). 1927. Observations on *Entamœba histolytica*. III. *Ann. Trop. Med. and Parasit.*, 21: 281-292.

YOSHIDA (K.). 1920. Reproduction in vitro of *Entamœba tetragena* and *Entamœba coli* from their cysts. *Journ. Exp. Med.*, 32: 357-379.

II. HELMINTHOLOGY

1. BOOKS AND JOURNALS

a. Books on Helminthology (in whole or in part)

BAYLIS (H. A.) and DAUBNEY (R.). 1926. *A synopsis of the Families and Genera of Nematoda*. 277 pp. London.

BAYLIS (H. A.). 1929. *A Manual of Helminthology*. 303 pp. London.

BRAUN (M.). 1925. *Die Tierschen Parasiten des Menschen*. 608 pp. Leipzig.

BRUMPT (E.). 1936. *Précis de Parasitologie,* 5th ed. 2139 pp. Paris.

CAMBRIDGE NATURAL HISTORY. Vol. II, 1922. London.

CHANDLER (A.). *Introduction to Human Parasitology*. 1936. 5th edition. 661 pp. New York and London.

CHITWOOD (B. G.) and CHITWOOD (M. B.). 1937. *An Introduction to Nematology*. Baltimore.

CRAIG (C. F.) and FAUST (E. C.). 1937. *Clinical Parasitology*. 733 pp. Philadelphia.

DOCK (G.) and BASS (C. C.). 1910. *Hookworm Disease*. 250 pp. St. Louis.

FAUST (E. C.). 1929. *Human Helminthology*. 616 pp. Philadelphia.

GRASSI (B.) and ROVELLI (G.) 1892. *Ricerche Embriologiche sui Cestodi*. 110 pp. Catania.

HALL (M. C.). *Diagnosis and Treatment of Internal Parasites,* 2nd ed. 102 pp. Chicago.

HEGNER (R. W.), CORT (W. W.), and ROOT (F. M.). 1923. *Outlines of Medical Zoölogy,* 175 pp. New York.

HUTYRA (F.) and MAREK (J.). 1926. *Special Pathology and Therapeutics of the Diseases of Animals*. 3 vols. Chicago.

JOEST (E.). 1923. *Spezielle Pathologische Anatomie der Haustiere*. 410 pp. Berlin.

LANGERON (M.) ET RONDEAU DU NOYER (M.). 1930. *Coprologie Microscopique*. 180 pp. Paris.

LEPAGE (G.). 1937. *Nematodes Parasitic in Animals*, 163 pp. London.

LEUCKART (R.). 1879-1901. Die Parasiten des Menschen und die von ihnen herrührenden Krankheiten, Leipzig, 856-897.

LEUCKART (R.). 1886. *The Parasites of Man*. 771 pp. Philadelphia.

MALLORY (F. B.). 1914. *Principles of Pathologic Histology*. 677 pp. Philadelphia.

MANSON-BAHR (P.). 1926. *Manson's Tropical Diseases*. 895 pp. New York.

MEGGITT (F. J.). 1924. *The Cestodes of Mammals*. 282 pp. London.

MÖNNIG (H. O.). 1934. *Veterinary Helminthology and Entomology*. 402 pp. London.

NAUYN (B.). 1862. *De Echinococci Evolutione*. 35 pp. Berolini.

NEVEU-LEMAIRE (M.). 1936. *Traité d'Helminthologie Médical et Vétérinaire*. 1514 pp. Paris.

RILEY (W. A.) and CHRISTENSON (R. O.). 1930. *Guide to the Study of Animal Parasites*. 127 pp. New York.

STAÜBLI (C.). 1909. *Trichinosis*. 295 pp. Wiesbaden.

STRONG (R. P.), SANDGROUND (J. H.), BEQUAERT (J. C.) and OCHOA (M. M.). 1934. *Onchocerciasis with Special Reference to the Central American Form of the Disease*. 234 pp. Cambridge, Mass.

WARD (H. B.) and WHIPPLE (G. C.). 1918. *Fresh-Water Biology*. 1111 pp. New York.

YORKE (W.) and MAPLESTONE (P. A.). 1926. *The Nematode Parasites of Vertebrates*. 536 pp. Philadelphia.

b. Journals that Contain Contributions on Helminthology

Acta Pathologica et Microbiologica Scandinavica. Copenhagen. Vol. 1. 1924.

American Journal of Hygiene. Baltimore. Vol. 1. 1921.

American Journal of Tropical Diseases and Preventive Medicine. New Orleans. Vol. 1. 1913.

American Journal of Tropical Medicine. Baltimore. Vol. 1. 1921.

Annales de la Société Belge de Médecine Tropical. Brussels. Vol. 1. 1920.

Annales de Parasitologie Humaine et Comparée. Paris. Vol. 1. 1923.

Annals of Tropical Medicine and Parasitology. Liverpool. Vol. 1. 1907.

Archiv für Schiffs-und Tropenhygiene. Leipzig. Vol. 1. 1897.

Archives de l'Institut Pasteur de Tunis. Tunis. Vol. 1. 1906.
Australian Journal of Experimental Biology and Medical Science. Adelaide. Vol. 1. 1924.
Bulletin de la Société de Pathologie Exotique. Paris. Vol. 1. 1908.
Bulletins of the Bureau of Animal Industry. Washington. 1890.
Bulletins of the Hygienic Laboratory. Washington. 1900.
Centralblatt für Bakteriologie, Parasitenkunde, und Infectionskrankheiten. Jena. Vol. 1. 1887.
Chinese Medical Journal. Shanghai. Vol. 1. 1887.
Comptes Rendus hebdomadaires des séances de l'Académie des Sciences. Paris. Vol. 1. 1835.
Comptes Rendus hebdomadaires des séances de la Société de Biologie. Paris. Vol. 1. 1849.
Helminthological Abstracts. St. Albans. Vol. 1. 1931.
Illinois Biological Monographs. Urbana. Vol. 1. 1914.
Indian Journal of Medical Research. Calcutta. Vol. 1. 1913.
Indian Medical Gazette. Calcutta. Vol. 1. 1866.
Japan Medical World. Tokyo. Vol. 1. 1921.
Journal of Agricultural Research. Washington. Vol. 1. 1913.
Journal of the American Veterinary Medical Association. Detroit. Vol. 1. 1877.
Journal of Experimental Medicine. Baltimore. Vol. 1. 1896.
Journal of Helminthology. London. Vol. 1. 1923.
Journal of the London School of Tropical Medicine. London. Vol. 1. 1911. Vol. 2. 1913.
Journal of Parasitology. Lancaster. Vol. 1. 1914.
Journal of the Royal Army Medical Corps. London. Vol. 1. 1903.
Journal of Tropical Medicine and Hygiene. London. Vol. 1. 1898.
Kitasato Archives of Experimental Medicine. Tokyo. Vol. 1. 1917.
Memorias do Instituto Oswaldo Cruz. Rio de Janeiro. Vol. 1. 1909.
Monographs of the Rockefeller Institute for Medical Research. New York. No. 1. 1910.
Onderstepoort Journal of Veterinary Science and Animal Industry. Onderstepoort. Vol. 1. 1933.
Parasitology. Cambridge. Vol. 1. 1908.
Philippine Journal of Science. Section B. Manila. Vol. 1. 1906.
Proceedings of the Royal Society of London. Series B. London. 1907.
Puerto Rico Journal of Public Health and Tropical Medicine. San Juan. Vol. 1. 1925.
Research Memoirs of the London School of Tropical Medicine London. No. 1. 1912.

Revista de Medicina Tropical y Parasitologia Bacteriologia, Clinica y Laboratorio. Havana. Vol. 1. 1935.
Revue Suisse de Zoölogie. Geneva. Vol. 1. 1893.
Revue de Zoologie et de Botanique Africaines. Brussels. Vol. 1. 1911.
Rivista di Parassitologia. Rome. Vol. 1. 1937.
Sinensia. Nanking. Vol. 1. 1929.
Transactions of the American Microscopical Society. Urbana. Vol. 1. 1892.
Transactions of the Royal Society of Tropical Medicine and Hygiene. London. Vol. 1. 1907.
Tropical Diseases Bulletin. London. Vol. 1. 1911.
Tropical Veterinary Bulletin. London. Vol. 1. 1912.
University of California Publications in Zoölogy. Berkeley. Vol. 1. 1902.
Zeitschrift für Infektionskrankheiten. Berlin. Vol. 1. 1906.

2. ARTICLES ON HELMINTHOLOGY IN JOURNALS

a. *Trematoda*

AFRICA (C. M.), DE LEON (W.) and GARCIA (E. Y.). 1936. Heterophydiasis. IV. Lesions found in the myocardium of eleven infested hearts including three cases with valvular involvement. *Philippine Journ. Pub. Health,* 3: 1-27.
ALVEY (C. H.). 1936. The morphology and development of the monogenetic trematode *Sphyranura oligorchis* (Alvey, 1933) and the description of *Sphyranura polyorchis* n. sp. *Journ. Parasitol.,* 28: 229-253.
AMEEL (D. J.). 1934. *Paragonimus,* its life history and distribution in North America and its taxonomy (Trematoda: TROGLOTREM-ATIDÆ). *Amer. Journ. Hyg.,* 19: 279-317.
ANDERSON (M. G.). 1935. Gametogenesis in the primary generation of a digenetic trematode, *Proterometra macrostoma* Horsfall, 1933. *Trans. Amer. Microscop. Soc.,* 54: 271-279.
ASKANAZY (M.). 1904. Die Aetiologie und Pathologie der Kaatzenegelerkrankung des Menschen. *Deutsche med. Wchnschr.,* 30: 689-691.
BARLOW (C. H.). 1925. The life cycle of the human intestinal fluke, *Fasciolopsis buski* (Lankester). *Amer. Journ. Hyg. Monog. Series,* 4: 98 pp.
BILHARZ (T.). 1852. Fernere Beobachtungen über das die Pfortader des Menschen bewohnende *Distomum hæmatobium* und sein

Verhältnis zu gewissen pathologischen Bildungen. *Zeitschr. f. wiss. Zoöl.*, 4:72-76.

BROOKS (F. G.). 1930. Studies on the germ cycle of trematodes. *Amer. Journ. Hyg.*, 12:299-340.

BROWN (N. W.). 1917. The FASCIOLOPSINÆ of China. A study of two species from Chekiang Province. *Johns Hopkins Hosp. Bull.*, 28:322-329.

BRUMPT (E.). 1931. *Cercaria ocellata*, determinant la dermatite des nageurs, provient d'une bilharzie des canards. *Compt. Rend. Acad. d. Sci.*, 193:612.

CAMERON (T. W. M.). 1931. Experimental infection of sheep with *Dicrocœlium dendriticum. Journ. Helminth.*, 9:41-44.

CHANDLER (A.). 1928. The prevalence and epidemiology of hookworm and other helminthic infections in India. Part XII. General Summary and Conclusions. *Ind. Journ. Med. Res.*, 15:695-740.

CHEN (H. T.). 1934. a. Helminths of dogs in Canton, with a list of those occurring in China. *Ling. Sci. Journ.*, 13:75-87. b. Helminths of cats in Fukien and Kwangtung Provinces with a list of those recorded from China. *Ibid.*, 261-273.

CH'EN PANG. 1923. A comparative study of *Clonorchis sinensis* (Cobbold). *Trans. Fifth Biennial Congress F.E.A.T.M.*, 434-446.

CHEN (PIN-DJI). 1937. The germ cell cycle in the Trematode, *Paragonimus kellicotti* Ward. *Trans. Amer. Mic. Soc.*, 56:208.

CONYNGHAM (H.). 1904. A new Trematode of man (*Amphistoma watsoni*). *Brit. Med. Journ.*, 2:663.

CORT (W. W.). 1917. Homologies of the excretory system of the forked-tailed cercariæ. *Journ. Parasitol.*, 4:49-57.

CORT (W. W.). 1936. Studies on schistosome dermatitis. 1. Present status of the subject. *Amer. Journ. Hyg.*, 23:349-371.

DAY (H. B.). 1937. Pulmonary bilharziasis. *Trans. Roy. Soc. Trop. Med. and Hyg.*, 30:575-582.

DUBOIS (G.). 1938. Monographie des STRIGEIDA (TREMATODA). *Mémoires de la Société Neuchateloise des Sciences Naturelles,* No. 6.

ERHARDT (A.). 1932. Chemotherapeutische Untersuchungen an der Opisthorchiasis der Katzen. *Arch. f. Schiffs-u. Tropen Hyg.*, 36:22-31.

FAIRLEY (N. H.). 1920. A comparative study of experimental bilharziasis in monkeys, contrasted with the hitherto described lesions in man. *Journ. Path. Bact.*, 23:289-314.

FAUST (E. C.). 1919. The excretory system in DIGENEA. II. Observations on the excretory system in distome cercariæ. *Biol. Bull.,* 36: 322-339.

FAUST (E. C.) and CHUNG-CHANG (TANG). 1936. Notes on new Aspidogastrid series, with a consideration of the phylogeny of the group. *Journ. Parasitol.,* 28: 487-501.

FAUST (E. C.) and HOFFMAN (W. H.). 1934. Studies on schistosomiasis mansoni in Puerto Rico. III. Biological studies. 1. The extra-mammalian phases of the life cycle. *Puerto Rico Journ. Pub. Health and Trop. Med.,* 10: 1-97.

FAUST (E. C.) and KHAW (OO-KEH). 1927. Studies on *Clonorchis sinensis* (Cobbold). *Amer. Journ. Hyg., Monographic Series,* No. 8, 284 pp.

FAUST (E. C.) and MELENEY (H. E.). 1924. Studies on schistosomiasis japonica. *Amer. Journ. Hyg., Monographic Series,* No. 3. 399 pp.

FISHER (A. C.). A study of the schistosomiasis of the Stanleyville District of the Belgian Congo. *Trans. Roy. Soc. Trop. Med. and Hyg.,* 28: 277-306.

FUHRMANN (O.). 1928. Zweite Klasse des Cladus Plathelminthes. TREMATODA. Handbuch der Zoölogie (Kükenthal) 11. (Berlin und Leipzig), 1-140.

FUJINAMI (A.) and NAKAMURA (H.). 1909. The route of infection and the development of the parasite of Katayama disease (schistosomiasis japonica) and the infected animal. *Kyoto Igaku Zasshi* 6: (Japanese text).

GALLIEN (L.). 1933. Transformations histologiques corrélative du cycle sexual chez *Polystomum integerrimum* Froelich. *Compt. Rend. Acad. d. Sci.,* 196: 426-428.

GARRISON (P. E.). 1908. A new intestinal trematode of man (*Fascioletta ilocana* G. N., S. N.) *Philippine Journ. Sci.,* 3: 385-393.

GODDARD (F. W.). 1919. A parasite of man as seen in Shaohsing. China. *Journ. Parasit.,* 4: 141-163.

GORDON (R. M.), DAVEY (T. H.) and PEASTON (H.). 1934. The transmission of bilharziasis in Sierra Leone, with an account of the life cycle of the schistosomes concerned, *S. mansoni* and *S. hæmatobium. Ann. Trop. Med. and Parasitol.,* 28: 323-418.

HILARIO (J. S.) and WHARTON (L. D.). 1917. *Echinostoma ilocanum* (Garrison): A report of five cases and a contribution to the anatomy of the fluke. *Philippine Journ. Sci.,* 12: Sec. B. 203-213.

HOEPPLI (R.). 1933. a. Parasites and tumor growth. *Chinese Med. Journ.*, 47: 1075-1111. b. Histological changes in the liver of fifty-six Chinese infected with *Clonorchis sinensis*. *Ibid.*, 1125-1141.

INGLES (L.). 1933. Studies on the structure and life-history of *Ostiolum oxyorchis* (Ingles) from the California red-legged frog, *Rana aurora draytoni*. *Univ. Cal. Pub. on Zoöl.*, 39: 135-156.

JOHNSON (J. C.). 1920. The life cycle of *Echinostoma revolutum* (Froelich). *Univ. Cal.*, 19: 335-388.

JOYEUX (CH.). 1922. Recherches sur les Notocotyles. *Bull. de la Soc. de Pathol. Exotique*, 15: 331-343.

KATHARINER (L.). 1904. Über die Entwicklung von *Gyrodactylus elegans* v. Nrdm. *Zoöl. Jb. Suppl.*, 7: 519-551.

KATSURADA (F.). 1912. On the genus *Heterophyes* in Japan. *Journ. Okagama Med. Assn.*, p. 268.

KAWAI (T.) and YUMATO (Y.). 1936. On the distribution of the encysted cercariæ of *Clonorchis sinensis* in the second intermediate host, *Pseudorasbora parva* (Temminck and Schlegel), and the rate of their infections to the mammalian hosts. *Journ. Med. Assoc. Formosa*, 35: 880.

KERBERT (C.). 1878. Zur Trematoden Kenntnis. *Zoöl. Anz.*, 1: 271-273.

KHALIL (M.). 1922. On the susceptibility of the egg masses of *Planorbis* to drying, chemical fertilizers, etc., and its bearing on the control of bilharzia disease. *Journ. Trop. Med. and Hyg.*, 25: 67-69.

KHALIL (M.). 1933. Life history of the human trematode parasite, *Heterophyes heterophyes* in Egypt. *Lancet*, 2: 537.

KHAW (O. K.). 1930. Remarks on the species of *Paragonimus*. With special references to the questions on their identity and distribution. *Nat. Med. Journ. of China*, 16: 93-115.

KOBAYASHI (H.). 1919. Studies on the lung-fluke in Korea. Structure of the adult worm with two plates. *Mitteilungen der Medizinischen Hochschule zu Keijo.*

KOBAYASHI (H.). 1923. A distomid infesting the Egyptian mullet. *Journ. Helminth.*, 1: 97-98.

KRULL (W.). 1930. The life history of two North American frog lung flukes. *Journ. Parasitol.*, 14: 207-212.

KRULL (W.). 1931. Life history studies on two frog lung flukes, *Pneumonœces medioplexus* and *Pneumobites parviplexus*. *Trans. Amer. Mic. Soc.*, 50: 215-277.

KRULL (W.) and PRICE (H. F.). 1932. Studies on the life history of *Diplodiscus temperatus* Stafford from the frog. *Occasional papers of the Museum of Zoölogy, U. of Michigan,* No. 237.

KRULL (W.). 1933. Studies on the life history of a frog lung fluke, *Hæmatolœchus complexus* (Seely, 1906) Krull, n. comb. *Zeit. f. Parasit.,* 6: 192-206.

KRULL (W.). 1934. Some additional notes on the life history of a frog lung fluke, *Hæmatolœchus complexus* (Seely, 1906) Krull. *Trans. Amer. Mic. Soc.,* 53: 196-199.

KRULL (W.). 1934. Life history studies on *Cotylophoron cotylophorum* (Fischoeder, 1901) Stiles and Goldberger, 1910. *Journ. Parasit.,* 20: 171-180.

LANE (C.). 1915. *Artyfechinostomum sufrartyfex,* a new Echinostome of man. *Indian Journ. Med. Res.,* 2: 977-983.

LEIPER (R. T.). 1911. A new Echinostome parasite in man. *Journ. London. School Trop. Med.,* 1: 27-28.

LEIPER (R. T.). 1918. Report on the results of the Bilharzia mission in Egypt. London. 140 pp.

LEWIS (T. R.) and McCONNELL (J. F.). 1876. *Amphistoma hominis* n. sp., a new parasite affecting man. *Proc. Asiatic Soc. Bengal.,* 8: 182-186.

LOOSS (A.). 1892. *Amphistomum subclavatum* Rud., und seine Entwickelung. *Leuckart's Festschr.,* pp. 147-167.

LOOSS (A.). 1894. Bemerkungen zur Lebensgeschichte der *Bilharzia hæmatobium* im Anschlusse an G. Sandison Brocks Arbeit über denselben Gegenstand. *Centralbl. f. Bakteriol. u. Parasitenk.,* 16: 286.

LOOSS (A.). 1896. Not. z. Helminth. Ægypt *Central f. Bakteriol.,* Abt. I., 20: 836-870.

LOOSS (A.). 1899. Weitere Beiträge zur Kenntnis der Trematoden-Fauna Aegyptens; Zugleich Versuch einer natürlichen Gliederung des Genus *Distomum,* Retzius. *Zoöl. Jahr., Jena. Abt. f. Syst.,* 12: (5-6), 564.

LOOSS (A.). 1907. On some parasites in the museum of the School of Tropical Medicine, Liverpool. *Ann. Trop. Med. Parasit.,* 1: 123-153.

LOOSS (A.). 1908. What is "*Schistosomum mansoni*" Sambon, 1907. *Ann. Trop. Med. Parasitol.,* 2: 153-191.

LÜHE (MAX). 1909. Parasitische Plattwürmer. I. Trematodes. *Die Süsswasserfauna Deutschlands.,* 17: 1-217.

LUTZ (A.). 1919. On *Schistosomum mansoni,* a Schistosomatose segundo observaçoes feitas no Brazil. *Men. Inst. Oswaldo Cruz,* 11: 121-155.

Macy (R. W.). 1934. Studies on the taxonomy, morphology and biology of *Prosthogonimus macrorchis* Macy, a common oviduct fluke of domestic fowls in North America. *U. of Minn. Agri. Exp. Sta. Tech. Bull. 98.*

Manson (Patrick). 1880. *Distoma ringeri* and parasitical hæmoptysis. *China Imperial Maritime Customs. Med. Reports, 22:* 55-62.

Maxwell (J. L.). 1931. Paragonimiasis in China. *China Med. Journ.,* 45: 43-49.

McConnell (J. F. P.). 1875. Remarks on the anatomical and pathological relations of a new species of liver fluke. *Lancet,* 2: 271-274.

Miyairi (K.) and Suzuki (M.). 1913. Contribution to the development of *Schistosoma japonicum. Tokyo Iji Shinshi (Tokyo Med. Weekly)* No. 1836. (Japanese text.)

Musgrave (W. E.). 1907. Paragonimiasis in the Philippine Islands. *Philippine Journ. Sci.,* Section B, 2: 16-63.

Nakagawa (K.). 1919. Further notes on the study of the human lung distome, *Paragonimus westermani. Journ. Parasitol.,* 6: 39-43.

Nakagawa (K). 1922. The development of *Fasciolopsis buski* (Lankester). *Journ. Parasit.,* 8: 161-165.

Narabayashi (H.). 1914. On prenatal infection with *Schistosoma japonicum. Verhandl. d. Jap. Path. Gesellsch.,* No. 4. (Japanese.)

O'Connor (P. W.). 1919. Helminth ova in human stools. Expeditionary Force Sinai Peninsula. *Journ. Trop. Med. and Hygiene,* 22: 166.

Odhner (T.). 1911. *Echinostomum ilocanum* (Garrison), ein neuer Menschenparasit aus Ostasien. *Zoöl. Anz.,* 38: 65-68.

Odhner (T.). 1911. Zum natürlichen System der digenen Trematoden. IV. *Zoöl. Anz.,* 38: 513-531.

Odhner (T.). 1912. Die hemologien der Weiblichen Genitalwege bei den Trematoden und Cestoden. Nebst Bemerkungen zum natürlichen System der monogenen Trematoden. *Zoöl. Anz.,* 39: 337-351.

Odhner (T). 1913. Ein zweites *Echinostomum* aus dem Menschen in Ostasien. (*Ech. malayanum* Leiper.) *Zoöl. Anz.,* 41: 577-582.

Onsey (Anis Bey). 1937. The pathogenesis of endemic (Egyptian) splenomegaly. *Trans. Roy. Soc. Trop. Med. and Hyg.*, 30: 583-600.

PEARSE (A. S.). 1936. Zoölogical Names. A list of phyla, classes and orders. *Duke University Press*, 1-24.

POCHE (F.). 1926. Das System der PLATODARIA. *Archiv. f. Natur-geschichte*, 91: 1-458.

PRICE (E. W.). 1937. North American monogenetic trematodes. The superfamily GYRODACTYLOIDEA. *Journ. Wash. Acad. Sci.*, 27: 114-130.

PRICE (H. F.). 1931. Life history of *Schistosomatium douthitti* (Cort). *Amer. Journ. Hyg.*, 13: 685-727.

RAILLIET (A.), HENRY (A.), and JOYEUX (C.). 1912. Sur deux Trematodes des Primates. *Bull. Soc. Path. Exot., Paris*, 5: 833-837.

RILEY (W. A.) and KERNKAMP (H. C. H.). 1924. Flukes of the genus *Collyriclum* as parasites of turkeys and chickens. *Amer. Vet. Med. Journ.*, 64: 1-9.

RÜFFER (M. A.). 1910. Note on the presence of *"Bilharzia hæma-tobium"* in Egyptian mummies of the twentieth dynasty (125-1000 B.C.). *Brit. Med. Journ.*, 1: 16.

SAMBON (L. W.). 1907. Remarks on *Schistosomum mansoni*. *Journ. Trop. Med. and Hyg.*, 10: 303-304.

SAMBUC (E.) and BAUJEAN (R.). 1913. Un cas de cachexie ac-queuse chez l'homme (Distomatose hepatipancreatique, avec syn-drome pseudo-beriberique). *Bull. soc. med. chirurg. de l'Indo-chine*, 4: 425-429.

SEWELL (R. B. S.). 1922. Cercariæ Indicæ. *Indian Journ. Med. Research*, 10 (Supplement No.) : 1-370.

SHIPLEY (A. E.). 1905. *Cladorchis watsoni* (Conyngham) : a human parasite from Africa. *Thompson Yates Lab. Rept.*, Liverpool, 6: 129-135.

STILES (C. W.) and GOLDBERGER (J.). 1910. A study of *Watsonius watsoni* of man. *U. S. Hygiene Lab. Bull.*, No. 17: 66.

STILES (C. W.) and HASSALL (A.). 1910. The lung fluke (*Para-gonimus westermanii*) in swine and its relation to parasitic hæmoptysis in man. *Am. Rept. Bur. An. Ind.*, 16: 560-611.

STILES (C. W.). 1926. Key-Catalogue of the worms reported for man. *Hyg. Lab. Bull.*, No. 142, Washington.

SWALES (W. E.). 1936. Further studies on *Fascioloides magna* (Bassi, 1875) Ward, 1917, as a parasite of ruminants. *Canad. Journ. Research. Zoöl. Sci.*, 14: 83-95.

TUBANGUI (M. A.) and PASCO (A. M.). 1933. The life history of the human intestinal fluke, *Euparyphium ilocanum* (Garrison, 1908). *Philippine Journ. Sci.*, 51 : 581-606.

VAN HAITSMA (J. P.). 1931. Studies on the trematode family *Strigeidæ* (*Holostomidæ*) No. XXIII : *Diplostomum flexicaudum* (Cort and Brooks) and stages in its life history. *Papers of the Mich. Acad. Sci., Arts and Letters,* 13 : 483-516.

VERDUN (R.) et Bruyant (S.). 1908. Sur la dualité spécifique de la douve de Chine (*Clonorchis sinensis* Cobbold), *Archiv. de Parasitologie,* 12 : 99-124.

VEVERS (G. M.). 1923. Observations on the genus Paragonimus Braun with a re-description of *P. compactus* (Cobbold, 1859) 1899. *Journ. Helminthology,* 1 : 9-19.

VOGEL (H.). 1929. Beobachtungen ueber *Cercaria vitrina* und deren Beziehung zum Lanzettegelproblem. *Arch. f. Schiffs-u. Trop.-Hyg.,* 33 : 474-489.

VOGEL (H.). 1932. Ueber den ersten Zwischenwirt und die Zerkarie von *Opisthorchis felineus* Riv. *Arch. f. Schiffs-u. Trop.-Hyg.,* 36 : 558-561.

WARD (H. B.). 1908. Data for the determination of human Entozoa. II. *Trans. Amer. Mic. Soc., 28* : 177-202.

WARD (H. B.) and HIRSCH (E.). 1915. The species of *Paragonimus,* and their differentiation. *Am. Trop. Med. Parasitol.,* 9 : 109-162.

WILLEY (C. H.). 1930. Studies on the lymph system of digenetic trematodes. *Journ. Morph. and Physiol.,* 50 : 1-37.

WOODHEAD (ARTHUR E.). 1931. The germ cycle in the trematode family, BUCEPHALIDÆ. *Trans. Amer. Mic. Soc.,* 50 : 169-187.

YOKOGAWA (S.). 1919. Studien über die Uebergangs-und Verbreitungswege des *Paragonimus westermani* kerbert (*Distoma pulmonale* Baelz) im Koerper des Endwirtes. Formosa Government Publication.

YOUNG (S.). 1936. Studies on the final host of *Fasciolopsis buski* and its development in the intestine of the pig. *Journ. Shankhai Sci. Inst.,* 2 : 225-236.

YUMOTO (Y.). 1936. On the minute structure of the egg-shells of *Clonorchis sinensis,* and on its abnormal eggs. *Journ. Med. Assoc. of Formosa,* 35 : 1836-1846.

b. *Cestoda*

ANDERSON (MARLOW). 1934. The validity of *Tænia confusa* Ward, 1896. *Journ. Parasit.,* 20 : 207-218.

BIRKELAND (I. W.). 1932. "Bothriocephalus anemia." *Medicine*, 11: 1-39.

BONNAL (G.), JOYEUX (C.) and BOSCH (P.). 1933. Un cas de cénurose humaine dû à *Multiceps cerialis* (Gervais). *Bull. Soc. Path. Exot.*, 26: 1060.

BULLOCK (F. D.). and CURTIS (M. R.). 1920. The experimental production of sarcoma of the liver of rats. *Proc. N. York. Path. Soc.*, 20: 149-175.

CASONI (T.). 1912. La diagnosi biologica dell' echinococcosi umana mediante l'intradermoreazione. *Folia Clin. Chim. et Micros.*, pp. 4, 5-16.

CHEN (H. T.). 1934. Reactions of *Ctenocephalides felis* to *Dipylidium caninum*. *Ztschr. f. Parasitenk*, 6: 603-637.

CHRISTENSEN (REED O.). 1931. An analysis of reputed pathogenicity of *Thysanosoma actinioides* in adult sheep. *Journ. Agric. Research*, 42: 245-249.

DENNIS (E. W.). 1937. A stable, concentrated, purified antigen for immunological study of hydatid disease. *Journ. Parasit.*, 23: 62-67.

DEW (H. R.). 1925. Daughter cyst formation in hydatid disease: Some observations on its causation and effects. *Med. Journ. Australia*, Oct. 24, p. 497.

DEW (H. R.). 1926. The mechanism of daughter cyst formation in hydatid disease. *Med. Journ. Australia*, Apr. 24, 32 pp.

DEW (H. R.). 1937. Some aspects of echinococcus disease. *Surgery*, 2: 363-380.

DIASTRE (A.) and STASSANO (H.). 1903. (a) Existence d'une antikinase chez les parasites intestinaux. *Compt. Rend. Soc. de Biol.*, 55: 130-132. (b) Antikinase des macerations d'*Ascaris* et de *Tænia*. *Ibid.*, pp. 254-256.

DIXON (H. B. F.) and SMITHERS (D. W.). 1935. Cysticercosis (*Tænia solium*). *Journ. Roy. Arm. Med. Corps*, April-August.

ESSEX (H. E.). 1927. Early development of *Diphyllobothrium latum* in northern Minnesota, *Journ. Parasitol.*, 14: 106-109.

FAIRLEY (K. D.). 1924. Hydatid disease of the liver. *Med. Journ. Australia*, 1: 177-186.

FAIRLEY (N. H.). 1922. The complement fixation test for hydatid disease and its clinical value. *Med. Journ. Australia*, 1: 341-346.

FUHRMANN (O.). 1931. Dritte Klasse des Cladus Plathelminthes. CESTOIDEA. *Handbuch der Zoölogie* (Kükenthal), II, Berlin und Leipzig, 141-416.

GRASSI (B.). 1888. Beiträge zur Kenntnis des Entwicklungsgeschichte von fünf Parisiten des Hundes (*Tænia cucumerina*, Goeze, *Ascaris marginata* Rud., *Spiroptera sanguinolenta* Rud., *Filaria immitis* Leidy und Hæmatozoön Lewis). *Centralb. f. Bakteriol. u. Parasitenk.*, 10: 282-285.

HALL (M. C.). 1919. The adult tænioid cestodes of dogs and cats, and of related carnivores in North America. *U. S. Nat. Museum*, 55: No. 2258.

HALL (M. C.). 1928. Parasite problems of live stock industry in the United States and Central America. *Cornell Veterinarian*, 28.

HALL (M. C.) and SCHILLINGER (J. E.). 1924. Some critical tests of arecoline hydrobromide as an anthelmintic. *Journ. Amer. Vet. Med. Assoc.*, 63: 454-463.

IWATA (S.). 1933. Some experimental and morphological studies on the post-embryonal development of Manson's tapeworm, *Diphyllobothrium erinacei* (Rudolphi). *Jap. Journ. Zoöl.*, 5: 209-247.

JANICKI (C.) and ROSEN (F.). 1917. Le Cycle évolutif du *Bothriocephalus latus*. Recherches expérimentales et observations. *Bull. Soc. Neuchâtel des Sci. Nat.*, 42: 19-53.

JONES (M.) and HORSFALL (M. W.). 1936. The life history of a poultry cestode. *Science*, 83: 303-304.

JOYEUX (C.). 1920. Cycle évolutif de quelques Cestodes. *Bull. Biol. de France et de Belgique*, 219 pp.

JOYEUX (C.) and BAER (J.). 1929. Les cestodes rares de l'homme. *Bull. Soc. de Path. Exot.*, 22: 114-136.

JOYEUX (C.), HOUDEMER (E.) and BEAR (J.). 1934. Recherches sur la biologie des *Sparganum* et l'étiologie de la sparganose oculaire. *Bull. Soc. Path. Exot.*, 27: 70-78.

LÖRINCZ (F.). 1933. Die Rolle der Katze in der Verbreitung der Echinococcosis. *Zent. f. Bakt., Parasit. u. Infektionskrankheiten, Erst. Abt. Orig.*, 129: 1-11.

MAGATH (T. B.) and BROWN (P. W.). 1927. Standardized method of treating tapeworm infestation in man to recover the head. *Journ. Amer. Med. Assoc.*, 88: 1548-1549.

MAGATH (T. B.). 1937. Hydatid (echinococcus) disease in Canada and the United States. *Amer. Journ. Hyg.*, 25: 107-134.

MILLER (H. M., JR.). 1931. a. The production of artificial immunity in the albino rat to a metazoan parasite. *Journ. Prev. Med.*, 5: 429-452. b. Superinfection of cats with *Tænia tæniæformis*. *Ibid.*, 6: 17-29.

OKUMURA (T.). 1919. An experimental study on the life history of *Sparganum mansoni. Kit. Arch. Exp. Med.*, 3: 190-198.

PEARSE (A. S.). 1936. Zoological names. A list of phyla, classes and orders. *Duke University Press,* 1-24.

POCHE (F.). 1926. Das System der PLATODARIA. *Archiv f. Naturgeschichte,* 91 : 1-458.

RANSOM (B. H.). 1913. *Cysticercus ovis,* the cause of tapeworm cysts in mutton. *Journ. Agri. Research,* 1 : 15-58.

RILEY (W. A.). 1919. The longevity of the fish tapeworm of man, *Dibothriocephalus latus. Journ. Parasitol.,* 5 : 193.

SAMBON (L.). 1924. The elucidation of cancer. *Journ. Trop. Med. and Hyg.,* 27 : 124-174.

SCHWARTZ (B.). Helminthological Society of Washington, Records of the 107th Meeting. Note 2, *Tænia solium* in dogs. *Journ. Parasit.,* 14 : 197-203.

SHORB (D. A.). 1932. Host-parasite relations of *Hymenolepis fraterna* in the rat and the mouse. *Amer. Journ. Hyg.,* 18 : 74-113.

SOUTHWELL (T.). 1925. A monograph on the TETRAPHYLLIDEA with notes on related cestodes. *Memoir of the Liverpool School of Trop. Med.,* N. S., No. 2.

SOUTHWELL (T.). 1930. CESTODA. *The fauna of British India, including Ceylon and Burma,* 2 : 1-262.

STILES (C. W.). 1908. The occurrence of a proliferating cestode larva (*Sparganum proliferum*) in man in Florida. *U. S. Pub. Health and Marine Hosp. Service, Hygienic Lab. Bull.,* No. 40.

STUNKARD (H. W.). 1937. The life cycle of *Moniezia expansa. Science,* 86 : 312.

TURNER (C. L.), BERBERIAN (D. A.) and DENNIS (E. W.). a. 1936. The production of artificial immunity in dogs against *Echinococcus granulosus. Journ. Parasit.,* 22 : 14-28. b. 1937. The production of artificial immunity against hydatid disease in sheep. *Ibid.,* 23 : 43-61.

VERGEER (T.). 1928. *Diphyllobothrium latum* (Linn., 1758), the broad tapeworm of man. *Journ. Amer. Med. Assoc.,* 90 : 673-678.

WELSH (D. A.), CHAPMAN (H. G.), and STOREY (J. C.). 1909. Some applications of the precipitin reaction in the diagnosis of hydatid disease. *Lancet,* p. 1103.

WOODLAND (W. N. F.). 1924. *Hymenolepis nana* and *H. fraterna. Lancet,* pp. 922-923.

YOSHIDA (S.). 1922. On the morphology of the adult worm of *Sparganum mansoni* found in the frog and other animals. *Tokyo Iji. Shinshi.,* Nos. 2271 and 2272.

c. *Nematoda*

ACKERT (J. E.). 1921. Investigations on the control of hookworm disease. IV. The relation of the domestic chicken to the spread of hookworm disease. *Amer. Journ. Hyg.*, 2: 26-38.

ACKERT (J. E.). 1923. On the habitat of *Ascaridia perspicillum* (Rud.). *Journ. Parasitol.*, 10: 101-103.

ACKERT (J. E.). 1924. Notes on the longevity and infectivity of hookworm larvæ. *Amer. Journ. Hyg.*, 4: 222-225.

ACKERT (J. E.). and PAYNE (F. K.). 1921. Investigations on the control of hookworm disease. V. The domestic pig and hookworm disease. *Amer. Journ. Hyg.*, 2: 39-50.

ACKERT (J. E.). 1923. Investigations on the control of hookworm disease. XII. Studies on the occurrence, distribution and morphology of *Necator suillus,* including descriptions of the other species of *Necator. Amer. Journ. Hyg.*, 3: 1-24.

ACKERT (J. E.), McILVAINE (M. F.) and CRAWFORD (N. Z.). 1931. Resistance of chickens to parasitism affected by vitamin A. *Amer. Journ. Hyg.*, 13: 320.

AFRICA (C.) and GARCIA (E.). 1936. A new nematode parasite (*Cheilospirura* sp.) of the eye of man in the Philippines. *Journ. Phil. Ids. Med. Assoc.*, 16: 603-607.

ALICATA (J. E.). 1935. The tail structure of the infective Strongyloides larvæ. *Journ. Parasitol.*, 21: 450-451.

ANDERSON (JOHN). 1924. Filariasis in British Guiana. *London School of Trop. Med., Research Memoir Series,* No. 7.

ARREZA-GUZMAN (A.). 1937. Recherches expérimentales sur le traitement de la strongyloidose murine. *Ann. de Parasit., Humaine et Comparée,* 15: 125-145.

ASHFORD (B. K.) and GUTIERREZ (P.). 1911. Uncinariasis in Porto Rico. *Senate Document No. 808, 61st Congress, 3d Session,* Washington, 335 pp.

AUCHINLOSS (H.). 1920. A new operation for elephantiasis. *Puerto Rico Journ. Pub. Health and Trop. Med.*, 6: 149-150.

AUGUSTINE (D. L.). 1937. Observations on living "sheathed" microfilariæ in the capillary circulation. *Trans. Roy. Soc. Trop. Med. and Hyg.*, 31: 55-60.

AUGUSTINE (D. L.), HELMY (M.), NAZMI (M.), and McGAVRAN (G.). 1928. The ova-parasite ratio for *Ancylostoma duodenale* and *Ascaris lumbricoides. Journ. Parasitol.*, 15: 45-51.

AUGUSTINE (D. L.) and SMILLIE (W. G.). 1926. The relation of the type of soil of Alabama to the distribution of hookworm disease. *Amer. Journ. Hyg.*, 6: 36-62.

AUGUSTINE (D. L.) and THEILER (H.). 1932. Precipitin and skin tests as aids in diagnosing trichinosis. *Parasitology*, 24: 60-86.

BACHMAN (G.) and GONZÁLEZ (J. O.). 1937. Immunization in rats against *Trichinella spiralis*. *Proc. Soc. Exp. Biol. and Med.*, 35: 215-217.

BAERMAN (G.). 1917. Über Ankylostomiasis deren Ausbreitungs-bedingungen durch die Bodeninfection und deren Bekaempfung. *Geneeskundig Tijdschrift voor Nederlandsch-Indie*, 57: 579-673.

BERNARD (P. N.) and BAUCHE (J.). 1914. Influence du mode de pénétration, cutanée au buccale de *Stephanurus dentatus* sur les localisations de ce nématode dans l'organisme du porc et sur son évolution. *Ann. de l'Inst. Pasteur*, 28: 450-469.

BLACKLOCK (D. B.). 1926. The development of *Onchocerca volvulus* in *Simulium damnosum*. *Ann. Trop. Med. and Parasitol.*, 20: 1-40.

BLICKHAHN (W. L.). 1893. Case of ankylostomiasis. *Med. News, Phil.*, 63: 662-663.

BBOWN (H.). 1927. Human Ascaris as a household infection. *Journ. Parasitol.*, 13: 206-212.

BROWN (H. W.) and CORT (W. W.). 1927. The egg production of *Ascaris lumbricoides*. *Journ. Parasitol.*, 14: 88-90.

CALDWELL (F. C.) and CALDWELL (E. L.). 1926. Are *Ascaris lumbricoides* and *Ascaris suilla* identical? *Journ. Parasitol.*, 13: 141-145.

CALDWELL (F. C.), CALDWELL (E. L.) and DAVIS (G. E.). 1930. Some aspects of the epidemiology of infestation with *Trichuris* and *Ascaris* as revealed in a study at hospitals for the insane and the home for mentally defective children in the State of Alabama. *Amer. Jour. Hyg.*, 2: 619-651.

CHANDLER (A.). 1924. Animals as disseminators of hookworm eggs and larvæ. *Ind. Med. Gaz.*, 59: 533-537.

CHANDLER (A.). 1925. The species of *Strongyloides* (Nematoda). *Parasitology*, 17: p. 426.

CHANDLER (A.). 1928. The prevalence and epidemiology of hook-worm and other helminthic infections in India. *Indian Journ. Med. Research*, 15: 695-743.

CHU (TSO-CHIH). 1936. Studies on the life history of *Rhabdias fuscovenosa* var. *catanensis* (Rizzo, 1902). *Journ. Parasitol.*, 22: 140-160.

COBB (N. A.). 1890. Two new instruments for biologists. *Proc. Linn. Soc. N. S. Wales*, 5: 157-167.

COBB (N. A.). 1914. Nematodes and their relationships. *Yearbook U. S. Dept. Agri.*, pp. 457-490.

CONNAL (A.) and CONNAL (S. L. M.). 1921. A preliminary note on the subject of *Loa loa* (Guyot) *Chrysops silacea* (Austen). *Trans. Roy. Soc. Trop. Med. and Hyg.*, 15: 131-134.

CORT (W. W.). 1931. Recent investigations on the epidemiology of human ascaris. *Journ. Parasit.*, 17: 121-144.

CORT (W. W.), ACKERT (J. E.), AUGUSTINE (D. L.) and PAYNE (F. K.). 1922. The description of an apparatus for isolating infective hookworm larvæ from soil. *Amer. Journ. Hyg.*, 2: 1-17.

CORT (W. W.), GRANT (J. B.), and STOLL (N. R.). 1926. Researches on hookworm in China. *Amer. Journ. Hyg.*, *Monographic Series*, No. 7, 398 pp.

CRAM (E. B.). 1925. The egg-producing capacity of *Ascaris lumbricoides*. *Journ. Agri. Research*, 30: 977-983.

CRAM (E. B.). 1931. Developmental stages of some nematodes of the SPIRUROIDEA parasitic in poultry and game birds. *Tech. Bull. No. 227, U. S. Dept. Agri.*

DAVEY (D. G.). 1938. Studies on the physiology of nematodes of the alimentary canal of sheep. *Parasitology*. (In press.)

DELBET (P.). 1936. Sur la nocivité du pain blanc. *Bull. Acad. Med.*, 115: 267-271.

DRINKER (C. K.). 1936. The relation of lymph circulation to streptococci infection. *Medical papers dedicated to Dr. Henry A. Christian*.

EPSTEIN (A.). 1892. Über die Übertragung des menschlichen Spulwurms (*Ascaris lumbricoides*). *Verk. d. 9, vers. d. Gessellsch. f. Kinderheilkunde*, Wiesbaden.

FAUST (E. C.). 1933. Experimental studies on human and primate species of *Strongyloides* in the experimental host. *Amer. Journ. Hyg.*, 18: 114.

FAUST (E. C.). 1935. Experimental studies on human and primate species of *Strongyloides*. IV. The pathology of *Strongyloides* infection. *Arch. of Path.*, 19: 769-806.

FAUST (E. C.) and KAGY (E. S.). 1933. Experimental studies on human and primate species of *Strongyloides*. I. The variability and instability of types. *Amer. Journ. Trop. Med.*, 13: 47-65.

FAUST (E. C.), WELLS (J. W.), ADAMS (C.) and BEACH (T. D.). 1934. Experimental studies on human and primate species of

Strongyloides. III. The fecundity of *Strongyloides* females of the parasitic generation. *Arch. of Path.,* 18:605-625.

FIBIGER (J.). 1913. Über eine Nematoden (*Spiroptera* sp. n.) hervorgerufene papillomatöse und carcinomatöse Geschmulstsbildung im Magen der Ratte, *Berl. klin. Wchnschr.,* 50: 289-298.

FOSTER (A. O.) and CROSS (S. X.). 1934. The direct development of hookworms after oral infection. *Amer. Journ. Trop. Med.,* 14: 565-573.

FOSTER (A. O.) and LANDSBERG (J. W.). 1934. The nature and cause of hookworm anemia. *Amer. Journ. Hyg.,* 20: 259-290.

FRANCIS (E.). 1919. Filariasis in the Southern United States. *U. S. Public Health Service, Hygienic Lab. Bull.,* No. 117, 34 pp.

FÜLLEBORN (F.). 1914. Untersuchungen über den Infektionsweg bei *Strongyloides* und *Ankylostomum* und die Biologie dieser Parasiten. *Arch. f. Schiffs-u. Tropen-Hyg.,* Beih, 5: 26-80.

FÜLLEBORN (F.). 1920. Über die Anpassung der Nematoden an den Parasitismus und den Infektionsweg bei Askaris und anderen Fadenwürmern des Menschen. *Arch. f. Schiffs. u. Tropenhyg.,* 24: 340-347.

FÜLLEBORN (F.). 1921. Über Askaridenlarven in Gehirn. *Arch. f. Schiffs. u. Tropenhyg.,* 25: 62-63.

FÜLLEBORN (F.). 1925. Über die Durchlässigkeit der Blutkapillaren für Nematodenlarven. *Arch. f. Schiffs. u. Tropenhyg.,* 29: 5-100.

FÜLLEBORN (F.). 1926. Eine seit 20 Jahren bestehende der "Creeping eruption" ähnliche wandernde Hautaffektion aus Ostafrika. *Arch. f. Schiffs. und Tropenhyg.,* 30: 702-704.

FÜLLEBORN (F.). 1926. Hautquaddeln und "Autoinfektion" bei Strongyloidesträgern. *Arch. f. Schiffs-u. Tropenkrankheiten,* 30: 721-732.

GAGE (J. G.). 1910. Larvæ of *Strongyloides intestinalis* in human lungs. *Journ. Med. Res.,* 23: 177-183.

GAGE (J. G.). 1911. A case of *Strongyloides intestinalis* with larvæ in the sputum. *Arch. Int. Med.,* 7: 560-579.

GOLDEN (R.). and O'CONNOR (F. W.). 1934. The roentgen treatment of filariasis. I. Chyluria. II. Lymphangitis. *Trans. Roy. Soc. Trop. Med. and Hyg.,* 27: 385.

GOODEY (T.). 1924. The anatomy and life history of the nematode *Rhabdias fuscovenosa* (Railliet) from the grass snake *Tropidonotus matrix. Journ. Helminth.,* 2: 51-64.

GOODEY (T.). 1926. Observations on *Strongyloides fülleborni* von Linstow, 1905, with some remarks on the genus *Strongyloides. Journ. Helminthology,* 4: 75-86.

GRACE (A. W.) and GRACE (F. G.). 1931. Researches in British Guiana 1926-1928 on the bacterial complications in filariasis and the endemic nephritis, with a chapter on epidemic abscess and cellulitis in St. Kitts, British West Indies. *No. 3, Memoir Ser., London School of Hyg. and Trop. Med.*

GRAHAM (G. L.), ACKERT (J. E.) and JONES (R. W.). 1934. Studies on an acquired resistance of chickens to the nematode *Ascaridia lineata* (Schneider). *Am. Journ. Hyg.,* 15 : 726.

GRASSI (G.). 1883. Anchilostomi e Anguillule. *Giorn. R. Accad. med. Torino.,* 31 : 119.

GRAYBILL (H. W.). 1921. Data on the development of *Heterakis papillosa. Journ. Exp. Med.,* Vol. 34.

HALL (M. C.). 1921. Carbon tetrachloride for the removal of parasitic worms, especially hookworms. *Journ. Agri. Research,* 21 : 157-175.

HALL (M. C.). 1923. Pinworm infection in man and its treatment. *Therap. Gazette,* Sept. 1-14.

HALL (M. C.). 1923. Notes on the present status of anthelmintic medication. *U. S. Naval Med. Bull.,* 18 : No. 6.

HALL (M. C.). 1937. Studies on oxyuriasis. I. Types of anal swabs and scrapers, with a description of an improved type of swab. *Amer. Journ. Trop. Med.,* 17 : 445-453.

HALL (M. C.) and SHILLINGER (J.). 1925. Tetrachlorethylene, a new anthelmintic for worms in dogs. *North Amer. Vet.,* 6 : 41-51.

HARRIS (W. H.) and BROWNE (D. C.). 1925. *Oxyuris vermicularis* as a causative fact in appendicitis. *Journ. Amer. Med. Assoc.,* 84 : 650-654.

HASEGAWA (T.). 1924. Beitrag zur Entwicklung von *Trichocephalus* im Wirte. *Arch. f. Schiffs. u. Tropenhyg.,* 28 : 337-340.

HIRAISHI (T.). 1927. Experimental ascariasis of young pigs with special reference to A. avitaminosis. *Jap. Med. World,* 7 : 79.

HUNG-SEE-LU and HOEPPLI (R.). 1923. Morphologische und histologische Beiträge zur Strongyloides-Infektion der Tiere. *Arch. f. Schiffs. u. Tropenhyg.,* 27 : 118-129.

KALJUS (W. A.). 1936. On the practical value of the intradermal reaction with trichinelliasis antigen for the diagnosis of trichinelliasis in man. *Puerto Rico Journ. Pub. Health and Trop. Med.,* 11 : 768-789.

KIRBY-SMITH (J. L.), DOVE (W. E.), and WHITE (G. F.). 1926. Creeping Eruption. *Archives of Dermatology and Syphilology,* 13 : 137-173.

Koino (S.). 1922. Experimental infections on human body with Ascarides. *Japan Med. World*, 2: 317-320.

Kotlán (S.). 1919. Beitrag zur Helminthologie Ungarns. 1. Neue Sclerostomiden aus den Pferden. *Centralfl. f. Bakt.*, 83: 559.

Kouri (P.) and Sellek (A.). 1936. Sobre et traitamiento de la strongyloidosis por el violeta de genciana. *Rev. Parasit., Clin. y Lab.*, 2: 7-16.

Kreis (H. A.). 1932. Studies on the genus *Strongyloides* (Nematoda). *Amer. Journ. Hyg.*, 16: 450.

Lane (C.). 1937. Bancroftian filariasis and the recticuloendothelial system. *Trans. Roy. Soc. Trop. Med. and Hyg.*, 31: 61.

Lane (C.). 1937. Hookworm anemia. An outline in basic of present knowledge and opinion. *Trop. Dis. Bull.*, 34: 1-14.

Lane (C.). 1936. What drug best kills hookworms? *Amer. Journ. Digestive Dis. and Nutrition*, 3: 770-772.

Leiper (R. T.). 1913. Metamorphosis of *Filaria loa*. *Journ. Trop. Med. and Hyg.*, 16: 59-60.

Leuckart (R.). 1882. Lebensgeschichte der sog, *Anguillula stercoralis*, u. deren Beziehung zu d. sog *A. intestinalis*, Bericht math. phys. Cl. k. Sächs. Gesellsch. Also in *Die menschlichen Parasiten und die von ihnen herruhrenden Krankheiten*. I, Leipzig, 1863; II, Leipzig, 1876.

Looss (A.). 1911. The anatomy and life history of *Agchylostoma duodenale* Dub. Part. I. The anatomy of the adult worm. Part. II. The development in the free state. *Ministry of Education, Egypt, Records of the School of Medicine*, Vols. 3 and 4, 613 pp.

Lucker (J.). 1936. Comparative morphology and development of infective larvæ of some horse strongyles. *Proc. Helminth. Soc. of Washington*, 3: 22-25.

Magath (T. B.). 1916. Nematode technique. *Trans. Amer. Mic. Soc.*, 35: 245-256.

McCoy (O. R.). 1934. The effect of vitamin A deficiency on the resistance of rats to infection with *Trichinella spiralis*. *Amer. Journ. Hyg.*, 20: 169.

McRae (A.). 1935. The extra-corporeal hatching of *Ascaris* eggs. *Journ. Parasit.*, 21: 222-223.

Moorthy (V. N.). 1932. An epidemiological and experimental study of dracontiasis in Chitaldrug District. *Ind. Med. Gaz.*, 67: 498.

Moorthy (V. N.). 1937. A redescription of *Dracunculus medinensis*. *Journ. Parasit.*, 23: 220-225.

Nishigori (M.). 1928. The factors which influence the external development of *Strongyloides stercoralis* and on autoinfection with this parasite. *Journ. Form. Med. Soc.*, 277: 1-56.

O'Connor (F. W.). 1923. Report on the results of the expedition sent from the London School of Tropical Medicine to the Ellice, Tokelau, and Samoan Islands in 1921-1922. *Research Memoirs of the London School of Trop. Med.*, 4: 57 pp.

O'Connor (F. W.). 1932. The etiology of the disease syndrome in *Wuchereria bancrofti* injections. *Trans. Roy. Soc. Trop. Med. and Hyg.*, 26: 13-47.

O'Connor (F. W.). 1935. Studies in filariasis. *Puerto Rico Journ. Pub. Health and Trop. Med.*, 11: 167-272.

O'Connor (F. W.). and Beatty (H.). 1936. The early migrations of *Wuchereria bancrofti* in *Culex fatigans. Trans. Roy Soc. Trop. Med. and Hyg.*, 30: 125-127.

O'Connor (F. W.), Golden (R.) and Auchinloss (H). 1930. The roentgen demonstration of calcified *Filaria bancrofti* in human tissues. *Amer. Journ. Roent. and Rad. Therapy*, 23: 494-502.

O'Connor (F. W.) and Hulse (C. R.). 1932. Some pathological changes associated with *Wuchereria (Filaria) bancrofti* infection. *Trans. Roy. Soc. Trop. Med. and Hyg.*, 25: 445-454.

Otto (G. F.). and Cort (W. W.). 1934. The distribution and epidemiology of human ascariasis in the United States. *Amer. Journ. Hyg.*, 19: 657-712.

Payne (F. K.), Ackert (J. E.), and Hartman (E.). 1925, The question of the human and pig *Ascaris. Amer. Journ. Hyg.*, 5: 90-101.

Pearse (A. S.). 1936. Zoological Names. A list of phyla, classes and orders. *Duke Univ. Press.*

Pēna Chavarria (A.) and Rotter (W.). 1935. Untersuchungen über die Hakenwurmanämie. *Arch f. Schiffs. u. Tropen-Hyg.*, 39: 505-516.

Penso (G.). 1932. Presence des oeufs d'oxyures en pleine muquense intestinal et biologie des oxyures. *Ann. Parasit. Humaine et Comparée*, 10: 271-275.

Penso (G.). 1933. Nouvelles considerations sur la biologie des oxyures. *Ibid.*, 11: 268-270.

Pintner (T.). 1927. Kritische Beiträge zum System der tetra-rhynchen. *Zoöl. Jahrb. Syst.*, 53: 559-590.

Poche (F.). 1926. Das System der platodaria. *Archiv. f. Naturgeschichte*, 91: 1-458.

RANSOM (B. H.). 1915. Trichinosis. *Rep. U. S. Live Stock San. Assoc.*, pp. 147-165.

RANSOM (B. H.). 1921. The prevention of intestinal worms in pigs. *Journ. Amer. Vet. Med. Assoc.*, 59:711-715.

RANSOM (B. H.) and CRAM (E. B.). 1921. Course of migration of *Ascaris* larvæ from the intestine to the lung. *Anat. Rec., Phila.*, 20:207., *Amer. Journ. Trop. Med.*, 1:129-159.

RANSOM (B. H.) and HALL (M. C.). 1915. The life history of *Gongylonema scutatum*. *Journ. Parasitol.*, 2:80-86.

RANSOM (B. H.) and HALL (M. C.). 1920. Parasitic diseases in their relation to the live stock industry of the southern United States. *Journ. Amer. Vet. Med. Assoc.*, Vol. 10.

RANSOM (B. H.), SCHWARTZ (B.) and RAFENSPERGER (H. B.). 1920. Effects of pork-curing processes on trichinæ. *U. S. Dept. Agri. Bull.*, No. 880.

RHOADS (C. P.), CASTLE (W. B.), PAYNE (G. C.), and LAWSON (H. A.). 1934. Observations on the etiology and treatment of anemia associated with hookworm infection in Puerto Rico. *Medicine*, 13:317-375.

RILEY (W. A.) and FITCH (C. P.). 1921. The animal parasites of foxes. *Journ. Amer. Vet. Med. Assoc.*, 59:294-305.

ROCKEFELLER FOUNDATION, INTERNATIONAL HEALTH BOARD. 1922. Bibliography of hookworm disease. *Publication No. 11.*

SANDGROUND (J. H.). 1926. Biological studies on the life-cycle in the genus *Strongyloides* Grassi, 1879. *Amer. Journ. Hyg.*, 6:337-388.

SANDGROUND (J. H.). 1931. Studies on the life history of *Ternidens deminutus,* a nematode parasite of man, with observations on its incidence in certain regions of Southern Africa. *Ann. Trop. Med. and Parasit.*, 25:147-184.

SAYAD (W. Y.), JOHNSON (V. M.) and FAUST (E. C.). 1936. Human parasitization with *Gordius robustus*. *Journ. Amer. Med. Assoc.*, 106:461.

SCHWARTZ (B.). 1925. *Ascaridia lineata*, a parasite of chickens in the United States. *Journ. Agri. Research*, 30:763-772.

SCHWARTZ (B.). 1926. Specific identity of whipworms from swine. *Journ. Agri. Research*, 33:311-316.

SEURAT (L. G.). 1919. Contributions nouvelles des formes larvaires de Nématodes parasites hétéroxènes. *Bull. Biol. de France et Belg.*, No. 52.

SHIMAMURA (T.) and FUJII (H.). 1917. Über das askaron, einen Toxischen Bestandteil der Helminthen besonders der Askariden und seine Biologische Wirkung. *Journ. Col. Agri. Imp. Univ., Tokyo,* 3: 189-258.

SHIMURA (S.) and OGAWA (T.). 1920. On the filariform larvæ found in the vomit of a patient infected with *Strongyloides stercoralis. Tokyo Med. News.* No. 2197, pp. 1829-1863. (Japanese text.) Review in *Trop. Dis. Bull.,* 1922, 19: No. 3, 223.

SMILLIE (W. G.) and AUGUSTINE (D. L.). 1926. The effect of varying intensities of hookworm infestation upon the development of school children. *South. Med. Journ.,* 19: 19-28.

SMILLIE (W. G.) and SPENCER (C. R.). 1926. Mental retardation in school children infested with hookworms. *Journ. Educational Psychology,* 17: 314-321.

SPINDLER (L. A.). 1937. Skin penetration experiments with the infective larvæ of the swine kidney worm, *Stephanurus dentatus. Journ. Parasit.,* 20: 76-77.

SPINK (W. W.). 1937. *Trichinella* antigen. Further observations on its use in the diagnosis of trichinosis. *New Eng. Journ. Med.,* 216: 508.

STEWARD (F. H.). 1916. On the life history of *Ascaris lumbricoides. Brit. Med. Journ.,* 2: 5-7, 486-488, 753-754.

STEWARD (F. H.). 1921. On the life history of *Ascaris lumbricoides. Parasitology,* 13: 37-47.

STILES (C. W.). 1903. Report upon the prevalence and geographic distribution of hookworm disease (Uncinariasis or anchylostomiasis) in the United States. *U. S. Pub. Health Serv., Hyg. Lab. Bull.,* No. 10.

STOLL (N. R.). 1923. Investigations on the control of hookworm disease. XV. An effective method of counting hookworm eggs in feces. *Amer. Journ. Hyg.,* 3: 59-70.

STOLL (W. R.) and HAUSHEER (W. C.). 1926. Concerning two options in dilution egg counting. *Amer. Journ. Hyg.,* 6: March Supplement.

SVENSSON (R. M.) and KESSEL (J. F.). 1926. Morphological differences between *Necator* and *Anchylostoma* larvæ. *Journ. Parasit.,* 13: 146.

TAYLOR (E. L.). 1935. *Syngamus trachea.* The longevity of the infective larvæ in the earthwork. Slugs and snails as intermediate hosts. *Journ. Path. and Ther.,* 48: 149-156.

THEILER (H.) and AUGUSTINE (D. L.) and SPINK (W. W.). 1935. On the persistence of eosinophila, and on immune reactions in human trichinosis, several years after recovery. *Journ. Parasit.,* 27: 345.

THIRA (T). 1919. Studien über *Strongyloides stercoralis, Mitt, Med. Gesellsch Tokio*, 33 : 2-3. (Review in *Trop. Dis. Bull.*, 1924.)

TYZZER (E. E.). 1926. *Heterakis vesicularis* Froelich 1791 : A vector of an infectious disease. *Proc. Soc. Exp. Biol. and Med.*, 23 : 708-709.

TYZZER (E. E.), FABYAN (M.), and FOOT (N. C.). 1921. Further observations on "Blackhead" in turkeys. *Journ. Infect. Diseases*, 29 : 268-286.

URIBE (C.). 1922. Observations on the development of *Heterakis papillosa* Bloch in the chicken. *Journ. Parasitol.*, 8 : 167-176.

VAN CLEAVE (H. J.). 1936. The recognition of a new order in the ACANTHOCEPHALA. *Journ. Parasit.*, 22 : 202-206.

VAN COTT (J. M.). and LINTZ (W.). 1914. Trichinosis. *Journ. Amer. Med. Assoc.*, 62 : 680.

VAN DURME (P.). 1902. Quelques notes sur les embryons de *Strongyloides intestinalis* et leur pénétration par la peau. *Thompson Yates Lab. Report, Liverpool*, 4 : 471-474.

WARD (H. B.). 1916. *Gongylonema* in the rôle of a human parasite. *Journ. Parasitol.*, 2 : 119-124.

WEHR (E. E.). 1937. Observations on the development of the poultry pageworm, *Syngamus trachea. Trans. Amer. Mic. Soc.*, 56 : 72-78.

WHARTON (L. D.). 1915. The development of the eggs of *Ascaris lumbricoides. Phil. Journ. Science*, 10 : 19-23.

WHITE (G. F.) and DOVE (W. E.). 1928. The causation of creeping eruption. *Journ. Amer. Med. Assoc.*, 90 : 1701-1704.

WINFIELD (G. F.) and YAO (TZU-NING). 1937. Studies on the control of fecal-borne diseases of North China. IV. Vegetables as a factor in the spread of *Ascaris lumbricoides. Chinese Med. Journ.*, 51 : 919-926.

YOKOGAWA (S.). 1920. On the migratory course of *Trichosomoides crassicauda* (Bellingham) in the body of the final host. *Journ. Parasitol.*, 7 : 80-84.

YOSHIDO (S.). 1919. On the development of *Ascaris lumbricoides. Journ. Parasitol.*, 5 : 105-115.

III. ARTHROPODS OF PARASITOLOGICAL IMPORTANCE

1. BOOKS AND JOURNALS

a. Books on Arthropods (in whole or in part)

ALCOCK (A.). 1920. *Entomology for Medical Officers*. 380 pp. London.

750 PARASITOLOGY

ALDRICH (J. M.). 1905. *A catalogue of North American Diptera.* *Smithsonian Misc. Coll.,* Vol. 46. 680 pp. Washington.

ALDRICH (J. M.). 1910. *Sarcophaga and allies in North America.* *Thomas Say Foundation of the Ent. Soc. of Am.* 302 pp. La Fayette, Ind.

AUSTEN (E. E.). 1911. *A handbook of the Tsetse-flies.* 110 pp. London.

BERLESE (A.). Vol. I. 1909. Vol. II. 1925. *Gli insetti.* 1004, 992 pp. Milano.

BONNE (C.) and BONNE-WEBSTER (J.). 1925. *Mosquitoes of Surinam. Royal Colonial Inst. of Amsterdam, Contr. No. 21, Dept. of Trop. Hygiene No. 13.* 558 pp. Amsterdam.

BOYD (M. F.). 1930. *An introduction to malariology.* 437 pp. Cambridge, Mass.

BRUMPT (E.). 1936. *Précis de Parasitologie.* 2139 pp. Paris.

BUXTON (P. A.). 1927. *Researches in Polynesia and Melanesia. Parts I to IV. Medical Entomology.* 260 pp. London.

BYAM (W.) and ARCHIBALD (R. G.). 1921. *The practice of medicine in the tropics.* Vol. I. 855 pp. London.

CALMETTE (A.). 1908. *Venoms, venomous animals and antivenomous serum-therapeutics.* 403 pp. London.

CARPENTER (G. D. H.). 1920. *A naturalist on Lake Victoria.* 333 pp. London.

COMSTOCK (J. H.). 1924. *An introduction to Entomology.* 1044 pp. Ithaca, N. Y.

COVELL (G.). 1931. *Malaria control by anti-mosquito measures.* 148 pp. Calcutta.

CRAIG (C. F.) and FAUST (E. C.). 1937. *Clinical parasitology.* 733 pp. Philadelphia, Penn.

CURRAN (C. H.). 1934. *The Families and Genera of North American Diptera.* 512 pp. New York.

DA COSTA (B. F. B.), SANT' ANNA (J. F.), DOS SANTOS (A. C.) and ALVAREZ (M. G. DE A.). 1916. *Sleeping Sickness in Principe.* 261 pp. London.

DOANE (R. W.). 1910. *Insects and Disease.* 227 pp. New York.

DYAR (H. G.). 1928. *The Mosquitoes of the Americas. Carnegie Inst. Publications No. 387.* 616 pp. Washington.

EWING (H. E.). 1929. *A manual of external parasites.* 225 pp. Springfield, Ill.

FOLSOM (J. W.). 1909. *Entomology, with special reference to its biological and economic aspects.* 485 pp. Philadelphia.

FOX (C.). 1925. *Insects and disease of man.* 349 pp. Philadelphia.

GALTSOFF (P. S.), LUTZ (F. E.), WELCH (P. S.) and NEEDHAM (J. G.). 1937. *Culture methods for invertebrate animals.* 590, + XXXIII. Ithaca, N. Y.

GATER (B. A. R.). 1934. *Aids to the identification of Anopheline larvæ in Malaya.* 160 pp. Singapore.

GATER (B. A. R.). 1935. *Aids to the identification of Anopheline imagines in Malaya.* 242 pp. Singapore.

GRAHAM-SMITH (G. S.). 1914. *Non-bloodsucking Flies.* 389 pp. Cambridge.

HACKETT (L. W.). 1937. *Malaria in Europe, an ecological study.* 336 pp. London.

HARDENBURG (W. E.). 1922. *Mosquito Eradication.* 248 pp. New York.

HERMS (W. B.). 1915. *Medical and Veterinary Entomology.* 393 pp. New York.

HEWITT (C. G.). 1910. *The House-fly.* 196 pp. Manchester, England.

HINDLE (E.). 1914. *Bloodsucking Flies.* 389 pp. Cambridge, Eng.

HOWARD (L. O.). 1911. *The House Fly, disease carrier.* 312 pp. New York.

HOWARD (L. O.), DYAR (H. G.) and KNAB (F.). 1912-1917. *The Mosquitoes of North and Central America and the West Indies.* 4 Vols. *Carnegie Inst. of Washington, Contribution No. 159.*

IMMS (A. D.). 1925. *A general Textbook of Entomology.* 698 pp. London.

INTERNATIONAL HEALTH BOARD. 1924. *The use of fish for Mosquito Control.* 120 pp. New York.

JAMES (S. P.) and LISTON (W. G.). 1911. *The Anopheline Mosquitoes of India.* 128 pp. Calcutta.

KELLOGG (V. L.). 1905. *American Insects.* 674 pp. New York.

KLIGLER (I. J.). 1930. *The epidemiology and control of malaria in Palestine.* 240 pp. Univ. of Chicago Press.

LARROUSE (F.). 1921. *Étude systématique et médicales des Phlébotomes.* 106 pp. Paris.

MARTINI (E.). 1923. *Lehrbuch der medizinischen Entomologie.* 462 pp. Jena, Germany.

MATHESON (R.). 1932. *Medical Entomology.* 489 pp. Springfield, Ill.

MENSE (C.). 1924. *Handbuch der Tropen-Krankheiten.* 3d ed. Vol. I. 713 pp. Leipzig.

MÖNNIG (H. O.). 1934. *Veterinary Helminthology and Entomology.* pp. 402. Baltimore.

NEWSTEAD (R.). 1907. *Preliminary report on the habits, life-cycle and breeding places of the common House-fly.* 23 pp. Liverpool.

NEWSTEAD (R.). 1924. *Guide to the study of Tsetse-flies. Liverpool School of Trop. Med. Memoir (new series) No. I.* 294 pp. Liverpool.

NUTTALL (G. H. F.), WARBURTON (C.), COOPER (W. F.) and ROBINSON (L. E.). 1908-1926. *Ticks, a monograph of the Ixodoidea.* 1908. *Part I. Argasidæ.* pp. 1-104. 1911. *Part II. Classification of the genus Ixodes.* pp. 105-348. 1915. Part III. *The genus Hæmaphysalis.* pp. 349-550. 1926. *Part IV. The genus Amblyomma.* pp. 1-302. Cambridge, England.

OLMER (D. and J.). 1933. *Fièvre boutonneuse, fièvre exanthématique du littoral mediterranéen. No. 57. Collection médecine et chirurgie pratiques.* 108 pp. Paris.

PATTON (W. S.) and CRAGG (F. W.). 1913. *A Textbook of Medical Entomology.* 768 pp. Calcutta.

PATTON (W. S.) and EVANS (A. E.). 1929, 1931. *Insects, ticks, mites and venomous animals of medical and veterinary importance. Part I.* 1929. *Medical.* 785 pp. *Part II.* 1931. *Public Health.* 740 pp. Croydon, England.

PIERCE (W. D.). 1921. *Sanitary Entomology.* 518 pp. Boston.

PINTO (C.). 1925. *Ensaio monographico dos Reduvideos hematophagos ou "Barbieros."* 118 pp. Rio de Janeiro. Brazil.

RILEY (W. A.) and JOHANNSEN (O. A.). 1915. *Handbook of Medical Entomology.* 348 pp. Ithaca, N. Y.

RILEY (W. A.) and JOHANNSEN (O. A.). 1932. *Medical Entomology. A Survey of Insects and allied forms which affect the health of man and animals.* 476 pp. New York and London.

ROGERS (L.) and MEGAW (J. W. D.). 1935. *Tropical medicine.* 2nd ed. 547 pp. London.

ROSS (R.). 1910. *The prevention of Malaria.* 669 pp. New York.

SILER (J. F.), HALL (M. W.) and HITCHENS (A. P.). 1926. *Dengue. Phil. Bur. of Science Monograph 20.* 476 pp. Manila, P. I.

STRICKLAND (C.). 1915. *Short key to the identification of the larvæ of the common Anopheline Mosquitoes of the Malay Peninsula.* 18 pp. Kuala Lumpur, F. M. S.

STRONG (R. P.), SWIFT (H. F.), OPIE (E. L.), MACNEAL (W. J.), BAETJER (W.), PAPPENHEIMER (A. M.) and PEACOCK (A. D.). 1918. Trench Fever. *Report of Commission Med. Res. Comm. Amer. Red Cross.* 446 pp.

SWELLENGREBEL (N. H.). 1916. *De Anophelinen van Nederlandsch*

Oost-Indie. Colonial Institute of Amersterdam Contr. No. 7, Dept. of Trop. Hygiene No. 3, 182 pp. Amsterdam.

SWELLENGREBEL (N. H.) and RODENWALD (E.). 1932. *Die Anophelen von Niederländisch-Ostindien.* Jena.

TALIAFERRO (W. H.). 1929. *The immunology of parasitic infections.* 414 pp. N. Y., N. Y.

TEGONI (G.). 1926. *Indice bibliografico della malaria. Rivista di Malariologia.*

THEOBALD (F. V.). 1901-1910. *A Monograph of the Culicidæ of the World.* 5 vols. London.

WATSON (M.). 1915. *Rural Sanitation in the Tropics.* 320 pp. London.

WATSON (M.). 1921. *The prevention of malaria in the Federated Malay States.* 2d ed. 381 pp. New York.

WHITE (G. F.). 1937. *Rearing maggots for surgical use. Culture methods for invertebrate animals.* 418-427 pp. Ithaca, N. Y.

WILLISTON (S. W.). 1908. *Manual of North American Diptera.* 405 pp. New Haven, Conn.

WOLBACH (S. B.), TODD (J. L.) and PALFREY (F. W.). 1922. *The etiology and pathology of typhus.* 222 pp. Cambridge, Mass.

b. Journals that Contain Contributions on Arthropods

American Journal of Hygiene. Baltimore. Vol. 1. 1921.

American Journal of Tropical Medicine. Baltimore. Vol. 1. 1921.

Annales de l'Institut Pasteur. Paris. Vol. 1. 1887.

Annales de l'Institut Pasteur, Alger. Algers. Vol. 1, 1923.

Annales de Parasitologie humaine et comparée. Paris. Vol. 1, 1923.

Annals of Tropical Medicine and Parasitology. Liverpool. Vol. 1. 1907.

Archiv. für Schiffs- und Tropen-Hygiene. Leipzig. Vol. 1. 1897.

Bulletin de la Société de Pathologie Exotique. Paris. Vol. 1. 1908.

Bulletin of Entomological Research. London, Vol. 1. 1910-1911.

Entomological News. Philadelphia. Vol. 1. 1890.

Indian Journal of Medical Research. Calcutta. Vol. 1. 1913-1914.

Journal of Economic Entomology. Geneva, N. Y. Vol. 1. 1908.

Journal of Hygiene. Cambridge, England. Vol. 1. 1901.

Journal of Parasitology. Lancaster, Pa. Vol. 1. 1914.

Journal of Tropical Medicine and Hygiene. London. Vol. 1. 1898.

Memorias do Instituto Oswaldo Cruz. Rio de Janeiro, Brazil. Vol. 1. 1909.

Parasitology. Cambridge, England. Vol. 1. 1908.

Puerto Rico Journal of Public Health and Tropical Medicine. San
Juan, P. R. Vol. 1. 1925.
Review of Applied Entomology. Section B. London. Vol. 1. 1913.
Rivista di Malariologia. Rome. Vol. 1. 1922.
Rivista di Parassitologia. Rome. Vol. 1. 1937.
*Transactions of the Royal Society of Tropical Medicine and Hy-
giene.* London. Vol. 1. 1907-1908.
Tropical Diseases Bulletin. London. Vol. 1. 1911.
Zentralblatt für Bakteriologie und Parasitenkunde. Jena. Vol. 1.
1887.

2. ARTICLES ON ARTHROPODS OF PARASITOLOGICAL IMPORTANCE IN JOURNALS

ADLER (S.) and THEODOR (O.). 1925. The experimental transmission of cutaneous Leishmaniasis to man from Phlebotomus
papatasii. *Ann. Trop. Med. and Parasit.,* 19: 365-372.
ALDRICH (J. M.). 1923. Notes on the dipterous family Hippobos-
cidæ. *Insecutor Inscitiæ Menstruus,* 11 : 75-79.
ANDERSON (J. F.) and FROST (W. H.). 1912. Transmission of polio-
myelitis by means of the stable-fly (Stomoxys calcitrans). *Public
Health Reports,* 27: 1733-1735.
ANDERSON (J. F.) and FROST (W. H.). 1912. Further attempts to
transmit the disease through the agency of the stable-fly (Stom-
oxys calcitrans). *Public Health Reports,* 28: 833-837.
ARAGÃO (H. DE B.). 1923. Ornithodorus brasiliensis n. sp. *Brazil-
Mexico,* 37 : 20.
ASHBURN (P. M.) and CRAIG (C. F.). 1907. Experimental investi-
gations regarding the etiology of dengue fever. *Journ. Infect.
Dis.,* 4 : 440-475.
BACOT (A. W.). 1914. A study of the bionomics of the common
rat fleas and other species associated with human habitations,
etc. *Journ. of Hygiene,* 13: Plague Supplement III : 447-654.
BACOT (A. W.) and MARTIN (C. J.). 1914. Observations on the
mechanism of the transmission of plague by fleas. *Journ. of
Hygiene,* 13: Plague Supplement III : 423-438.
BAHR (P. H.). 1912. Filariasis and Elephantiasis in Fiji. *Journal of
the London School of Trop. Med.,* Supplement I. 192 pp. Lon-
don.
BAKER (C. F.). 1904. A revision of the American Siphonaptera.
Proc. U. S. Nat. Mus., 28: 365-469.
BAKER (C. F.). 1905. The classification of the American Siphonap-
tera. *Proc. U. S. Nat. Mus.,* 29: 121-170.

BANKS (N.). 1904. A treatise on the Acarina or mites. *Proc. U. S. Nat. Mus.*, 28: 1-114.

BANKS (N.). 1908. A revision of the Ixodoidea or Ticks of the United States. *U. S. Dept. of Agr., Bur. of Ent., Technical Series*, No. 15. 60 pp. Washington.

BANKS (N.). 1912. The structure of certain dipterous larvæ with particular reference to those in human foods. *U. S. Dept. of Agr., Bur. of Ent., Technical Series*, No. 22. 44 pp. Washington.

BANKS (N.). 1915. The Acarina or mites. *U. S. Dept. of Agr., Bur. of Ent., Report*, No. 108. 153 pp. Washington.

BARBER (M. A.). 1918. Observations and experiments on Malayan Anopheles with special reference to transmission of Malaria. *Phil. Journ. Science*, 13 B: 1-47.

BARBER (M. A.) and RICE (J. B.). 1936. Methods of dissecting and making permanent preparations of the salivary glands and stomachs of Anopheles. *Amer. Journ. of Hygiene*, 24: 32-40.

BARRAND (P. G.). 1928. The distribution of Stegomyia fasciata in India, with remarks on dengue and yellow fever. *Ind. Journ. of Med. Res.*, 16: 377-388.

BARRAUD (P. J.). 1923-1927. A revision of the Culicine mosquitoes of India. Parts I to XXII. *Ind. Journ. of Med. Res.*, Vols. 10 to 14.

BASTIANELLI (G.), BIGNAMI (A. E.) and GRASSI (B.). 1898. Coltivazione delle semilune malariche dell' nomo nell' Anopheles claviger Fabr. Nota preliminar. *Real. Accad. dei Lincei.*, Nov. 28.

BATES (L. B.), DUNN (L. H.) and ST. JOHN (J. H.). 1921. Relapsing Fever in Panama. *Am. Journ. Trop. Med.*, 1: 183-210.

BAUER (J. H.). 1928. The transmission of yellow fever by mosquitoes other than Aëdes ægypti. *Am. Journ. Trop. Med.*, 8: 261-282.

BEDFORD (G. A. H.) and COLES (J. D. W. A.). 1933. The transmission of Ægyptianella pullorum Carpano to fowls by means of ticks belonging to the genus Argas. *Onderstp. Journ. Vet. Sci. and Anim. Indust.*, 1: 15-18.

BEEUWKES (H.), KERR (J. A.), WEATHERSBEE (A. A.) and TAYLOR (A. W.). 1933. Observations on the bionomics and comparative prevalence of the vectors of yellow fever and other domestic mosquitoes of West Africa, and the epidemiological significance of seasonal variations. *Trans. Roy. Soc. Trop. Med. & Hyg.*, 26: 425-447.

BENGTSON (I. A.). 1933. Seasonal acute conjunctivitis occurring in the Southern States. *U. S. Public Health Rept.*, 48:917-926.

BEZZI (M.). 1927. Some Calliphoridæ (Diptera) from the South Pacific islands and Australia. *Bull. Ent. Res.*, 17:231-247.

BISHOPP (F. C.). 1915. Flies which cause myiasis in man and animals—Some aspects of the problem. *Journ. Econ. Ent.*, 8:317-329.

BISHOPP (F. C.). 1915. Fleas. *U. S. Dept. of Agr. Bull.*, No. 248. 31 pp. Washington.

BISHOPP (F. C.). 1916. Flytraps and their operation. *U. S. Dept. of Agr., Farmer's Bull.*, No. 734. 16 pp. Washington.

BISHOPP (F. C.) and LAAKE (E. W.). 1921. Dispersion of flies by flight. *Journ. Agr. Research*, 21:729-766.

BISHOPP (F. C.), MITCHELL (J. D.) and PARMAN (D. C.). 1917. Screw-worms and other maggots affecting animals. *U. S. Dept. of Agr., Farmer's Bull.*, No. 857. 20 pp. Washington.

BLACKLOCK (D. B.). 1926. The development of Onchocerca volvulus in Simulium damnosum. *Ann. Trop. Med. and Parasit.*, 20:1-48.

BLACKLOCK (D. B.). 1926. The further development of Onchocerca volvulus Leuckart in Simulium damnosum Theob. *Ann. Trop. Med. and Parasit.*, 20:213-218.

BLACKLOCK (D. B.) and GORDON (R. M.). 1927. The experimental production of immunity against metazoan parasites. *Lancet*, Apr. 30, p. 923.

BLACKLOCK (B.) and THOMPSON (M. G.). 1923. A study of the Tumbu-fly. Cordylobia anthropophaga Grünberg, in Sierra Leone. *Ann. Trop. Med. and Parasit.*, 17:443-510.

BLAIZOT (L.), CONSEIL (E.) and NICOLLE (C.). 1913. Etiologie de la fievre récurrente, son mode de transmission par les poux. *Ann. Inst. Pasteur*, 27:204-225.

BLANC (G.) and CAMINOPETROS (J.). 1930. La transmission des varioles aviaires par les moustiques. *C. R. Acad. Sci.*, 190:954-956.

BLANC (G.) and CAMINOPETROS (J.). 1930. Recherches expérimentales sur la dengue. *Ann. Inst. Past.*, 44:367-436.

BOGEN (E.). Arachnidism. *Arch. Int. Med.*, 38:623-632.

BOYD (M. F.). 1936. Studies of the epidemiology of malaria in the coastal lowlands of Brazil. *Am. Journ. of Hygiene, Monographic Series*, No. 5. 261 pp. Baltimore, Md.

BOYD (M. F.), KITCHEN (S. F.) and MULRENNAN (J. A.). 1936. On the relative susceptibility of the inland and coastal varieties of A. crucians to P. falciparum. *Am. Journ. Trop. Med.*, 16: 159-161.

BRADLEY (G. H.). 1936. On the occurrence of Anopheles walkeri Theobald in Florida. *Sou. Med. Journ.*, 29: 857-859.

BRADLEY (G. H.). 1936. On the identification of the mosquito larvæ of the genus Anopheles occurring in the United States. *Sou. Med. Journ.*, 29: 859-861.

BRUCE (D.). 1895. Tsetse-fly disease or Nagana in Zululand. Preliminary Report. Bennett & Davis, Field St. Durban.

BRUCE (D.). 1897. Further report on the tsetse-fly disease or nagana in Zululand. Umbobo, May 29, 1896. London.

BRUES (C. T.). 1913. The relation of the stable-fly (Stomoxys calcitrans) to the transmission of infantile paralysis. *Journ. Econ. Ent.*, 6: 101-109.

BRUG (S. L.). Filariasis in the Dutch East Indies. *Proc. R. Soc. Med.*, 24: 23-33.

BRUMPT (E.). 1926. Transmission du Treponema crociduræ par deux Ornithodorus (O. moubata et O. marocanus). *C. R. Acad. Sci.*, 183: 1139-1141.

BRUMPT (E.). 1930. Transmission de la fièvre exanthematique de Marseille par la tique méridionale du chien, Rhipicephalus sanguineus. *C. R. Acad. Sci.*, Nov. 10.

BRUMPT (E.). 1931. Transmission d'Anaplasma marginale par Rhipicephalus bursa et par Margaropus. *Ann. d. Parasit.*, 9: 4-9.

BRUMPT (E.). 1933. Transmission de la fièvre pourprée des montagnes rocheuses par la tique americaine Amblyomma cayennense. *C. R. Seance d. l. Soc. Biol.*, 114: 416-419.

BRUMPT (E.). 1936. Etude experimentale du Plasmodium gallinaceum parasite de la poule domestique. Transmission de ce germe par Stegomyia fasciata et Stegomyia albopicta. *Ann. de Parasit. hum. et comp.*, 14: 597-620.

BULL (C. G.) and KING (W. V.). 1923. The identification of the blood meal of mosquitoes by means of the precipitin test. *Am. Journ. of Hygiene*, 3: 491-496.

BULL (C. G.) and ROOT (F. M.). 1923. Preferential feeding experiments with Anopheline mosquitoes. I. *Am. Journ. of Hygiene*, 3: 514-520.

BULL (C. G.) and REYNOLDS (B. D.). 1924. Preferential feeding experiments with Anopheline mosquitoes. II. *Am. Journ. of Hygiene*, 4: 109-118.

BUXTON (P. A.). 1921. On the Sarcoptes of man. *Parasit.*, 13: 146-151.

CAMERON (A. E.). The life-history and structure of Hæmatopota pluvialis, Linné (Tabanidæ). *Trans. R. Soc. Edinburgh,* 58: 211-250.

CANNON (P. R.) and McCLELLAND (P. H.). 1928. Rôle of ectoparasites in Bartonella infection of albino rats. *Proc. Soc. Exp. Biol. and Med.,* 26: 157-158.

CANNON (P. R.) and McCLELLAND (P. H.). 1929. The transmission of Bartonella infection in albino rats. *Journ. Inf. Dis.,* 44: 56-61.

CARTER (H. F.). 1921. A revision of the genus Leptoconops Skuse. *Bull. Ent. Res.,* 12: 1-28.

CARTER (H. F.). 1925. The Anopheline mosquitoes of Ceylon. *Ceylon Journ. of Science,* Sect. D., 1. 57-97.

CARTER (H. F.), INGRAM (A.) and MACFIE (J. W. S.). 1920. Observations on the Ceratopogonine midges of the Gold Coast. Part I. Introduction. Part II. Culicoides. *Ann. Trop. Med. and Parasit.,* 14: 187-210, 211-274.

CHAGAS (C.). 1909. Nova tripanozomiaze humana. (Ueber eine neue Trypanosomiasis des Menschen.) *Mem. do Instituto Oswaldo Cruz.,* 1: 159-218.

CHRISTOPHERS (S. R.). 1913. Contributions to the study of Colour Marking and other variable characters of Anophelinæ. *Ann. Trop. Med. and Parasit.,* 7: 45-100.

CHRISTOPHERS (S. R.). 1915. The male genitalia of Anopheles. *Ind. Journ. of Med. Res.,* 3: 371-394.

CHRISTOPHERS (S. R.). 1916. A revision of the nomenclature of Indian Anophelini. *Ind. Journ. of Med. Res.,* 3: 454-488.

CHRISTOPHERS (S. R.). 1922. The development and structure of the terminal abdominal segments and hypopygium of the mosquito. *Ind. Journ. of Med. Res.,* 10: 530-572.

CHRISTOPHERS (S. R.). 1923. The structure and development of the female genital organs and hypopygium of the mosquito. *Ind. Journ. of Med. Res.,* 10: 698-720.

CHRISTOPHERS (S. R.). 1924. Provisional list and reference catalogue of the Anophelini. *Ind. Med. Res. Memoirs,* No. 3. 105 pp. Calcutta.

CHRISTOPHERS (S. R.), SINTON (J. A.) and COVELL (G.). 1927. Synoptic table for the identification of the Anopheline mosquitoes of India. *Health Bulletin No. 10 Malaria Bureau No. 2,* 22 pp. Calcutta.

CLELAND (J. B.), BRADLEY (B.) and MACDONALD (W.). 1919.

Further experiments in the etiology of Dengue fever. *Journ. of Hygiene*, 18: 217-254.

CONNAL (A.) and CONNAL (S. L. M.). 1922. The development of Loa loa (Guyot) in Chrysops silacea (Austen) and in Chrysops dimidiata (Van der Wulp). *Trans. Roy. Soc. Trop. Med. and Hygiene*, 16: 64-89.

CONNOR (M. E.). 1924. Suggestions for developing a campaign to control Yellow Fever. *Am. Journ. of Trop. Med.*, 4: 277-307.

COOLEY (R. A.). 1936. Ornithodorus parkeri, a new species on rodents. *Public Health Reports*, 51: 431-433.

COVELL (G.). 1927. Anti-mosquito measures. *Govt. of India. Health Bulletin No. 11, Malaria Bureau No. 3.* 24 pp. Calcutta.

COVELL (G.). 1927. The distribution of Anopheline mosquitoes in India and Ceylon. *Ind. Med. Res. Memoirs*, No. 5. 85 pp. Calcutta.

COVELL (G.). 1927. A critical review of the data recorded regarding the transmission of malaria by the different species of Anopheles. *Ind. Med. Res. Memoirs*, No. 7. 117 pp. Calcutta.

COX (G. L.), LEWIS (F. C.) and GLYNN (E. E.). 1912. The number and varieties of bacteria carried by the common Housefly. *Journ. of Hygiene*, 12: 290-319.

CRAGG (F. W.). 1921. Geographical distribution of the Indian rat-fleas as a factor in the epidemiology of Plague. *Ind. Journ. of Med. Res.*, 9: 374-398.

CRAGG (F. W.). 1923. Further records of the distribution of Indian rat fleas. *Ind. Journ. of Med. Res.*, 10: 953-961.

CREEL (R. H.) and FAGET (F. M.). 1916. Cyanide gas for the destruction of insects. *Public Health Reports*, 31: 1464-1475.

CUMMINGS (B. F.). 1918. The Bed-bug. *Brit. Mus. (Nat. Hist.). Economic Series*, No. 5. 20 pp. London.

CURRY (D. P.). 1925. Some observations on mosquito control in the Canal Zone, with especial reference to the genus Anopheles. *Am. Journ. of Trop. Med.*, 5: 1-16.

DAMPF (A.). 1936. Los Ceratopogónidos o Jejenes como transmisores de filiarias. *Medicina no. 268.* 7 pp. Mexico.

DARLING (S. T.). 1910. Factors in the transmission and prevention of malaria in the Panama Canal Zone. *Ann. Trop. Med. and Parasit.*, 4: 179-224.

DARLING (S. T.). 1911. Murrina, a trypanosomal disease of equines in Panama. *Journ. Inf. Dis.*, 8: 467-485.

DARLING (S. T.). 1911. The probable mode of infection and the methods used in controlling an outbreak of equine trypanosomiasis (Murrina) in the Panama Canal Zone. *Parasit.*, 4:83-86.

DARLING (S. T.). 1912. Experimental infection of the mule with Trypanosoma hippicum by means of Musca domestica. *Journ. Exp. Med.*, 15:365.

DARLING (S. T.). 1926. Mosquito species control of malaria. *Am. Journ. of Trop. Med.*, 6:167-179.

DAVIES (F. C.) and WELDON (R. P.). 1917. A preliminary contribution on "P. U. O. Trench Fever." *Lancet*, 1:183-184.

DAVIS (N. C.). 1925. A field study of mountain malaria in Brazil. *Am. Journ. of Hygiene*, 6:119-138.

DAVIS (N. C.). 1928. A study of the transmission of Filaria in Northern Argentina. *Am. Journ. Hygiene*, 8:457-466.

DAVIS (N. C.). 1931. A note on the malaria-carrying Anophelines in Belém, Pará, and in Natal, Rio Grande do Norte, Brazil. *Revist. di Malariologia*, 10:43-51.

DAVIS (N. C.). 1933. Attempts to transmit yellow fever virus with Triatoma megista (Burmeister). *Journ. of Parasit.*, 19:209-214.

DAVIS (N. C.). 1933. Transmission of yellow fever virus by Culex fatigans. *Ann. Entom. Soc. of Amer.*, 26:491-494.

DAVIS (N. C.) and SHANNON (R. C.). 1929. Studies on yellow fever in South America. Transmission experiments with certain species of Culex and Aëdes. *Journ. Exp. Med.*, 50:803-808.

DAVIS (N. C.) and SHANNON (R. C.). 1931. Studies on yellow fever in South America. Attempts to transmit the virus with certain Aëdine and Sabethine mosquitoes and with Triatomes. *Am. Journ. Trop. Med.*, 11:21-29.

DAVIS (N. C.) and SHANNON (R. C.). 1931. Further attempts to transmit yellow fever with mosquitoes of South America. *Am. Journ. of Hygiene*, 14:715-722.

DAVIS (N. C.) and KUMM (H. W.). 1932. Further incrimination of Anopheles darlingi Root as a transmitter of Malaria. *Am. Journ. Trop. Med.*, 12:93-95.

DAVIS (N. C.), LLOYD (W.) and FROBISHER (M. JR.). 1932. The transmission of neurotropic yellow fever virus by Stegomyia mosquitoes. *Journ. Exp. Med.*, 56:853-865.

DE BOISSEZON (P.). 1929. Expériences au sujet de la maturation des œufs chez les Culicides. *Bull. d. l. Soc. Path. Exot.*, 22:683-688.

DE BUCK (A.). 1935. Beitrag zur Rassenfrage bei Culex pipiens. *Zeitschr. f. Angew. Entom.*, 22:242-252.

DINGER (J. E.), SCHÜFFNER (W. A. P.), SNIJDERS (E. P.) and

SWELLENGREBEL (N. H.). 1929. Onderzock van gele koorts in Nederland. *Nederl. Tijdschrift. voor Geneeskunde.* 73rd year: 3255-3257 and 5982-5991.

DOERR (R.), FRANZ (K.) and TAUSSIG (S.). 1909. Das Pappatacifieber. Leipzig and Wien.

DOVE (W. E.). 1918. Some biological and control studies of Gastrophilus hæmorrhoidalis and other bots of horses. *U. S. Dept. of Agr., Bull.,* No. 597. 51 pp. Washington.

DOVE (W. E.), HALL (D. G.), HULL (J. B.). 1932. The salt marsh sand fly problem. *Ann. Entom. Soc. Amer.,* 25: 505-527.

DOVE (W. E.) and SHELMIRE (B.). 1931. Tropical rat mites, Liponyssus bacoti Hirst, vectors of endemic typhus. *Journ. Amer. Med. Assoc.,* 97: 1506-1510.

DOVE (W. E.) and SHELMIRE (B.). 1932. Some observations on tropical rat mites and endemic typhus. *Journ. Parasit.,* 18: 159-168.

DUTTON (J. E.) and TODD (J. L.). 1905. The nature of human tick fever in the eastern part of the Congo Free State, with notes on the distribution and bionomics of the tick. *Liverpool School of Trop. Med. Mem.,* 17: 18 pp. (See also *Brit. Med. Journ.,* II: 1259-1260.)

DYAR (H. G.). 1918. Notes on American Anopheles. *Insecutor Inscitiæ Menstruus.,* 6: 141-151.

DYAR (H. G.). 1922. The mosquitoes of the United States. *Proc. U. S. Nat. Mus.,* 62: Art. 1: 1-119.

DYAR (H. G.). 1925. The mosquitoes of Panama. *Insecutor Inscitiæ Menstruus.,* 13: 101-195.

DYAR (H. G.) and SHANNON (R. C.). 1924. The subfamilies, tribes and genera of American Culicidæ. *Journ. Wash. Acad. of Sci.,* 14: 472-486.

DYAR (H. G.) and SHANNON (R. C.). 1924. The American Chaoborinæ. *Insecutor Inscitiæ Menstruus.,* 12: 201-216.

DYAR (H. G.) and SHANNON (R. C.). 1927. The North American two-winged flies of the family Simuliidæ. *Proc. U. S. Nat. Mus.,* 69: Art. 10: 1-54.

DYER (R. E.), BADGER (L. F.) and RUMREICH (A.). 1931. Rocky mountain spotted fever (Eastern type) transmission by the American dog tick (Dermacentor variabilis). *Public Health Reports,* 46 (1483): 1403-1413.

EDWARDS (F. W.). 1912. A synopsis of the species of African Culicidæ other than Anopheles. *Bull. Ent. Res.,* 3: 1-53.

EDWARDS (F. W.). 1912. A key for determining the African species of Anopheles. *Bull. Ent. Res.,* 3 : 241-250.

EDWARDS (F. W.). 1912. Revised keys to the known larvæ of African Culicinæ. *Bull. Ent. Res.,* 3 : 373-385.

EDWARDS (F. W.). 1915. On the British species of Simulium. *Bull. Ent. Res.,* 6 : 23-42.

EDWARDS (F. W.). 1921. On the British species of Simulium. II. The early stages. *Bull. Ent. Res.,* 11 : 211-246.

EDWARDS (F. W.). 1920. The nomenclature of the parts of the male hypopygium of Diptera Nematocera, with special reference to mosquitoes. *Ann. Trop. Med. and Parasit.,* 14 : 23-40.

EDWARDS (F. W.). 1921. A revision of the mosquitoes of the Palæarctic region. *Bull. Ent. Res.,* 12 : 263-351.

EDWARDS (F. W.). 1922. On some Malayan and other species of Culicoides, with a note on the genus Lasiohelea. *Bull. Ent. Res.,* 13 : 161-167.

EDWARDS (F. W.). 1922. The carriers of Filaria bancrofti. *Journ. Trop. Med. and Hyg.,* 25 : 168-170.

EDWARDS (F. W.). 1922. A synopsis of adult Oriental Culicine (including Megarhinine and Sebethine) mosquitoes. *Ind. Journ. of Med. Res.,* 10 : 249-294, 430-475.

EDWARDS (F. W.). 1924. A synopsis of the adult mosquitoes of the Australasian region. *Bull. Ent. Res.,* 14 : 351-401.

EDWARDS (F. W.). 1926. On the British biting midges. *Trans. Entom. Soc. London,* 74 : 389-426.

EDWARDS (F. W.). 1932. Diptera. Family Culicidæ. (Wytsman's *Genera Insectorum,* Fasc., 194 : 258 pp.)

ELIOT (C. P.). 1936. The insect vector for the natural transmission of Eperythrozoon coccoides in mice. *Science,* 84 (2183) : 397.

ELIOT (C. P.) and FORD (W. W.). 1929. Further observations of the virus of rat anemia with special reference to its transmission by the rat louse, Polyplax spinulosa. *Am. Journ. Hygiene,* 10 : 635-642.

ENDERLEIN (G.). 1904. Lause-studien. *Zoöl. Anz.,* 28 : 121-147.

ESKEY (C. R.). 1934. Epidemiological study of plague in the Hawaiian Islands. *Public Health Bull.,* No. 213. 70 pp.

ESKEY (C. R.). 1936. Plague infection discovered in fleas and lice taken from marmots in Western Montana and in a marmot in Utah. *U. S. Public Health Reports,* 51 : 1159-1160.

EVANS (A. M.). 1927. A short illustrated guide to the Anophelines of Tropical and South Africa. *Liverpool School of Trop. Med., Memoir* (new series) No. 3. 54 pp. Liverpool.

EWING (H. E.). 1920. The genus Trombicula Berlese in America and the Orient. *Ann. Ent. Soc. of Am.,* 13 : 381-390.

EWING (H. E.). 1921. Studies on the biology and control of Chiggers. *U. S. Dept. of Agr., Bull.,* No. 986. 19 pp. Washington.

EWING (H. E.). 1922. The Dermanyssid mites of North America. *Proc. U. S. Nat. Mus.,* 62 : Art. 13 : 1-26.

EWING (H. E.). 1923. Our only common North American chigger. *Journ. Agr. Res.,* 26 : 401-403.

EWING (H. E.). 1924. On the taxonomy, biology and distribution of the biting lice of the family Gyropidæ. *Proc. U. S. Nat. Mus.,* 63 : Art. 20 : 1-42.

EWING (H. E.). 1926. A revision of the American lice of the genus Pediculus. *Proc. U. S. Nat. Mus.,* 68 : Art. 19 : 1-30.

EWING (H. E.). 1926. Key to the known adult Trombiculas (adults of chiggers) of the New World. *Ent. News,* 37 : 111-113.

EWING (H. E.). 1926. The common Box-turtle, a natural host for chiggers. *Proc. Biol. Soc. of Wash.,* 39 : 19-20.

EWING (H. E.). 1938. The scientific name of the common North American chigger preoccupied. *Proc. Helm. Soc. of Wash.,* 39 : 19-20.

EYSELL (A.). 1924. Die Krankheitsüberträger und Krankheitserreger unter den Arthropoden. In Mense (C.). *Handbuch der Tropenkrankheiten.* 3d ed. Vol. 1. pp. 1-454.

FAUST (E. C.) and MAXWELL (T. A.). 1930. The finding of the larva of Chigœ, Tunga penetrans, in scrapings from human skin. Report of a case. *Arch. Derm. & Syph.,* 22 (1) : 94-97.

FELT (E. P.). 1904. Mosquitoes or Culicidæ of New York State. *N. Y. State Mus. Bull.,* No. 79. 400 p. Albany, N. Y.

FENG (L. C.). 1933. A brief mosquito survey in some parts of China. *Chinese Med. Journ.,* 47 : 1347-1358.

FERRIS (G. F.). 1920-23. Contributions toward a monograph of the sucking lice, Parts I-IV. *Stanford Univ. Publ., Univ. Series, Biol. Sci.,* Vol. 2, Nos. 1-4.

FIELDING (J. W.). 1926. Australasian Ticks. *Comm. of Austr., Dept. of Health, Service Publ. (Trop. Div.)* No. 9. 114 pp. Melbourne.

FINLAY (C.). 1886. Yellow Fever : its transmission by means of the Culex mosquito. *Am. Journ. of Med. Science,* 92 : 395-409.

FISKE (W. F.). 1920. Investigations into the bionomics of Glossina palpalis. *Bull. Ent. Res.,* 10 : 347-463.

FOX (C.). 1914. The taxonomic value of the copulatory organs of the females in the order Siphonaptera. *Hygienic Lab. Bull.*, No. 97. 31 pp. Washington.

FRACKER (S. B.). 1913. A systematic outline of the Reduviidæ of North America. *Proc. Iowa Acad. Sci.*, 19: 217-252.

FRANÇA (C.). 1921. Phlébotomes du Nouveau Monde. *Bull. Soc. Port. Sci. Nat.*, 8: 3-24.

FRANÇA (C.) and PARROT (L.). 1920. Introduction à l'étude systématique des Diptères du genre Phlebotomus. *Bull. Soc. Path. Exot.*, 13: 695-708.

FRANCIS (E.). 1919. Filariasis in southern U. S. *Hygienic Lab. Bull.*, No. 117. 36 pp. Washington.

FRANCIS (E.). 1922. Tularæmia, a new disease of man. *Journ. Am. Med. Assn.*, 78: 1015-1018.

FRANCIS (E.). 1922. Tularæmia. *Hygienic Lab. Bull.*, No. 130. 87 pp. Washington.

FRANCIS (E.) and MAYNE (B.). 1921. Tularæmia. II. Experimental transmission by the fly, Chrysops discalis. *U. S. Public Health Reports*, 36 (30) : 1728-1746.

FREEBORN (S. B.). 1924. The terminal abdominal structures of male mosquitoes. *Am. Journ. of Hygiene*, 4: 188-212.

FREEBORN (S. B.). 1926. The mosquitoes of California. *Univ. of Calif. Publ., Technical Bulletins, Entomology*, 3: 333-460.

FREEBORN (S. B.) and ATSATT (R. F.). 1918. The effects of petroleum oils on mosquito larvæ. *Journ. Econ. Ent.*, 11: 299-398.

FÜLLEBORN (F.). 1908. Über Versuche an Hundefilarien und deren Übertragung durch Mücken. *Arch. f. Schiffshyg*, 12 (8) : 1-43.

FÜLLEBORN (F.). 1929. Filarosen des Menschen. *Handb. d. Path. Mikroorganismen*, 6: 1043-1224.

FÜLLEBORN (F.) and MAYER (M.). 1908. Ueber die moglichkeit der Uebertragung pathogenen Spirochæten durch verschiedene Zeckenarten. *Arch. f. Schiffs- u. Trop. Hyg.*, 12: 31-32.

GALLIARD (H.) and GASCHEN (H.). 1937. Parasitisme d'Anopheles hyrcanus par les Culicoides au Tonkin. *Ann. de Parasit. hum. et comp.*, 15: 320-322.

GOETGHEBUER (M.) and LENZ (F.). 1933. Heleidæ (Ceratopogonidæ). Die Fliegen der Palæarktischen Region. Lief., 77, 78. Stuttgart. 133 pp.

GORDON (W. S.), BROWNLEE (A.), WILSON (D. R.) and MACLEOD (J.). 1932. Studies in Louping-Ill. I. *Journ. Comp. Path. and Therap.*, 45: 106-140.

GRAHAM-SMITH (G. S.). 1916. Observations on the habits and parasites of common flies. *Parasit.*, 8: 440-544.

GRAHAM-SMITH (G. S.). 1930. The Oscinidæ as vectors of conjunctivitis, and the anatomy of their mouthparts. *Parasit., 22*: 457-467.

GREEN (H. W.). 1924. The effect of oil upon Anopheles mosquito larvæ. *Am. Journ. of Hygiene,* 4: 12-22.

GREEN (R.). 1932. A malarial parasite of Malayan monkeys and its development in anopheline mosquitoes. *Trans. Roy. Soc. Trop. Med. Hyg.,* 25: 455-477.

GREENE (C. T.). 1925. The puparia and larvæ of Sarcophagid flies. *Proc. U. S. Nat. Mus.,* 66: Art. 29: 1-26.

GRUBBS (S. B.) and HOLSENDORF (B. E.). 1913. Fumigation of vessels for the destruction of rats. *Public Health Reports,* 28: 3-18.

HADWEN (S.). 1913. On "Tick Paralysis" in sheep and man following bites of Dermacentor venustus. *Parasit.,* 6: 283-297.

HADWEN (S.). 1915. Warble Flies. *Parasit.,* 7: 331-338.

HALL (M. C.). 1929. Arthropods as intermediate hosts of helminths. *Smithsonian Miscellaneous Collections,* 81 (15): 1-77.

HALL (M. C.) and MUIR (J. T.). 1913. A critical study of a case of myiasis due to Eristalis. *Arch. Intern. Med.,* 11: 193-203.

HARRIS (R. H. T. P.). 1931. Trapping Tsetse as a means for the control of Trypanosomiasis (Nagana). *Journ. S. Afr. Vet. Med. Assn.,* 2: 26-30.

HARRIS (R. H. T. P.). 1932. Some facts and figures regarding the attempted control of Glossina pallidipes in Zululand. *S. Afr. Journ. Sci.,* 29: 495: 507.

HARRISON (L.). 1916. The genera and species of Mallophaga. *Parasit.,* 9: 1-154.

HEADLEE (T. J.). 1921. The mosquitoes of New Jersey and their control. *N. J. Agr. Exp. Sta. Bull.,* No. 348. 229 pp. New Brunswick, N. J.

HELM (R.). 1924. Beitrag zum Anaplasmen-problem. *Ztschr. Infektionskrank. u. Hyg. Haustiere,* 25: 199-226.

HERMS (W. B.). 1926. Hippelates flies and certain other pests of the Coachella Valley, California. *Journ. Econ. Entom.,* 19 (2): 692-695.

HERMS (W. B.) and HOWELL (D. E.). 1936. The Western Dog Tick, Dermacentor occidentalis Neum, a vector of bovine anaplasmosis in California. *Journ of Parasit.,* 22: 283-288.

HERMS (W. B.), WHEELER (C. M.), HERMS (H. P.). 1934. Attemps to transmit equine encephalomyelitis by means of blood-sucking insects, especially mosquitoes. *Journ. Econ. Entom.*, 27 : 987-998.

HERMS (W. B.) and WHEELER (C. M.). 1936. Ornithodorus hermsi Wheeler as a vector of relapsing fever in California. *Journ. of Parasit.*, 22 : 276-282.

HEWITT (C. G.). 1912. Fannia canicularis Linn. and F. scalaris Fab. *Parasit.*, 5 : 161-174.

HILDEBRAND (S. F.). 1921. Top minnows in relation to malaria control. *U. S. Public Health Service, Public Health Bull.*, No. 114. 34 pp. Washington.

HINE (J. S.). 1903. Tabanidæ of Ohio. *Papers, Ohio State Acad. of Sci.*, No. 5. 55 pp. Columbus, Ohio.

HINE (J. S.). 1906. Habits and life histories of some flies of the family Tabanidæ. *U. S. Dept. of Agr., Bur. of Ent., Technical Series*, No. 12, Part 2. 38 pp. Washington.

HINMAN (E. H.). 1933. The use of insects and other arthropods in medicine. *Journ. Trop. Med. and Hyg.*, 36 : 128-134.

HINTON (M. A. C.). 1920. Rats and mice as enemies of mankind. *Brit. Mus. (Nat. Hist.), Economic Series*, No. 8. 67 pp. London.

HOARE (C. A.). 1923. An experimental study of the sheep-trypanosome and its transmission by the sheep-ked. *Parasit.*, 15 : 365-424.

HOFFMAN (W. A.). 1925. A review of the species of Culicoides of North and Central America and the West Indies. *Am. Journ. of Hygiene*, 5 : 274-301.

HOFFMAN (W. A.). 1927. Irritation due to insect secretion. *Journ. Am. Med. Assn.*, 88 : 145-146.

HOOKER (W. A.), BISHOP (F. C.) and WOOD (H. P.). 1912. The life history and bionomics of some North American ticks. *U. S. Dept. of Agr., Bur. of Ent. Bull.*, No. 106. 239 pp. Washington.

HOWARD (L. O.). 1900. A contribution to the study of the insect fauna of human excrement. *Proc. Wash. Acad. of Sci.*, 2 : 541-604.

HU (S. M. K.). 1931. Studies on host-parasite relationships of Dirofilaria immitis Leidy and its Culicine intermediate hosts. *Am. Journ. of Hygiene*, 14 : 614-629.

HUFF (C. G.). 1927. Studies on the infectivity of Plasmodia of birds for mosquitoes. *Am. Journ. of Hygiene*, 7 : 706-734.

HUFF (C. G.). 1929. Color inheritance in larvæ of Culex pipiens Linn. *Biol. Bull.*, 57 : 172-175.

HUFF (C. G.). 1929. Ovulation requirements of Culex pipiens Linn. *Biol. Bull.*, 56 : 347-350.

HUFF (C. G.). 1931. The inheritance of natural immunity to Plasmodium cathemerium in two Species of Culex. *Journ. Prev. Med.* 5: 249-259.

HUFF (C. G.). 1932. Further infectivity experiments with mosquitoes and bird malaria. *Am. Journ. of Hygiene,* 15: 751-754.

HUFF (C. G.). 1932. Studies on Hæmoproteus of Mourning Doves. *Am. Journ. of Hygiene,* 16: 618-623.

HUFF (C. G.). 1938. Studies on the evolution of some disease-producing organisms. *Quart. Rev. of Biology.* (In press).

HULL (J. B.), DOVE (W. E.), PRINCE (F. M.). 1934. Seasonal incidence of sand fly larvæ (*Culicoides dovei*) in salt marshes. *Journ. Parasit.,* 20: 162-172.

HUTCHINSON (R. H.). 1915. A maggot trap in practical use. *U. S. Dept. of Agr., Bull.,* No. 200. 15 pp. Washington.

INGRAM (A.) and MACFIE (J. W. S.). 1924. Notes on some African Ceratopogoninæ—Species of the genus Lasiohelea. *Ann. Trop. Med. and Parasit.,* 18: 377-392.

JENNINGS (A. H.) and KING (W. V.). 1913. One of the possible factors in the causation of pellagra. *Journ. Am. Med. Assn.* 60: 271-274.

JENNINGS (A. H.). 1914. Summary of two years' study of insects in relation to pellagra. *Journ of Parasit.,* 1: 10-21.

JOHNSTON (T. H.) and HARDY (G. H.). 1923. A revision of the Australian Diptera belonging to the genus Sarcophaga. *Proc. Linn. Soc. New South Wales,* 48: 94-129.

JORDAN (K.). 1933. A survey of the classification of the American species of Ceratophyllus s. lat. *Novitates Zoölogicæ,* 39 (1): 70-79.

JORDON (K.) and ROTHSCHILD (N. C.). 1908. Revision of the non-combed, eyed Siphonaptera. *Parasit.,* 1: 1-100.

KELLOGG (V. L.). 1913. Distribution and species-forming of ecto-parasites. *Am. Naturalist,* 47: 129-158.

KELLOGG (V. L.). 1914. Ectoparasites of mammals. *Am. Naturalist.* 48: 257-279.

KELLOGG (V. L.) and FERRIS (G. F.). 1915. The Anoplura and Mallophaga of North American mammals. *Stanford Univ. Publ., Univ. Series,* 74 pp. Stanford Univ., Calif.

KELSER (R. A.). 1933. Mosquitoes as vectors of the virus of equine encephalomyelitis. *Journ. Am. Vet. Med. Assn.,* 82: 767-771.

KEMP (H. A.), MOURSUND (W. H.), and WRIGHT (H. E.). 1934.

Relapsing fever in Texas IV. Ornithodorus turicata Duges: a vector of the disease. *Am. Journ. Trop. Med.*, 14: 479-489.

KEPHART (C. F.). 1914. The poison glands of the larva of the browntail moth (Euproctis chryssorrhœa). *Journ. Parasit.*, 1: 95-103.

KERR (J. A.). 1932. Studies on the transmission of experimental yellow fever by Culex thalassius and Mansonia uniformis. *Ann. Trop. Med. and Parasit.*, 26: 119-127.

KING (A. F. A.). 1883. Insects and disease—mosquitoes and malaria. *Pop. Sci. Mont.*, 23: 644-658.

KING (W. V.) and BULL (C. G.). 1923. The blood feeding habits of malaria-carrying mosquitoes. *Am. Journ. of Hygiene*, 3: 497-513.

KLIGLER (I. J.), MUCKENFUSS (R. S.), and RIVERS (T. M.). 1929. Transmission of fowl-pox by mosquitoes. *Journ. Exp. Med.*, 49: 649-660.

KNIPLING (E. F.). 1936. A comparative study of the first-instar larvæ of the genus Sarcophaga (Calliphoridæ, Diptera) with notes on the biology. *Journ. of Parasit.*, 22: 417-454.

KNOWLES (R.), NAPIER (L. E.) and SMITH (R. O.). 1924. On a Herpetomonas found in the gut of the sandfly Phlebotomus argentipes fed on kala-azar patients. *Ind. Med. Gaz.*, 59: 593-597.

KOFOID (C. A.) and DONAT (F.). 1933. South American trypanosomiasis of the human type—occurrence in mammals in the United States. *Calif. and West. Med.*, 38: 245.

KOFOID (C. A.) and WHITAKER (B. G.). 1936. Natural infection of American human trypanosomiasis in two species of Cone-nosed bugs, Triatoma protracta Uhler and Triatoma uhleri Neiva, in the Western United States. *Journ. of Parasit.*, 22: 259-263.

KOMP (W. H. W.). 1926. Observations on Anopheles walkeri and Anopheles atropos. *Insecutor Inscitiæ Menstruus*, 14: 168-176.

KUMM (H. W.). 1931. The geographical distribution of the yellow fever vectors. *Am. Journ. of Hygiene Monograph Series*, No. 12.

KUMM (H. W.). 1936. The Jamaican species of Hippelates and Oscinella. *Bull. Entomol. Res.*, 27: 307-329.

KUMM (H. W.) and TURNER (T. B.). 1936. The transmission of yaws to rabbits by an insect vector, Hippelates pallipes Loew. *Am. Journ. Trop. Med.*, 16: 245-272.

LAMBORN (W. A.). 1922. Some problems of the breeding-places of the Anophelines of Malaya. *Bull. Ent. Res.*, 13: 1-23.

LAMBORN (W. A.). 1922. The bionomics of some Malayan Anophelines. *Bull. Ent. Res.*, 13: 129-149.

LANTZ (D. E.). 1909. How to destroy rats. *U. S. Dept. of Agr., Farmer's Bull.*, No. 369. 20 pp. Washington.

LANTZ (D. E.). 1909. The brown rat in the United States. *U. S. Dept. of Agr., Biol. Survey Bull.*, No. 33. 54 pp. Washington.

LARROUSSE (F.). 1927. Etude biologique et systematique du genre Rhodnius Stal. *Ann. Parasit. hum. et comp.*, 5: 62-88.

LEESON (H. S.). 1931. Anopheline mosquitoes in Southern Rhodesia, 1926-1928; a report of investigations made during researches on Blackwater Fever by Dr. G. R. Ross. *Lond. Sch. Hyg. and Trop. Med.*, Memo. Series, No. 4: 1-55.

LEIPER (R. T.). 1912. Metamorphosis of Filaria loa. *Brit. Med. Jour.*, Jan. 4: 39-40.

LUTZ (A.). 1910. Zweiter Beitrag zur Kenntnis der Brasilianischen Simuliumarten. *Mem. Inst. Oswaldo Cruz.*, 2: 213-267.

LUTZ (A.). 1912-1913. Beiträge zur Kenntnis der blutsaugenden Ceratopogoninen Brasiliens. *Mem. Inst. Oswaldo Cruz.*, 4: 1-33, 5: 45-73.

LUTZ (A.). 1913-1915. Tabaniden Brasiliens und einiger Nachbarstaaten. *Mem. Inst. Oswaldo Cruz.*, 5: 142-191; 7: 51-119.

MACALISTER (C. J.). 1912. A new cell proliferant: its clinical application in the treatment of ulcers. *Brit. Med. Journ.*, 1: 10-12.

MACGREGOR (M. E.). 1914. The posterior stigmata of dipterous larvæ as a diagnostic character. *Parasit.*, 7: 176-188.

MACKIE (F. P.). 1907. The part played by Pediculus corporis in the transmission of relapsing fever. *Brit. Med. Journ.*, (Dec. 14): 1706-1709.

MALLOCH (J. R.). 1913. American black-flies or buffalo-gnats. *U. S. Dept. of Agr., Bur. of Ent., Tech. Bull.*, No. 26. 72 pp. Washington.

MALLOCH (J. R.). 1915. The Chironomidæ or midges of Illinois. *Bull. Ill. State Lab. of Nat. Hist.*, 10: Art. 6: 275-543.

MALLOCH (J. R.). 1915. Some additional records of Chironomidæ for Illinois. *Bull. Ill. State Lab. of Nat. Hist.*, 11: Art. 4: 305-363.

MANSON (P.). 1884. The metamorphosis of Filaria sanguinis hominis in the mosquito. *Trans. Linn. Soc. Zoöl.*, 11: 10 and 367.

MARCHAND (W.). 1920. The early stages of Tabanidæ (Horse-flies). *Monographs of the Rockefeller Institute for Medical Research,* No. 13. 203 pp. New York.

MARCHOUX (E.) and SALIMBENI (A.). 1903. La spirillose des poules. *Ann. l'Inst. Pasteur.,* 17: 569-580.

MARTINI (E.). 1920. Ueber Stechmücken. *Arch. f. Schiffs- und Tropen-Hygiene,* 24: Beiheft 1: 267 pp. Leipzig.

MARTINI (E.). 1923. Ueber einige für das System bedeutungsvolle Merkmale der Steckmücken. *Zoöl. Jahrb., Syst.,* 46: 517-590.

MARTINI (E.) and TEUBNER (E.). 1933. Über das verhalten von Stechmücken besonders von Anopheles maculipennis bei verschiedenen tempaturen und luftfeuchtigkeiten. *Arch. f. Schiffs-und Tropen-Hygiene Path. und Therap. Exot. Krankh.,* 37: 1-80.

MATHESON (R.), BRUNETT (E. L.) and BRODY (A. L.). 1931. The transmission of fowl-pox by mosquitoes. *Poultry Science,* 10: 211-223.

MATHESON (R.). 1935. Three news species of Ticks, Ornithodorus (Acarina, Ixodoidea). *Journ. of Parasit.,* 21: 347-353.

MATHESON (R.), BOYD (M. F.) and STRATMAN-THOMAS (W. K.). 1933. Anopheles Walkeri Theobald, as a vector of Plasmodium vivax. *Am. Journ. of Hygiene,* 17: 515-516.

MATHESON (R.) and SHANNON (R. C.). 1923. The Anophelines of northeastern America. *Insecutor Inscitiæ Menstruus,* 11: 57-64.

MAVER (M. B.). 1911. Transmission of spotted fever by other than Montana and Idaho ticks. *Journ. Infect. Dis.,* 8: 327-332.

McIVOR (B. C.). 1937. A new species of Ornithodorus tick from California. *Journ. Parasit.,* 23: 365-367.

MELENY (H. E.) and HARWOOD (P. D.). 1935. Human intestinal myiasis due to the larvæ of the Soldier fly, Hermetia illucens. *Am. Journ. Trop. Med.,* 15: 45-49.

MERRILL (M. H.), LACAILLADE (C. M. JR.), TENBROECK (C.). 1934. Mosquito transmission of equine encephalomyelitis. *Science,* 80: 251-252.

MILLER (W. W.). 1908. Hepatozoön perniciosum (n. g., n. sp.), a hæmogregarine pathogenic for white rats; with a description of the sexual cycle in the intermediate host, a mite (Lælaps echidninus). *Hygienic Lab. Bull.,* No. 46. 51 pp. Washington.

MITZMAIN (M. B.). 1910. General observations on the bionomics of rodent and human fleas. *U. S. Pub. Health Serv., Public Health Bull.,* No. 38. 34 pp. Washington.

MITZMAIN (M. B.). 1914. Collected studies on the insect transmission of Trypanosoma evansi, and Summary of experiments in the transmission of Anthrax by biting flies. *Hygienic Lab. Bull.,* No. 94. 53 pp. Washington.

MÖLLERS (B.). 1907. Experimentelle Studien über die Uebertragung des Rückfallfiebers durch Zecken. *Zeitsch. f. Hygiene und Infekt.-Krankh.* 58 : 277-285.

MOORE (W.) and HIRSCHFELDER (A. D.). 1919. An investigation of the louse problem. *Res. Publ. of the Univ. of Minn.,* 8 : 4 : 86 pp.

MOOSER (H.). 1932. Ornithodorus nicollei sp. n. *Anales del Instituto de Biologia, Mexico,* 3 : 127-131.

NAGAYO (M.), MIYAGAWA (Y.), MITAMURA (T.), TAMIYA (T.) and TENJIN (S.). 1921. Five species of Tsutsugamushi and their relation to the Tsutsugamushi disease. *Am. Journ. of Hygiene,* 1 : 569-590.

NATIONAL MALARIA COMMITTEE. 1936. Malaria control for engineers. 81 pp. (mimeog.). Washington.

NEIVA (A.) and GOMEZ (J. F.). 1917. Biologia da mosca do Berne (Dermatobia hominis) observada em todas as suas phases. *Annæs Paulistas de Med. e Cirurgia,* 8 : 197-209.

NEWSTEAD (R.). 1911. The Papataci flies (Phlebotomus) of the Maltese Islands. *Bull. Ent. Res.,* 2 : 47-78.

NICOLLE (C.), BLAIZOT (L.), and CONSEIL (E.). 1912. Conditions de transmission de la fièvre récurrente par le pou. *Compt. rend. Acad. Sci.,* 155 : 481-483.

NICOLLE (C. N.), BLAIZOT (L.), and CONSEIL (E.). 1912. Etiologie de la fièvre récurrente son mode de transmission par le pou. *Compt. rend. Acad. Sci.,* 154 : 1936-1938.

NICOLLE (C.), COMTE (C.), and CONSEIL (E.). 1909. Transmission experimentale du typhus exanthimatique par le pou du corps. *Compt. rend. Acad. Sci.,* 149 : 486-489.

NOGUCHI (H.), SHANNON (R. C.), TILDEN (E. B.) and TYLER (J. R.). 1928. Phlebotomus and Oroya Fever and Verruga Peruana. *Science,* 68 : 493-495.

NONO (A. M.). 1932. Avian malaria studies. VI. Susceptibility of Lutzia fuscana to avian malaria. *Phil. Journ. Sci.,* 49 : 225-229.

NORDENSKÏOLD (E.). 1908. Zur anatomie und Histologie von Ixodes reduvius. *Zool. Jahrb.,* 25 : 637-674.

NUTTALL (G. H. F.). 1914. "Tick Paralysis" in man and animals. *Parasit.,* 7 : 95-104.

NUTTALL (G. H. F.). 1916. Ticks of the Belgian Congo and the diseases they convey. *Bull. Ent. Res.,* 6 : 313-352.

NUTTALL (G. H. F.). 1917. Bibliography of Pediculus and Phthirus. *Parasit.,* 10: 1-42.

NUTTALL (G. H. F.). 1917. The part played by Pediculus humanus in the causation of disease. *Parasit.,* 10: 43-79.

NUTTALL (G. H. F.). 1917. The biology of Pediculus humanus. *Parasit.,* 10: 80-195.

NUTTALL (G. H. F.). 1918. Combating lousiness among soldiers and civilians. *Parasit.,* 10: 411-586.

O'CONNOR (F. W.). 1922. Some results of medical researches in the western Pacific. *Trans. Roy. Soc. Trop. Med. and Hyg.,* 16: 28-52.

O'ROKE (E. C.). 1930. The morphology, transmission, and life-history of Hæmoproteus lophortyx O'Roke, a blood parasite of the California Valley Quail. *Univ. Calif. Pub. Zoöl.,* 36: 1-50.

O'ROKE (E. C.). 1930. The incidence, pathogenicity, and transmission of Leucocutozoon anatis of ducks. *Journ. Parasit.,* 17: 112. abs.

PARKER (R. R.). 1916. Dispersion of Musca domestica under city conditions in Montana. *Journ. Econ. Ent.,* 9: 325-354.

PARKER (R. R.) and DADE (J.). 1929. Tularemia: its transmission to sheep by the wood tick, Dermacentor andersoni Stiles. *Journ. Am. Vet. Med. Assn.,* 75: 173-191.

PATTON (W. S.). 1920. Mesopotamian house flies and their allies. *Ind. Journ. of Med. Res.,* 7: 751-777.

PATTON (W. S.). 1920. Chrysomyia bezziana Villeneuve, the common Indian Calliphorine whose larvæ cause cutaneous myiasis in man and animals. *Ind. Journ. of Med. Res.,* 8: 17-29.

PATTON (W. S.). 1921. Notes on the myiasis-producing Diptera of man and animals. *Bull. Ent. Res.,* 12: 239-261.

PATTON (W. S.). 1922. How to recognize the Indian myiasis-producing flies and their larvæ. *Ind. Journ. of Med. Res.,* 9: 635-653.

PHILIP (C. B.). 1929. Preliminary report of further tests with yellow fever transmission by mosquitoes other than Aedes aegypti. *Am. Journ. Trop. Med.,* 9: 267-269.

PHILIP (C. B.). 1930. Studies on transmission of experimental yellow fever by mosquitoes other than Aëdes. *Am. Journ. Trop. Med.,* 10: 1-16.

PHILIP (C. B.). 1930. Supplemental note regarding mosquito vectors of experimental yellow fever. *Science,* 72: 578.

POMEROY (A. W. J.). 1922. New species of African Simulidæ and further studies of the early stages. *Bull. Ent. Res.,* 12: 457-463.

REED (W.). 1900. The etiology of yellow fever. *Phila. Med. Journ.*, 6: 790-796.

REICHENOW (E.). 1932. Die Entwicklung von Proteosoma circumflexum in Theobaldia annulata nebst Beobachtungen über das Verhalten anderer Vogelplasmodien in Mücken. *Jenaische Zeit. Naturw.* (67 Festschr. Ludwig Plate): 434-451.

RICHARDSON (C. H.). 1917. The response of the house-fly to certain foods and their fermentation products. *Journ. Econ. Ent.*, 10: 102-109.

RICKETTS (H. T.). 1906. The transmission of Rocky Mt. spotted fever by the bite of the wood tick (Dermacentor occidentalis). *Journ. Am. Med. Assn.*, 57: 358.

RICKETTS (H. T.) and WILDER (R. M.). 1910. The transmission of the typhus fever of Mexico (tabardillo) by means of the louse, Pediculus vestimenti. *Journ. Am. Med. Assn.*, 54: 1304.

ROBINSON (W.). 1934. Literature relating to the use of maggots in the treatment of suppurative infections. *U. S. Bur. Ent. Circ.*, E-310.

ROBINSON (W.). 1935. Stimulation of healing in non-healing wounds by allantoin occurring in maggot secretions and of wide biologic distribution. *Journ. Bone and Joint Surg.*, 17: 267-330.

ROBLES (R.). 1919. Onchocercose humaine au Guatemala produisant la cécité et "l'erysipèle du littoral" (Erisipela de la costa). *Bull. Soc. Path. Exot.*, 12: 442-463.

ROOT (F. M.). 1921. Experiments on the carriage of intestinal protozoa of man by flies. *Am. Journ. of Hygiene*, 1: 131-153.

ROOT (F. M.). 1922. The larvæ of American Anopheles mosquitoes. *Am. Journ. of Hygiene*, 2: 379-393.

ROOT (F. M.). 1923. Notes on larval characters in the genus Sarcophaga. *Journ. of Parasit.*, 9: 227-229.

ROOT (F. M.). 1923. The male genitalia of some American Anopheles mosquitoes. *Am. Journ. of Hygiene*, 3: 264-279.

ROOT (F. M.). 1924. The larval pilotaxy of Anopheles quadrimaculatus and Anopheles punctipennis. *Am. Journ. of Hygiene*, 4: 710-724.

ROOT (F. M.). 1926. The Anophelines of the Nyssorhynchus group. *Am. Journ. of Hygiene*, 6: 684-717.

ROOT (F. M.). 1927. Chagasia fajardoi. *Am. Journ. of Hygiene*, 7: 470-480.

ROOT (F. M.) and HOFFMAN (W. A.). 1937. The North American species of *Culicoides. Amer. Journ. Hyg.*, 25: 150-176.

ROSENAU (M. J.) and BRUES (C. T.). 1912. Some experimental

observations on monkeys concerning the transmission of polio-myelitis through the agency of Stomoxys calcitrans. *Mo. Bull. Mass. State Bd. of Health.* N. s., 7: 314-317.

Ross (I. C.). 1924. The bionomics of Ixodes holocyclus Neumann. *Parasit.,* 16: 365-381.

Ross (I. C.). 1926. An experimental study of tick paralysis in Australia. *Parasit.,* 18: 410-429.

Ross (R.). 1898. Pigmented cells in mosquitoes. *Brit. Med. Journ.,* Feb. 26: 550-551.

Ross (R. H.) and MILNE (A. D.). 1904. Tick fever. *Brit. Med. Journ.,* 2: 1453-1454.

ROTHSCHILD (N. C.). 1910. A synopsis of the fleas found on Mus norvegicus, Mus rattus and Musculus. *Bull. Ent. Res.,* 1: 89-98.

ROTHSCHILD (N. C.). 1914. On three species of Xenopsylla occurring on rats in India. *Bull. Ent. Res.,* 5: 83-85.

ROUBAUD (E.). 1920. Emploi du Trioxyméthylène en poudre pour la destruction des larves d'Anopheles. *C. R. hebdom. Acad. Sci. Paris,* 170: 1521-1522.

ROUBAUD (E.). 1926. L'emploi des poudres larvicides légères dans la lutte contre les moustiques. *Bull. Soc. Path. Exot.,* 19: 287-302.

RUSSELL (P. F.). 1925. Identification of the larvæ of the three common Anopheline mosquitoes of the southern United States. *Am. Journ. of Hygiene,* 5: 149-174.

RUSSELL (P. F.). 1932. Avian malaria studies. Plasmodium capistrani sp. nov., an avian malaria parasite in the Philippines. *Phil. Journ. Sci.,* 48: 269-287.

RUSSELL (P. F.) and EATON (L. S.). 1934. An automatic distributing machine for Paris green mixtures. *Phil. Journ. Sci.,* 53: 497-501.

SAMBON (L. W.) and Low (G.). 1900. The malaria experiments in the Campagna. *Brit. Med. Journ.,* 2: 1679-1682.

SANDERSON (E. D.). 1910. Controlling the black-fly in the White Mountains. *Journ. Econ. Ent.,* 3: 27-29.

SAWYER (W. A.) and HERMS (W. B.). 1913. Attempts to transmit poliomyelitis by means of the stable-fly (Stomoxys calcitrans). *Journ. Am. Med. Assn.,* 61: 461-466.

SCHULE (P. A.). 1922. Dengue Fever: Transmission by Aëdes ægypti. *Am. Journ. Trop. Med.,* 8: 203-213.

SCOTT (J. W.). 1922. Insect transmission of Swamp Fever or Infectious Anemia of Horses. *Univ. of Wyoming Agr. Exp. Sta. Bull.,* No. 133. 137 pp. Laramie, Wyo.

SENIOR-WHITE (R.). 1926. Physical factors in mosquito ecology. *Bull. Ent. Res.,* 16: 187-248.

SERGENT (ED. and ET.). 1906. Sur le second hôte de l'Hæmoproteus du pigeon. *C. R. Soc. Biol.,* 61: 494.

SERGENT (E.) and FOLY (H.). 1910. Recherches sur la fièvre recurrente et son mode de transmission, dans une epidémie algérienne. *Ann. Inst. Past.,* 24: 337-373.

SHANNON (R. C.). 1922. The bot-flies of domestic animals. *Cornell Veterinarian,* July, 1922.

SHANNON (R. C.). 1923. Genera of Nearctic Calliphoridæ, Blowflies, with revision of the Calliphorini. *Insecutor Inscitiæ Menstruus,* 11: 101-118.

SHANNON (R. C.). 1924. Nearctic Calliphoridæ, Lucilíini. *Insecutor Inscitiæ Menstruus,* 12: 67-81.

SHANNON (R. C.). 1924. Notes on Calliphoridæ. *Insecutor Inscitiæ Menstruus,* 12: 14.

SHANNON (R. C.). 1930. O apparecimento de uma especie africana de anopheles no Brasil. *Brasil-Medico,* 44: 515-516.

SHANNON (R. C.). 1931. On the classification of Brazilian Culicidæ with special reference to those capable of harboring the yellow fever virus. *Proc. Ent. Soc. of Wash.,* 33: 125-164.

SHANNON (R. C.). 1932. Anopheles gambiæ in Brazil. *Am. Journ. of Hygiene,* 15: 633-663.

SHANNON (R. C.) and DAVIS (N. C.). 1930. Observations on the Anophelini (Culicidæ) of Bahia, Brazil. *Ann. Ent. Soc. of Am.,* 23: 467-492.

SHARP (N. A. D.). 1928. Filaria perstans: its development in Culicoides austeni. *Trans. Roy. Soc. Trop. Med. and Hygiene,* 21: 371-396.

SHORTT (H. E.), BARRAUD (P. J.) and CRAIGHEAD (A. C.). 1926. An account of methods employed in feeding and re-feeding sandflies, Phlebotomus argentipes, for the second and third time on man and animals. *Ind. Journ. of Med. Res.,* 13: 923-942.

SILER (J. F.), HALL (M. W.) and HITCHENS (A. P.). 1925. Transmission of Dengue Fever by Mosquitoes. *Proc. Soc. Exp. Biol. and Med.,* 23: 197-201.

SILER (J. F.), HALL (M. W.) and HITCHENS (A. P.) 1926. Dengue: Its history, epidemiology, mechanism of transmission, etiology, clinical manifestations, immunity and prevention. *Phil. Journ. of Science,* 29: 1-304.

SIMOND (P.). 1898. La propagation de la peste. *Ann. de l'Inst. Past.,* 12: 625.

SIMMONS (J. S.). 1936. Anopheles (Anopheles) neomaculipalpus Curry experimentally infected with malaria plasmodia. *Science*, 84: 202-203.

SIMMONS (J. S.). 1936. Anopheles (Anopheles) punctimacula naturally infected with malaria plasmodia. *Am. Journ. Trop. Med.*, 16: 105-108.

SIMMONS (J. S.). 1937. Observations on the importance of Anopheles punctimacula as a malaria vector in Panama and report of experimental infections in A. neomaculipalpus, A. apicimacula, and A. eiseni. *Am. Journ. Trop. Med.*, 17: 191-212.

SIMMONS (J. S.), ST. JOHN (J. H.) and REYNOLDS (J. H. K.). 1930. Transmission of Dengue Fever by Aëdes albopictus Skuse. *Phil. Journ. Sci.*, 41: 215-239.

SIMMONS (J. S.), KELSER (R. A.) and CORNELL (V. H.). 1933. Insect transmission experiments with herpesencephalitis virus. *Science*, 78: 243-246.

SIMMONS (J. S.), REYNOLDS (F. H. K.), and CORNELL (V. H.). 1936. Transmission of the virus of equine encephalomyelitis through Aedes albopictus Skuse. *Am. Journ. Trop. Med.*, 16: 289-302.

SIMPSON (F.). 1913. Rat proofing. *Public Health Reports*, 28: 3-11.

SINTON (J. A.). 1924. Notes on some Indian species of the genus Phlebotomus. Part III. Provisional diagnostic table of the males of the species and varieties recorded from India and Ceylon. *Ind. Journ. of Med. Res.*, 11: 807-816.

SINTON (J. A.). 1925. The rôle of insects of the genus Phlebotomus as carriers of disease, with special reference to India. *Ind. Journ. of Med. Res.*, 12: 701-730.

SINTON (J. A.) and MULLIGAN (H. W.). 1933. A critical review of the literature relating to the identification of the malarial parasites recorded from monkeys of the families Cercopithecidæ and Colobidæ. *Rec. Malaria Survey of India*, 3: 381-443.

SMITH (R. O. A.). 1925. A note on a simple method of breeding sandflies. *Ind. Journ of Med. Res.*, 12: 741-742.

SMITH (T.) and KILBOURNE (F. L.). 1893. Investigations into the nature, causation, and prevention of Texas or Southern Cattle Fever. *U. S. D. A. Bur. Anim. Indust.* No. 1. 301 pp.

SNIJDERS (E. P.), DINGER (J. E.) and SCHÜFFNER (W.). 1931. On the transmission of Dengue in Sumatra. *Am. Journ. Trop. Med.*, 11: 171-197.

SOPER (F. L.). 1935. Rural and jungle yellow fever, a new public health problem in Colombia. Bogotá. pp. 1-42.

Soper (F. L.), Penna (H.), Cardoso (E.), Serafim (J.), Fro-
bisher (M.), Pinheiro (J.). 1933. Yellow fever without
Aëdes ægypti. Study of a rural epidemic in the Valle do
Canaan, Espirito Santo, Brazil, 1932. Am. Journ. Hyg., 18:
555-587.
Stanton (A. T.). 1915. The larvæ of Malayan Anopheles. Bull.
Ent. Res., 6: 159-172.
Stein (F.). 1853. Beiträge zur Entwicklungsgeschichte der Ein-
geweidewümer. Zeitschr. f. wiss. Zoöl., 4: 196-214.
Stewart (M. A.). 1934. The rôle of Lucilia sericata Meig. larvæ
in osteomyelitis wounds. Ann. Trop. Med. and Parasit., 28:
445-459.
Stiles (C. W.). 1910. The taxonomic value of the microscopic
structure of the stigmal plates in the tick genus Dermacentor.
Hygienic Lab. Bull., No. 62. 72 pp. Washington.
Stiles (C. W.) ·and Hassall (A.). 1927. Key-catalogue of the
Crustacea and Arachnoids of importance in Public Health.
Hygienic Lab. Bull., No. 148. 289 pp. Washington.
Stiles (C. W.) and Collins (B. J.). 1930. Ctenocephalides, new
genus of fleas, type Pulex canis. Public Health Reports, 45:
1308-1310.
Stokes (J. H.). 1914. A clinical, pathological and experimental
study of the lesions produced by the bite of the "black fly"
(Simulium venustum). Journ. of Cutan. Dis., 32: 751; 830.
Strong (R. P.), Sandground (J. H.), Bequaert (J. C.) and
Ochoa (M. M.). 1934. Onchocerciasis, with special reference
to the central American form of the disease. pp. 234. Cam-
bridge, Mass.
Surcouf (J.). 1921. Diptera, Family Tabanidæ. Genera Insectorum,
Fascicle 175. 182 pp. Brussels.
Swellengrebel (N. H.) and Swellengrebel-De Graaf (J. M.
H.). 1920. List of the Anophelines of the Malay Archipelago.
Bull. Ent. Res., 11: 77-92.
Swellengrebel (N. H.) and Swellengrebel-De Graaf (J. M.
H.). 1920. A malaria survey in the Malay Archipelago. Parasit.,
12: 180-198.
Syverton (J. T.) and Berry (G. P.). 1936. An arthropod vector
of equine encephalomyelitis, western strain. Science, 84: 186-
187.
Tao (S. M.). 1927. A comparative study of the early larval stages
of some common flies. Am. Journ. of Hygiene, 7: 735-761.
Tate (P.) and Vincent (M.). 1936. The biology of autogenous

and anautogenous races of Culex pipiens L. *Parasit.*, 28: 115-145.

TAUTE (M.). 1911. Experimentelle Studien über die Beziehungen der Glossina morsitans zur Schlafkrankeit. *Zeitschr. f. Hygiene*, 69: 553-558.

TEMPLE (I. U.). 1912. Acute ascending paralysis, or tick paralysis. *Medical Sentinel* (Portland, Ore.), Sept., 1912.

THEILER (A.). 1903. A new trypanosoma. *Journ. Comp. Path. and Therap.*, 16: 193.

TIEDEMAN (W. v. D.). 1927. Malaria in the Philippines. *Journ. Prev. Med.*, 1: 205-254.

TONNOIR (A. L.). 1925. Australasian Simuliidæ. *Bull. Ent. Res.*, 15: 213-255.

TOWNSEND (C. H. T.). 1913. The transmission of verruga by Phlebotomus. *Journ. Am. Med. Assn.*, 61: 1717.

TOWNSEND (C. H. T.). 1914. Progress of verruga work with Phlebotomus verrucarum. *Journ. Econ. Ent.*, 7: 357-367.

TOWNSEND (C. H. T.). 1917. A synoptic revision of the Cuterebridæ, with synonymic notes and the description of one new species. *Insecutor Inscitiæ Menstruus*, 5: 23-27.

TYZZER (E. E.). 1907. The pathology of the brown-tail moth dermatitis. *Journ. Med. Res.*, 16: 43-64.

URIBE (C.). 1926. A new invertebrate host of Trypanosoma cruzi Chagas. *Journ. Parasit.*, 12: 213-215.

VERJBITSKI (D. T.). The part played by insects in the epidemiology of plague. *Journ. of Hygiene*, 8: 162-208.

WALCH (E. W.). 1923. On Trombicula deliensis, probably carrier of the Pseudotyphus, and on other Trombicula species of Deli. *Kitasato Arch. of Exp. Med.*, 5: 63.

WALCH (E. W.). 1925. On the Trombiculæ, carriers of Pseudotyphus, and related species from Sumatra (Second Part). *Kitasato Arch. of Exp. Med.*, 6: 235-257.

WALKER (E. M.). 1920. Wohlfahrtia vigil as a human parasite. *Journ. of Parasit.*, 7: 1-7.

WALKER (E. M.). 1922. Some cases of cutaneous myiasis, with notes on the larvæ of Wohlfahrtia vigil. *Journ. of Parasit.*, 9: 1-5.

WARBURTON (C.). 1920. Sarcoptic Scabies in man and animals. *Parasit.*, 12: 265-300.

WARBURTON (C.). 1912. Notes on the genus Rhipicephalus. *Parasit.*, 5: 1-20.

WEBSTER (F. M.). 1910. A predaceous mite proves noxious to man.

U. S. Dept. of Agr., Bur. of Ent., Circular, No. 118. 24 pp. Washington.

WESENBERG-LUND (C.). 1920-1921. Contributions to the biology of the Danish Culicidæ. *Mem. Acad. Roy. Sci. et Lettres de Danemark.* Series 8, Vol. 7, No. 1. 210 pp. Copenhagen.

WHEELER (C. M.). 1935. A new species of tick which is a vector of relapsing fever in California. *Am. Journ. Trop. Med.,* 15: 435-438.

WHITAKER (B. G.). 1937. Two species of Triatoma (Reduviidæ) from Mexico naturally infected with Trypanosoma cruzi Chagas. *Journ. of Parasit.,* 23: 537 (abs.).

WILSON (P. W.) and MATHIS (M. S.). 1930. Observations on the epidemiology and pathology of yaws. *Journ. Am. Med. Assn.,* 94: 1289.

WOLBACH (S. B.). 1919. Studies on Rocky Mountain Spotted Fever. *Journ. Med. Res.,* 41: 1-193.

WOODWORTH (C. W.). 1924. Public Health activities in Nanking. *Health* (Shanghai), 1: 16-21.

YAMADA (S.). 1921. Descriptions of ten new species of Aëdes found in Japan, with notes on the relation between some of these mosquitoes and the larva of Filaria bancrofti Cobbold. *Annot. Zoöl. Japon,* 10: 45-81.

YAMADA (S.). 1924-1925. A revision of the adult Anopheline mosquitoes of Japan. *Sci. Repts. from the Govt. Inst. for Inf. Dis., Tokyo Imp. Univ.,* 3: 215-241, 4: 447-493.

ZELLER (H.) and HELM (R.). 1923. Versuche zur Frage der Ubertragbarkeit des Texas-Fiebers auf Deutsche Rinder durch die bei una vorkommenden Zecken Ixodes ricinus und Hæmaphysalis punctata cinnabarina. *Tierarztl. Wochnschr.,* 39: 1-4.

ZETEK (J.). 1913. Determining the flight of Mosquitoes. *Ann. Ent. Soc. of Am.,* 6: 5-21.

ZINSSER (H.) and CASTENEDA (M. R.). 1931. Studies on typhus fever. VIII. Ticks as a possible vector of the disease from animals to man. *Journ. Exp. Med.,* 54: 11-21.

INDEX OF AUTHORS

INDEX OF AUTHORS

All numbers refer to pages. Page numbers in the **bold-face** type indicate that the title of a contribution by the author will be found on that page.

A

Ackert, 385, 387, 397, **740**
Adie, 150, **704**
Adler, 174, **754**
Africa, 275, **729**, **740**
Alcock, **749**
Aldrich, 603, 605, 614, **750**, **754**
Alicata, **740**
Alvarez, **750**
Alvey, **729**
Ameel, 277, **729**
Anderson, J. F., 610, **740**, **754**
Anderson, M. G., 231, 346, 475, **729**, 736
Ando, 277, 283
Andrews, 51, 52, 70, 75, 83, 197, **704**
Arago, **754**
Archibald, **750**
Arreza-Guzman, **740**
Ashburn, **754**
Ashford, **740**
Askanazy, 264, **729**
Atchley, 206, **704**
Atsatt, 550
Auchinloss, **740**
Augustine, 387, 394, 399, 437, **740**, **741**
Austen, 611, **750**

B

Bachman, **741**
Bacot, 640, 699, **754**
Baer, 325, 332, 339, 345, 630
Baerman, **741**
Baetjer, **704**, **752**
Bahr, 569, **754**
Baker, **754**
Banks, **755**
Barber, 545, **755**
Barlow, 243, 331, **729**
Barrand, **755**
Barraud, **755**
Barret, 61, 74, **705**
Bass, 61, 170, 172, **705**

Bastianelli, **755**
Bates, **755**
Bauer, 566, **755**
Baujean, 213
Baylis, 385, 386, **726**
Beaujean, 253
Becker, 93, 94, 194, **701**, **705**
Bedford, 668, **755**
Beeuwkes, 567, **755**
Bengtson, 615, **756**
Bentley, **705**
Bequaert, 589, **756**
Berberian, 361
Bercovitz, **705**
Berlese, 497, **750**
Bernard, **741**
Berry, 681
Bezzi, **756**
Bilharz, 271, **729**
Birkeland, 329, **737**
Bishopp, 124, **705**, **756**
Blacklock, 174, 454, 589, 622, **701**, **705**, 706, **741**, **756**
Blaizot, **756**
Blanc, 568, **756**
Blanchard, 271
Bland, **706**
Blickhahn, **741**
Boeck, 51, 65, 74, **706**
Bogen, 692, **756**
Bonnal, 363, **737**
Bonne, **750**
Boyd, 533, 534, **750**, **756**
Boyers, **706**
Bradley, 528, **757**
Brailsford, 319, 360
Brandt, 84, **706**
Brau, 287
Braun, 236, 276, 323, **726**
Brody, 568, **757**, **770**
Brooks, 231, **730**
Brown, 387, 388, **730**, **741**
Bruce, 98, **706**, **757**
Brues, 610, **757**
Brug, 80, 83, 264, **706**, **757**

Brumpt, 90, 121, 306, 568, **701, 706, 707, 726, 730, 750, 757**
Brunett, 568, **770**
Bruyant, 251, 287
Bucy, 342
Buisson, 193, **707**
Bull, **757**
Bullock, 348, **737**
Bundesen, 58, **707**
Busk, 240
Bütschli, **701**
Buxton, 750, **757**
Byam, 701, **750**

C

Caldwell, 387, 392, **741**
Calkins, **701**
Calmette, **750**
Cameron, 262, 592, **730, 758**
Caminopetros, 568, **756**
Cannon, 650, **758**
Carpenter, **750**
Carter, **758**
Carus, 323
Casagrandi, 59
Casoni, **737**
Castellani, 80, 98, **701, 707**
Celli, 157
Chagas, **707, 758**
Chandler, 287, **726, 730, 741**
Chatton, 58, 203, **707**
Chen, H. T., 192, 231, 253, 372, 373, **730, 737**
Chen, Pin-Dji, **730**
Ch'en Pang, 252, **730**
Chiang, 83, **707**
Chitwood, 377, 385, 476, **726**
Christenson, 366, **737**
Christophers, 152, 522, **707, 758**
Chu, 63, 68, **741**
Clark, 55, 58, 190, **701**
Claus, 398
Cleland, **758**
Cleveland, 55, 76, 97, **707, 708**
Coatney, 150, **708**
Cobb, 374, 385, **742**
Cobbold, 241, 251, 277
Coles, 668, **758**
Collins, 638, **777**
Comstock, **750**
Connal, A., 595, **708, 759**
Connal, S. L. M., 595, **759**
Connor, **759**
Conyngham, 288, **730**
Cooley, **759**
Cooper, **752**
Cornell, 567, **776**

Cort, 224, 226, 227, 230, 233, 236, 303, 305, 385, 387, 392, **730, 742**
Councilman, 48, **708**
Covell, 522, **750, 759**
Coventry, 100, **708**
Cowdry, **708**
Cox, **759**
Cragg, 638, **752, 759**
Craig, 56, 57, 58, 75, **702, 708, 709, 726, 750**
Cram, 379, 380, 381, 387, 388, 465, **742**
Creel, **759**
Cummings, **759**
Cunha, **709**
Cunningham, 48, 59, 110, **709**
Curran, 505, 579, **750**
Curren, 286
Curry, **759**
Curtis, 348
Cutler, 74

D

Da Costa, 612, **750**
Daengsvang, 468
Dampf, 581, **759**
Darling, 19, 183, 617, **709, 759**
Das Gupta, 174
Dastidar, **709**
Daubney, 385, 386
Davaine, 388
Davey, 378
Davies, **760**
Davis, 392, 525, 534, 566, 760
Day, **730**
De Bary, **709**
De Boissezon, **760**
De Buck, **760**
DeLangen, **709**
Delbet, 463
Dennis, 152, 359, 361, **709, 737**
Descazeaux, 462
Deve, 355
DeVolt, **709**
Dew, 351, 354, 356, **737**
Diastre, **737**
Diesing, 323
Dinger, 566, **760**
Dixon, 337, **737**
Doane, **750**
Dobell, 52, 65, 76, **702, 709, 710**
Dock, **710, 726**
Doerr, **761**
Doflein, **702**
Donat, 657, **768**
Donovan, 110, **710**
Dos Santos, **750**
Dove, 683, **761**

Drbohlav, 63, 74, **710**
Drinker, **742**
Dubois, 236, **730**
Dujardin, 367
Dunn, 108, **710**
Dutton, 98, **710**, **761**
Dyar, 513, 588, **750**, **751**, **761**

E

Eaton, 152, **710**
Edwards, 513, 522, 557, 558, 577, 651
Eliot, 650, **762**
Elmassian, **710**
Enderlein, **762**
Entz, **710**
Epstein, 388, **742**
Erdmann, 183, **710**
Erhardt, 264, **730**
Eskey, 638, 650, **762**
Essex, 328, 331, **737**
Evans, 98, 108, 626, **710**, **752**, **762**
Ewing, 648, 662, 682, 684, 685, 686, **750**, **763**
Eysell, **763**

F

Fabyan, 395
Fairley, **730**, **737**
Fantham, 81, **710**
Faust, 224, 252, 253, 258, 259, 264, 296, 468, 488, 631, **710**, **726**, **730**, **731**, **742**, **750**, **763**
Felt, **763**
Feng, **763**
Ferris, 646, **763**
Fibiger, **743**
Fielding, **763**
Finlay, 566, **763**
Fisher, **731**
Fiske, **763**
Fletcher, **702**
Folsom, **750**
Fonseca, 127, **710**
Ford, 650, **762**
Forde, **710**
Foster, 388, **743**
Fox, 633, 634, **763**
Fracker, **764**
Franca, **764**
Franchini, 93
Francis, 595, **743**, **764**
Freeborn, **764**
Frost, 610, **754**
Fuhrmann, 236, 323, **731**, **737**
Fujii, 295, 390
Fujinami, 295, 296, **731**

Fülleborn, **743**, **764**
Fulton, 190, **711**

G

Gabaldon, 122, **711**
Gage, **743**
Galliard, 454, 455, 580, **764**
Gallien, **731**
Galtsoff, 699, **751**
Gamble, 236
Gardner, 388
Garrison, 268, **731**
Gaschen, 580, **764**
Gater, **751**
Gedoelst, 81
Geiman, **711**
George, 581
Giles, 286
Glaser, 93, **711**
Goddard, 241, 246, **731**
Goetghebuer, **764**
Goldberger, 288
Golden, **743**
Golgi, 157, **711**
Gonzalez, 296
Goodey, **743**
Goodrich, 63, **711**
Gordon, R. M., 622, **756**
Gordon, W. S., **764**
Gorgas, 566
Grace, **744**
Graham, 397, 744
Graham-Smith, **751**, **764**
Grassi, 59, 61, 157, 158, 175, 370, 702, **711**, **726**, **737**, **744**
Graybill, 396, **744**
Green, H. W., **765**
Green, R., 537, **765**
Greene, **765**
Gros, 61, **711**
Grubbs, **765**
Gruby, 98, **711**
Gunn, **711**

H

Hackett, 169, **751**
Hadwen, **765**
Hakansson, 68, **711**
Hall, 361, 391, 393, 394, 397, 399, 485, 693, **702**, **726**, **738**, **744**, **765**
Hardenburg, **751**
Harris, 613, **744**, **765**
Harrison, **765**
Hartmann, 83, 176, 387, **702**, **711**
Harwood, 626, **770**
Hasegawa, **744**

Hassall, 236, 271, 276
Haughwout, 712
Headlee, 765
Hecker, 63
Hegner, 54, 61, 63, 65, 68, 90, 94, 109, 121, 156, 176, 192, 230, 702, 712, 713, 726
Helm, 765
Hemmert-Halsweck, 474, 475, 477, 478, 479
Henry, 288
Herman, 155, 714
Herms, H. P., 567, 765
Herms, W. B., 567, 615, 669, 751, 765
Herrick, 480
Hesse, 181, 714
Hewitt, 176, 751, 766
Hilaria, 731
Hilton, 473
Hindle, 751
Hine, 766
Hinmann, 475, 690, 766
Hinshaw, 63, 122, 714
Hinton, 766
Hiraishi, 744
Hirsch, 276, 277
Hoare, 93, 714, 766
Hoeppli, 264, 731
Hoffman, 296, 691, 766
Hogue, 86, 714
Holmes, 83, 94, 714
Hooker, 766
Horsfall, 364
Houdemer, 332
Howard, 751, 766
Howitt, 714
Hu, 766
Huber, 59, 715
Huff, 165, 500, 501, 547, 568, 614, 649, 683, 715, 766, 767
Hull, 767
Hung-See-Lu, 744
Hutchinson, 767
Hutyra, 726

I

Ijima, 334
Imms, 751
Ingles, 268, 732
Ingram, 767
International Health Board, 751
Iturbe, 296
Iwata, 332, 738

J

James, 751
Janeway, 480
Janicki, 328, 330, 738

Jennings, 610, 767
Jepps, 67, 715
Joest, 264, 726
Johannsen, 752
Johns, 61
Johnson, 73, 269, 270, 370, 488, 715, 732
Johnston, 19, 715, 767
Jones, 364, 397, 738
Jordan, 767
Joyeux, 239, 288, 325, 332, 367, 370, 732, 738

K

Kaljus, 482, 744
Kartulis, 48, 56, 715
Kathariner, 732
Katsunuma, 715
Katsurada, 295, 732
Kawai, 257, 732
Keilin, 193, 715
Kellogg, 19, 644, 646, 751, 767
Kelser, 567, 767
Kemp, 669, 767
Kephart, 691, 768
Kerbert, 276, 732
Kernkamp, 285
Kerr, 567, 768
Kessel, 58, 61, 65, 67, 80, 385, 715, 716
Khalil, 273, 732
Khaw, 252, 253, 258, 259, 732
Kilbourne, 152
King, A. F. A., 768
King, W. V., 610, 768
Kirby-Smith, 744
Kitchen, 533, 768
Kiyono, 251, 276
Klebs, 157
Kligler, 568, 751, 768
Knab, 751
Knipling, 626, 768
Knowles, 174, 702
Kobayashi, 252, 258, 277, 732
Koch, 48, 716
Kofoid, 58, 657, 768, 716
Koino, 390, 744
Komp, 768
Kotlan, 745
Kouri, 745
Krabbe, 334
Kreis, 745
Krull, 268, 289, 290, 732, 733
Küchenmeister, 318
Kudo, 179, 180, 702, 716
Kuenen, 716
Kumm, 534, 615, 768

L

Laake, 617, 772
Labbe, 155, 717
Lacaillade, 567, 770
Lafleur, 48
La Font, 94, 717
Lamarre, 387
Lamborn, 769, 717
Lane, 733, 745
Langeron, 727
Lantz, 769
Larrouse, 751, 769
Larson, 717
La Rue, 224, 324
Laveran, 93, 110, 157, 702, 717
Lawson, 717
Leeson, 769
Leger, 717
Leidy, 84, 474, 717
Leiper, 271, 287, 288, 296, 466, 595, 733, 745, 769
Leishman, 110, 717
Lepage, 727
Le Roux, 304
Leuckart, 276, 287, 320, 343, 727, 733, 745
Lewis, 48, 59, 98, 286, 717, 733
Liebetanz, 717
Lintz, 480
Liston, 751
Loesch, 48, 717
Looss, 225, 251, 271, 295, 733, 745
Lörincz, 349, 738
Lucas, 718
Lucker, 745
Lühe, 323, 733
Lutz, 296, 699, 733, 751, 769
Lynch, 123, 702, 718

M

Macalister, 630, 769
MacArthur, 193, 337, 718
MacCallum, 158, 718
MacGregor, 769
Mackie, 769
MacKinnon, 84, 718
MacNeal, 109, 752
Macy, 266, 734
Magath, 65, 331, 349, 385, 718, 738, 745
Malloch, 577, 769
Mallory, 727
Manson, 158, 569, 718, 734, 769
Manson-Bahr, 702, 727
Manwell, 155, 718
Maplestone, 385

Marchand, 769
Marchiafava, 157, 718
Marchoux, 770
Martin, 388, 640, 754
Martini, 527, 718, 751, 770
Mast, 718
Matheson, 533, 568, 670, 751, 770
Mathews, 51
Maver, 679, 770
Maxwell, 278, 631, 734, 763
McClelland, 650, 768
McConnell, 251, 286, 734
McCullock, 94, 718
McDonald, 202, 206, 718
McFall, 719
McIvor, 670, 770
McNaught, 475
McRae, 388, 745
Megaw, 752
Meggitt, 727
Meleney, 51, 65, 67, 626, 719, 770
Mense, 751
Mercier, 719
Merrill, 566, 770
Mesnil, 110, 174, 719
Metcalf, 19, 719
Migone, 94, 719
Miller, 348, 682, 719, 738, 770
Mills, 719
Minchin, 101, 370, 702, 719
Minot, 479
Mitzmain, 610, 770
Miyairi, 277, 296, 734
Möllers, 668, 771
Monnig, 394, 727, 751
Montgomerie, 264
Monticelli, 323
Moore, 253, 771
Moorthy, 457, 745
Mooser, 771
Morris, 84, 719
Moseley, 63
Moursund, 669, 767
Muckenfuss, 568, 768
Mueller, 190, 334
Mühlens, 719
Muir, 625, 765
Mulligan, 537, 776
Mulrennan, 533, 756
Musgrave, 70, 719, 734
Muto, 252

N

Nagayo, 684, 685, 771
Nakagawa, 243, 277, 279, 734
Nakahama, 251, 276
Nakamura, 296

Nauyn, 355, 727
Needham, 699, 751
Negri, 183, 719
Neiva, 771
Nelson, 197, 206, 719
Neveu-Lemaire, 727
Newstead, 611, 752, 771
Nicoll, 370
Nicolle, 111, 155, 720, 771
Nieschulz, 63, 720
Nishigori, 275, 745
Nishio, 271, 273
Noguchi, 111, 720, 771
Nono, 568, 771
Nordenskiold, 771
Novy, 109, 720
Noyer, 345
Nuttall, 677, 752, 771, 772

O

O'Brien, 286
Ochoa, 589, 777
O'Connor, 63, 81, 271, 720, 734, 746, 772
Odhner, 236, 268, 734
Okumura, 738
Olfers, 369
Oliver, 343
Oliveria Castro, 568
Olmer, 752
Onji, 271, 273
Onsey, 734
Opie, 752
O'Roke, 151, 589, 614, 720, 772
Osler, 720
Otto, 392, 746
Owen, 473

P

Paget, 473
Palfrey, 753
Pappenheimer, 752
Parker, 617, 772
Pasco, 269
Pasteur, 181
Patton, 619, 621, 626, 752, 772
Paulson, 720
Payne, 387, 746
Peacock, 473, 752
Pearse, 236, 323, 735, 739, 746
Penna Chavarria, 746
Penso, 746
Pfeiffer, 184
Pintner, 323, 746
Pinto, 752
Poche, 236, 323, 735, 739, 746

Pomeroy, 772
Portchinski, 596
Price, 236, 290, 305
Prommas, 468
Prowazek, 65, 703, 720

Q

Queen, 475
Quincke, 720

R

Railliet, 288, 735
Ransom, 340, 388, 392, 463, 482, 739, 747
Ratcliffe, 161, 720
Reed, 566, 773
Rees, 206, 720
Reichenow, 174, 568, 721, 773
Reis, 721
Reuling, 721
Reynolds, 567, 721, 776
Rhoads, 747
Rice, 545, 755
Richardson, 773
Ricketts, 773
Riley, 285, 320, 349, 727, 735, 739, 747, 752
Rivas, 721
Rivers, 568, 768
Robinson, L. E., 678, 752
Robinson, W., 630, 773
Robles, 773
Rodenwalt, 753
Roehl, 176, 721
Rogers, 111, 703, 721, 752
Root, 119, 230, 533, 721, 773
Rosen, 328, 330
Rosenau, 610, 773
Ross, I. C., 774
Ross, R., 110, 158, 166, 546, 703, 721, 752, 774
Ross, R. H., 774
Rothschild, 774
Roubaud, 174, 462, 552, 774
Rovelli, 370
Row, 172, 721
Rozeboom, 534
Rudolf, 703
Rudolphi, 323
Rüffer, 294, 735
Russell, 552, 568, 774

S

Saito, 252
Sambon, 295, 735, 739, 774

Sambuc, 213, 253, 735
Sanders, 84, 152, 722
Sanderson, 774
Sandground, 589, 747, 777
Sant 'Anna, 750
Sawyer, 774
Sayad, 488, 747
Scalas, 57, 722
Schaudinn, 59, 70, 207, 722
Schüffner, 566, 760
Schule, 774
Schwartz, 338, 363, 397, 739, 747
Scott, 325, 610, 722, 774
Sellards, 48, 57, 58, 61, 722
Senior-White, 775
Sergent, 775
Seurat, 747
Sewell, 224, 735
Shannon, 522, 534, 566, 588, 603, 605, 775
Sharp, 581, 775
Shelmire, 683, 761
Shimamura, 390, 747
Shimura, 748
Shipley, 735
Shorb, 367, 739
Shortt, 93, 152, 722, 775
Siler, 752, 775
Simond, 775
Simmons, 533, 567, 776
Simpson, 776
Sinton, 172, 537, 722, 776
Skidmore, 150, 722
Smillie, 437, 748
Smith, 61, 67, 703, 722
Smith, R. O. A., 776
Smith, T., 776
Smithers, 337
Smyly, 723
Snijders, 566, 776
Soper, 575, 776, 777
Southwell, 323, 739
Spindler, 748
Spink, 480, 482, 748
Stabler, 192, 723
Stanton, 777
Staübli, 727
Stein, 777
Steinberg, 61
Stephens, 723
Steward, 748
Stewart, 630, 777
Stiles, 51, 65, 236, 271, 276, 288, 334, 388, 482, 673, 677, 735, 739, 748, 777
Stitt, 703
St. John, 76
Stokes, 777

Stoll, 748
Stratman-Thomas, 533, 756
Strickland, 752
Strong, 94, 115, 589, 723, 727, 777
Stunkard, 225, 739
Suga, 251, 276
Surcouf, 592, 777
Suzuki, 296
Svensson, 385, 748
Swales, 249, 735
Sweet, 457
Swellengrebel, 81, 566, 752, 753, 777
Swezey, 723
Swift, 752
Syverton, 681, 777

T

Taliaferro, 100, 176, 703, 723, 753, 777
Tanabe, 55, 206, 723
Tao, 626, 777
Tate, 777
Taute, 778
Taylor, 567, 748, 755
Tegoni, 753, 778
Temple, 778
Ten Broeck, 567, 770
Theiler, 156, 614, 723, 748, 778
Theobald, 753
Thira, 749
Thomas, 99, 724
Thomson, 59, 703, 724
Tiedemann, 473, 778
Todd, 753
Tonnoir, 778
Townsend, 778
Tsuchiya, 77
Tubangui, 269, 735
Turner, 361, 466, 615, 739, 768
Tyler, 724
Tyzzer, 83, 228, 307, 395, 396, 691, 724, 749, 778

U

Uhlenmeyer, 190, 724
Ujüe, 270
Underwood, 455
Uribe, 395, 396, 778

V

Valentine, 98
van Cleave, 489, 749
van Cott, 480, 749
van Durme, 749
van Haitsma, 292, 736
Verdun, 251, 736

Vergeer, 329, 331, 739
Verjbitski, 778
Vevers, 277, 736
Vianna, 111, 724
Vogel, 262, 736
von Jauregg, 172, 715
Von Jhering, 18
Von Siebold, 367

W

Wagener, 57, 724
Walch, 778
Walker, 48, 57, 61, 83, 724, 725, 778
Warburton, 677, 752, 778
Ward, 236, 276, 277, 463, 727, 736, 749
Watson, 253, 753
Weathersbee, 567, 755
Webster, 685, 778
Wehr, 749
Weidman, 485
Welch, 157, 699, 725, 739, 751
Wenrich, 51, 65, 67, 90, 189, 725
Wenyon, 63, 65, 193, 703, 725
Wesenberg-Lund, 779
Wharton, 268, 749
Wheeler, 567, 669, 779
Whitaker, 657, 779
White, 753, 749
Wichterman, 186, 725
Wight, 725

Willey, 225, 736
Williston, 753
Wilson, 70, 725, 779
Winfield, 749
Wolbach, 699, 753, 779
Woodbury, 325
Woodhead, 231, 293, 736
Woodland, 367, 739
Woodworth, 618, 779
Wright, 111, 455, 669, 725, 767

Y

Yamada, 779
Yamagata, 251, 276
Yamagiwa, 295
Yokogawa, 273, 277, 281, 486, 736, 749
Yorke, 51, 52, 385, 725, 726, 727
Yoshida, 61, 388, 726, 729, 749
Young, 243, 736
Yumoto, 257, 736

Z

Zeder, 323
Zeller, 779
Zenker, 474
Zetek, 779
Ziemann, 703
Zinsser, 779
Zschokke, 18

INDEX OF SUBJECTS

INDEX OF SUBJECTS

All numbers refer to pages. Words in *italics* are names of genera or species; divisions higher than generic rank are indicated by SMALL CAPITALS. Page numbers in **bold-face type** indicate that a figure will be found on that page.

A

Abramis brama, 260
Abortive treatment, 548
ACALYPTRATÆ, 505, 597
ACANTHOCEPHALA, 211, 212, 489
  general description, 489
  life-cycle, 489
Acanthocheilonema perstans, 456
  transmission, 581
Acanthoconops, 577
Acarapis, 685
ACARINA, 648
  keys to, 662
Acerina cernua, 329
ACINETARIA, 186
ACNIDOSPORIDIA, 134
ACTINOPODA, 43
Acuaria hamulosa, 465
  spiralis, **465**
ACUARIINÆ, 464, 461
Aëdeomyia, 563
Aëdes, 557
  ægypti, 561, 566, 567, 568, 570, **572**, 573
  africanus, 566
  albopictus, 566, 567, 568
  aldrichi, 571
  comments on, 561
  communis, 568
  dorsalis, 567, 571
  fluviatilis, 566
  koreicus, 570
  luteocephalus, 566
  mariæ, 568
  scapularis, 566
  scutellaris, 570
  simpsoni, 566
  sollicitans, 567
  squamiger, 571
  stokesi, 566
  tæniorhynchus, 571
  togoi, 570
  triseriatus, 568, 571

Aëdes (*cont.*)
  variegatus, 569
  vexans, 568, 571
  vittatus, 566
Aëdiomorphus, 561
Ægyptianella, 668
Africa, 465
Agriolimax, 364
Air-tube, 512
Allantoin, 630
Allassostoma magnum, 288
AMBLYCERA, 645
Amblyomma, 662, 678
Amebic liver abscess, 56
Amœba proteus, **44**-45
Amœbæ, birds, 83
  cockroach, 84, **85**
  concentration, 73
  coprozoic, 69
  cultivation, 74
  differential diagnosis, 78, 79
  doubtful species, 68
  food animals, 81
  free-living, 44
  frogs, 84
  genera, 46
  insects, 84
  laboratory animals, 83
  man, 46-79
  methods, 70
  monkeys, 80
  nuclei, **46**
  pets, 81
  reptiles, 84
Amœbotænia sphenoides, 373
Amphileptus, **188**, 189
Amphimerus noverca, 260
  pseudofelineus, 260
AMPHISTOMATA, 238, 286
Amphistomym hominis (See *Gastrodiscoides hominis*)
Amphistomum cervi, 288
Anal gills, 512
ANALGESIDÆ, 686

Anaplasma, **154**, 156
Anaplasmosis, transmission, 680
Anas platyrhynchos, 288
Ancylostoma duodenale, 218
Anisogamy, 35
Anisolabis annulipes, 370
Anisotarsus, 364
ANNELIDA, 6
Anopheles, 165
  adult characteristics, 515
  albimanus, 533
  albitarsis, 534, 570
  algeriensis, 570
  annularis, 536
  annulipes, 536
  apicamucula, 533
  asiaticus, 542
  atropus, 542
  avian malaria vectors, 568
  bachmanni, 534
  barberi, 542
  classification, 521
  claviger, 535
  crucians, 515, 531, 533, 542
  culicifacies, 515, 536
  darlingi, 532, 534
  dissection, 544
  eggs, 518, **535**
  epidemiological "index," 542
  experimental index, 543
  flavirostris, 536
  fluviatilis, 536
  funestus, 536, 570
  gambiæ, 522, 534, 536, 570
  geographical distribution, 521
  hyrcanus, 535, 570
  identification, 522, 526, 521
  intermedius, 533
  key to adults, 523-525
  key to larvæ, 528-531
  larvæ, **518**, 519-520, **526**
  litoralis, 536
  ludlowi, 536
  maculatus, 536, 542
  maculipalpis, **532**
  maculipennis, 531, 534, **535**
  male term nalis, 520
  minimus, 536
  natural index, 543
  neomaculipalpus, 533
  nimbus, 515
  notes on American, 531-534
  palmate hairs, **527**
  palpi, **517**
  parvus, **532**
  pharænsis, 536
  pseudomaculipes, **532**, 533
  pseudopunctipennis, 531, 532

Anopheles (*cont.*)
  punctimacula, 533
  punctipennis, 515, 531, 542
  pupæ, **519**
  quadrimaculatus, 515, 516, 531, 542
  resting attitude, 515, **516**
  sacharovi, **535**
  scutellar form, 517
  sinensis, 535
  stephensi, 536
  subpictus, 542, 568, 570
  sundraicus, 536
  superpictus, 536
  tarsimaculatus, 534, 570
  umbrosus, 536
  vector of avian malaria, 568
  walkeri, 531, 542
  wing pattern, 532
  wing spotting, 515
  wing venation, 510
Anopheline surveys, 541
  breeding places, 542
ANOPHELINI (See *Anopheles*), 515
Anoplocephala perfoliata, 366
ANOPLOCEPHALIDÆ, 336
Anoplophyra marylandensis, 38
ANOPLURA, 644-652
Antepygidial bristles, 633
ANTHOCORIDÆ, 691
Aphiochæta, 626
Aphodius, 364
  coloradensis, 463
  femoralis, 463
  fimentarius, 463
  granarius, 463
  vittatus, 463
Aponomma, 678
ARACHNIDA, 494, 692, 658-665
ARANEIDA, 692
Arcella, 42
Archigetes, 323
Arduenna strongylina, 464
ARDUENNINÆ, 461
Argas, **666**, 668
ARGASIDÆ, 668-670
  key, American species, 669
Arianta, 364
Arion, 364
Arista, 504
Armadillo, 108
Armadillidium vulgare, 465
Armigeres, 557
Arribalzagia, 524, **532**, 533
ARTHROPODA, 311, 493
Arthropods, relation to disease, 498
Artyfechinostomum sufrartyfex, 270
ARUDUENNINÆ, 462
Ascaridia lineata, **397**

ASCARIDÆ, 377, 386
Ascaris equorum, 393
 lumbricoides, 214, 215, 217, **230, 375,**
  379, 380, 381, 383, 388, 393, 399
 description, 386, **387, 388**
 epidemiology, 391
 life-cycle, 388
 pathogenesis, 390
 prevention, 392
 treatment, 391
 vitulorum, 393
ASCAROIDEA, 386
Aschiza, 597
Asopia farinalis, 370
Aspidogaster conchicola, **223,** 237
ASPIDOGASTREA, 235, 237
Assassin-bugs, **656,** 657
Astasia captiva, 90
 mobilis, 90
Atebrin, 171
Attagenus, 690
Auchmeromyia, 622
Australorbis glabratus, 297
Automeris, 691
Axostyle, **120, 128**

B

Babesia, transmission, 680-681
Babesia begemina, 151, 152, **153**
 canis, 152
BABESIDÆ, 149, 151-155
Bacillus malaria, 157
Balantidium, 38
 blattarum, 38
 caviæ, 39
 coli, **28,** 40, 196, 201-206
 binary fission, 202, **204**
 conjugation, 203-205, **204**
 cross infection, 197
 cultivation, 206
 cyst, **203**
 guinea-pig, 197
 life-cycle, 201
 monkey, 197
 neuromotor apparatus, 202
 pathogenesis, 206
 pig, 196
 sporulation, 203
 transmission, 205
 trophozoite, **28,** 201
Barbeiros, 657
Barbus barbus, 260
Bartonella, 650
Bed-bugs, 653-654
BELOSTOMIDÆ, 691
Benacus, 691
Bertilla studeri, 365

Bilharziasis, 294, 295
Bilharziella polonica, 306
Bird lice, 19
Bironella, 521
Bithynia fuchsiana, 256
BITHYNIINÆ, 256
Black-flies (See SIMULIIDÆ), 587
Blackhead (See *Histomonas melea-
 gridis*)
Black Widow spider, 692
Blanfordia formosana, 297
 nosophora, 297
Blaps, 690
Blastocystis hominis, **77**
Blatta orientalis, 464
Blattella germanica, 463, 464
Blepharoplast, **99, 128**
Blister beetles, 690
Blood fluke (See Schistosomiasis)
BODONIDÆ, 88
Bogeria, 624
Boöphilus, 156, **675,** 678
BOÖPIDÆ, 645
Borborus, 598
Bot-flies, 623
Boutonneuse fever, 679
BRACHYCERA, 505
Breathing trumpets, 513
Brown-tail moth, 691
BUCEPHALATA, 292
Bucephalus papilosus, 293
Budding, 34
Bulinus brochii, 297
 contortus, 297, 304
 dybowskyi, 297
 innesi, 297
Bütschlia, **193,** 194

C

CÆCULIDÆ, 683
Calathrus, 364
Calliphora, 625
CALLIPHORIDÆ, key to genera, 607
CALYPTRATÆ, 505, 597
CAMALLANIDÆ, 467
Camallanus ancylodirus, 467
 lacustris, 467
CANESTRINIIDÆ, 686
CANIDÆ, 284
Canthariasis, 690
Cantharidin, 690
Capillaria annulata, 485
 brevipes, 485
 hepatica, 485
Capitulum, 670
Carceag, 681
Carriers, 16

Carrion's disease, 585
Carrollia, 564
CARYOPHYLLÆIDÆ, 323
Case index, 539
Casoni test, 359
Catatropis filamentis, 239
  verrucosa, 239
Caterpillars, 691
Catostomus commersonii, 292
Cattle, protozoa of, 40
Caudamœba sinensis, 69
Cediopsylla, 638
Cepæa, 364
Cepedea, 191
Cephalont, 137
Cephalopsis, 624
Cephalothorax, 658
Cephenomyia, 624
CERATOPOGONIDÆ, 577, 578
  key to genera, 579
Ceratophyllus, 638
Cercaria douthitti, 233
  elvæ, 306
  inhabilis, 233
  isocotylea, 233
  megalura, 233
  trigonura, 233
  urbanensis, 233
Cerci, 511
Cercocebus fuliginosus, 298
CERCOMONADIDÆ, 88
Cercomonas, 127
Cercopithecus callitrichus, 288
  sabaeus, 298
CESTODA, 311
CESTODARIA, 311
CESTOIDEA, 211, 212, 311, 323
  general characteristics, 310
Chagasia, 521, 523
Channa formosana, 275
CHAOBORINÆ, 508
Cheilospirura sp., 465
Chiggers, 683
Chigœ flea, 635
Chilodon, 207
CHILOMASTIGIDÆ, 88
Chilomastix aulostomi, 119
  bettencourti, 39, 119
  capræ, 119
  caulleryi, 119
  cuniculi, 119
  gallinarum, 39, 119
  intestinalis, 39, 119
  mesnili, 117-119, 118, 132
  motellæ, 119
Chilomonas paramecium, 90
Chimpanzee, protozoa of, 40
CHIRONOMIDÆ, 577

Chlamydophrys stercorea, 70, 82
Choanotænia infundibulum, 373
Chæridium, 364
Cholera, 617
Chorioptes, 688
CHRYSOMONADIDA, 87
Chrysomyia, 623, 625
Chrysops, 594, 595
  dimidiatus, 214
  silacea, 214
CHYLETIDÆ, 683
CILIATA, 185
Ciliates, 185-207
  cattle, 193-195
  characteristics, 185
  classification, 185
  coprozoic, 207
  ectoparasitic, 188-190
  man, 201-207
  monkeys, 195-196
  mosquito larvæ, 192-193
  suctoria, 199-200
CIMICIDÆ, 653-654
Cimex, 653
Cirri, 29
Clarias batrachus, 468
Clinical periods, 12, 13
Clonorchiasis, 262
  pathology, 263
  symptoms, 264
  treatment, 264
Clonorchis sinensis, 213, 214, 230, 254,
    255, 256, 257, 260, 274, 275
  control, 258
  development in final host, 208
  distribution, 252
  entrance into final host, 258
  historical, 251
  life-cycle, 256
  longevity, 253
  morphology, 254
  position in host, 253
Clypeal hairs, 526
Cnemidocoptes, 688
CNIDOSPORIDIA, 178-184
Coarctate pupa, 604
Cobboldia, 623
COCCIDIA, 133, 140-148
  characteristics, 140-143
  lower animals, 144-145
  man, 140-143, 141
Cochlicella acuta, 262
Cochliomyia, 625
Cockroach, protozoa of, 38
CŒLENTERATA, 5
Collecting arthropods, 696
COLEOPTERA, 690
Collyriclum faba, 228, 284

Colpoda, 207
Comb, 512
Commensalism, 3
Complete metamorphosis, 499
Comstock-Needham venation, 510
Cone-nosed bugs, 658
Congo floor maggot, 622
Conjugation, 36
Contagion, 11
Control
  Aëdes ægypti, 574
  malaria, 548-555
  Phlebotomus, 586
Convalescent period, 12, **13**
Coolie itch, 686
Copra itch, 686
Copromonas subtilis, **90**
Coprozoic ciliates, 207
Copulation, 35
Corbicula producta, **270**
Cordylobia, 621
Coregonus albula, 329
  lavaretus, 329
Corizoneura, 594
Costa, 504
Costia necatrix, **95,** 96
Cotylophoron cotylophorum, **288,** 289,
  290
Councilmania lafleuri, 69
Crab-louse, 649
Crassius auratus, 257, 275
Cratacanthus, 364
Creeping disease, 468
Cricket, 40
Crithidia, 91, **92,** 93, 94
  gerridis, 41
Crop, 498
Cross-veins, 505
CRUSTACEA, 494
CRYPTOBIDÆ, 88
Cryptobia helicis, **95,** 96
CRYPTOMONADIDA, 87
Cryptosporidium muris, 39
Ctenidium, 631
Ctenocephalides, 632, **638**
  canis, 370, 372
Ctenopharyn-godon idellus, 257
Ctenophthalmus, 640
Ctenopsyllus, 639
CUCULLANIDÆ, 468
Cucullanus clitellaris, 468
Culex
  annulirostris, 569
  fatigans, 518, 564, 566, 568-570, 575
  fuscana, 568
  group, 557
  hortensis, 568
  mimeticus, 516

Culex (cont.)
  pipiens, 518, 568, 664
  posterior end, **260**
  salinarius, 564, 568
  tarsalis, 568
  territans, 564, 568
  vector of filariasis, 575
CULICIDÆ, 508
CULICINÆ, 508
  abdomen, 511
  adult structure, 508
  characteristics, 508
  classification, 513-514
  key to tribes, 514
  larval structure, 512
  legs, 511
  life history, 509, 511
  pupal structure, 513
  thorax, 509
  wing venation, 510
Culicine mosquitoes, 556
  relation to disease, 565
CULICINI
  air-tube, 519
  control, 511
  eggs, 518
  key to Amer. genera, 558
  key to groups, 514
  tribe, 556
CULICOIDES, 455, 456, **578,** 580
  austeni, 581
  furens, 580
  grahami, 581
  obsoletus, 580
Culter brevicauda, 257
Cuterebra, 624
CYCLOCŒLIDÆ, 238
Cyclo-developmental, 500
CYCLOPHYLLIDEA, 313, 317, 324
Cyclo-propagative, 500
Cyclops, 370, 383
  brevispinosus, 328
  prasinus, 328
CYCLORRHAPHA, 503, 505
Cynomyia, 625
Cyprinus carpio, 260, 275
Cysticercosis, 340
  diagnosis, 341
  prevention, 341
Cysticercus bovis, 345, 346
  cellulosæ, 213, 337, 340, 345, 346
  fasciolaris, **348**
  ovis, 347
  pisiformis, 319, 347
  tenuicollis, 347
Cystidicola stigmatura, 466
Cystobia irregularis, 137
Cytamœba bacterifera, 38, **154,** 155

CYTOLEICHIDÆ, 686
Cytoplasm, of protozoa, 27
Cytopyge, 28
Cytostome, 28, 120

D

Dacnitoides cotylophora, 468
Davainea proglottina, 364, 364
  life-cycle, 364
DAVAINEIDÆ, 336, 363, 364, 366
Deer-flies, 590
Definitive host, 33
Deinocerites, 557, 564
Delhi boil, 110
Demodex, 688
DEMODICOIDEA, 688
Dengue fever, 567
Depluming mite, 688
Dermacentor, 674, 677, 679, 680
DERMANYSSIDÆ, 682
Dermanyssus, 682
Dermatobia, 622
Deutomerite, 137
Diachlorus, 594
Diamanus, 639
Diaptomus gracilis, 328
Diatomineura, 594
Dichelacera, 594
DICROCŒLIIDÆ, 260
Dicrocœlium dendriticum, 261, 264
  hospes, 262
  macrostomum, 262
Dictyocaulus filaria, 383
Dientamœba fragilis, 67-68
  cyst, 68
  historical, 67
  host-parasite relations, 68
  incidence, 68
  morphology, 67
  nucleus, 46
  trophozoite, 68
DIGENEA, 224, 235, 237
Digramma brauni, 325
DILEPIDIDÆ, 336, 371
Dimastigamœba gruberi, 69, 70
DINENYMPHIDÆ, 88
Dinobryon sertularia, 90
DINOFLAGELLIDA, 87
Dioctophyme renale, 470, 471
  description, 470
  life-cycle, 471
DIOCTOPHYMIDÆ, 470
DIOCTOPHYMOIDEA, 470
DIOICOCESTIDÆ, 323
DIPELIDIDÆ, 373
DIPHYLLOBOTHRIIDÆ, 317, 325
DIPHYLLOBOTHRIINÆ, 325

Diphyllobothrium americanum, 334
  cirdatynm, 333
  decipiens, 332
Diphyllobothrium erinacei, 332-333
  description, 332
  historical, 332
  pathology, 333
Diphyllobothrium lateum, 214, 230, 317,
    320, 325-332, 328, 329, 330, 331,
    332
  control, 330
  description, 326
  distribution, 325
  epidemiology, 331
  frequency, 325
  life-cycle, 327
  pathogenicity, 329
  prevention, 330
Diphyllobothrium mansoni, 332
  mansonoides, 334
  okumurai, 332
  parvum, 333
  ranarum, 332
  reptans, 332
Diplodinium, 193, 194, 195
  ecaudatum, 40
Diplodiscus temperatus, 223, 288, 289,
    290
Diplogonoporus grandis, 335
DIPLOMONADIDA, 88
Diplopylidium acanthotetra, 373
Diplostomum flexicaudum, 292, 293
DIPTERA, 502
  antennæ, 503
  characteristics, 502, 505
  classification, 503
  importance, 502
  key to families, 506
  legs, 505
  wing venation, 504
Dipylidium, transmission, 638, 650
Dipylidium caninum, 317, 371-372, 373
  description, 371
  life-cycle, 372
Dirofilaria immitis, 454, 455
  vectors, 570
Dirofilaria magalhæsi, 455
Distoma crassum (See *Fasciolopsis
    buski*)
  heterophyes (See *Heterophyes hete-
    rophyes*)
  sinensis (See *Clonorchis sinensis*)
DISTOMATA, 238, 240
Distribution in host, 14
DIXINÆ, 508
Dracunculus medinensis, 383, 457, 458,
    459, 460
  description, 457

Dracunculus medinensis (*cont.*)
  distribution, 458
  life-cycle, 458
  pathology, 459
  prevention, 460
  treatment, 460
Drainage, 553
Drosophila, 598
Duck, 41
Dum-dum fever, 110
Dwarf tapeworm (See *Hymenolepis nana*)

E

Earthworm, protozoa of, 38
East Coast fever, transmission, 680
Echidnophaga, 635
Echinochasmus perfoliatus, 270
Echinococcosis, 349-361
  diagnosis, 358
  pathology, 358
  prevention, 361
  secondary, 356
  symptoms, 358
  transmission, 617
  treatment, 360
Echinococcus granulosus, 213, 349-362
  description, 349
  life-cycle, 349
Echinococcus multilocularis, 357
ECHINODERMATA, 5
Echinolælaps, 682
ECHINOPTHIRIIDÆ, 645
Echinorhynchus, 489
Echinostoma ilocanum, 268
  morphology, 269
  life-cycle, 269
Echinostoma revolutum, 268, 269, 270
ECHINOSTOMATIDÆ, 240, 268
Ectoparasite, 3, 17, 188
Ectoplasm, 28, 44
Eimeria, of lower animals, 145
  caviæ, 39
  meleagridis, 39
  miyiarii, 39, 144
  oxyspora, 141
  sardinæ, 141
  stiedæ, 40, 144, 145
  tenella, 39, 144, 145
  zürnii, 145
Eliochairs tuberosa, 245
EMBADOMONADIDÆ, 88
Embadomonas, 126
Empodium, 505
Endamœba anatis, 83
  apis, 84

Endamœba anatis (*cont.*)
  aulastomi, 84
  barreti, 84
  belostomæ, 84
  blattæ, 38, 82, 84, 85
  bovis, 40, 81
  capræ, 81
  cobayæ, 39, 83
Endamœba coli, 40, 59-61, 60
  chromatoid bodies, 60
  cyst, 60
  differential diagnosis, 78, 79
  excystation, 61
  historical, 59
  host-parasite relations, 60
  host-parasite specificity, 61
  incidence, 61
  infection, method, 60
  life-cycle, 59
  nucleus, 46
  precystic stage, 60
  trophozoite, 59
Endamœba cuniculi, 40, 83
  debliecki, 81
  dispar, 69
  equi, 81
  gallinarum, 38
Endamœba gingivalis, 40, 61-63, 62
  historical, 61
  host-parasite specificity, 63
  incidence, 62
  life-cycle, 61
  morphology, 62
  pathogenicity, 62
  transmission, 62
  trophozoite, 62
Endamœba histolytica, 40, 48-59
  carrier, 52
  chromatoid bodies, 49, 50
  clinical period, 53
  complement fixation, 57
  cultivation, 74
  cyst, 49, 50, 51, 52, 54
  differential diagnosis, 78, 79
  distribution in host, 53
  excystation, 54, 55
  historical, 48
  host-parasite adjustments, 57
  host-parasite relations, 50-58
  host-parasite specificity, 58
  immunology, 56
  incidence, 50
  intradermal reaction, 57
  life-cycle, 48
  localization in host, 53
  lower animals, 58
  morphology, 49
  nucleus, 46, 49, 50

Endamœba intestinalis, 81
  lagopodis, 83
  minchini, 84
  muris, 39, **82**, 83
  nuttalli, 80
  ovis, 81
  pitheci, 80
  polecki, 40, 81
  ranarum, 38, **82**, 84
  ratti, 83
  testudinis, **82**
  thomsoni, **82**
Endemic hematuria, 294
Endocyst, **135**
Endolimax blattarum, **82**
  caviæ, 39, **82**
  cynomolgi, 80
  gregariniformis, 38
Endolimax rana, 63-65
  cyst, **64**
  differential diagnosis, 78, 79
  historical, 63
  host-parasite relations, 64
  incidence, 65
  life-cycle, 64
  nucleus, **46**
  precystic stage, 64
  trophozoite, **64**
Endolimax reynoldsi, 86
Endoparasite, 3, 17, 18
Endoplasm, 28, **44**
English sparrow, protozoa of, 39
Enterobius vermicularis, 213, 214, **230**,
    381, 383, **398**
  description, 398
  distribution, 399
  habitat, 399
  life cycle, 399
Enteromonas hominis, **127**, 132
Entodinium, **193**, 194
Eperythrozoon coccoides, 650
  wenyoni, 681
Epicyst, **135**
Epidemiology, 10
Epimerite, 137
Epimeron, 496
Episternum, 496
Epithelioma contagiosum, 568
Equine encephalomyelitis, 567, 681
Eratyrus, 657
Erephopsis, 594
Eretmopodites, 557, 566
Eristalis, 625
ERYTHRÆIDÆ, 683
Esenbeckia, 594
Esox lucius, 329
Euglena, 88-**89**
Euglenamorpha hegneri, 38, **90**

EUGLENOIDIDA, 87
EUGREGARINIDA, 136
Euparyphium jassyense, 270
  malayanum, 270
Euproctis, 691
Eusimulium, 589
Eye-flies, 615
Eye worm (See *Loa loa*)

F

Fasciola hepatica, 247, 264
  life-cycle, 249
Fascioliasis, 250
FASCIOLIDÆ, 240
Fascioloides magna, 249
Fasciolopsis buski, **230**, 240, **241**, **242**,
    244, **248**, 249
  description, 242
  distribution, 241
  epidemiology, 247
  historical, 240
  life-cycle, 243
  morphology, 248
  symptoms, 245
  treatment, 246
Fasciolopsis goddardi, 241
  rathouisi, 241
  spinifera, 241
Fat-body, 498
Ficalbia, 557
Ficus glabrata, 485
FILARIIDÆ, 214, 384
Filling, 553
Fimbriaria fasciolaris, 370
Finlaya, 561
Fish tapeworm (See *Diphyllobothrium
    latum*)
Flagellar segments, 508
Fleas, 631-643
Flies (see DIPTERA), 502
Fontaria virginica, 370
FORAMINIFERA, 42, **43**, 45
Fork cells, 510
Fossaria modicella, 289
Fowl, protozoa of, 38
Fowl-pox, 567
Fracticipita, 633
Free-living organisms, 1
Frit-flies, 615
Frog, protozoa of, 38
Frontal lunule, 503
  suture, 504

G

Galba plicifera silicula, 284
Gallsickness, 681

Galumna, 366
Gambusia affinis, 275
Gametocyte, 136, **159**, 161, **163**, 164
 carriers, 539
Gasterophilus, 623
GASTRODISCIDÆ, 286
Gastrodiscoides hominis, 286, **287**
 description, 287
 historical, 286
 life cycle, 288
 position in host, 287
GASTROPHYLACIDÆ, 286, 289
Gedœlstia, 624
Gene's organ, 661
Geotrupes sylvaticus, 370
Giardia agilis, 38, **130**, 131
 ardeœ, 41
 caviœ, 39, **130**, 131
 duodenalis, 40, **130**, 131
Giardia lamblia, 40, 127-130, **128**
 characteristics, 128, 132
 cysts, **128**, 129
 life-cycle, 127
 pathogenicity, 129
 transmission, 129
 trophozoite, **128**
Giardia microti, 41
 muris, 39, **130**, 131
Glossina, 611-613, **612**
 morsitans, 611
 pallidipes, 613
 palpalis, 99, 612
 swynnertoni, 611
 tachinoides, 611
Glyciphagus, 686
Gnathostoma hispidium, 468
 horridum, 468
 sociale, 468
 spinigerum, 468
GNATHOSTOMIDÆ, 468
Gongylonema, invertebrate hosts, 695
 ingluvicola, 463
 neoplasticum, 216, 463
 pulchrum, 462, **463**
 life cycle, 463
 scutatum, 384
Gonospora minchina, 137
Gordius robustus, 488
GORDIACEA, 211, 212
 general description, 487
 life cycle, 487
Gorgodera minima, **223**
Grabhamia, 562
Gregarina, 137, **138**
 blattarum, 38
 locustœ, 40
 oviceps, 40
Gregarines, 136-139

Gregarines (*cont.*)
 acephaline, 137
 cephaline, 137
 schizogregarines, 139
GREGARINIDA, 133
Grocer's itch, 686
Guinea-pig, protozoa of, 39
Gyrodactylus elegans, 235, 236
GYROPIDÆ, 645
Gyrostigma, 623

H

Habronema, transmission, 617
Habronema megastoma, 461
 description, 461
 life cycle, 461
Habronema microstoma, 462
 muscœ, 462
Hæmagogus, 562
Hæmaphysalis, **667**, 677, 679
Hæmatobia, 610
HÆMATOMYZIDÆ, 646
Hæmatopinus, 646
Hæmatopota, 593
Hæmocoele, 497
Hæmodipsus, 646, 650
Hæmoflagellates, 98-115
Hæmogamasus, 682
Hæmogregarines, 145-148, **147**
Hæmogregarina, 147
HÆMOPROTEIDÆ, 149
Hæmoproteus, 149-**150**
 transmission, 614
Hæmoproteus columbœ, 39
HÆMOSPORIDIA, 149-156, 133
Hair-tufts, 512
Hair worms (See GORDIACEA)
Haller's organ, 661
HAPLOSPORIDIA, 134, 184
Harara, 585
Hard ticks (IXODIDÆ), 670
Harpalus, 364
Harpyrynchus, 683
Hartmannella hyalina, **69**, 70
Harvest mites, 683
Heartwater, 681
HECTOPSYLLIDÆ, 635
Hegneria leptodoctyli, 90
Heizmannia, 557
Helicella candidula, 262
 itala, 262
HELIOZOA, **43**, 45
Helisoma trivalvis, 290
Helminths, 211
 biology, 212
 distribution and incidence, 212
 effects on host, 214

Helminths (*cont.*)
  general classification, 211
Hemerocampa, 691
Hemibia hupensis, 297
HEMIPTERA, 652, 657, 690
Hepatozoön canis, transmission, 681
Hepatozoön muris, 145-147, **146**
  transmission, 682
Hereditary transmission, 11, 181
Hermetia, 626
Hermiculter kneri, 257
Heron, 41
Herpesencephalomyelitis, 567
Herpetomonas, 91, **92**, 94
Herpetomonas muscarum, 40
HETERAKIDÆ, 377, 386, 394
Heterakis gallinæ, **395**
  description, 395
  life cycle, 396
Heterodera radicicola, 230
Heterophyes heterophyes, 271, 272
  description, 272
  distribution, 271
  life cycle, 273
  position in final host, 272
Heterophyes nocena, 271
HETEROPHYIDÆ, 240, 270
HETEROTRICHIDA, 186
Hexamita intestinalis, 38
  muris, 39, **95**, 96, **131**
Himasthla mühlensi, 270
Hippelates, 615, **624**
HIPPOBOSCIDÆ, 613
Histomonas meleagridis, 39, **95**, 396
History index, 539
HOLOTRICHIDA, 185
HOMOPTERA, 651
Hookworm, 19, 418-437
Hoplodontophorus, 398
Hoplopsyllus, 639
Horse, 41
Horse-flies, 590
Horse hair snakes (See GORDIACEA)
Host, 3
Host-parasite relations, 10
Host-parasite specificity, 6
House fly, 40, 616
Howardina, 561
Humeral cross-vein, 510
Hyalomma, 676, 678, 679
  accidental, 7
  casual, 7
  definitive, 3
  first intermediate, 3
  foreign, 7
  intermediate, 3, 11
  natural, 7
  provisional, 7

Hyalomma (*cont.*)
  refractory, 7
  resistance, passive, 14
  second intermediate, 3
  susceptibility, 6
  temporary, 7
  tolerant, 7
  transitory, 7
  types, 3
Hydatid cyst, 350-351, 353, **354, 355,**
    356, 360
  alveolar, 356
  diagnosis, 358
  pathology, 358
  prevention, 360
  symptoms, 358
  treatment, 360
  unilocular, 356
Hydatid sand, 353
Hydra, 189
  protozoa of, 40
HYDRACHNOIDEA, 685
HYMENOLEPIDIDÆ, 366, 336, 317
Hymenolepis diminuta, 230, 317, 370,
    369
  historical, 369
  life cycle, 369
  transmission, 638, 695
Hymenolepis fraterna, 367
Hymenolepis nana, 214, 230, 320, 323,
    366, 367
  description, 367
  historical, 367
  life cycle, 368
  prevention, 369
  transmission, 617
HYMENOPTERA, 691
HYPERMASTIGIDA, 88
Hypopleura, 496
Hypopygium, 498, 511
Hypothalmichthys nobilis, 257
HYPOTRICHIDA, 186
Hyrax, 398
HYSTRICHOPSYLLIDÆ, 639

I

Ichthyophthirius, 199
Idus idus, 472
  melanotus, 260
Incomplete metamorphosis, 498
Incubation period, 12, 13
  malaria, 166
Infective stage, 10
INFUSORIA, 30
Insects, external structure, 495
  internal structure, **496**
  life histories, 498

Integricipita, 634
Intermediate host, 3
Intestinal flagellates, 116-132
Iodamœba suis, 40
Iodamœba williamsi, 65-67
  cyst, **66**
  differential diagnosis, 78, 79
  excystation, 67
  historical, 65
  host-parasite relations, 67
  incidence, 67
  life-cycle, 65
  nucleus, **46**
  precystic stage, 66
  trophozoite, **66**
ISCHNOCERA, 644
Isle of Wight disease, 685
Isogamy, 35
Isospora bigemina, 141
  felis, 134, **142**
  hominis, 140-143, **141**
  lacazii, 39
  of lower animals, 145
Isostomyia, 564
Isotricha, **193,** 194
Itch mites, 687
Ixodes, **672,** 677
IXODIDÆ, 670-681
  key to genera, 673
IXODOIDEA, 666

J

Janthinosoma, 561
Jungle yellow fever, 575

K

Kala Azar, 111
  transmission, 585
Karyamœbina falcata, 69
Karyolysus, 147-148
  lacertarum, 38
Katayama disease, 294, 295
Kerona, **189**
Kerteszia, 525, 534
Keys to
  ACARINA, 662-663
  Amer. adult female ANOPHELINI,
    523-525
  Amer. anopheline larvæ, 528-531
  Amer. ARGASIDÆ, 669
  Amer. CULICINI
    by adults, 558
    by larvæ, 560
  ANOPHELINI, 521
  families of
    PARASITOIDEA, 663

Keys to (*cont.*)
  families of
    SARCOPTOIDEA, 664-665
    TARSONEMOIDEA, 664
    TROMBIDOIDEA, 664
  genera of
    CALLIPHORIDÆ, 607
    CERATOPOGONIDÆ, 579
    IXODIDÆ, 667
    MUSCIDÆ, 606
    muscoid flies, 628
    OESTRIDÆ, 607
    REDUVIIDÆ, 657
    SARCOPTIDÆ, 686
    SIPHONAPTERA, 634
    SIPHUNCULATA, 646
    TABANIDÆ, 593
Kirkioestrus, 624

L

Labeo Jordani, 257
Lælaps, 682
Lagoa, 691
Lagochilascaris minor, 393
Lambornella, 192
Lankesterella ranarum, 38
Lankesteria culicis, 137
Lasiohelea, **578,** 580
Latency, 16
Latent period, 12, **13**
Latrodectus, 692
Leidyana erratica, **138**
Lepidoselaga, 594
Leishman-Donovan bodies, **110**
Leishmania, 91, 93, 110-115
  historical, 110
  kala-azar, 111
  lower animals, 114
  morphology, 111
  oriental sore, 113
  South American, 114
  transmission, 112
Leishmania braziliensis, 111, 114
Leishmania donovani, **110, 111-113**
  control, 113
  cultivation, 113
  diagnosis, 113
  geographical distribution, 111
  host-parasite relations, 112
  life-cycle, 111
Leishmania infantum, 111
  tarentolæ, 115
  tropica, 113-114
Leishmaniasis, South American, 114
LEPIDOPTERA, 691
Leptoconops, **578,** 580
Leptomonas, 91, **92,** 93

Leptopsylla, 639
  musculi, 370
Lethocercus, 691
Leucocytozoön, 150-151
  transmission, 589
Leucocytozoön anatis, 41
Lice, 644-651
LIGULINÆ, 325
Limax, 364
Linognathus, 646
Liponyssus, bacoti, **683**
  bursa, 682
  saurarum, 683
  sylviarum, 682
Lipoptena, 614
LISTROPHORIDÆ, 686
Liver fluke (See *Clonorchis sinensis*)
Lizard, protozoa of, 38
Loaisis, transmission, 594
Loa loa, 214
Locust, 40
Lophomonas blattarum, 38, **95**, 96
Lota maculosa, 329
  vulgaris, 329
Louping ill, 681
Loxa, 691
Lucilia, 625, 630
Lung fluke (See *Paragonimus wester-
  mani*)
Lutzia, 557
LYGÆIDÆ, 691
Lygus, 691
LYMANTRIIDÆ, 691
Lymnæa limosa, 306
  palustris, 305
  reflexa, 305
  stagnalis, 306
  stagnalis appressa, 305
  stagnalis perampla, 304
Lynchia, 614

M

Macracanthorhynchus hirudinæceus,
  488, 489
  invertebrate hosts, 695
Macrogametocyte, 136, **159, 163,** 164
Malaria, 157-177
  abortive treatment, 548
  asexual cycle, 158-164
  birds, **175-176**
  carriers, 170, 534
  clinical periods, 166
  control, 171
  cultivation, 172
  differential diagnosis, 167
  discovery, 157
  epidemiology, 546
  estivo-autumnal, 162

Malaria (*cont.*)
  fertilization, **159,** 164
  gametogenesis, **159,** 164
  immunity, 169
  latency, 169
  life-cycle, 137
  lower animals, 177
  monkeys, 174
  mosquitoes, 515
  parasitological periods, 166
  pathology, 168
  prevention, 171
  quartan, 162
  relapse, 170
  sexual cycle, **159,** 164-166
  sporogony, 165
  staining, 173
  surveys, 538
  symptoms, 168
  tertian, 158-162
  therapeutic, 171
  transmission, 166
  treatment, 170
Male terminalia, **520**
Malignant jaundice, transmission, 681
MALLOPHAGA, 644
Mange, 688
Mangrove flies, 590
Mansonella ozzardi, 456
Mansonia, 557, 563, 566, 570
Manubrium, 633
Margaropus, 152
Margeana californiensis, **224, 226, 227**
Mastigina hylæ, **95**
MASTIGOPHORA, 30, 87-97
Maurer's dots, 162, **163**
Measly pork (see *Tænia solium*), 340,
  342, 343
Melania gottschei, 279
Mechanical transmission, 500
Medical entomology, 493
Megalopyge, 691
MEGARHININI, 556
Melania libertina, 274, 279
  obliquegranosa, 275
  reiniana, 275
Melanoconion, 564
Melanoplus differentialis, 465
  femurrubrum, 465
Meloë, 690
MELOIDÆ, 690
Melolontha melolontha, **488**
Melophagus, **614**
MENOPONIDÆ, 645
Merozoite, 136, 161
Mesopleura, 496
Metagonimus yokogawai, **230, 274,** 275
  historical, 273

METAZOA, 27, 211, 212
Microculex, 564
Microgametocyte, 136, 159, 163, 164
Microlynchia, 614
MICROSPORIDIA, 134, 180-182
Microtus pennsylvanicus, 304
Miescher's tubes, 183
MIRIDÆ, 691
Mites, 682-688
Mitosis, 29
Mochlostyrax, 564
MOLLUSCA, 6
MONADIDÆ, 88
Moniezia benedeni, 365
  expansa, 364
  life cycle, 365, 366
Moniliformis moniliformis, 489
  invertebrate hosts, 695
Monkey, protozoa of, 20-22, 40
Monocystis, 38, 134, 135, 137
MONOGENEA, 235, 236
MONOPISTHOCOTYLEA, 236
Monopsyllus, 639
Monorchotrema taichui, 271, 275
  taihokui, 275
MONOSTOMATA, 238
Morellia, 627, 628
Morphology, of protozoa, 27
Mosquito, natural enemies, 552
  reduction, 550
  surveys, 538
Mosquitoes (See CULICINÆ), 508
  nuisance, 570
Moult, 498
Mouse, protozoa of, 39
Mouthbrushes, 511
Mugil cephalus, 273
  japonicus, 273
Multiceps multiceps, 361, 362
  description, 362
  life cycle, 362
  pathogenesis, 363
Multiceps serialis, 363
Musca, 602, 615-620
Musca domestica, 364, 461
MUSCIDÆ, blood-sucking, 609
  key to genera, 606
  non-blood-sucking, 615
Muscoid flies, key to genera, 628
Mutualism, 3
MYCETOZOA, 42, 43
Myiasis, 621-630
Mylabris, 690
MYRIAPODA, 494
MYXOSPORIDIA, 133, 178-180
  species, 180
Myzomyia, 534, 536
Myzorhynchella, 525, 533

N

Nairobi disease, 681
NEMATOCERA, 505
Natrix, 334
Necator americanus, 213, 218
Necturus maculosus, 237
NEMATHELMINTHES, 211, 212
NEMATMORPHA, 211
NEMATODA, 211, 212, 374
  general characteristics, 374
Nematodes, 374
  bionomics, 374-385
  classification, 385
  collection of, 384
  preservation of, 384
Nematodirus filicollis, 383
Neoechinorhynchus, 489
Newt, 41
Nomenclature, rules of, 22-23
Nosema apis, 181
  bombycis, 180
Nosopsyllus, 636, 639, 641
  fasciatus, 370
NOTOCOTYLIDÆ, 238, 239
Notocotylus attenuatus, 239
  quinqueserialis, 223, 239
Notœdres, 687, 688
NOTONECTIDÆ, 691
Notum, 496
Nuisance mosquitoes, 570
NYCTERIBIIDÆ, 613
Nycticorax nycticorax, 274, 275
Nyctotherus cordiformis, 38, 186-188, 187
  faba, 207
  ovalis, 38, 188
Nyssorhynchus, 525, 532, 533

O

Ochlerotatus, 561
Œdamagena, 624
ŒSTRIDÆ, key to genera, 607
  myiasis, 623
Œstrus ovis, 625
Oiling, 550
Onciola canis, 489
Onchocerca, transmission, 581, 589
Onchocerca cæcutiens, 454, 455
  cervicalis, 455
  flexuosa, 455
  gibsoni, 455
  volvulus, 454
Onthophagus hecate, 463
  pennsylvanicus, 463
Oöcyst, 135, 136, 141, 159, 165

Oökinete, 153, 154, 159, 165
OPALINIDÆ, 190-192
Opalina, 191
  ranarum, 38
Ophicephalus striatus, 468
Ophthalmia, 617
Opifex, 557
OPISTHORCHIIDÆ, 240, 250
Opisthorchis felineus, 259, 260
  viverrini, 260
Oriental sore, transmission, 585
Ornithodorus, 668
Oropsylla, 639
Oroya fever, 585
Orthopodomyia, 557, 563
ORTHORRAPHA, 503, 505, 590
Ostertagia marshalli, 383
Ostiolum medioplexus, 220, 265, 267
  life cycle, 267
Oswaldocruzia auricularis, 383
Otodectes, 688
Ovipositor, 496
Oxyspirura mansoni, 466, 467
OXYURIDÆ, 377, 386, 398
Oxyuris incognita, 230

P

Paddles, 513
Pœderus, 690
Palpi, 495
Panama larvicide, 551
Pangonia, 544
Pansporoblast, 181, 182
Panstrongylus, 657
PANTASTOMATIDA, 87
Papataci fever, 585
Parabasal body, 99, 128
Parafossarulus striatulus, 252, 256
Paragonimus compactus, 277
  kellicotti, 277
  ringeri, 277
Paragonimus westermani, 230, 276,
  278, 279, 282
  course in final host, 280
  distribution, 277
  life cycle, 279
  morphology, 278
  pathology, 282
  position in final host, 280
  prevention, 283
  symptoms, 283
Parametorchis complexus, 260
  moveboracensis, 260
PARAMPHISTOMIDÆ, 286, 288
Paramphistomum cervi, 289
Paramonostomum parvum, 239
Parasa, 691

Parasimulium, 588
Parasite, definition, 3
  distribution in host, 14
  erratic, 3
  escape from host, 16
  facultative, 3
  incidental, 3
  index, 539
  infectivity, 8
  localization in host, 14
  man, 21
  method of attack, 15
  monkey, 20-22, 40
  obligatory, 4
  pathogenic, 4, 15
  periodic, 4
  permanent, 4
  resistance, 14
  temporary, 4
PARASITIDÆ, 682
Parasitism, 1
  definition, 1
  effects of, on parasite, 4
  in animal kingdom, 5
  origin and evolution, 17
  relation to host distribution, 18
  types, 2
PARASITOIDEA, key to families, 663,
  682
Parasitological periods, 12, 13
Paris Green, 551
Patagiamyia, 531, 532
Patent period, 12, 13
Pathogenic parasite, 4, 15
Pecten, 512, 528
PEDICULIDÆ, 646
Pediculoides, 685
Pediculus, 648
Pelomyxa, 42, 43
PENTATOMIDÆ, 691
Pentatrichomonas, 120
Perca flavescens, 488
  fluviatilis, 329
PERITRICHIDA, 186
Petiole, 510
Phagocytes, in malaria, 169
PHILOMETRIDÆ, 456
PHILOPTERIDÆ, 644
Phthirus, 648, 649
Phlebotomus, 583-586, 584
Phormia, 625, 630
Physa ancillaria parkeri, 305
  occidentalis, 269
Physaloptera caucasica, 466
  constricta, 466
  mordens, 466
  rara, 466
  truncata, 466

PHYSALOPTERINÆ, 461, 466
Physocephalus sexulatus, 464
Physopsis africana, 296, 297, 304
  globosa, 297, 304
PHYTOMONADIDA, 87
Phytomonas, 91, **92,** 93, 94
PHYTOMASTIGINA, 87
Pig, protozoa of, 40
Pigeon, protozoa of, 39
Pigment, in malaria, 159, **163**
Pink eye, 615
Pinworms (See *Enterobius vermicula*)
Piophila, 626
Pirenella conica, 273
PIROPLASMIDÆ, 151
Piroplasmoses, transmission, 680
PLAGIORCHIIDÆ, 240, 265
Plagiorhynchus formosus, 489
Plague, 640, 650
Planorbis adowensis, 297
  boissyi, 297
  corneus, 306
  dufouri, 297
  exustus, 304
  guadelupensis, 297
  olivaceous, 297
  pfeifferi, 297
  rotundatus, 239
  schmackeri, 244
Plasmochin, 171
PLASMODIDÆ, 149
Plasmodium cathemerium, 39
  falciparum, 162, **163,** 167
  inui, 174
  knowlesi, 174
  malariæ, 162, **163,** 167
  præcox, **175**
Plasmodium vivax, 158-162
  asexual cycle, 158-162
  differential diagnosis, 167
  exflagellation, **159,** 164
  fertilization, **159,** 164
  gametocytes, **159, 163,** 164
  gametogenesis, **159,** 163, 164
  macrogametocyte, **159, 163,** 164
  merozoite, **159**
  microgametocyte, **159, 163**
  oöcyst, **159,** 165
  oökinete, **159,** 165
  pigment, **163**
  sexual cycle, 164-166
  schizogony, **159,** 160, **163**
  schizont, **159,** 160, **163**
  Schüffner's dots, 160, **163**
  sporogony, **159,** 165
  sporozoite, **159, 160,** 165
  trophozoite, 158, **159**
  zygote, **159,** 165

Plasmotomy, 179
PLATYHELMINTHES, 211, 212, 236, 323, 379
Plecoglossus altivelis, 274
Pleural membranes, 496
Pleuron, 496
Podapolipus, 685
Poisons, contact, 550
  stomach, 550
Polar filament, **179,** 180
Polymastix melalonthæ, 96
POLYMONADIDA, 88
POLYOPISTHOCYTYLEA, 236
Polyplax, 646, 650
Polystoma integerrimum, 235, 237
  megacotyle, **223**
Pomatiopsis lapidaria, 279
Ponding, 554
Porcellio scaber, 465
PORIFERA, 5
Pork tapeworm in man (See *Tænia solium*)
Postscutellum, 496
Potamon abtusipes, 277
Prepatent period, 12, **13**
Prescutum, 496
Preserving insects, 697-699
Proboscis, 508
Proboscis-worms (See ACANTHOCEPHALA)
Propagative transmission, 500
Prosimulium, **588**
PROSOSTOMATA, 237, 238, 240, 286, 292
Prosthogonimus, invertebrate hosts, 695
  macrorchis, **265**
  life-cycle, 266
  pathology, 266
  symptoms, 266
Protocalliphora, 622
PROTOMONADIDA, 88
Protoopalina, 190, **191**
Protospirura gracilis, 461
PROTOZOA, asexual reproduction, 34
  biology, 27-41
  blood-inhabiting, 37
  circulation, 32
  classification, 30
  excretion, 33
  intestinal, 36
  locomotion, **28,** 32
  lower animals, 38
  maintenance of individual, 31
  maintenance of race, 33
  man, 36
  morphology, 27
  motion, 32
  nuclei, **29**

PROTOZOA (*cont.*)
  nutrition, 32
  protection, 31
  reproduction, 33
  respiration, 33
  response to stimuli, 31
  secretion, 33
  sexual reproduction, 35
  syngamy, 35
  parasitological periods, 53
  pathogenesis, 56
  precipitin test, 57
  precystic stage, 50
  prevention and control, 58
  pseudopodia, **49**, 50
  sites of infection, **55**
  transmission, 51
  trophozoite, **49**
PROTRACHEATA, 494
Prowazekella lacertæ, 38, 96
PROWAZEKELLIDÆ, 88
Pseudolynchia, **613**, 614
Pseudoparasite, 4, **77**
PSEUDOPHYLLIDEA, 313, 317, 316, 325, 336
Pseudorasbora parva, 257, 275
Pseudosuccinea columella, 249
Psorophora, **509**, 561, 622
Psoroptes, 687, **688**
Psychoda, 582, **583**
PSYCHODIDÆ, 582-586
Pteropleura, 496
Ptilinum, 503, 605
Pulex, **636**
  irritans, 370
PULICIDÆ, 636-639
Pulvilli, 505
Pupa, 499
Puparium, 503
Pygidium, 633

Q

Quinine, 171

R

Rabbit, protozoa of, 40
RADIOLARIA, **43**, 45
Raillietina asiatica, 364
  celebensis, 364
  madagascariensis, 364
  (*Skrjabinia*) *cesticellus*, 364
  (*Raillietina*) *echinobothrida*, 364
  (*Raillietina*) *tetragona*, 364
Rainey's corpuscles, **183**
Rana pipiens, 267
Rat, 641
  protozoa of, 39

Rat-tailed maggot, 625
Rearing arthropods, 699
"Red-bugs," 683
REDUVIIDÆ, 656
  key to genera, 657
Redwater fever, transmission, 680
Relapse, 12, **13**, 16
Relapsing fever, epidemic (European), 649
  endemic (African), 668
Retortamonas, 39
  blattæ, 38
  caviæ, 39
  cuniculi, 40
  in lower animals, 126-127
  intestinalis, **126**, 132
Rhabdias bufonis, 382
  fuscovenosa, 382
RHABDIASIDÆ, 382
RHABDITIDÆ, 386
Rhinœstrus, 623
Rhipicephalus, 152, 676, 677
RHIZOPODA, 42
Rhodeus ocellatus, 275
Rhodnius, 655, 656
Rocky Mountain spotted fever, 678

S

Sabethes, 557
Sabethoides, 562
Salmo umbla, 329
Sand-flies (CERATOPOGONIDÆ), 577
Sao Paulo fever, 679
Sappinia diploidea, **69**, 70
Sarcocystin, 184
Sarcocystis muris, 39
SARCODINA, 42-45, **43**
  classification, 30, 42
  parasitic, 45
  types, **43**
Sarcophaga, 625
Sarcoptes, 687
SARCOPTIDÆ, 686
SARCOPTOIDEA, 686
  key to families, 664
SARCOSPORIDIA, 134, 182-184, **183**
  species, 184
SIPHUNCULATA, 645
  key to genera, 646
Siphunculina, 615
Site of infection, **14**
Sleeping sickness, 98
Soft ticks (ARGASIDÆ), 668
Spanish fly, 690
Sparganum proliferum, 334
Sphyranura aligorchis, 237
Spiders, 692

Spineheaded worms (See ACANTHO-
    CEPHALA)
Spinitectus gracilis, 467
Spinning mites, 683
Spinose ear-tick, 669
Spiracles, 498
Spirocerca sanguinolenta, 464
Spirochætosis, fowl, 668
SPIRURIDÆ, 461
Spleen index, 540
Sponges, 5
Spore, **135, 141, 179**
Sporoblast, **135,** 136
Sporocyst, 136
Sporogony, 136, **159,** 165
Sporont, 137, **138**
Sporoplasm, **179,** 182
SPOROZOA, 30, 133-139
    classification, 133
    life-cycles, 134-139
Sporozoite, 134, **135, 141,** 158, **159**
Spotted fever, 679
Squama, 505
Stamnosoma armatum, 274, 275
    formosanum, 274, 275
Stegomyia, 561
Stenolophus, 364
Stephanofilaria dedœsi, 456
    stilesi, 456
Stephanoprora gelberti, 223
Sternellum, 496
Sternopleura, 496
Sternum, 496
Stizostedeon canadense - griseum,
    329
    vitreum, 329, 468
Stomach (of insects), 498
Stomach worm (See *Ascaris lumbri-*
    coides)
Stomoxys, 609, 610
    calcitrans, 456
    irritans, 462
STREBLIDÆ, 613
Streblomastix strix, **97**
STRIGEATA, 292
STRIGEATOIDEA, 237, 292
Strongyloides stercoralis, 216, 218,
    381, 382
Stylets, 509
Subcosta, 504
SATURNIDÆ, 691
Scab mites, 687
Scaly-leg, 688
Scenopinus, 504
Schellackia, transmission, 683
Schistosoma, 294-310
    bovis, 304
    geographical distribution, 300

Schistosoma (cont.)
    hœmatobium, 216, **230,** 297, 295, 296,
        298, 300, **301,** 306
    indicum, 304
    intercalatum, 296
    japonicum, 213, **230,** 296, 297, 298,
        299, 300, **303,** 306
    life history, 300
    mansoni, **230,** 295, 297, **296, 298,**
        300, **302,** 306
    position in host, 297
    spindale, 304
SCHISTOSOMATA, 234, 292, 294
SCHISTOSOMATIDÆ, 225, 294
Schistosomatium douthitti, 223, 304,
        305
    pathlocopticum, 305
Schistosomiasis, 294, 295
    historical, 294
    methods of infection, 303
    pathology, 306
    prophylaxis, 308
    symptoms, 307
    treatment, 310
Schizocystis, 139
Schizogony, 34, 136, **159,** 160, **163**
Schizogregarines, 139
SCHIZOPHORA, 597
Schüffners granules, 160, **163**
Sclerites, 495
SCORPIONIDA, 692
Screening, 549
Screw-worms, 625
Scutellum, 496
Scutum, 496
Seat worm (see *Enterobius vermicu-*
    laris)
Segmentina nitedellus, 244
Selenophorus, 364
Sepsis, 598
Seroot, 590
Setaria equina, 456
    labiato-papillosa, 456
Sibine, 691
Silvius, 594
Simian malaria, vectors of, 537
Simulium, **586,** 587-589
    avidum, 454
    damnosum, 454
    mooseri, 454
    ochraceum, 454
SIPHONAPTERA, 631-643
    key to genera, 634
Subpatent, 12, **13**
SUCTORIA, 186
Survey, anopheline, 540
    malaria, 538
Sutures, 496

Sylvatic plague, 640
Sylvilagus floridanus, 319
Symbiosis, 3, 97
Symptoms, 12, 13
Syngamy, 35
Synopsylla, 640
Syzygy, 137, 138

T

TABANIDÆ, 590, 591
  key to genera, 593
Tabanus, 592, 593
Tænia antarctica, 348
  balaniceps, 348
  brachysoma, 348
  brauni, 348
  cervi, 348
  confusa, 346
  crassicollis, 348
  diminuta, 369
  fenestrata, 345
  fusa, 345
  hydatigena, 347
  krabbei, 348
  nana, 367, 368
  ovis, 347
  piseformis, 318, 319, 320, 337, 347
Tænia saginata, 214, 230, 317, 320, 321,
  343-347, 344
  description, 343
  historical, 343, 344, 346
  life-cycle, 346
  prevention, 347
Tænia solium, 214, 230, 317, 321, 336-
  343, 345, 346
  description, 337
  historical, 336
  life-cycle, 338
Tænia tæniæformis, 216, 348
TÆNIIDÆ, 317, 336
TÆNIOIDEA, 336
Tadpole, protozoa of, 38
Tapeworms, 311-373
  bionomics, 310-321
  classification, 323
  collection of, 322
  cyclophyllidean, 336
  dog-sheep, prevention of, 347
  general characteristics, 311
  preservation of, 322
  pseudophyllidean, 325-335
  treatment, 322
  types of larvæ, 318
TARSONEMOIDEA, 685
  key to families, 663
TELOSPORIDIA, 133
Tenebrio molitor, 370, 464

Tergite, 496
Termite flagellates, 41, 96, 97
Tetrameres americana, 465
  crami, 466
Tetramorium cæspitum, 364
TETRANYCHID, 683
Tetranychus, 683
Tetrapetalonema, transmission, 581
TETRAPHYLLIDEA, 324
Texas fever, 152
  transmission, 680
Theileria, 154-155
  transmission, 680
Thelazia californiensis, 467
  callipæda, 466, 467
THELAZÜNÆ, 461, 466
Thelohania, 181
Theobaldia, 563, 568
Theobaldia-Mansonia group, 557
Threadworms (See NEMATODA)
Thymallus vulgaris, 329
Thysanosoma actinioides, 365
Tick fever, 681
Tick paralysis, 677, 680
Ticks (IXODOIDEA), 666
Tinca tinca, 260
Top-minnows, 552
Torus, 508
Toxocara canis, 393, 394
  mystax, 394
Toxoplasma, 154, 155
  paddæ, 39
Trachea, 498
Tracheal mite, 685
Tracheophilus cymbius, 238
Transmission, 10
Trapa natans, 245
TREMATODA, 211, 212, 224, 236, 237
Transmission, 10
  by contamination, 11
  by inoculation, 11
  classification of, 500
  direct, 11
  epidemiology, 10
  hereditary, 11
  prenatal, 11
Trench fever, 649
Triatoma, 655, 656
Tricercomonas, 127
Trichina worm (See *Trichinella spi-*
  ralis)
Trichinella spiralis, 213, 214, 215, 218,
  342, 384, 473, 474, 475, 476,
  477, 478, 479
  diagnosis, 480
  distribution, 475
  historical, 473
  life-cycle, 476

Trichinella spiralis (*cont.*)
    prevention, 482
    symptoms, 479
    treatment, 482
TRICHINELLIDÆ, 473
TRICHINELLINÆ, 473, 377
TRICHINELLOIDEA, 473
Trichinosis (see *Trichinella spiralis*)
Trichobilharzia ocellata, 306
Trichodectes, 650
    canis, 372
TRICHODECTIDÆ, 644
Trichodina, 189, 190
    pediculus, 38, 40
TRICHOMONADIDÆ, 88
Trichomonas augusta, 38
    buccalis, 122
    caviæ, 39
    columbæ, 39, 124, 125
    elongata, 120, 122-123, 132
    fœtus, 40, 124, 126
    gallinarum, 39
Trichomonas hominis, 40, 119-122, 120
    characteristics, 120, 132
    host-parasite relations, 121
    life-cycle, 119
    morphology, 120
Trichomonas lacertæ, 38
    muris, 39
    parva, 39
    ruminantium, 40
    suis, 40
    termopsidis, 97
    vaginalis, 40, 120, 123-124, 132
Trichonympha campanula, 97
TRICHOSOMOIDINÆ, 473, 486
Trichosomoides crassicauda, 383, 486
Trichostrongylus orientalis, 230
TRICHURINÆ, 483
Trichuris ovis, 485
    suis, 485
Trichuris trichiura, 214, 230, 377, 383, 483, 484
    description, 483
    life-cycle, 484
    pathogenesis, 484
    prevention, 485
Trichuris vulpis, 485
Triphleps, 691
Tritrichomonas, 120
    fecalis, 125
    muris, 131
Troglodytella, 195
    abrassarti, 40
Troglotrema salmincola, 284
TROGLOTREMATIDÆ, 240
    historical, 276

Trombicula, 684, 685
TROMBIDIIDÆ, 683
TROMBIDOIDEA, 683-685
    key to families, 663
Trophozoite, 135, 136, 158, 159, 163
Tropical rat mite, 683
Trutta lacustris, 329
    vulgaris, 329
Trypanoplasma borreli, 96
Trypanosoma, 91, 93, 98-110
    brucei, 107, 108
Trypanosoma cruzi, 105-106
    diagnosis, 106
    host-parasite relations, 106
    invertebrate host, 105
    life-cycle, 105
    transmission, 106, 657
    vertebrate host, 105
Trypanosoma diemyetyli, 41, 107, 109
    equinum, 107, 108
    equiperdum, 107, 108
    evansi, 107, 108, 595
Trypanosoma gambiense, 102-104, 103
    course of infection, 103
    diagnosis, 102
    host-parasitic relations, 102
    host-parasitic specificity, 104
    invertebrate host, 102
    life-cycle, 102
    prevention and control, 104
    transmission, 102, 612
    vertebrate host, 102
Trypanosoma hippicum, 108
    lewisi, 39, 100-102, 101
    melophagium, 108, 614
    noctuæ, 109
    paddæ, 108
Trypanosoma rhodesiense, 104-105
    transmission, 612
Trypanosoma rotatorium, 38, 107, 109
    simiæ, 108
Trypanosoma theileri, 108
    transmission, 614
Trypanosoma vivax, 108
Trypanosomes, 98-110
    amphibia, 109
    birds, 108
    cultivation, 109
    fish, 109
    lower animals, 106-109
    mammals, 107
    man, 102-106
    rat, 100-102
    reptiles, 109
TRYPANOSOMIDÆ, 88, 91, 92-94
Tsutsugamushi disease, 684
Tularemia, 595, 650, 680
Tunga penetrans, 365

TUNGIDÆ (see HECTOPSYLLIDÆ), 635
TURBELLARIA, 212, 219, 220
Turkey, protozoa of, 39
Tussock moth, 691
Typhocœlum cucumerinum, 238
Typhoid fever, 617
Typhus fever, epidemic, 649
  endemic, 640, 683
TYROGLYPHOIDEA, 686

U

Uranotænia, 557
Undulating membrane, 99, 120
Uronema, 207
UROPODIDÆ, 682
Urospora seanurides, 137

V

Vahlkampfia patuxent, 86
Vampire bat, 108
Vampyrella, 45
Vector, 500
Ventral brush, 513
Verruga peruana, 585
Vertebrata, 6
Veterinary entomology, 493
Viverra mungos, 277

W

Warble flies, 623
Water mites, 683
Water strider, 41
Watsonius watsoni, 288
Whipworm (See *Trichuris trichiura*)
Wohlfahrtia, 623
Wuchereria bancrofti, 217, 455, 456
  vectors, 569, 570

X

Xenopsylla, 636, 637, 638, 641
  cheopis, 370

Y

Yaws, 615, 617
Yellow fever, 565

Z

Zebrina detrita, 262
Zelleriella, 19, 190, 191
ZOÖMASTIGINA, 87
ZOÖXANTHELLÆ, 45
Zygocotyle ceratosa, 288
Zygote, 135, 136, 159, 165